PEDIATRIC SURGERY SECRETS

PHILIP L. GLICK, MD, FAAP, FACS
Surgeon-in-Chief
Children's Hospital of Buffalo
Professor, Department of Surgery, Pediatrics, and Obstetrics/Gynecology
State University of New York
Buffalo, New York

RICHARD H. PEARL, MD, FAAP, FACS
Surgeon-in-Chief
Children's Hospital of Illinois, Peoria
Professor, Departments of Surgery and Pediatrics
University of Illinois College of Medicine
Peoria, Illinois

MICHAEL S. IRISH, MD, FAAP, FACS
Administrative Chief Resident
Department of Pediatric Surgery
Children's Hospital of Buffalo
Buffalo, New York

MICHAEL G. CATY, MD
Senior Attending Surgeon
Children's Hospital of Buffalo
Associate Professor of Surgery and Pediatrics
State University of New York
Buffalo, New York

HANLEY & BELFUS, INC. / Philadelphia

Publisher: HANLEY & BELFUS, INC.
                    Medical Publishers
                    210 South 13th Street
                    Philadelphia, PA 19107
                    (215) 546-7293; 800-962-1892
                    FAX (215) 790-9330
                    Web site: http://www.hanleyandbelfus.com

Note to the reader: Although the information in this book has been carefully reviewed for the correctness of dosage and indications, neither the authors nor the editors nor the publisher can accept any legal responsibility for any errors or omissions that may be made. Neither the publisher nor the editors make any warranty, expressed or implied, with respect to the material contained herein. Before prescribing any drug, the reader must review the manufacturer's current product information (package inserts) for accepted indications, absolute dosage recommendations, and other information pertinent to the safe and effective use of the product described.

Library of Congress Cataloging-in-Publication Data

Pediatric surgery secrets / edited by Philip L. Glick . . . [et al.]
        p.   cm. — (The Secrets Series®)
    Includes bibliographical references and index.
    ISBN 1-56053-317-X (alk. paper)
      1. Children—Surgery—Examinations, questions, etc.   I. Glick, Philip L.   II. Series.
    [DNLM: 1. Surgical Procedures, Operative—Child—Examination Questions.
    2. Surgical Procedures, Operative—Infant—Examination Questions.   WO 18.2 P371 2000]
RD137.P445 2001
617.99'8'0076—dc21

                                                                            00-027594

Printed and bound by CPI Group (UK) Ltd, Croydon, CR0 4YY

Transferred to digital print 2012

PEDIATRIC SURGERY SECRETS   ISBN 1-56053-317-X

Dedication

This book is dedicated to David Tapper, MD, FACS, FAAP and James E. Allen, MD, FACS, FAAP, who dedicated their careers to caring for the surgical needs of children, educating students, residents, fellows, and colleagues, and training the next generation of pediatric surgeons. We, the editors of this book, want to gratefully acknowledge these Herculean contributions and say thanks.

Philip L. Glick, MD
Michael S. Irish, MD
Richard H. Pearl, MD
Michael G. Caty, MD

CONTENTS

CONTRIBUTORS

Ashraf Abdel-Monem, MD
Fellow, Department of Pediatric Hematology/Oncology, State University of New York, Buffalo; Fellow, Roswell Park Cancer Institute, Buffalo, New York

Samuel Matthew Alaish, MD
Assistant Professor, Department of Surgery, Columbia University College of Physicans and Surgeons, New York; Attending Surgeon, New York Presbyterian Hospital, New York, New York

Kathryn D. Anderson, MD
Professor of Surgery, University of Southern California; Surgeon-in-Chief, Children's Hospital of Los Angeles, Los Angeles, California

Marjorie J. Arca, MD
Pediatric Surgery Resident, Department of Pediatric Surgery, University of Michigan Medical School, Ann Arbor, Michigan

Douglas G. Armstrong, MD, FRCS(C), FACS
Clinical Assistant Professor, Department of Orthopedic Surgery, State University of New York and the University of Buffalo, Buffalo, New York

Kenneth S. Azarow, MD, LTC MC
Assistant Professor, Department of Surgery, Uniformed Services University of the Health Sciences, Bethesda, Maryland; Chief, Department of Pediatric Surgery, Madigan Army Medical Center, Tacoma, Washington

James Backstrom, MD
Attending Radiologist, Devos Children's Hospital, Grand Rapids, Michigan

Patrick Vance Bailey, MD
Assistant Professor, Departments of Surgery and Pediatrics, University of Tennessee, Knoxville; Attending Physician, University of Tennessee Medical Center, Knoxville, Tennessee

Douglas Barnhart, MD
Pediatric Surgery Resident, Department of Pediatric Surgery, University of Michigan Medical School, Ann Arbor, Michigan

Denis D. Bensard, MD
Assistant Professor, Department of Pediatric Surgery, University of Colorado Health Sciences Center, Denver, Colorado

Drucy Borowitz, MD
Associate Professor, Department of Clinical Pediatrics, State University of New York, Buffalo; Chief, Division of Pediatric Pulmonology, Children's Hospital, Buffalo, New York

Scott C. Boulanger, PhD, MD
Fellow, Division of Pediatric Surgery, State University of New York, Buffalo, New York

Rebeccah L. Brown, MD
Assistant Professor, Department of Pediatric Surgery, University of Cincinnati, Cincinnati, Ohio

Thomas A. Brown, MD, MAJ MC
Staff Surgeon, Ireland Army Community Hospital, Fort Knox, Kentucky

Steven W. Bruch, MD
Pediatric Surgery Fellow, Department of Pediatric General Surgery, The Hospital for Sick Children, Toronto, Ontario, Canada

John G. Buchlis, MD
Clinical Assistant Professor, Department of Pediatrics, Children's Hospital of Buffalo, Division of Endocrinology/Diabetes, State University of New York School of Medicine, Buffalo, New York

Anthony A. Caldamone, MD
Professor of Surgery and Pediatrics, Department of Urology, Brown University School of Medicine, Providence, Rhode Island

Michael G. Caty, MD
Senior Attending Surgeon, Children's Hospital of Buffalo; Associate Professor of Surgery and Pediatrics, Department of Surgery, State University of New York, Buffalo, New York

Steven C. Chen, MD
Assistant Professor, Department of Surgery, University of California, Los Angeles; Associate Director, Pediatric Surgery, Cedars-Sinai Medical Center, Los Angeles, California

Douglas E. Coplen, MD
Fellow, Department of Pediatric Surgery, Sick Children's Hospital, Toronto, Ontario, Canada

Arnold G. Coran, MD
Professor, Department of Pediatric Surgery, University of Michigan Medical School; Surgeon-in-Chief, C.S. Mott Children's Hospital, Ann Arbor, Michigan

Kent Crickard, MD
Associate Professor, Emeritus, Department of Obstetrics/Gynecology, State University of New York, Buffalo, New York

Alfred A. de Lorimier, MD
Professor of Surgery, Emeritus, University of California, San Francisco; Chief, Department of Pediatric Surgery, California Pacific Medical Center, San Francisco, California

Jean-Claude Desmangles, MD
Assistant Clinical Professor, Department of Pediatrics, Children's Hospital of Buffalo, Division of Endocrinology/Diabetes, State University of New York School of Medicine, Buffalo, New York

Mark S. Dias, MD
Associate Professor, Department of Neurosurgery, State University of New York, Buffalo; Chief of Pediatric Neurosurgery, Children's Hospital, Buffalo, New York

Karen Diefenbach, MD
Chief Surgical Resident, Department of Surgery, University of Illinois College of Medicine, Peoria, Illinois

Robert C. Dukarm, MD
Assistant Professor, Department of Pediatrics, State University of New York, Buffalo, New York

Robert M. Filler, MD
Professor, Department of Surgery and Pediatrics, University of Toronto, Toronto; Director of Telehealth and External Medicine Affairs, The Hospital for Sick Children, Toronto, Ontario, Canada

Steven J. Fishman, MD
Department of Surgery, Harvard University Medical School, Boston, Massachusetts

Henri R. Ford, MD
Associate Professor, Department of Surgery, Children's Hospital of Pittsburgh, Pittsburgh, Pennsylvania

Lou Ann Gartner, MD
Clinical Assistant Professor, Department of Pediatric Endocrinology, Children's Hospital of Buffalo, Buffalo, New York

James Duncan Geiger, MD
Assistant Professor, Department of Pediatric Surgery, University of Michigan, Ann Arbor, Michigan

Philip L. Glick, MD, FAAP, FACS
Surgeon-in-Chief, Children's Hospital, Buffalo; Professor, Department of Surgery, Pediatrics, and Obstetrics/Gynecology, State University of New York, Buffalo, New York

Benjamin P. Green, MD
Associate Clinical Professor, Department of Psychiatry, University of Colorado Health Sciences Center, Denver, Colorado

Daniel M. Green, MD
Professor, Department of Pediatrics, State University of New York, Buffalo; Attending Physician, Roswell Park Cancer Institute, Buffalo, New York

Holly L. Hedrick, MD
Clinical Instructor, Department of Surgery, University of Pennsylvania School of Medicine; Schnaufer Senior Surgical Fellow, Children's Hospital of Philadelphia, Philadelphia, Pennsylvania

Bonnie B. Hudak, MD
Department of Pediatrics, Nemours Children's Clinic, Jacksonville, Florida

Michael S. Irish, MD, FAAP, FACS
Administrative Chief Resident, Department of Pediatric Surgery, The Children's Hospital of Buffalo, Kaleida Health, Buffalo, New York

Thomas Jaksic, MD, PhD
Associate Professor, Department of Pediatric Surgery, Harvard University, Boston, Massachusetts

Chatt A. Johnson, MD, MAJ, MC USA
Senior Surgery Resident, Madigan Army Medical Center, Tacoma, Washington

J. B. Joo, MD
Chief Surgical Resident, Department of Surgery, University of Illinois College of Medicine, Peoria, Illinois

Frederick M. Karrer, MD
Associate Professor, Department of Pediatric Surgery, University of Colorado Health Sciences Center, Denver, Colorado

Robert E. Kelly, Jr., MD
Assistant Professor of Clinical Surgery and Pediatrics, Eastern Virginia Medical School, Norfolk; Chief, Department of Surgery, Children's Hospital of the King's Daughters, Norfolk, Virginia

Peter C. W. Kim, MD
Assistant Professor, Department of Surgery, Division of Pediatric Surgery, The Hospital for Sick Children, Toronto, Ontario, Canada

Michael P. La Quaglia, MD
Chief, Department of Pediatric Surgery, Memorial Sloan-Kettering Cancer Center, New York; Professor, Department of Surgery, Weil-Cornell Medical School, New York

Jacob C. Langer, MD
Chief of Pediatric Surgery, Sick Children's Hospital, Toronto; Professor of Surgery, University of Toronto, Toronto, Ontario, Canada

Eric Loren Lazar, MD
Assistant Professor, Department of Surgery, Columbia University College of Physicians and Surgeons, New York; Attending Surgeon, New York Presbyterian Hospital, New York, New York

Marc A. Levitt, MD
Fellow, Division of Pediatric Surgery, State University of New York, Buffalo, New York

Veetai Li, MD
Assistant Professor, Department of Neurosurgery, State University of New York, Buffalo, New York

Margaret H. MacGillivray, MD
Professor, Department of Pediatrics, Children's Hospital of Buffalo; Chief, Division of Endocrinology/Diabetes, State University of New York School of Medicine, Buffalo, New York

J. Stephen Marshall, MD
Assistant Professor, Department of Surgery, University of Illinois College of Medicine, Peoria, Illinois

David Martin, MD
Attending Radiologist, Children's Hospital of Buffalo, Buffalo, New York

Amanda J. McCabe, FRCS
Pediatric Research Fellow, Children's Hospital of Buffalo, State University of New York, Buffalo, New York

Jerome M. McDonald, MD
Chief Resident, Department of Surgery, Madigan Army Medical Center, Tacoma, Washington

Evan P. Nadler, MD

William C. Olivero, MD
Associate Professor of Neurological Surgery and Pediatrics, University of Illinois College of Medicine, Peoria, Illinois

Charles N. Paidas, MD
Associate Professor, Department of Pediatric Surgery, Johns Hopkins University School of Medicine, Baltimore; Associate Professor, Johns' Hopkins Hospital, Baltimore, Maryland

Richard H. Pearl, MD, FACS, FAAP, FRCS(C)
Surgeon-in-Chief, Children's Hospital of Illinois, Peoria; Professor, Departments of Surgery and Pediatrics, University of Illinois College of Medicine, Peoria, Illinois

Nikola Kaylar Puffinbarger, MD
Chief Resident, Division of Pediatric Surgery, Babies' and Children's Hospital, New York, New York

William Ray Puffinbarger, MD
Clinical Assistant Professor, Department of Orthopedic Surgery and Rehabilitation, University of Oklahoma Health Sciences Center, Oklahoma City, Oklahoma

Churphena A. Reid, MD
Clinical Instructor, Departments of Surgery and Pediatrics, University of Illinois School of Medicine, Peoria, Illinois

Jorge Reyes, MD, FACS, FAAP
Professor, Department of Surgery, University of Pittsburgh; Chair, Pediatric Transplantation, Thomas F. Starzl Transplantation Institute, Pittsburgh; Director, Pediatric Transplantation Surgery, Children's Hospital, Pittsburgh, Pennsylvania

Henry E. Rice, MD
Assistant Professor, Division of Pediatric Surgery, Duke University Medical Center, Durham, North Carolina

Bradley M. Rodgers, MD
Professor and Chief, Division of Pediatric Surgery, University of Virginia Health System, Charlottesville, Virginia

Ray Thomas Ross, MD
Resident, Memorial Health University Medical Center, Department of Surgical Education, Mercer University, Savannah, Georgia

Steven S. Rothenberg, MD, FACS
Chief of Pediatric Surgery, The Hospital for Infants and Children at Presbyterian/St. Luke's Hospital, Denver; Assistant Clinical Professor, Department of Surgery, University of Colorado, Denver, Colorado

David P. Roye, Jr., MD
Livingston Professor of Pediatric Orthopedic Surgery, Columbia University College of Physicians and Surgeons, New York, New York

Joel Shilyansky, MD
Assistant Professor, Departments of Surgery and Pediatrics, University of Chicago, Chicago; Attending Surgeon, University of Chicago Children's Hospital, Chicago, Illinois

Sharon H. Smith, MD
Assistant Professor, Department of Pediatric Hematology/Oncology, State University of New York, Buffalo, New York

Perry W. Stafford, MD
Assistant Professor, Department of Surgery, University of Pennsylvania School of Medicine; Director, Trauma and Surgical Critical Care, Children's Hospital of Philadelphia, Philadelphia, Pennsylvania

Mark C. Stovroff, MD, FACS, FAAP
Clinical Associate Professor, Department of Surgery, Morehouse School of Medicine, Atlanta, Georgia

Carl St. Remy, MD
Department of Orthopedic Surgery, Columbia University College of Physicians and Surgeons, New York, New York

Steven Stylianos, MD
Associate Professor of Clinical Surgery and Pediatrics, Department of Surgery, Columbia University College of Physicians and Surgeons, New York; Director, Pediatric Trauma Program, Babies' and Children's Hospital, New York, New York

Leslie D. Tackett, MD
Chief Resident, Department of Urology, Brown University, Providence, Rhode Island

William Blair Tisol, MD
Senior Surgical Resident, Department of Surgery, University of Illinois College of Medicine, Peoria, Illinois

Jeffrey S. Upperman, MD
Fellow, Department of Pediatric Surgery, University of Pittsburgh, Pittsburgh, Pennsylvania

Robert J. Waldinger, MD
Assistant Professor, Department of Psychiatry, Harvard Medical School, Boston, Massachusetts

Julian Wan, MD
Attending Pediatric Urologist, Department of Pediatric Urology, Children's Hospital of Buffalo, Buffalo, New York

Wayne R. Waz, MD
Chief, Pediatric Nephrology, Children's Hospital, Buffalo; Assistant Professor, Department of Pediatrics, State University of New York, Buffalo, New York

David E. Wesson, MD
Professor, Department of Pediatric Surgery, Baylor College of Medicine, Houston, Texas

PREFACE

The title "Pediatric Surgical Secrets" is a misnomer. The information in this book is intended to be anything but secret. In fact, it should be considered additional core knowledge for medical students, pediatric and surgical residents, pediatric surgical trainees, pediatric nurse practitioners, primary care pediatricians, family practitioners, med-peds practitioners, and pediatric surgeons. The intent of this book is not to replace the information in a standard pediatric surgical textbook, but to supplement it. These pearls of wisdom should help all the previously mentioned pediatric caretakers provide better care for their patients. The authors of the various chapters were charged with the task of providing contemporary, state-of-the-art knowledge based on physiologic principles, literature review, and clinical experience. The authors have met this challenge. We thank them for a superb job.

This is the fifth writing project that this editorial team has completed in the last 5 years. With the changes in medicine caused by managed care, it has been more and more difficult to find the time. We could not have completed this project without our support team. We would like to acknowledge our administrative staff, Ms. Cindy Messina, Ms. Susan Reick, Ms. Mary Beth Saba, Ms. Carol Frosbink, and Ms. Paula Vallianatos, who helped this book to come to fruition. We also would like to acknowledge the help, guidance, and patience provided by the staff at Hanley and Belfus, Inc., including Mr. Bill Lamsback and Ms. Jacqueline Mahon. And, most importantly, the senior members of the editorial team (PLG, RP, and MGC) want to thank Dr. Michael Irish for his energy and enthusiasm on this project, without which this book would not be a reality. Lastly, we would like to acknowledge the support and understanding of our spouses and children, who have "allowed" us the time to write significant portions and edit the remainder of this book in our "spare time."

Philip L. Glick, MD
Michael S. Irish, MD
Richard H. Pearl, MD
Michael G. Caty, MD
EDITORS

I. General

1. EVALUATION OF THE PEDIATRIC SURGICAL PATIENT

Philip L. Glick, M.D., Michael S. Irish, M.D., and Michael G. Caty, M.D.

1. Why are pediatric patients not just small adults?

In addition to their size, infants, toddlers, preschoolers, children, and adolescents have unique disease processes, physiology, and physical and psychological responses to illnesses. As a result of these unique characteristics, optimal care requires specifically trained pediatric primary care practitioners (pediatricians, family practitioners, and med-peds) and pediatric specialists (medical and surgical).

2. Discuss the unique aspects of the relationship between the pediatric surgeon and the patient/family.

Many patients are either preverbal or unable to articulate their specific chief complaints or give a detailed history of their present illness. Therefore, it is essential to include the patient's parents, grandparents, guardians, home-care nurses, or other significant caretakers to obtain the proper history of the present illness. A mother's, grandmother's, or nurse's intuition often provides the most useful clues to the child's current illness or status change in a chronic illness.

3. What unique aspects of the history should a pediatric surgeon investigate?

- Many disease processes that pediatric surgeons confront actually begin in utero during fetal development. Therefore, a thorough understanding of the infant's development and the mother's pregnancy is crucial. Specifically, questions should be asked about routine prenatal care, prenatal testing, birth defects, interventions, and adverse outcomes.
- Because of the genetic basis for many diseases treated in infancy and childhood, a careful family pedigree should be elicited by the pediatric surgeon. Specifically, are any siblings or other relatives, living or deceased, affected by the same disease?
- In children with complicated medical histories, it is imperative to obtain all previous medical records and to take a team approach to their prospective care.

4. What are the unique aspects of the physical exam of an infant?

- Because an infant can become hypothermic easily, even in a well-heated exam room, it is imperative to complete the history before undressing the infant for a thorough physical exam.
- A thorough physical exam is crucial not only for complete assessment of the current problem but also for routine screening of illnesses for which infants are at risk. Examples include abdominal masses, hernias, hydroceles, cryptorchid testis, hypospadias, ectopically located anus, brachial cleft remnants, thyroglossal duct remnants, and vascular malformations.

5. What techniques can be used to overcome "white coat syndrome" in toddlers?

Don't wear a white coat! Obsessive-compulsive surgeons who see their patients in a white coat must gain trust in other ways. For instance, attempt to complete the physical exam with the parent holding the child. If this approach precludes a thorough exam, at least keep the mother by the exam table in direct vision of the child.

6. If you refer a healthy child to a pediatric surgeon for an inguinal hernia repair, what routine preoperative tests should be ordered?

None. Studies have shown that healthy infants, toddlers, preschoolers, children, and adolescents require no routine preoperative testing before elective surgery.

7. Are there any exceptions to this policy?

For healthy pediatric patients, the only exception is routine pregnancy testing for all female adolescents going to the operating room for an anesthetic.

8. What steps help to improve the physician-patient-parent relationship during office or hospital visits?

Many easy steps can be taken to strengthen the physician-patient-parent relationship and to allay many of the fears that parents experience when their children are ill. Make every attempt to sit down and talk to the parents eye to eye. This approach is considerably less intimidating than standing and looking down at the parents. Sitting down also gives the impression that you are less hurried. Even though you may spend the same 5 minutes with the family, their perception is that you spent much longer. Ask open-ended questions when taking the history and allow the parents to express all of their insights. When you have a better idea of the problems, help the parents focus their thoughts. Drawing simple pictures of anatomy and planned procedures often helps to communicate complicated details in an understandable fashion. Considering that many parents are young with variable educational backgrounds, use simple language to articulate your thoughts and plans. Avoid "med-speak."

9. How do you deal with parents who show up in your office with reams of Internet material or a list of detailed, complicated questions?

Take advantage of their concern. Take the time to review the materials and to answer the questions thoroughly. Be certain that the parents are not concerned about a problem that their child in fact does not have. Several families in our practice with children with complicated chronic illnesses (e.g., Hirschprung's disease, tracheoesophageal fistula, VATER-associated anomalies, congenital diaphragmatic hernia) belong to disease-specific Internet listserves and are sources of a plethora of information. As with most material on the web, such sites are not peer-reviewed, and the information must be viewed with this limitation in mind. However, parents often have spent hours acquiring such materials; they believe that the information helps them to deal with their child's illness and should be embraced. Reeducation, when appropriate, may be necessary. On more than one occasion, Internet sources have provided practical solutions to problems and have been greatly appreciated.

2. FLUIDS, ELECTROLYTES, AND NUTRITION FOR THE PEDIATRIC SURGERY PATIENT

Henry E. Rice, M.D.

1. What is the total body water content of a newborn? How does it change after birth?

The total body water content of a newborn is 75–80% at term gestation. During the first week of life, total body water decreases by 4–5%, which is reflected as a normal loss in body weight.

2. What is the risk of fluid overload in preterm infants?

Preterm infants with an excess of total body fluids have an increased incidence of patent ductus arteriosus, left ventricular failure, respiratory distress syndrome, and necrotizing enterocolitis.

3. How does renal fluid physiology differ in newborns and adults?

The glomerular filtration rate (GFR) of the term newborn is 25% that of the adult. The GFR rapidly rises during the first week of life and then slowly increases to adult levels by 2 years of age. Despite this low GFR, the newborn can handle large water loads, because the newborn kidney has a low concentrating capacity.

4. What is deficit fluid therapy?

Deficit fluid therapy refers to the management of the fluid losses that occurred before the patient's presentation. Deficit therapy has two essential components: (1) an accurate estimation of the severity of dehydration and (2) development of an approach to repair the deficit.

5. What are the typical signs of dehydration in a child?

The severity of dehydration is estimated from the patient's history and physical condition. No single piece of laboratory data can predict the severity of dehydration. In children with mild dehydration (1–5% total body fluid volume), the usual history is 12–24 hours of vomiting and diarrhea with minimal findings on exam. Children with moderate dehydration (6–10%) have a history of abnormal fluid losses plus physical findings that include tenting of the skin, weight loss, sunken eyes and fontanel, slight lethargy, and dry mucous membranes. With severe dehydration (11–15%), the patient develops skin mottling, cardiovascular instability (tachycardia, hypotension), and neurologic involvement (irritability, coma). Dehydration over a protracted period may be more severe than is clinically evident.

6. What are typical maintenance fluid requirements for a child?

AGE, (WT)	FLUIDS
Newborn day 1	50–60 ml/kg/day of $D_{10}W$
Newborn day 2	100 ml/kg/day of $D_{10} \frac{1}{4}$ NS
Newborn day > 7	100–150 ml/kg/day of $D_{5-10} \frac{1}{4}$ NS
Older child (0–10 kg)	100 ml/kg/day (4 ml/kg/hr)
Older child (10–20 kg)	1000 ml/day + 50 ml/kg/day) (40 ml/hr + 2 ml/kg/hr)
Older child (> 20 kg)	1500 ml/day + 25 ml/kg/day (60 ml/hr + 1 ml/kg/hr)

$D_{10}W$ = 10% aqueous dextrose solution, D10 $\frac{1}{4}$ NS = 10% dextrose in one-fourth normal saline solution, D_{5-10} = 5–10% dextrose solution.

7. How do normal fluid requirements (losses) change for the sick infant?

Normal fluid losses are composed of two parts: (1) evaporative losses (33% of total losses) and (2) urinary losses (66% of total losses). Evaporative losses are free water losses through the skin and lungs and are used for thermal regulation and to humidify inspired air. The ambient humidity and temperature affect the magnitude of evaporate losses, and patients receiving humidified air have a reduction in fluid requirements. Similarly, patients with hyperthermia or tachypnea have exaggerated evaporative losses. Urinary losses are affected by various conditions. Infants with diabetes insipidus and premature infants have an obligatory production of dilute urine, and appropriate increases in the volume of maintenance fluids must be made. In conditions of excessive secretion of antidiuretic hormone or physiologic stress, the patient may not be able to decrease urine osmolality, and the volume of fluids must be decreased.

8. What is the typical dehydration of a child with pyloric stenosis?

Dehydration with pyloric stenosis is based on loss of both fluid and electrolytes, with large losses of hydrogen and chloride ions from gastric secretions. The degree of dehydration can be estimated by physical exam and serum electrolytes. After progressive acid and fluid losses, the child develops hypokalemic, hypochloremic metabolic alkalosis. The degree of dehydration can be estimated by serum chloride and bicarbonate levels.

9. Explain paradoxical aciduria.

In children with severe dehydration, the urine pH often demonstrates a paradoxical aciduria, because the renal mechanisms for acid resorption are lost in an attempt to retain both sodium and potassium ions. The deficit in renal acid resorption contributes to metabolic alkalosis, and this cycle can be broken only by adequate fluid and electrolyte replacement. Surgery for pyloric stenosis should be deferred until the child is adequately rehydrated.

10. How many calories does a newborn infant require?

Most term infants are fed 90–120 kcal/kg/day. Increased calories are necessary in newborns with increased metabolic demands (e.g., prematurity, increased work of breathing, congenital heart disease). The overall best measure of adequate caloric support is weight gain (goal of 1%/day). Gavage feeds may be necessary in tachypneic infants.

11. How do you pick the right food for the right baby?

In general, breast milk is the best choice for most infants. When breast milk is not available, standard formulas (e.g., Enfamil, Similac) are the cheapest, most widely available alternatives and should be used unless there are other concerns. Premature infants require a special premature formulation. Soy formulas (e.g., Prosoybee, Isomil) are lactose-free and use soy for the protein source; they are used for infants who are intolerant of milk protein (with malabsorptive symptoms). Elemental formulas (e.g., Nutramigen, Pregestimil) are lactose-free and have predigested proteins (hydrolyzed casein); they are used for infants with malabsorption, short bowel, and cystic fibrosis.

12. What are the major components of total parenteral nutrition?

When possible, enteral feeds are preferable to total parenteral nutrition (TPN). TPN provides fluids, calories (in the form of carbohydrates and fat), electrolytes, and protein. Each of these components must be structured carefully for the child requiring parenteral nutrition.

13. How should you monitor a child on TPN?

As the child begins TPN, hyperglycemia is poorly tolerated and requires a reduction in glucose infusion: Routine electrolytes, lipid levels, and liver function tests are mandatory. The major risk to long-term TPN use is cholestatic liver failure.

14. What risk is associated with overfeeding a sick child?

Overfeeding calories or substrate in excess of metabolic demands may result in respiratory compromise, hepatic dysfunction, and an increased risk of dying from a particular condition.

BIBLIOGRAPHY

1. Bell E, Warburton D, Stonestreet B, et al: Effect of fluid administration on the development of symptomatic patent ductus arteriosus and congestive heart failure in premature infants. N Engl J Med 302:598, 1980.
2. Cosnett JE: The origins of intravenous fluid therapy. Lancet i:768, 1989.
3. Letton RW, Chwals WJ: Fluid and electrolyte metabolism. In Oldham KT, Colombani PM, Foglia RP (eds): Surgery of Infants and Children: Scientific Principles and Practice. Philadelphia, Lippincott-Raven, 1997, pp 83–116.
4. Marchini G, Stock S: Thirst and vasopressin secretion counteract dehydration in newborn infants. J Pediatr 130:736, 1997.
5. Tammela OK: Appropriate fluid regimens to prevent bronchopulmonary dysplasia. Eur J Pediatr 154(8 Suppl 3):515, 1995.
6. Travis LB: Disorders of water, electrolyte, and acid-base physiology. In Rudolph AM, Hoffman JIE, Rudolph CD (eds): Rudolph's Pediatrics, 20th ed. Stamford, CT, Appleton & Lange, 1996, p 1319.

II. Critical Care

3. SHOCK

Karen Diefenbach, M.D., and Richard H. Pearl, M.D.

1. How is shock defined?
The purest definition of shock is an acute state of oxygen deficiency at the cellular level.

2. What physical signs are associated with shock?
Shock, regardless of etiology, is associated with several physical signs that reflect the body's attempt to compensate for decreased oxygen delivery to the tissues. They include tachycardia, peripheral vasoconstriction (leading to delayed capillary refill, diminished pulses, and decreased skin temperature), hypotension, tachypnea, and decreased urine output.

3. What is MODS?
MODS stands for **m**ultiple **o**rgan **d**ysfunction **s**yndrome and may be associated with shock of any etiology. Acute respiratory failure, renal failure, hepatic dysfunction, pancreatitis, coagulopathies, gastrointestinal hemorrhage, immunologic dysfunction, and endocrine and metabolic abnormalities may result from inadequate tissue oxygenation. The diagnosis of MODS indicates organ dysfunction to the degree that homeostasis cannot be maintained without intervention. Older textbooks may use the acronym MOSF (**m**ultiple **o**rgan **s**ystem **f**ailure).

4. What is SIRS?
SIRS, an acronym for **s**ystemic **i**nflammatory **r**esponse **s**yndrome, is defined as a major inflammatory response to a variety of severe clinical insults such as sepsis, trauma, and burns. It results in activation of common pathogenic pathways, both molecular and cellular, with common clinical manifestations. It is diagnosed by the presence of two or more of the following conditions:
- Temperature < 36°C or > 38°C
- Heart rate > 90 beats/min (adults; variable increase in children)
- Respiratory rate > 20 breaths/min (adults) or partial pressure of carbon dioxide in arterial blood < 32 mmHg
- White blood cell count > 12,000, < 4,000, or > 10% bands

5. What is ARDS?
Known as **a**cute or adult **r**espiratory **d**istress **s**yndrome, ARDS is acute respiratory failure due to injury to the alveolar capillary unit; it results in increased permeability and pulmonary edema. ARDS may be associated with a variety of insults but most frequently is associated with shock, sepsis, near-drowning, massive transfusions, or aspiration.

6. What are some of the clinical sequelae of shock?
Metabolic acidosis, multiple organ dysfunction syndrome, disseminated intravascular coagulation, and death.

7. When and how is the metabolic acidosis associated with shock treated? Why?
Metabolic acidosis in shock results from inadequate tissue perfusion, which causes cellular hypoxia. Hypoxia results in the accumulation of acid products of anaerobic metabolism (lactic acidosis). It usually resolves as oxygenation of tissues and renal function improve. However, correction with sodium bicarbonate (in addition to volume resuscitation) is indicated when the arterial blood pH is less than 7.2. To avoid overcorrection, aggressive correction of the acidosis

should stop when the pH is greater than 7.3. The reason for quickly correcting the acidosis is to alleviate the myocardial depression and increased systemic and pulmonary vascular resistance that undermine resuscitative efforts in patients with shock.

8. What are the four determinants of oxygen delivery?

Oxygen delivery (DO_2) depends on heart rate (HR), stroke volume (SV), hemoglobin (Hgb), and arterial oxygen saturation (SaO_2), as indicated by the following equations:
(1) $DO_2 = CO \times CaO_2$, where CO = cardiac output and CaO_2 = arterial oxygen content
(2) $CO = HR \times SV$
(3) $CaO_2 = (SaO_2 \times Hgb \times 1.34)$ ($Hgb \times 1.39 \times SaO_2$) + ($0.003 \times PaO_2$), where PaO_2 = partial pressure of oxygen

9. What is SvO_2? How is it helpful in monitoring the patient in shock?

SvO_2 refers to mixed venous oxygen saturation in a sample taken from the right atrium. It is determined by the following equation:

$$SvO_2 = 1 - VO_2/DO_2$$

where VO_2 = volume of oxygen utilization. The determinants of SvO_2 are oxygen consumption, hemoglobin, cardiac output, and oxygen saturation. Other than oxygen consumption, these factors can be manipulated during resuscitation to maximize oxygen delivery to the tissues. Monitoring of SvO_2 allows minute-to-minute assessment of interventions in cardiorespiratory support and resuscitation. SvO_2 is affected by increasing Hgb with transfusions; support of cardiac output with volume, vasopressors, or cardiotropic drugs; and increased oxygen delivery.

10. List the four major types of shock.
1. Hypovolemic   3. Neurogenic
2. Cardiogenic   4. Septic

11. How do the hemodynamic variables compare in the different types of shock?

	CO	SVR	MAP	PAWP	CVP
Hypovolemic	↓	↑	N or ↓	↓↓↓	↓↓↓
Cardiogenic	↓↓	↑↑↑	N or ↓	↑↑	↑↑
Neurogenic	↑↑	↓↓↓	N or ↓	N or ↓	N or ↓
Septic					
Early	↑↑↑	↓↓↓	N or ↓	↓	↓
Late	↓↓	↓↓	↓↓	↑	↑ or N

CO = cardiac output, SVR = systemic vascular resistance, MAP = mean arterial pressure, PAWP = pulmonary artery wedge pressure, CVP = central venous pressure, N = normal.

12. What are the primary goals of shock management, regardless of etiology?

For all forms of shock, treating the underlying cause is mandatory. Always remember the ABCs: assess airway and breathing, and supply supplemental oxygen to ensure adequate circulation and oxygenation. Intubation for airway control and management should be done in all cases of shock that are not readily reversible. Establishment of intravenous access and stabilization of systemic arterial blood pressure, followed by careful monitoring and repeated physical exams to assess the response to therapeutic interventions, are necessary. Central venous monitoring and Foley catheter measurement of urine output often are required.

13. What type of shock is encountered most frequently in children?

Regardless of the cause (hemorrhage, plasma losses, or water and electrolyte losses), hypovolemic shock is the most common type of shock in children. It is defined as a clinical state characterized by decreased venous return to the heart and subsequent diminished left ventricle filling (decreased stroke volume), resulting in insufficient oxygen delivery to the tissues.

14. For patients with hypovolemic shock, what is the initial order for resuscitation?

The first line of therapy is a 20-ml/kg bolus of crystalloid solution, which may be repeated at least twice or until clinical improvement is seen. The use of colloids such as albumin and blood products, when indicated for acute hemorrhage or coagulopathy, is recommended when overall fluid deficit exceeds 15–25%.

15. What is the 4-2-1 rule for intravenous fluids?

The 4-2-1 rule refers to a method for determining the patient's maintenance fluid requirements. The patient requires 4 ml/kg/hr for the first 10 kg of body weight, 2 ml/kg/hr for the second 10 kg of body weight, and 1 ml/kg/hr for every kg over 20 kg. For example, a child who weighs 33 kg requires (4 ml/kg/hr × 10 kg) + (2 ml/kg/hr × 10 kg) + (1 ml/kg/hr × 13 kg) = 40 ml/hr + 20 ml/hr + 13 ml/hr = 73 ml/hr.

16. What percent of body weight must be lost as a result of dehydration before an average healthy child becomes hypotensive?

Decreased blood pressure usually is not seen until about 15% of body weight is lost.

17. How do you calculate the fluid deficit for a child who is hypovolemic and now weighs 18 kg, given that the previous weight was 20 kg?

The patient has lost 2 kg and is therefore 10% dehydrated (2 kg of 20 kg). One liter is 1 kg. Therefore, a 2-kg weight loss translates to a 2000-ml deficit.

18. How should the fluids be administered to resuscitate the patient in question 17, assuming no ongoing losses?

The patient should be resuscitated over 24 hours, and the usual rule of thumb for replacement of losses is one half of the deficit over the first 8 hours and the other half over the next 16 hours. The patient's calculated fluid deficit is 2000 ml. In addition, the patient has a maintenance requirement of 60 ml/hr. Every patient receives an initial bolus of 20 ml/kg (= 400 ml). Therefore, the deficit to be replaced over the next 24 hours is now 1600 ml. The rate in ml/hr for the first 8 hours is 800 ml/8 hr = 100 ml/hr + maintenance = 160 ml/hr. The rate for the next 16 hours is 800 ml/16 hr = 50 ml/hr + maintenance = 110 ml/hr. Electrolyte composition after intravenous flush is determined and adjusted according to the results of serum electrolytes and laboratory tests.

19. What is the estimated blood volume for a term infant? For a child?

The estimated blood volume for a term infant is 90 ml/kg. An average child has an estimated blood volume of 80 ml/kg.

20. What are the characteristics of the four different classifications of hemorrhagic shock?

	I	II	III	IV
Estimated blood volume deficit	10–15%	20–25%	30–35%	> 40%
Pulse (beats/min)	> 100	> 150	> 150	> 150
Respirations	Normal	Increased	Tachypneic	Tachypneic/apneic
Capillary refill (sec)	< 5	5–10	10–15	> 20
Blood pressure	Normal	Decreased pulse pressure	Decreased	Severely decreased
Mentation	Normal	Anxious	Confused	Unconscious
Orthostatic hypotension	+	++	+++	+++
Urine output (ml/kg)	1–3	0.5–1	< 0.5	None

21. What is cardiogenic shock?

A clinical state characterized by abnormalities of cardiac rhythm or function, which result in abnormal oxygen delivery to the tissues and pump failure.

22. What are the most common causes of cardiogenic shock?
Congenital heart disease, cardiomyopathy, cardiac tamponade, arrhythmias, metabolic disorders, and connective tissue disorders can be associated with cardiogenic shock. The common denominator is depressed cardiac output.

23. What physical findings are associated with cardiogenic shock?
Patients with cardiogenic shock are tachycardic, diaphoretic, oliguric, acidotic, and hypotensive. Hepatomegaly, jugular venous distention, rales, and peripheral edema also may be observed. Cardiac output is decreased; CVP, PAWP, and SVR are elevated.

24. What are the clinical signs of cardiac tamponade?
Low cardiac output, pulsus paradoxus, jugular venous distention, narrowed pulse pressure, and muffled heart tones.

25. What diagnostic testing should be done in a patient suspected of having cardiogenic shock?
All patients with suspected cardiogenic shock should have a chest radiograph, an electrocardiogram, and an echocardiogram. CVP determination and urine output are helpful in management decisions.

26. What pathophysiology is associated with neurogenic shock?
Neurogenic shock is characterized by hypotension secondary to decreased or absent sympathetic activity and the subsequent loss of vascular tone after central nervous system trauma. In essence, the size of the vascular bed is drastically changed with no change in blood volume; the result is distributional hypovolemic shock.

27. What injury is associated most frequently with neurogenic shock? How is it diagnosed?
The classical description is hypotension after transection of the spinal cord in the cervicothoracic region. The diagnosis is made by physical exam demonstrating neurologic injury, hypotension that does not respond to fluid resuscitation, and a high index of clinical suspicion. A rectal exam demonstrating absent sphincter tone is virtually diagnostic.

28. How is neurogenic shock treated?
In addition to placing the patient in the Trendelenburg position (when possible) and continuing fluid resuscitation, the mainstay of therapy is administration of vasopressors, most commonly neosynephrine.

29. What is the mechanism of hypovolemia in septic shock?
Septic shock typically is associated with an abnormal distribution of volume due to peripheral vasodilatation and venous pooling as well as an absolute intravascular volume loss secondary to increased microvascular permeability, which leads to a loss into the interstitial spaces. In essence, every cell in the body "leaks," causing intracellular hypovolemia and extracellular water excess, a combination resulting in total body edema.

30. Which two inflammatory mediators have the most significance in the development of septic shock?
Tumor necrosis factor alpha and interleukin (IL)-1 are the most clinically relevant. However, research also has linked IL-6, IL-8, platelet-activating factor, cytokines, kinins, and nitric oxide to the inflammatory response associated with septic shock.

31. Which pathogens most often cause septic shock in neonates, infants, and children?
Neonates: group B beta-hemolytic streptococci, Enterobacteriaceae, *Listeria monocytogenes*, *Staphylococcus aureus*, herpes simplex

Infants: *Haemophilus influenzae, Streptococcus pneumoniae, S. aureus*
Children: *S. pneumoniae, Neisseria meningitidis, S. aureus,* Enterobacteriaceae, *H. influenzae*
Immunocompromised: Enterobacteriaceae, *S.aureus,* Pseudomonadaceae, *Candida albicans*

BIBLIOGRAPHY

1. Giroir BP, Levin DL, Perkin RM: Shock. In Levin DL, Morriss FC (eds): Essentials of Pediatric Intensive Care, 2nd ed. New York, Churchill Livingstone, 1997, pp 280–301.
2. McConnell MS, Perkin RM: Shock states. In Fuhrman BP, Zimmerman JJ (eds): Pediatric Critical Care, 2nd ed. St. Louis, Mosby, 1998, pp 293–306.
3. Nichols DG, Yaster M, Lappe DG, Haller JA (eds): Golden Hour: The Handbook of Advanced Pediatric Life Support, 2nd ed. St. Louis, Mosby, 1996.
4. Tobin JR, Wetzel RC: Shock and multi-organ system failure. In Rogers MC, Nichols DG, Ackerman AD, et al (eds): Textbook of Pediatric Intensive Care, 3rd ed. Baltimore, Williams & Wilkins, 1996, pp 555–605.

4. EXTRACORPOREAL MEMBRANE OXYGENATION

Patrick V. Bailey, M.D.

1. What is extracorporeal membrane oxygenation?

Extracorporeal membrane oxygenation (ECMO) is a technique of prolonged, nonpulsatile, partial cardiopulmonary bypass achieved via extrathoracic cannulation.

2. Who developed the technique?

ECMO was developed by Robert H. Bartlett, Professor of Surgery at the University of Michigan. It was originally developed in the hope of providing support and improving outcome for adults with "shock lung" or adult respiratory distress syndrome. However, a trial sponsored by the National Institutes of Health in 1979 showed no improvement in survival for adults. Subsequently, the technique was applied to newborns with respiratory failure and found to improve outcome dramatically.

3. When is the use of ECMO considered?

In general, ECMO should be considered to provide support to infants and occasionally older children with potentially reversible cardiac or pulmonary failure that is refractory to less invasive, more conventional medical techniques. Respiratory failure in newborns, unlike that in adults, is rarely associated with damage to the lung parenchyma and is therefore reversible. ECMO provides temporary support during which the lungs can rest and recover without being subjected to iatrogenically induced damage of increased ventilator pressures and high FiO_2.

4. What are the specific indications for ECMO?

Meconium aspiration syndrome
Persistent pulmonary hypertension (PPHN)/persistent fetal circulation (PFC)
Respiratory distress syndrome
Group B streptococcal pneumonia/sepsis
Congenital diaphragmatic hernia
Barotrauma/air leak syndrome
Postoperative cardiac failure (after repair of congenital heart defect)

5. How is the decision made to place a patient on ECMO?

The use of ECMO depends on meeting both eligibility criteria and selection criteria. A patient must be "eligible" to be "selected." Eligibility criteria include:

- Weight > 2 kg
- Gestational age > 34 wk
- No evidence of intracranial hemorrhage
- No evidence of systemic bleeding
- Absence of congenital heart disease
- Absence of major congenital anomaly or chromosomal abnormality
- Reversible lung disease

The weight and gestational age criteria were established to limit the occurrence of significant bleeding complications, specifically intracranial hemorrhage. Because systemic anticoagulation is necessary, sonographic evidence of intracranial hemorrhage or other systemic bleeding disqualifies a patient from consideration. An echocardiogram is used to exclude congenital cardiac disease, some forms of which may mimic persistent pulmonary hypertension. It also identifies patients with noncorrectable heart defects. Nearly all lung disease in newborns is reversible. If there are no contraindications based on the above criteria, the patient may be selected for ECMO. Discussion has centered mainly on the selection of patients and the appropriate time to use ECMO. Numerous studies have attempted to establish criteria to predict the need for ECMO support. Examples of such criteria are as follows:

- Oxygenation index (OI) > 40 on 3 of 5 blood gas analyses obtained 30–60 minutes apart. The oxygenation index is calculated as follows:

$$OI = MAP \times FiO_2 \times 100/postductal\ PaO_2$$

where MAP = mean airway pressure, FiO2 = fractional concentration of oxygen in inspired gas, and PaO_2 = partial pressure of oxygen in arterial blood.
- Alveolar-arterial oxygenation difference (Aa-DO_2) > 610 for more than 8 hours.
- For patients with congenital diaphragmatic hernia, a ventilatory index (VI) > 1000 with a partial pressure of carbon dioxide in arterial blood ($PaCO_2$) > 40 mmHg. The VI is calculated as the product of mean airway pressure × ventilator rate (MAP × rate).
- Severe barotrauma with 4 of the following 7 conditions: pneumothorax, pneumoperitoneum, pneumopericardium, interstitial emphysema, subcutaneous emphysema, MAP >15 cm H_2O, and persistent air leak.

6. How is the patient cannulated?

Cannulation is performed at the bedside in the intensive care unit. The large vessels of the neck (i.e., the carotid and the jugular) are most commonly chosen for cannulation with venoarterial bypass. Local anesthetic and/or intravenous narcotics may be used to provide analgesia during the procedure. Before beginning the procedure, both a shoulder roll and an x-ray plate are placed beneath the patient, and the head is turned to the left. Either a longitudinal or transverse incision may be used. The vessels are identified after retracting the sternocleidomastoid muscle. Manipulation of the vessels should be minimized to prevent vasospasm. Proximal and distal control of both the artery and vein is obtained with vessel loops or suture.

Cannulas of appropriate size are then chosen. Selection of the largest cannula possible facilitates drainage of blood from the body and minimizes resistance to its return. Typically, 8- to 14-French cannulas are chosen for newborns. Pursestring sutures may be placed at the site of cannulation to facilitate later repair at decannulation. Before ligating the vessels distally, a loading dose of heparin (100 U/kg) is administered. Ligation of the carotid artery causes understandable concern. However, the collateral circulation in infants is such that the risk of cerebral ischemia is minimal.

Venotomy and arterotomy are then performed and the cannulas inserted. The tip of the venous cannula is positioned in the right atrium and the tip of the arterial cannula at the junction of carotid with the aortic arch. After securing the cannulas in place and removing all air from them, especially the arterial cannula, they are connected to the circuit and flow is instituted. The wound is then closed.

Throughout the procedure, careful attention is directed toward hemostasis with the liberal use of electrocautery, thrombin, and Gelfoam. With venovenous bypass, a double-lumen cannula is typically inserted in the jugular vein. Alternatively, the blood may be drained from the jugular cannula and returned via another large systemic vein such as the femoral vein.

7. What are the components of the circuit? How does it work?

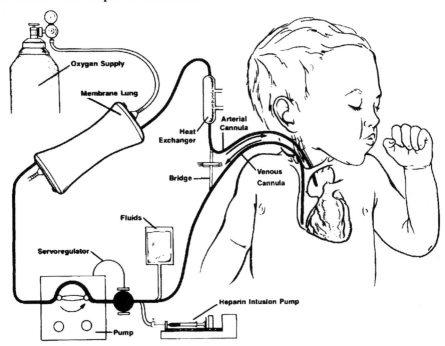

Components of the venoarterial circuit.

Venous blood drains by gravity through a collapsible venous reservoir or bladder onto the roller pump. The roller pump circulates the blood through the circuit. The mechanism of propulsion is compression and displacement of the blood within the tubing. Servoregulation prevents negative pressure from being applied to the venous cannula by interrupting the flow by the roller pump if venous return is not adequate (i.e., the bladder collapses). Next the blood is pumped through the membrane oxygenator for gas exchange. Oxygenation occurs down a large gradient between that of the desaturated venous blood and the FiO_2 of the sweep gas. Oxygenation is directly related to the pump flow rate and the oxygen gradient between the sweep gas and the desaturated venous blood. Carbon dioxide exchange occurs down a much smaller gradient but is approximately 6 times more efficient. It is primarily related to the surface area of the membrane lung. Before being returned to the body via the arterial cannula, the blood passes through a heat exchanger for warming.

8. How is the circuit managed after cannulation?

After cannulation initial flow rates are set at approximately 100 cc/kg/min or 80% of cardiac output. ECMO flow is adjusted according to the oxygen saturation in venous (SvO_2) and arterial blood (SaO_2). The flow is increased or decreased to maintain an $SvO_2 > 65\%$ and an $SaO_2 > 90\%$. Once there is evidence of improved lung function, the flow can be weaned. Because most patients receive a significant amount of fluid in attempts at resuscitation before ECMO is used, diuresis usually is necessary after cannulation. Most patients accomplish diuresis on their own, beginning 24 hours after cannulation. Lasix or other diuretics are used to augment the diuresis. Occasionally, placement of a hemofilter in the circuit is necessary to facilitate the diuresis. Because enteral feedings are poorly tolerated by patients on ECMO, it is necessary to institute parenteral nutrition via the circuit within 24 hours of cannulation.

9. How is the ventilator managed while the patient is on ECMO?
The establishment of ECMO flow allows the lungs to be put at rest, meaning that the ventilator settings are dramatically decreased. The FiO_2 is reduced to 21–30%, the peak inspiratory pressure (PIP) is set at 18–22, positive end-expiratory pressure (PEEP) is set at 3–5, and the respiratory rate is decreased to 10–16. A PEEP of 12–14 has been reported to be useful in increasing dynamic compliance, which may lead to a shorter course of ECMO. Typically, it is necessary to increase the PIP, PEEP, and FiO_2 to more moderate settings as the patient is weaned from the circuit.

10. What is the difference between venoarterial and venovenous bypass?
ECMO flow may be instituted in one of two ways, either venoarterial (VA) or venovenous (VV) bypass. In a VA circuit, blood is drained from the internal jugular vein, passed through the circuit, and then returned to the body via the carotid artery. With a VV circuit, the blood is drained from the jugular vein, but after gas exchange it also is returned to the venous circulation via a double-lumen jugular catheter or separate cannula in another large systemic vein. Total cardiopulmonary bypass may be achieved with VA bypass. However, flow is usually established at approximately 80% of cardiac output (80–120 cc/kg/min). With VV bypass, the blood from the circuit is mixed in the right atrium with blood from the systemic circulation. In addition, some of the blood undergoes "recirculation" back into the ECMO circuit. Therefore, a higher flow rate is required for adequate oxygen delivery. In addition, VV bypass has no effect on cardiac output and therefore can provide only respiratory support. The major advantages to VV bypass are that carotid artery ligation is not necessary and that air or particulate matter in the circuit can embolize only as far as the pulmonary circulation.

11. How is clotting of the circuit prevented?
In a word, heparin. Anticoagulation is necessary to overcome the activation of the coagulation cascade whenever the blood comes into contact with a foreign surface such as silastic, polyurethane, or polycarbonate. Without heparin-induced anticoagulation, thrombosis of the circuit results. Before cannulation, a loading dose of heparin of approximately 100 U/kg is administered. In addition, a continuous infusion of heparin is given via the circuit (25–75 U/kg/hr). Whole blood activated clotting time (ACT) is monitored and the heparin infusion modified to maintain an ACT of 180–200 seconds, approximately 1.5–2 times normal. Heparin is excreted in the urine and is bound to platelets. Therefore, it may be necessary to increase infusion during diuresis or platelet transfusion. Heparin alone is adequate to prevent thrombosis. Therefore, platelet counts and procoagulant levels are maintained at near-normal levels to prevent bleeding complications.

12. What criteria are used for weaning the patient from the circuit? How is weaning accomplished?
Patients may be weaned from the circuit once their pulmonary function begins to show signs of improvement. Examples of such signs include: (1) improved lung compliance on serial measurements, (2) clearing of the chest radiograph, and (3) increasing mixed venous oxygen saturation or PaO_2 or decreasing $PaCO_2$ without change in the ventilator settings or ECMO flow rate. The method by which weaning is accomplished depends on whether VA or VV bypass is used. With VA bypass, once there is evidence of improved lung function, the flow rate is gradually decreased in increments, usually 10–30 ml per change. Once flow is approximately 25% of the initial rate, a "trial-off" period may be attempted. During these trials, the ventilator is increased to moderate settings and the lines to the patient are clamped. The circuit continues to flow across a bridge and therefore bypasses the clamped lines to the patient. Successful trials indicate the ability of the patient to tolerate decannulation.

VV bypass weaning is accomplished by simply decreasing the FiO_2 going to the circuit. The flow does not need to be changed. Again, the ventilator is adjusted to more moderate settings as weaning begins. Once the patient is able to tolerate a circuit FiO_2 of 21–30% on moderate ventilator settings, ECMO may be discontinued.

13. What are the potential complications of ECMO?

Complications of ECMO fall into the three broad categories: (1) the underlying disease process, (2) medical issues specific to the use of the technology, and (3) technical issues related to the cannulas or circuit. Failure of the lung to recover enough physiologic function for adequate exchange of oxygen and carbon dioxide, recurrent persistent pulmonary hypertension after successful weaning from ECMO, and disease progression despite ECMO are relatively infrequent. By contrast there are approximately 1.5 medical complications per patient. Of these, neurologic complications such as seizures and cerebral infarction are the most frequent (24%). Hemorrhagic complications secondary to the required anticoagulation are almost as common at 21%. Intracranial bleeds are the most clinically significant. However, other reported sites of bleeding include the cannulation site, chest tubes sites, other surgical wounds, and the gastrointestinal and urinary tracts. Technical complications such as malpositioning of the cannulas, rupture of the circuit, or malfunction of the oxygenator are much less common (0.3 complications per patient).

14. What are the long-term outcomes for neurologic and developmental function?

Cannulation for VA bypass necessitates ligation of the carotid artery. Subsequent attempts at repair have had mixed success. Thus, there has been much concern about the long-term neurologic and developmental outcome for patients placed on ECMO. Because ECMO has been frequently used only since the mid 1980s, good long-term data have become available only recently. These data indicate normal neurologic function in 70–80% of patients, which is comparable to the outcome for cohorts of similar patients treated by conventional means only. This finding suggests that impairment of neurologic and developmental function may be related to events that occur before cannulation, such as hypoxia and hypotension, as opposed to carotid artery ligation.

15. Are all patients successfully weaned from the circuit?

No. Unfortunately, in some patients the lung is unable to recover adequate physiologic function despite the use of ECMO. In such cases, it becomes necessary to discontinue support, knowing that the patient will die. Such action is considered after a complication that necessitates discontinuing therapy or after a prolonged course during which multiple attempts at weaning have failed. Infants usually are not kept on ECMO for longer than 10–14 days.

16. What are the results for the various indications?

In a 1995 report from the Extracorporeal Life Support Organization, an 81% survival rate was reported in nearly 10,000 patients. The results for the various diagnoses are as follows:

Meconium aspiration syndrome	94%
PPHN/PFC	84%
Respiratory distress syndrome	84%
Pneumonia/sepsis	76%
Air leak syndrome	73%
Congenital diaphragmatic hernia	58%

BIBLIOGRAPHY

1. Anderson HL, Snedecor SM, Otsu T, et al: Multicenter comparison of conventional venoarterial access versus venovenous double-lumen catheter access in newborn infants undergoing extracorporeal membrane oxygenation. J Pediatr Surg 28:530–535, 1993.
2. Bartlett RH: Surgery, science and respiratory failure. J Pediatr Surg 32:1401–1407, 1997.
3. Bartlett RH, Andrews AF, Toomasien JM, et al: Extracorporeal membrane oxygenation (ECMO) for newborn respiratory failure: 45 cases. Surgery 92:425–433, 1982.

4. Bartlett RH, Gazzaniga AB, Huxtable RF, et al: Extracorporeal circulation (ECMO) in neonatal respiratory failure. J Thorac Cardiovasc Surg 74:826–833, 1977.
5. Bartlett RH, Gazzaniga AB, Toomasien JM, et al: Extracorporeal membrane oxygenation (ECMO) in neonatal respiratory failure: 100 cases. Ann Surg 204:236–245, 1986.
6. Bohn DJ, James I, Filler RM, et al: The relationship between $PaCO_2$ and ventilatory parameters in predicting survival in congenital diaphragmatic hernia. J Pediatr Surg 19:666–671, 1984.
7. Cilley RE: Respiratory physiology and extracorporeal life support. In Oldham KT, Colombani PM, Foglia RP (eds): Surgery of Infants and Children. Philadelphia, Lippincott-Raven, 1997, pp 183–222.
8. Hirschl RB, Bartlett RH: Extracorporeal life support in cardiopulmonary failure. In O'Neill JA, Rowe MI, Grosfeld JL, et al (eds): Pediatric Surgery, 5th ed. St. Louis, Mosby, 1998, pp 89–102.
9. Hofkosh D, Thompson AE, Nozza RJ, et al: Ten years of extracorporeal membrane oxygenation: Neurodevelopmental outcome. Pediatrics 87:549–555, 1991.
10. Klein MD, Shaheen KW, Whittlesey GC, et al: Extracorporeal membrane oxygenation for the circulatory support of children after repair of congenital heart disease. J Thorac Cardiovasc Surg 100:498–505, 1990.
11. Krummel TM, Greenfield LJ, Kirkpatrick BV, et al: Alveolar-arterial oxygen gradients versus the neonatal pulmonary insufficiency index for prediction of mortality in ECMO candidates. J Pediatr Surg 19: 380–384, 1984.
12. Morton A, Dalton H, Kochanek P, et al: Extracorporeal membrane oxygenation for pediatric respiratory failure: Five-year experience at the University of Pittsburgh. Crit Care Med 22:1659–1667, 1994.
13. Rowe MI, O'Neill JA, Grosfeld JL, et al: Respiratory considerations. In Rowe MI, O'Neill JA, Grosfeld JL, et al (eds): Essentials of Pediatric Surgery. St. Louis, Mosby, 1995, pp 47–61.
14. Schumacher RE, Palmer TW, Roloff DW, et al: Follow-up of infants treated with extracorporeal membrane oxygenation for newborn respiratory failure. Pediatrics 87:451–457, 1991.
15. Zwischenberger JB, Nguyen TT, Upp RJ, et al: Complications of neonatal extracorporeal membrane oxygenation. Collective experience from the extracorporeal life support organization. J Thorac Cardiovasc Surg 107:838–849, 1994.

5. MECHANICAL VENTILATION

Scott C. Boulanger, M.D., Ph.D., Vivian Lindfield, M.D., Michael G. Caty, M.D., and Philip L. Glick, M.D.

1. What are the indications for mechanical ventilation?

Indications can be classified in three categories: inability to oxygenate (hypoxia), inability to ventilate (hypercapnia), and inability to protect the airway.

2. Define tidal volume, total lung capacity, vital capacity, functional residual capacity, and closing capacity.

Tidal volume: the volume of gas moved into and out of the lungs during a single breath.
Total lung capacity: the total volume of gas in the lungs during maximal inflation.
Vital capacity: the maximal amount of gas in the lungs available for respiration.
Functional residual capacity: the volume of gas left in the lung after a normal breath.
Closing capacity: the volume of gas left in the lung when small airways begin to collapse.

3. Define work of breathing. Why is it important?

Work of breathing is the amount of work performed by the respiratory muscles during respiration. Increased airway resistance or decreased compliance leads to greater work of breathing and ultimately to respiratory failure.

4. Define peak inspiratory pressure and mean airway pressure.

Peak inspiratory pressure (PIP) is the highest pressure reached during inspiration. In pressure-controlled ventilation the PIP is preset, whereas in volume-controlled ventilation it is variable. Mean airway pressure (MAP) is the average pressure exerted on the airway and lung during the respiratory cycle. MAP is important for both oxygenation and ventilation. MAP is affected by volume, PIP, flow, and positive end-expiratory pressure (PEEP) as well as other factors.

5. What is dead space?
Dead space is the volume of gas in the lungs that does not participate in gas exchange and the volume of gas in the ventilator tubing.

6. How do lung compliance and airway resistance affect lung inflation?
Lung compliance is defined as the change in lung volume per change in pressure. The elasticity of lungs, airways, and chest wall contributes to lung compliance. Normally, lung compliance is high due, in part, to the action of pulmonary surfactant. For example, lung compliance decreases in respiratory distress syndrome. Airway resistance is the resistance to gas flow by the airway. Increases in resistance lead to decreased lung inflation. The most important determinant of flow is the radius of the tubes (i.e., Poiseuille's law).

7. How do you calculate minute ventilation?
Minute ventilation is the product of tidal volume times respiratory rate in 1 minute.

8. How are ventilator settings determined for neonates?
Tidal volume: for patients with normal lung compliance a reasonable goal is an effective tidal volume of 8–10 ml/kg.

Respiratory rate: depends on age and disease. For infants with normal lungs respiratory rate is set at 15–20 breaths per minute.

Oxygen concentration: initially set at 50–100% and reduced to keep partial pressure of oxygen in arterial blood (PaO_2) within an acceptable range (60–80 mm).

Inspiratory/expiratory (I:E) ratio: 1:4–6.

PEEP: at least 2–4 cmH_2O (physiologic PEEP).

Pressure: 25/5 cmH_2O.

9. What are the two types of positive-pressure ventilators?
Positive-pressure ventilators deliver a constant flow of oxygen across the patient's airway with intermittent breaths under positive pressure. In contrast, negative-pressure ventilators (i.e., the iron lung) more closely duplicate normal respiratory physiology. Positive-pressure ventilators can be classified as pressure-controlled or volume-controlled. Pressure-controlled ventilators deliver a breath that is terminated when a preselected pressure is reached, whereas volume-controlled vents deliver a preselected tidal volume.

10. What is the difference between controlled mechanical ventilation, intermittent mandatory ventilation, and assisted control ventilation?
Controlled mechanical ventilation refers to a mode of ventilation in which a given tidal breath is delivered regardless of the patient's effort. In contrast, intermittent mandatory ventilation (IMV) gives a certain number of tidal breaths but also allows spontaneous breathing. IMV can be synchronized with the patient's own breathing (SIMV). Assist control ventilation delivers a certain number of preset breaths and will deliver a breath in response to the patient's breath. This means of ventilation is not often used in neonates.

11. What is pressure support ventilation?
The patient's spontaneous effort is augmented with a preset amount of positive pressure. Inspiration is terminated when a preset flow is reached.

12. Define continuous positive airway pressure and positive end-expiratory pressure.
Continuous positive airway pressure (CPAP) is the maintenance of continuous positive airway pressure during a patient's breathing without the delivery of a breath. CPAP can be

applied via endotracheal tube, nasal prongs, and facemask. CPAP can recruit alveoli and may prevent the need for mechanical ventilation. It also has been used as a means of ventilator weaning. PEEP is the maintenance of positive pressure at the airway opening at the end of expiration. This technique also can effectively recruit alveoli, leading to a reduction in ventilation-perfusion mismatch.

13. What is auto-PEEP?

Auto-PEEP is the inadvertent development of PEEP as a result of incomplete exhalation during positive pressure breathing (i.e., stacked breaths). Auto-PEEP can lead to hypotension and barotrauma.

14. Define barotrauma and volutrauma.

Barotrauma refers to lung injury as a result of high inspiratory pressures. Barotrauma can manifest as pneumomediastinum, pneumothorax, pneumopericardium, or air embolism.

Volutrauma or ventilator-induced lung injury is the result of overdistention of alveoli. This overdistention may be a more important factor than pressure per se.

15. What is the most common complication of mechanical ventilation?

The most common complication is due to positive pressure (i.e., barotrauma). Increased airway pressure leads to rupture of the alveoli, which in turn leads to pneumomediastinum or pneumothorax. Other complications include cardiovascular compromise, infection, airway trauma, and malposition, accidental removal, or blockage of the endotracheal tube.

16. How do you manage patient agitation on the ventilator?

Patient agitation is a sign of a ventilator problem or change in medical condition. Common ventilator problems include inadvertent disconnection or inadequate ventilator setting. Changes in medical condition include inadequate sedation, pneumonia, mucus plugging, pneumothorax, and pulmonary embolism.

17. What noninvasive means of mechanical ventilation is available?

CPAP can be applied without intubation. It is useful for patients with respiratory failure and sometimes raises the partial pressure of oxygen sufficiently to prevent intubation.

18. Is inhaled nitric oxide of value in mechanical ventilation?

Perhaps. Inhaled nitric oxide increases oxygenation in pulmonary hypertension of the newborn. At present it remains investigational but may prove useful for congenital diaphragmatic hernia and postoperative cardiac patients.

19. What is high-frequency ventilation?

High-frequency ventilation (HFV) is a technique in which ventilation is achieved using low tidal volumes and high respiratory rates. Tidal volumes approximate dead space volume and respiratory rates are greater than 60 breaths per minute.

20. How do high-frequency jet ventilation and high-frequency oscillatory ventilation differ?

High-frequency jet ventilation (HFJV) involves delivery of a forced jet of gas into the trachea. Rates exceed 100 cycles/min and can reach 400 cycles/min.

High-frequency oscillatory ventilation (HFOV) uses a piston to develop alternating positive and negative airway pressure. Oscillation frequencies are generally 900–3600 cycles/min, and tidal volumes range from 1 to 3 ml/kg.

21. How does gas exchange occur in HFV?

The mechanism is still not clearly understood. One possibility is oscillation of lung parenchyma. High frequencies of ventilation cause the airways to oscillate, which in turn may result in motion of the neighboring parenchyma. The end result is intra- and interparenchymal gas mixing.

22. What are the clinical uses of HFV?

The main advantage of HFV is ventilation with low airway pressures and volumes, thus decreasing the risk of barotrauma. HFV has been used in neonates with respiratory distress syndrome (RDS), although recent trials have not shown an advantage over conventional ventilation. HFV may prove to be advantageous in children with acute RDS. HFOV has been used as rescue therapy for infants with congenital diaphragmatic hernia, decreasing the number of infants requiring extracorporeal membrane oxygenation (ECMO).

23. How do you control HFOV?

Controlled parameters include frequency, amplitude, and inspiratory time. Amplitude is the total change in pressure around the MAP as a result of displacement of the piston. The selected amplitude usually provides good shaking of the thoracic cavity. Frequencies generally are set at 5–10 hz. For a given amplitude, lower frequencies result in improved gas exchange. Inspiratory time is usually set at 33% of the cycle time.

24. When do you terminate mechanical ventilation and start ECMO?

The main indication of ECMO is cardiorespiratory failure unresponsive to mechanical ventilation. Specific criteria vary from center to center, but usually preterm or low-birth-weight infants are excluded because of the risk of intracranial hemorrhage.

25. What is liquid breathing?

The ability to extract oxygen from liquid. Although liquid breathing is an obvious characteristic of fish, even mice have a limited ability to extract oxygen from liquids with high oxygen solubility for short periods. Based on these phenomena, a means of ventilation has been developed using a mechanical ventilator and a synthetic liquid instilled into the lung.

26. How is liquid ventilation administered?

Tidal or total liquid ventilation (TLV) involves filling the lungs with liquid and using a specially designed mechanical ventilator that circulates the liquid between the lungs and the machine, allowing oxygenation of the fluid and removal of carbon dioxide. In 1970, Shaffer and Moskowitz created a type of demand ventilation that allows animals to control the movement of fluid in and out of the lungs while breathing spontaneously.

Time-cycled, pressure-limited, and/or volume limited liquid ventilation was developed more recently. Its advantage is uniform distribution of the liquid in the lung, which allows complete elimination of surface tension and, therefore, alveolar recruitment at lower alveolar pressures. The major disadvantage is the necessity for specially designed ventilators and the consequent increase in cost.

Several years after the initial studies with TLV, Schaffer and colleagues developed perflourocarbon-associated gas exchange (PAGE), a type of liquid ventilation that used a standard gas ventilator. In this method, now called partial liquid ventilation (PLV), the lungs are not filled to capacity with fluid but rather to a volume equal to functional residual capacity. The fluid is not exchanged; instead, the ventilator delivers gas to the airway, allowing the exchange of oxygen and carbon dioxide.

27. What type of ventilator settings are required?

The strategy of ventilator timing for TLV is different from that of gas ventilation. A rate of 3–8 breaths per minute, a tidal volume of 15–30 ml/kg, and an I:E ratio of 1:2 or 1:3 are used. All of these factors determine how long the liquid remains in the lungs. Optimal ventilation requires sufficient time for diffusion of gases to and from the liquid.

28. What are the advantages of liquid ventilation over gas ventilation?

Elimination of the gas–liquid interface in the liquid-filled lung decreases surface tension, allowing recruitment of alveoli that otherwise would be collapsed and ventilation with lower alveolar pressures. Liquid ventilation thus decreases the incidence of barotrauma associated with traditional gas ventilation, whereas in gas ventilation pulmonary vascular pressure varies with hydrostatic gradients. In addition, distribution of blood flow in the liquid-filled lung is uniform, allowing better ventilation-perfusion matching. The liquid also can be used to lavage the lung and cleanse it of debris.

29. What is perflubron? Why is it used in liquid ventilation?

Perflubron (perfluorooctyl bromide) is the only medical-grade perfluorocarbon available for clinical use. Perfluorocarbons (PFCs) have several qualities that make them suitable for liquid ventilation, including high solubility for oxygen and carbon dioxide, poor systemic absorption, and poor solvency for surfactant. PFCs are clear, colorless, odorless, inert, and chemically and physiologically stable. They dissolve about 20 times the amount of oxygen and more than 3 times the amount of carbon dioxide than water.

30. Can PFCs be used for adjuvant therapies?

Yes. PFC administration is an effective way to deliver drugs directly into the lungs, including surfactant, antibiotics, steroids, chemotherapeutics, and bronchodilators, while protecting nontargeted organs. PFCs are also radiopaque, making them useful contrast media. They provide a good way to evaluate pulmonary structure and function without the problems associated with existing contrast media. Because PFCs do not have hydrogen ions, they do not produce a magnetic signal and are useful as an oral agent for magnetic resonance imaging. They also are useful as bronchogenic contrast agents to allow navigation of the distal airways that are not usually reachable with standard bronchoscopy.

31. Does liquid ventilation have an anti-inflammatory benefit?

Several studies have shown that liquid ventilation with PFCs can reduce pulmonary hemorrhage, alveolar permeability, and edema. They also decrease neutrophil infiltration.

32. How does liquid ventilation affect the cardiovascular system?

During traditional gas ventilation, elevated PEEP can impair venous return, leading to decreased cardiac output and decreased mean arterial pressure. These same events occur in liquid ventilation if the functional residual capacity or volume becomes elevated in the liquid-filled lung. Recent studies with improved equipment and techniques have reported fewer episodes of compromised cardiac function. The improved ventilation-perfusion matching and oxygenation and the decreased oxygen tension allow increased pulmonary flow and decreased right-to-left ductal shunting. Echocardiograms and Doppler exams of cardiovascular function show that left ventricular-output, heart rate, and systemic arterial pressure remain unchanged compared with gas ventilation.

33. How are patients weaned from PFC liquid ventilation?

PFC rapidly evaporates from the lung, requiring replacement at about 1–2 ml/kg/hr. Liquid ventilation is stopped simply by stopping this replacement and allowing the PFC to evaporate completely. Once the liquid is removed, the patient is placed on traditional ventilation and weaned and extubated by standard means.

34. What strategies are used to wean patients from mechanical ventilation?

Numerous strategies are used for weaning from the ventilator, including IMV, which was developed as a technique for weaning the ventilator, and pressure support. In infants, continuous flow ventilation has been shown to be effective.

35. Why should oxygen concentration in inspired air be less than 50%?

Exposure to high concentrations of oxygen can cause lung injury from creation of reactive oxygen species and lead to DNA damage, inactivation of proteins, activation of inflammatory pathways, and lipid peroxidation. There is also a relationship between high oxygen concentration and retinopathy of prematurity. For these reasons, hyperoxia should be avoided in premature infants.

36. What is respiratory distress syndrome?

RDS, also called hyaline membrane disease, is acute respiratory failure in newborns as a result of surfactant deficiency. RDS is a disease of prematurity; 95% of cases occur in infants born before 36 weeks gestation. RDS presents as grunting, retractions, cyanosis, and increased oxygen requirement. Signs and symptoms begin within 6 hours of birth. Surfactant is started once the diagnosis is made.

37. What are the common strategies for treating RDS in children?

Common strategies include conservative indications for mechanical ventilation, low peak inspiratory pressures, moderate levels of PEEP (3–5 cmH$_2$O), permissive hypercapnia, use of sedation and paralysis as needed, and aggressive vent weaning.

38. What is bronchopulmonary dysplasia? Is it related to mechanical ventilation?

Bronchopulmonary dysplasia (BPD), also known as chronic lung disease of the newborn, is a complication of RDS. Almost all patients are premature or very-low-birth-weight infants treated with mechanical ventilation.

39. Is acute RDS the same as RDS?

No. Acute RDS is not the result of surfactant deficiency; it has multiple causes that result in pulmonary edema. Acute RDS and RDS are similar in that both diseases are nonhomogeneous in the lung and result in ventilation-perfusion mismatch. The same ventilation strategies are used for both diseases, including low PIP, permissive hypercapnia, and adequate sedation. Liquid ventilation also has been used as therapy for acute RDS.

40. What is permissive hypercapnia?

In permissive hypercapnia, PaO$_2$ levels are allowed to increase in an effort to limit the amount of pressure needed to ventilate patients with acute RDS or RDS. Studies of newborns with RDS suggest a higher incidence of BPD after ventilator strategies that result in hypercapnia.

41. Does patient position affect ventilation in acute RDS?

Yes. In fact, the prone position has been shown to have benefits in ventilating patients with acute RDS, in part because ventilation of dependent lung segments is improved.

42. What is the respiratory quotient? How does it affect nutrition in ventilated children?

Respiratory quotient refers to the amount of carbon dioxide produced by oxidation of fat, carbohydrates, and proteins. For example, oxidation of fat produces less carbon dioxide than oxygenation of glucose. Less carbon dioxide to clear may be beneficial to patients with compromised lung function.

43. What are the hemodynamic effects of mechanical ventilation?

Positive-pressure mechanical ventilation can result in a decrease in venous return to the heart because of elevated intrathoracic pressure. It may lead to a decrease in cardiac output and, potentially, hypotension.

BIBLIOGRAPHY

1. Adamkin DH: Issues in the nutritional support of the ventilated baby. Clin Perinatol 25:79, 1998.
2. Clark RH, Gertsman DR: Controversies in high-frequency ventilation. Clin Perinatol 25:113, 1998.
3. Fuhrman BP, Hernan LJ, Papo MC, Steinhorn DM: Perfluorocarbon liquid ventilation. In Fuhrman BP, Zimmerman JJ (eds): Pediatric Critical Care, 2nd ed. St. Louis, Mosby, 1998.
4. Kallas HJ: Non-conventional respiratory support modalities applicable in the older child. Crit Care Clin 14:655, 1998.
5. Mariani GL, Carlo WA: Ventilatory management in neonates: Science or art? Clin Perinatol 25:33, 1998.
6. Venkataraman ST, Orr RA: Mechanical ventilation and respiratory care. In Fuhrman BP, Zimmerman JJ (eds): Pediatric Critical Care, 2nd ed. St. Louis, Mosby, 1998.

III. Thoracic

6. CHEST WALL DEFORMITIES

Amanda J. McCabe, FRCS, and Philip L. Glick, M.D.

1. Outline the development of the sternum.
A pair of mesenchymal vertical bands (sternal bars) develop ventrolaterally in the body wall. They move medially and fuse craniocaudally, forming cartilaginous models of the manubrium, sternebrae (segments of the sternal body), and xiphoid process. Centers of ossification appear craniocaudally in the sternum before birth, except for the xiphoid process, which appears during childhood.

2. Outline the development of the ribs.
The ribs develop from the mesenchymal costal processes of the thoracic vertebrae. They become cartilaginous during the embryonic period and ossify during the fetal period. Costovertebral plane synovial joints replace the union of the costal processes with the vertebrae. Seven pairs of ribs (true ribs) attach through their own cartilages to the sternum. Five pairs of false ribs (8–12) attach to the sternum via the cartilages of another rib(s). The last two pairs of ribs do not attach to the sternum (floating ribs).

3. Name five categories of congenital chest wall deformity.
Pectus excavatum (funnel chest), pectus carinatum (pigeon chest), Poland's syndrome, sternal defects, and miscellaneous dysplasias.

4. What is pectus excavatum?
Pectus excavatum, an anterior chest wall deformity characterized by posterior depression of the sternum and lower costal cartilages, occurs more frequently in boys than girls (3:1) and usually is noted within the first year of life. It progresses through childhood, and regression is rare. It is believed to occur in as many as 1 in 400 births but is uncommon in black and Hispanic populations.

5. What causes pectus excavatum?
The cause is not yet established. Theories include intrauterine pressure, rickets, and abnormalities of the diaphragm that cause posterior traction on the sternum. Its association with other musculoskeletal abnormalities suggests a role for abnormal connective tissue. Increased levels of zinc and decreased levels of magnesium and calcium have been demonstrated in some studies. The deformity may result from an imbalance of growth in the costochondral regions, thus explaining the asymmetrical appearance in some cases and the completely opposite deformity of pectus carinatum. A family history of chest wall deformity in 37% of cases also supports a genetic predisposition.

6. What musculoskeletal abnormalities are associated with pectus excavatum?
Approximately 20% of pectus excavatum cases are associated with other musculoskeletal abnormalities. The most common association is scoliosis. Other associations include kyphosis, Marfan's syndrome, Poland's syndrome, Pierre-Robin syndrome, prune-belly syndrome, neurofibromatosis, cerebral palsy, tuberous sclerosis, and congenital diaphragmatic hernia.

7. What is Marfan's syndrome?
Marfan's syndrome is an autosomal dominant connective tissue disorder in which patients are characteristically tall and slender with hyperextensibility of the joints, arachnodactyly, dislocation of the lenses of the eye, and chest wall deformity such as pectus excavatum and carinatum. Patients also present with spontaneous pneumothorax and dissecting aortic aneurysms or mitral valve prolapse.

8. What clinical signs can be demonstrated in a case of pectus excavatum?

Depression deformities. The spectrum of depression deformities ranges from mild to severe cases in which the sternum almost abuts the vertebral bodies. The depression is a combination of posterior angulation of the body of the sternum beginning just below the insertion of the second costal cartilage and posterior angulation of the costal cartilages to meet the sternum. Older patients also may have angulation of the anterior portion of the osseous ribs.

Cardiac murmurs. Congenital heart disease was identified in 1.5% of children undergoing chest wall correction. The anterior compression of the heart may deform the mitral valve annulus or the ventricular chamber and produce mitral valve prolapse. Such patients may have an intermittent history of palpitations, which indicates transient atrial arrhythmias.

9. What is the physiologic impact of pectus excavatum?

This topic has led to much debate. Some authors contend that no cardiovascular or pulmonary impairment is associated with pectus excavatum. Many patients, however, report increased stamina and level of activity after surgical repair. Pathologic studies of patients with pectus excavatum demonstrate compression of the heart between the vertebral column and the depressed sternum. The left lung was compressed more often than the right because of the asymmetry of the lesion. Conventional pulmonary function tests at rest are usually within normal limits in children with pectus excavatum, but it is difficult to obtain good measurements in children under 7 years. Cardiac output measurements using right ventricular catheterization have demonstrated diminished outputs in preoperative patients during upright exercise. This finding has not been repeated in supine cases at rest. Cahill et al. used the cycle ergometer to assess patients before and after surgery. They found that exercise performances were improved as measured both by total exercise time and by maximal oxygen consumption. After repair, patients showed a lower heart rate and higher minute ventilation compared with preoperative values. Thus, restricted cardiac stroke volume and increased work of breathing can be ameliorated by operative repair.

10. What are the indications for surgical correction of pectus excavatum?

Because most children with pectus excavatum are asymptomatic, careful clinical observation and physiological testing are necessary to assess any form of chest wall deformity. Many pediatric surgeons recommend that patients with a moderate-to-severe depression and demonstrated physiologic impairment should undergo surgical correction. Others believe that the abnormality is of cosmetic rather than physiologic significance and operate to improve the appearance of the chest because the deformity interferes with the child's self-image and psychosocial development. This issue has not been formally assessed.

11. What surgical options have been used in the treatment of pectus excavatum?
- Chondrosternal resection. First reported in 1911 by Meyer, this technique resulted in paradoxical respiration and left the heart unprotected.
- External traction. Popular in the 1920s and 1930s, this approach was abandoned because of the impractical nature of the apparatus and lethal infections in the preantibiotic era.
- Cartilage resection and sternal osteotomy. In 1949 Ravitch described a technique that involved excision of all deformed costal cartilages with the perichondrium, division of the xiphoid from the sternum, division of the intercostal bundles from the sternum, and transverse sternal osteotomy, displacing the sternum anteriorly with Kirschner wires or silk sutures. A later modification preserved the perichondrial sheaths. Other groups have used posterior sternal osteotomy with posterolateral division of the normal cephalad cartilages.
- Metallic struts. Rehbein and Wernicke developed struts that can be anchored into the marrow cavity of the ribs at the costochondral junction. An arch then is formed by the struts, anterior to the sternum, and the sternum is secured to this arch.
- Retrosternal elevation. This technique also has been used in association with multiple chrondrotomies for flexibility.
- Sternal turnover. A free sternal graft is rotated through 180° and secured to the cartilages from which it was previously divided.

• Silastic mold in the subcutaneous space. This approach does not address the primary chest wall defect and is purely cosmetic.

13. What is the minimally invasive Nuss repair for pectus excavatum?
A convex steel bar is inserted under the sternum through small bilateral thoracic incisions under direct thoracoscopic vision. The bar is inserted with the convexity facing posteriorly. When it is in a suitable position, the bar is turned through 180°, thereby correcting the deformity. After 2 years, when permanent remolding has occurred, the bar is removed.

14. What rationale supports the Nuss approach to pectus excavatum correction?
Adult patients who suffer from chronic obstructive lung disease undergo a remodeling of the chest into the classic barrel shape. This remodeling occurs long after the skeleton has matured and calcified. Therefore, it was thought that it should be possible to remodel the chest wall in children whose ribs and cartilages are still soft and pliable without resorting to rib cartilage incision, resection, or sternal osteotomy. This result has been observed clinically with cases treated with the Nuss repair.

15. What is pectus carinatum?
Pectus carinatum is a protrusion deformity of the chest. It is approximately 10 times less common than pectus excavatum and occurs more frequently in boys than girls (4:1). This deformity usually is not appreciated until the rapid growth of early adolescence. Pectus carinatum has a more variable presentation than pectus excavatum, but there are two basic patterns: **chondromanubrial**, in which the protuberance is maximal in the upper portion of the sternum, and **chondrogladiolar**, in which the protuberance is sited at the xiphisternum.

16. What causes pectus carinatum?
The cause remains uncertain. However, there seems to be a genetic predisposition, with 26% of patients having a family history of chest wall deformity. In addition, 15% of patients have scoliosis, indicating a diffuse abnormality in connective tissue development.

17. What features characterize the pectus carinatum deformity?
The typical feature is symmetrical protrusion of the sternal body and costal cartilages. A common association is lateral depression of the ribs (Harrison's grooves), which has been likened to crushing the chest from each side. In some cases the protrusion is asymmetric, producing a keel-like deformity. A mixed deformity has both protrusion and depression elements, and the sternum rotates posteriorly toward the depressed side.

18. How is the pectus carinatum deformity corrected?
Because the appearance varies greatly, the surgical approach is unique to each case. The basic principles are similar to those of the traditional open repair of pectus excavatum. The most severely affected costal cartilages are resected, leaving the perichondrium intact. A transverse osteotomy is made across the anterior table of the upper sternum, and the resultant wedge is filled with a piece of costal cartilage to secure it in a more downward posterior position. A substernal bar may be required to stabilize the chest wall temporarily.

19. What is Poland's syndrome?
Poland's initial observation (made as a medical student in 1841) grouped absent pectoralis major and minor muscles with syndactyly. Subsequent reports have added absent ribs, chest wall depression, athelia or amastia, absence of axillary hair, and limited subcutaneous fat to the spectrum of anomalies.

20. What is the pentalogy of Cantrell?
• Ectopia cordis
• Ventral diaphragmatic defect
• Midline abdominal defect or omphalocele
• Pericardial defect allowing communication with the peritoneal cavity
• Cardiac anomaly

21. What sternal defects have been described?

- Thoracic ectopia cordis: classic "naked heart." The heart has no overlying somatic structures, and the apex is situated anteriorly. Intrinsic cardiac anomalies are frequent.
- Cervical ectopia cordis: similar to thoracic ectopia cordis but with superior displacement of the heart. Often the heart is fused to the mouth, and other craniofacial defects may be present.
- Thoracoabdominal ectopia cordis: the heart is covered by a membrane or thin pigmented skin with an inferiorly placed cleft sternum. This defect is associated almost invariably with abdominal wall, anterior diaphragmatic, pericardial defects, and cleft or bifid sternum.

22. What anomalies have been reported with a cleft sternum?

A band-like scar from the umbilicus or chin to the sternal defect, hemangiomas, diastasis of the recti, cleft mandible (gnathoschisis), microcephaly or severe cranial anomalies, hydrocephalus, and coarctation of the aorta have been reported. No cardiac anomalies are included.

23. What chest wall deformities are associated with congenital diaphragmatic hernia (CDH) survivors?

Musculoskeletal growth of the chest may be affected by the pathophysiology of CDH as well as treatment of the disease. About 20% of patients with CDH develop a pectus excavatum deformity, possibly due to the increased work of breathing. In addition, one series reports a 10% occurrence of thoracic scoliosis in patients with CDH.

24. Describe the variety of rib abnormalities that are seen incidentally on chest radiograph.

Complete absence or partial development of the ribs is the characteristic finding. A rib may be bifurcated, and one component may articulate or fuse with a hypoplastic adjacent rib. If the costal defects are extensive, they may cause a noticeable cosmetic deformity or even physiologic embarrassment. Severe fusion can cause progressive kyphoscolosis or serious compression of the lungs with resultant ventilatory disturbance.

25. What is Jeune's syndrome?

This rare autosomal disorder is characterized by osseous dysplasia, fetal respiratory distress, and renal failure later in life. It also is known as asphyxiating thoracic dystrophy and was initially described in 1954. The most prominent features are a narrow, bell-shaped thorax and protuberant abdomen. The ribs are short and wide, and the splayed costochondral junctions barely reach the anterior axillary line. Other skeletal abnormalities include short stubby extremities with relatively short and wide bones, clavicles in a fixed and elevated position, and small, hypoplastic pelvis with square iliac bones. The syndrome has variable expression and degree of pulmonary involvement. Autopsy cases have revealed normal bronchial development but fewer alveolar divisions. Patients surviving the neonatal period are later at risk of developing renal failure, which is thought to be secondary to nephronophthisis. One such patient who had undergone renal transplant reportedly developed a sarcoma in the soft tissue of the chest wall, the principal site of dysplasia.

26. What is Sprengel's deformity?

The scapula is hypoplastic and fixed in an elevated position to the vertebral column by fibrous bands, cartilage, or bone. This deformity causes limitation of movement around the shoulder joint. The scapula also may appear winged; this appearance also may result from traumatic or operative injury to the long thoracic nerve (C6–C7).

27. What is Jarcho-Levin syndrome?

This autosomal recessive deformity, also known as spondylothoracic dysplasia, is associated with multiple vertebral and rib malformations. Death often occurs in early infancy from respiratory failure and pneumonia. Multiple hemivertibrae affect both the thoracic and lumbar spine. Multiple posterior fusions of the ribs result in a crablike radiographic appearance of the chest. The syndrome commonly is associated with cardiac and renal anomalies. There have been no attempts at surgical correction.

BIBLIOGRAPHY

1. Cahill JL, Lees GM, Robertson HT: A summary of preoperative and postoperative respiratory performance in patients undergoing pectus excavatum and carinatum repair. J Pediatr Surg 19:430, 1984.
2. Glick PL, Irish MS, Holm BA (eds): Insights into the Pathophysiology of Congenital Diaphragmatic Hernia. Philadelphia, W.B. Saunders, 1996.
3. Moore KL, Persaud TVN: The Developing Human, 6th ed. Philadelphia, W.B. Saunders, 1998.
4. Nuss D, Kelly RE, Croitoru DP, Katz ME: A 10-year review of a minimally invasive technique for the correction of pectus excavatum. J Pediatr Surg 33:545–552, 1998.
5. O'Neill JA, Rowe MI, Gorsfeld JL, et al (eds): Pediatric Surgery, 5th ed. St. Louis, Mosby, 1998.
6. Redmond J, Richter MP, Stein HD, et al: Primitive neuroectodermal tumor of the chest wall in a patient with Jeune's syndrome and renal transplant. Am J Kidney Dis 21:449–451, 1993.
7. Ring E, Zobel G, Ratschek M, et al: Retrospective diagnosis of Jeune's syndrome in two patients with chronic renal failure. Child Nephrol Urol 10(2):88–91, 1990.
8. Rowe MI, O'Neill JA, Grosfeld JL, et al (eds): Essentials of Pediatric Surgery. St. Louis, Mosby, 1995.
9. Shamberger RC, Welch KJ: Sternal defects. Pediatr Surg Int 5:156–164, 1990.

7. DIAPHRAGMATIC HERNIAS

Amanda J. McCabe, FRCS, and Philip L. Glick, M.D.

1. What four embryologic elements combine to form the diaphragm?

The septum transversum forms the anterior central tendon, the pleuroperitoneal membranes form the dorsolateral portions, the esophageal mesentery forms the dorsal crura, and the thoracic intercostal muscle groups form the peripheral muscular portion of the diaphragm.

2. What are the four stages of fetal lung development?

- **Embryonic** (0–7 weeks). A foregut diverticulum appears at the caudal end of the laryngotracheal groove. The trachea and two lung buds form by the fourth week, and the buds develops into defined bronchopulmonary segments by the sixth week.
- **Pseudoglandular** (8–16 weeks). Lung airway differentiation establishes all bronchial passages by the end of this phase. Differentiation of the airway epithelium results in four of the eight epithelial cell types seen in the adult lung-ciliated, non-ciliated (pre-Clara cells), secretory, and early basal types.
- **Canalicular** (17–24 weeks). Crude air sacs form. Type I pneumocytes begin to differentiate, and the precursors of type II pneumocytes, which are responsible for surfactant production, begin to appear.
- **Saccular** (24 weeks to term). Remodeling of air space dimensions and maturation of surfactant synthesis capabilities continue.

Further alveolar maturation and multiplication continues from birth until approximately 8 years of age.

3. What mechanical forces act on the growing fetal lung?

- Lung liquid. Fluid actively secreted by the pulmonary epithelium expands the fetal lungs. Fluid production increases toward term; then, under the action of the labor stress hormones, it decreases. The upper airway (i.e., the glottis) appears to regulate the volume and pressure within a narrow range.
- Amniotic fluid volume. Conditions that lead to oligohydramnios, including renal agenesis and urinary tract obstruction, are associated with pulmonary hypoplasia. The explanation for this observation is unclear. Paradoxically, the most severe pulmonary hypoplasia in cases of congenital diaphragmatic hernia (CDH) is seen in association with polyhydramnios.
- Intrathoracic size/mass. Experiments in which balloons were progressively inflated inside a fetal chest resulted in small lungs with decreased compliance. This preparation mimics CDH.

• Fetal breathing. Episodic movements of the diaphragm occur late in gestation and result in increased lung liquid efflux. Abolition of these movements in experimental animal models resulted in smaller lungs with decreased compliance.

4. How does normal pulmonary vascular development progress?

The developing lung buds branch into mesenchyme containing a vascular network. These vessels accompany developing airways as they differentiate into arteries and then join the larger pulmonary arteries that originate from the sixth branchial arch. Airway and vessel branching appears to be synchronized, indicating that both may respond to common mediators or exchange messenger molecules. The veins arise separately from the loose mesenchyme of the lung septa and subsequently connect to the developing left atrium. The muscular coat of the vessels is apparent in the canalicular stage of development. The muscularization begins in the more central arteries and progresses toward the periphery, reaching the terminal bronchi by term. Control of the proliferation is not fully understood, but transforming growth factor β, fibroblastic growth factors, and platelet-derived growth factor have all been implicated.

5. What congenital defects can occur in the diaphragm?

• Bochdalek hernia: a posterolateral defect. The most common type of CDH, it ranges from a small defect to almost complete agenesis of the diaphragmatic tissue.
• Morgagni hernia: an anteromedial defect, approximately 20 times less common than the classical Bochdalek lesion.
• Diaphragmatic eventration: a central weakening of the diaphragm.

6. What is the incidence of CDH?

The reported incidence of CDH is 1 in 2000–4000 births. The incidence in stillbirths is less well documented, but approximately 8% of infants with CDH are stillborn. Death usually is due to associated fatal congenital anomalies. Eighty percent occur on the left side, 19% on the right side, and 1% are bilateral. About 2% of cases are of the Morgagni type.

7. How does a CDH occur?

Failure of the pleuroperitoneal canals to close at 8–10 weeks in human development leads to a defect in the dorsolateral region of the diaphragm. Bowel loops returning from the embryonic yolk sac may herniate through this defect into the chest. The exact mechanism of closure failure remains unclear, but studies with the rat nitrofen model of CDH have revealed several clues. The growth of the liver is in sequential balance with an area of mesenchyme termed the posthepatic mesenchymal plate (PHMP), and its caudal and lateral growth finally leads to closure of the pleuroperitoneal canal. The PHMP appears to use the liver surface as a matrix for normal development. In the experimental rat model the balance of growth is disturbed, as an abnormal cluster of cells appears at the lower border of the PHMP. The liver cells in the vicinity of this abnormal cluster readily invade the thoracic cavity. An interesting pattern of cell death in cervical somites (C2–C4) in the rat model also has been demonstrated.

8. Do genetic factors play a role in the etiology of CDH?

Approximately one-third of patients with CDH have a known chromosomal defect or a combination of anomalies. Trisomy 13, 18 and 21 have been associated with cases of CDH. Other genetic translocations (8q22.3), deletions (Turner syndrome XO), and mutations (WT1) have been suggested and investigated, but no single association has been demonstrated. The male-to-female ratio is approximately 1:1 but changes to 2:1 when familial cases are considered. Familial cases account for 2% of all diaphragmatic hernias, and current data from these groups suggest a multifactorial mode of genetic transmission.

9. What environmental factors are implicated in the etiology of CDH?

The cause of CDH remains largely unknown, but various chemicals, such as polybrominated diphenyls, thalomide, nitrofen, quinine, and phenmetrazine, have been found to induce CDH in various animal models. There are also reports that maternal use of phenmetrazine, thalomide, or quinine results in the birth of siblings with CDH. Nitrofen long has been used to induce the defect in fetal rats. Because it interacts with and disturbs thyroid hormone homeostasis, much research has been directed to the effects of the thyroid on lung development. As yet, no firm conclusions have been made. A vitamin A-deficient diet also has been noted to induce the lesion in certain strains of rat.

10. Which three prenatal features identify fetuses with CDH who are likely to have a poor outcome with conventional treatment after birth?

Liver herniation into the hemithorax, low lung-to-head ratio, and diagnosis before 25 weeks gestation. In one center such patients have undergone one of three treatment options: standard postnatal care, fetal tracheal occlusion via open hysterotomy, or tracheal occlusion via a videofetoscopic technique. Survival rates were 38%, 15%, and 75%, respectively. In experienced hands, these high-risk neonates may benefit from temporary tracheal occlusion performed fetoscopically but not by open fetal surgery. However, prospective, randomized human trials need to be performed to confirm this observation.

11. What other action can be taken prenatally in the treatment of a fetus with CDH?

Prenatal counseling of the parents is important so that they can make informed decisions about management options. Counseling should involve discussion about prenatal therapies, such as glucocorticoids, and possible fetal therapy. The counseling is carried out by a multidisciplinary team that includes an obstetrician, neonatologist, pediatric surgeon, geneticist, ethicist/clergy, and social worker. The future management of the pregnancy and subsequent vaginal delivery are planned and organized so that the birth takes place in a tertiary center, where clinical management and comprehensive multidisciplinary care can be provided.

12. What anomalies are associated with CDH?

The incidence of associated anomalies is approximately 40%. This figure approaches 100% when only the stillborn group is considered. In the stillborn group, neural tube defects such as anencephaly, myelomeningocele, hydrocephalus, and encephaloceles predominate. When patients with CDH are considered as a whole, cardiac defects are the second most common group of anomalies, including ventriculoseptal defects, vascular rings, and coarctation of the aorta. Pulmonary sequestration, genitourinary anomalies, malrotation, and duodenal atresia are recognized associations. In addition, midline defects such as esophageal atresia, omphalocele, and cleft palate also have been described.

13. Describe the structural parenchymal abnormalities of the CDH lung.

Airways: reduced number of bronchial divisions. Division is arrested at 12–14 bronchial divisions in the ipsilateral lung and 16–18 in the contralateral lung. The normal lung has 23 divisions.

Alveoli: decrease in gas exchange area. With fewer bronchi only a finite number of alveoli and air sacs can be supported. In addition, the lungs are less mature and arrested in the saccular phase of development. There are fewer septae and thus fewer mature alveoli. The septae that are present contain more interstitium; therefore, there is a greater distance between the capillary and air interface. This significantly impairs gas exchange in CDH lungs.

Pneumocytes: not fully differentiated. The thin type I pneumocytes that usually line the alveoli retain a cuboid configuration in the CDH lung, as seen in the saccular phase of development. The type II pneumocytes (type I precursors) are more numerous in CDH lungs and in the nitrofen rat model appear to contain more glycogen than usual, which is a sign of immaturity. The lamellar bodies of the type II cells (responsible for surfactant storage) are less frequently seen in the CDH lung and appear to have a more disorganized structure (another sign of cell immaturity). All of these changes are evident in both right and left lungs.

14. What is surfactant?

Surfactant is a mixture of phospholipids (90% by weight) and surfactant-associated proteins (5–10% by weight). It is synthesized and stored in alveolar type II cells. The primary function of surfactant is to facilitate the variation of alveolar surface tension during lung expansion and de-flation. Its action promotes alveolar stability, reduces atelectasis, and decreases edema formation, thus minimizing the work of breathing.

15. Describe the pulmonary vascular abnormalities of the CDH lung.

The number of arterial branches in CDH is dramatically reduced. The vessel walls are thick-ened as a result of smooth muscle hyperplasia, and a significant increase in pulmonary artery muscle mass has been demonstrated. As a result, the total cross-sectional area of the pulmonary vascular bed is reduced, and persistent pulmonary hypertension subsequently develops. Cardiac catheterization studies have demonstrated the presence of a persistent pattern of fetal circulation in some patients with CDH, giving a right-to-left shunt of blood. These anatomic limitations are further compounded by functional inadequacies of the vasculature, which have been shown to be hyperreactive to mediators of pulmonary vasoconstriction (hypoxia, hypercarbia, acidemia). A broad spectrum of drugs has been used to combat this hypertension. Tolazoline (an alpha recep-tor blocker) has been most useful in lowering pulmonary vascular resistance in neonates with hy-poxemia and respiratory failure, but its efficacy in neonates with CDH is marginal. Patients who respond to a test dose warrant further treatment with the drug, but only with cautious monitoring for the major side effects of systemic hypotension and tachyphylaxis.

16. How does nitric oxide play a role in the management of CDH?

Nitric oxide (NO) is a potent mediator of vasodilatation, and as a highly diffusible gas it is par-ticularly suited for delivery to the pulmonary vasculature. It improves oxygen saturations in neonates with respiratory failure due to persistent pulmonary hypertension. Results of its clinical effectiveness have been variable in cases of CDH. The NO-cyclic guanosine monophosphate pathway of vasodi-latation has been found to be abnormal in the near-term fetal lamb with CDH. These abnormalities are most marked in the pulmonary veins and may reflect abnormal NO synthase activity or content in the isolated vessels of the lamb model of CDH. Surfactant therapy also facilitates NO delivery.

17. What typical physical features are demonstrated in a neonate with left-sided CDH?

Obvious respiratory distress and cyanosis are common, along with a scaphoid abdomen, prominence of the ipsilateral chest, cardiac apex beat under the sternum or right side of chest, prominent heart sounds in the right chest, diminished breath sounds and possible bowel sounds in the left side of the chest.

18. What is involved in the immediate management of a neonate with a prenatal diagnosis of CDH?

Ideally, the neonate should be transported in utero to a perinatal high-risk center, where the delivery should be planned and the appropriate neonatal, obstetric, and pediatric surgical person-nel alerted. An endotracheal tube is placed in the delivery room along with a nasogastric tube. On delivery, the neonate is dried and wrapped with as little stimulation as possible, and the nasogas-tric tube is inserted and placed on suction to decompress the stomach. Endotracheal intubation follows to facilitate ventilation and oxygenation and to allow surfactant to be administered before the first breath. All efforts to avoid bowel distention from mask ventilation should be made. Ventilatory pressure is adjusted as required, keeping it as low as possible (ideally, < 30 mmHg). A rapid ventilatory rate of 40–60 breaths/minute is used. Meanwhile, venous and arterial lines are obtained peripherally and at the umbilicus so that fluids and sedation can be administered. In addition, pre- and postductal oxygen saturations can be measured to assess the degree of arterial oxygenation and ductal shunting.

19. Outline the physiologic parameters used to assess the neonate with CDH.

Arterial blood gas measures (pre- and postductal) are used to assess the degree of right-to-left shunting. These measures have been further manipulated to establish predictive criteria. For example, the alveolar-arterial oxygen gradient ($AaDO_2$) initially was used to determine entry into extracorpo-real membrane oxygenation treatment regimens. The following indices include ventilatory data:

- Ventilatory index (VI)

$$VI = RR \times MAP \times PaCO_2$$

where RR = respiratory rate, MAP = mean airway pressure, and $PaCO_2$ = partial pressure of carbon dioxide in arterial blood. When the $PaCO_2$ could be reduced below 40 mmHg with a ventilatory index less than 1000, all patients survived.
- Modified ventilatory index (MVI)

$$MVI = RR \times PIP \times PaCO_2/1000$$

where PIP = peak inspiratory pressure. In patients with an MVI less than 40, the survival rate was found to be 96% using conventional therapy. All infants died if MVI was greater than 80.
- Oxygen index (OI)

$$OI = MAP \times FiO_2 \times 100/PaO_2$$

where FiO_2 = fractional concentration of oxygen in inspired gas and PaO_2 = partial pressure of oxygen in arterial blood. An OI less than 6 was associated with a survival rate of 98%, whereas an OI greater than 17 had no survivors.

The predictive power of these parameters in conjunction with such therapies as ECMO, high-frequency oscillation, surfactant, and NO has not yet been determined.

20. What ventilatory options are considered in the management of a neonate with CDH?

Most infants initially are managed with conventional ventilation, using a combination of high respiratory rates (80–100 breaths/min) and *modest* peak airway pressures (18–22 H_2O). The goal is to obtain preductal partial pressure of oxygen greater than 60 torr (oxygen saturation in arterial blood 90–100%) with an associated partial pressure of carbon dioxide of less than 60 torr. The hypoplastic lungs of the neonate with CDH are not structurally sound enough to withstand high peak pressures. In the event of hypoxemia and hypercarbia, high-frequency techniques with a jet or oscillating ventilator can be used to recruit alveoli while limiting iatrogenic barotrauma (also known as gentle ventilation). These techniques are particularly useful in removing carbon dioxide but have not been shown to improve overall outcome. Further efforts to stabilize such neonates may involve ECMO, as outlined in question 23.

21. Why should surfactant therapy be considered in the neonate with CDH?

Evidence suggests that the surfactant system develops abnormally in CDH. Autopsy studies of infants dying of CDH show a decreased phospholipid fraction in the bronchoalveolar lavage (BAL) of the ipsilateral lung compared with the contralateral lung. Histologic, morphologic, and quantitative biochemical similarities have been shown between the fetus/newborn with CDH and the surfactant-deficient newborn with respiratory distress syndrome. Studies using the lamb model of CDH have demonstrated a quantitative and qualitative reduction in surfactant phospholipids (especially the major bioactive phospholipid, phosphatidylcholine), surfactant proteins, and surfactant function. Exogenous surfactant replacement studies in the lamb model of CDH also show improved oxygenation and ventilation. By recruiting alveoli, surfactant decreases pulmonary vascular resistance, increases pulmonary blood flow, and decreases pulmonary artery pressure.

22. What is the honeymoon period?

The honeymoon period is a time when some neonates with CDH demonstrate adequate oxygenation and ventilatory parameters in the absence of maximal medical therapy. It is independent of subsequent deterioration, but it suggests that pulmonary tissue and function may be compatible with life. The pathophysiology of this phenomenon is complex but may relate to iatrogenic ventilatory barotrauma and/or oxygen-induced injury via free radical release. Antioxidant enzyme system deficiency, as demonstrated in the lamb model of CDH, may help to explain this well-recognized clinical course.

23. What is ECMO?

ECMO is a form of cardiopulmonary bypass that aims to maintain oxygen delivery for an extended period during which the pulmonary vasculature is given time to recover from its hypertensive state. It is achieved using either a venoarterial route or venovenous route with a double-lumen catheter. ECMO can be complicated by bleeding, but it also produces significant tissue edema. As a result, repair can be difficult in terms of tissue handling and dissection of the potentially bloody posterior diaphragmatic rim area. The United Kingdom Collaborative ECMO Trial Group have reported that ECMO support in the treatment of cardiorespiratory failure in CDH appears to be beneficial for patients with intermediate severity of disease. If the ventilation indices predict severe pulmonary hypoplasia, the chance of success with ECMO therapy alone is small.

24. When is the optimal time for surgery in a neonate with CDH?

At present, nobody knows the best time to operate. Historically, CDH was regarded as a surgical emergency, and newborn infants were rushed to the operating room for anatomic correction. In 1987 Bohn et al. proposed a period of medical stabilization and delayed surgical repair in an attempt to improve the overall condition of the neonate. This strategy has not lowered the survival rate, and increasing physiologic evidence favors a waiting period. As a result, the period of preoperative stabilization has increased, and some serial echocardiographic measures have shown slow normalization of pulmonary artery pressures.

25. Describe the traditional surgical repair of a CDH.

Most surgeons favor an initial left subcostal approach, which allows the gentle replacement of the herniated abdominal viscera and correction of the associated malrotation. The posterior rim of the diaphragm, which is covered with peritoneum or pleura, is dissected free of the retroperitoneal tissue, and, if the anterior and posterior lips of the defect can be easily opposed, a primary repair with interrupted sutures is performed. If the defect is too large for primary closure, a transversus abdominis muscle flap or synthetic patch can be used to bridge the gap. However, in addition to the risk of infection, the prosthetic patch closure is also at risk of dislodgment and subsequent re-herniation. If the abdomen cannot accommodate the replaced viscera comfortably, a ventral hernia and silo can be fashioned; otherwise the subcostal incision is closed in layers.

In the repair of a right-sided defect, the liver is often the only organ in the chest. Liver replacement in the abdomen can be complicated by kinking of the hepatic veins and the superior vena cava (SVC), causing a marked decrease in venous return and profound hypotension. Careful evaluation and dissection of the fibrous attachments of the SVC to the medial side of the diaphragmatic defect usually provide sufficient length to ameliorate the problem and allow the fragile fetal liver to be replaced below the diaphragm.

26. What is the long-term outlook for infants born with CDH?

The overall survival rate varies widely among studies but has remained at approximately 50% despite the use of new management strategies. Survival rates of 80–100% have been reported in some small, nonrandomized studies. Long-term survivors may have chronic lung problems, but they seem to improve with time. Nonpulmonary morbidity, such as developmental delay, has been described in patients requiring aggressive management. Other neurologic problems include visual disturbance, hearing loss, seizures, and abnormal brain imaging. There is a high incidence of gastroesophageal reflux and foregut dismotility, which must be treated aggressively to ensure optimal growth and development. Skeletal defects such as pectus excavatum or carinatum and scoliosis also have been reported.

27. How does a Morgagni hernia present?

The defect is situated anteriorly at the point where the internal mammary and epigastric vessels traverse the diaphragm. It is rarely symptomatic in neonates and typically presents in older children or adults. The hernia may present as an incidental finding of a mass or air-fluid level on chest radiograph. Symptoms may include episodic coughing, choking, vomiting, and epigastric complaints. Occasionally the defect is associated with the pentalogy of Cantrell (ectopia cordis, ventral diaphragmatic defect, midline abdominal defect or omphalocele, pericardial defect allowing communication with the peritoneal cavity, and cardiac anomaly).

28. What is an eventration of the diaphragm?

Eventration, an abnormal elevation of the diaphragm, may be congenital or secondary to phrenic nerve damage. Congenital defects usually are due to a muscularization abnormality, and most patients are asymptomatic, requiring only observation. The acquired lesion is due to a lack of diaphragmatic innervation, and most children develop significant respiratory symptoms. Other symptoms include wheezing, frequent respiratory infections, and exercise intolerance. The elevation can rise as high as the third intercostal space and result in physiologic consequences similar to those of CDH. The diagnosis is made using fluoroscopy or real-time ultrasound with the demonstration of paradoxic movement of the diaphragm. A small eventration may be left untreated, but when a functional deficit is demonstrated, repair is necessary to ensure maximal development of both lungs. The surgical approach is usually a low thoracotomy through which the diaphragm can be plicated with nonabsorbable sutures.

BIBLIOGRAPHY

1. Bohn D, Tamura M, Perrin D, et al: Ventilatory predictors of pulmonary hypoplasia in congenital diaphragmatic hernia, confirmed by morphologic assessment. J Pediatr 111:423–431, 1987.
2. Collaborative UK ECMO Trial: Follow-up to 1 year of age. Pediatrics 101:690, 1988.
3. Glick PL, Irish MS, Holm BA (eds): New Insights into the Pathophysiology of Congenital Diaphragmatic Hernia. Philadelphia, W.B. Saunders, 1996.
4. Harrison MR, Mychaliska GB, Albanese CT, et al: Correction of congenital diaphragmatic hernia in utero. IX. Fetuses with poor prognosis (liver herniation and low lung-to-head ratio) can be saved by fetoscopic temporary tracheal occlusion. J Pediatr Surg 33:1017–1023, 1998.
5. Holm BA, Kapur P, Irish MS, Glick PL: Physiology and pathophysiology of lung development. J Obstet Gynaecol 17:519–527, 1997.
6. Irish MS, Glick PL, Russel J, et al: Contractile properties of intralobar pulmonary arteries and veins in the fetal lamb model of congenital diaphragmatic hernia. J Pediatr Surg 33:921–928, 1998.
7. O'Neill JA, Rowe MI, Grosfeld JL, et al (eds): Pediatric Surgery, 5th ed. St. Louis, Mosby, 1998.
8. O'Toole SJ, Davis CF: UK Collaborative ECMO Trial: The CDH story. Presented at the 45th Annual International Congress of the British Association of Paediatric Surgeons, Bristol, England, 1998.

8. SURGICAL ANATOMY, EMBRYOLOGY, AND PHYSIOLOGY OF THE ESOPHAGUS

Marc A. Levitt, M.D., and Michael G. Caty, M.D.

1. What anatomic landmarks define the path of the esophagus as it travels through the mediastinum?

The esophagus passes through the neck, thorax, and abdomen. It starts at the inferior end of the pharynx at the level of the cricoid cartilage (sixth cervical vertebrae) and ends at the cardiac orifice of the stomach (eleventh thoracic vertebrae). It enters the mediastinum and lies between the trachea and vertebral column, passing posterior to the left mainstem bronchus. It descends posteriorly and to the right of the aortic arch and posterior to the pericardium and left atrium. At its most caudal extent, the esophagus deviates to the left and passes through the posterior part of the diaphragm, anterior to the descending thoracic aorta.

2. Name four areas of anatomic narrowing of the esophagus. Why are they important?
- At the level of the cricopharyngeus
- In the area of the aortic arch
- At the level of the left mainstem bronchus
- At the level of the diaphragm

Foreign bodies are more likely to lodge in these areas of narrowing.

3. How do the esophagus and trachea form?

At 22 days of gestation, the esophagus and trachea originate from a median ventral foregut diverticulum, which is composed of endoderm and mesoderm. The esophagus forms from the area between the tracheal diverticulum and stomach dilatation. The tracheal diverticulum becomes a groove in the floor of the esophagus, and both structures begin to lengthen. The tracheal bud (future trachea and lungs) and the esophagus separate as a result of proliferation at approximately the 36th day of gestation; full esophageal length is attained by the 7th week. A newborn's esophagus is 10 cm long from cricoid cartilage to gastroesophageal junction.

4. Describe the arterial blood supply of the esophagus.

The cervical esophagus is supplied mainly by the inferior thyroid artery with small branches from the common carotid and subclavian arteries. Bronchial arteries arising from the distal aortic arch supply the proximal intrathoracic esophagus. The distal esophagus and the intraabdominal portion are supplied by the left gastric and inferior phrenic arteries.

5. What is the importance of the blood supply as it relates to the repair of esophageal atresia?

In operating on an infant with esophageal atresia, it is a pediatric surgical principle to mobilize the proximal esophageal pouch, while trying not to mobilize the distal pouch. The proximal esophagus can be mobilized because of its superior intramural blood supply. Mobilizing the distal pouch can disrupt the tenuous bronchial arterial supply and lead to ischemia of the anastomosis.

6. How do esophageal duplications, webs, and rings form?

The esophageal lumen forms through a process of endodermally derived mucosal proliferation. Vacuoles form and subsequently coalesce, leading to a lumen. Incomplete recanalization or vacuole resolution leads to the formation of esophageal duplications, webs, and rings.

7. What is the embryologic basis for esophageal atresia with tracheoesophageal fistula?

Normal embryogenesis requires separate organ-forming fields on opposite sides of the foregut. These fields control differentiation of the endoderm. The tracheal mucosa forms anteriorly, and the esophageal mucosa forms posteriorly. When a disproportionate amount of endoderm becomes organized into the trachea, an inadequate amount of endoderm is left from which to form the esophagus. This portion falls under the influence of the tracheal mesoderm, and a short section of the foregut becomes entirely trachea, with a fistula to the upper or lower portion of the esophagus.

8. What are the muscular components of the upper and lower esophageal sphincters?

The upper esophageal sphincter (UES) is composed of the cricopharyngeus and thyropharyngeus. The lower esophageal sphincter (LES) is made up of the distal esophageal and esophagogastric sling fibers. The length of the esophagus is composed of an inner circular and an outer longitudinal muscle layer. Striated muscles in both layers gradually become smooth muscle, ending in a tight spiral of smooth muscle distally.

9. Describe the normal motility of the esophagus during swallowing.

The UES remains contracted in the resting state. During deglutition it begins to relax and opens for less than 1 second, contracting again for 1 second before returning to its resting tone. The UES prevents esophageal distention during inspiration and prevents aspiration of gastric contents. The esophageal body has a resting pressure of –5 mm to –15 mmHg during inspiration and –2 to +5 mmHg during expiration, while the resting pressure of the stomach is +5 mmHg. The peristaltic wave progresses at 3 cm per second, increases to 5 cm per second in the middle esophagus, and slows to 2 cm per second in the distal esophagus. The LES is a high-pressure zone of contraction at the esophagogastric junction. It relaxes during peristalsis and lets food into the stomach. The LES relaxes within 2 seconds of deglutition and lasts for about 10 seconds, allowing time for esophageal peristalsis to carry found to the stomach.

10. What causes disorders of esophageal motility?

Diffuse esophageal spasm occurs when the smooth muscle of the esophageal body has high-amplitude, repetitive, and nonperistaltic contractions. It has been treated with smooth muscle relaxants such as nitrates, anticholinergics, calcium-channel blockers, and hydralazine. Pneumatic dilatation and esophagomyotomy are used if medical treatment fails.

Patients who have undergone repair of **esophageal atresia** experience symptoms related to esophageal dysmotility such as regurgitation, heartburn, vomiting, dysphagia, and chronic respiratory disorders. It is unclear whether problems with motility are associated with esophageal atresia or result from neurologic damage after surgical repair. Incomplete UES relaxation, incomplete LES relaxation, and decreased LES pressure are common as well as abnormalities in the amplitude or coordination of peristaltic waves.

In patients with **scleroderma** esophageal depositions of collagen and connective tissue components can lead to decreased LES pressure, low-amplitude contractions, or abnormal peristalsis. Esophageal dysmotility is common in patients with other collagen vascular diseases such as polymyositis, dermatomyositis, and systemic lupus erythematosus.

Patients with **achalasia** have failure of relaxation of the distal esophagus and esophagogastric junction. Contrast radiography demonstrates a smooth distal esophageal narrowing with no stricture and may show a dilated tortuous esophagus. Manometry demonstrates failure of LES relaxation with swallowing. Low-amplitude, nonprogressive, or absent peristaltic waves are seen in the esophageal body. Treatment involves medications that relax smooth muscle or mechanical means of disrupting the nonrelaxing distal esophagus such as pneumatic dilatation or a surgical esophagocardiomyotomy (Heller procedure).

Gastroesophageal reflux results from failure of the distal esophagus to contract in response to increased intragastric pressure. Transient relaxation of the esophagogastric junction leads to acid reflux episodes or vomiting, which usually occur after feedings, while awake, and during acute illnesses. Treatment is with fundoplication, which creates pressure at the gastroesophageal junction when the stomach and its wrapped fundus is distended.

BIBLIOGRAPHY

1. Albertucci M, Ferdinand FD: Anatomy of the esophagus. In Nyhus LM, Baker RJ, Fischer JE (eds): Mastery of Surgery, 3rd ed. Boston, Little, Brown, 1997, pp 721–726.
2. Gray SW, Skandalakis JE: Embryology for Surgeons: The Embryological Basis for the Treatment of Congenital Defects. Philadelphia, W.B. Saunders, 1972, pp 63–100.
3. Jolley SG, Baron HI: Disorders of esophageal function. In O'Neill JA, Rowe MI, Grosfeld JL, et al (eds): Pediatric Surgery, 5th ed. St. Louis, Mosby, 1998, pp 997–1005.
4. Moore KI: Clinically Oriented Anatomy, 2nd ed. Baltimore, Williams & Wilkins, 1995, pp 131–142.

9. ESOPHAGEAL ATRESIA WITH OR WITHOUT TRACHEOESOPHAGEAL FISTULA

Douglas C. Barnhart, M.D., Marjorie J. Arca, M.D., and Arnold G. Coran, M.D.

1. What is the incidence of esophageal atresia?

The incidence of esophageal atresia is between 1:2500 and 1:10,000. There is a slight male preponderance.

2. Is a second child at risk if the parents already have a child with esophageal atresia?

There is a 0.5–2% risk of having a second child with esophageal atresia.

3. How do the esophagus and trachea develop?

Although the process is poorly understood, the foregut is thought to be divided into the trachea and esophagus by development of a septum through invagination of the lateral longitudinal ridges. Anomalies such as esophageal atresia and tracheoesophageal fistula result from a failure of this process.

4. What are the types of esophageal atresia and tracheoesophageal fistula? What is the frequency of each form?

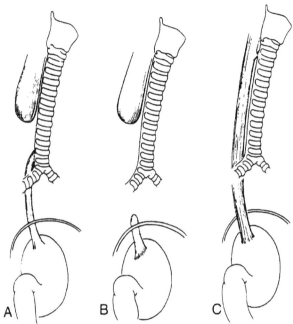

A, Proximal esophageal atresia with distal tracheoesophageal fistula (TEF) (85–90%). B, Isolated esophageal atresia (5–7%). C, TEF without esophageal atresia (2–6%). Rare forms of this anomaly include atresia with proximal TEF (< 1%) and esophageal atresia with both proximal and distal TEF (< 1%). (Adapted from Coran AG, Behrendt DM, Weintraub WH, Lee DC: Surgery of the Neonate. Boston, Little, Brown, 1978.)

5. What prenatal ultrasound findings are suggestive of esophageal atresia?

Small or absent gastric bubble and polyhydramnios.

6. How do infants with esophageal atresia typically present?

Esophageal atresia is symptomatic within the first hours of life. Findings include excessive salivation, respiratory distress, cyanosis, and inability to pass a nasogastric tube. Attempts at feeding cause choking, coughing, and regurgitation.

7. What is the characteristic presentation of a child with TEF without esophageal atresia?

Isolated TEF presents in the first several months after birth with choking and coughing with feeding. Delayed presentations with recurrent episodes of pneumonia are seen with isolated TEFs.

8. How can plain radiographs be used to confirm the diagnosis of esophageal atresia and demonstrate the presence of a distal TEF?

Plain radiographs demonstrate the upper esophageal pouch if an oral tube is placed and insufflated with a few milliliters of air. Air within the stomach and bowel on plain abdominal radiograph confirms the presence of a distal TEF.

9. What anomalies are associated with esophageal atresia?

Other anomalies occur in 50–70% of infants with esophageal atresia. Associated anomalies are most common with esophageal atresia and distal TEF. Common types of anomalies are cardiovascular, genitourinary, gastrointestinal, and skeletal malformations. Cardiac defects account for the majority of deaths in infants with esophageal atresia.

10. What is the VACTERL association?

The VACTERL association consists of vertebral, anorectal, cardiac, tracheoesophageal, renal, and radial limb abnormalities. It is not correlated with a known chromosomal abnormality or syndrome.

11. What preoperative studies are routinely performed in infants with esophageal atresia?

In addition to a careful physical examination, evaluation for associated anomalies should include echocardiography, renal ultrasonography, and chromosomal analysis. Some pediatric surgeons also perform a pouchogram (insertion of $1\frac{1}{2}$ ml of thin barium cut onto the upper pouch) to detect a proximal fistula.

12. How is an infant with esophageal atresia managed preoperatively?

A sump tube is placed in the upper esophageal pouch and maintained on low suction to reduce the risk of aspiration of saliva. The infant should be placed in the upright sitting position to minimize gastroesophageal reflux and chemical pneumonitis due to gastric acid.

13. Should infants with esophageal atresia and TEF routinely receive endotracheal intubation?

No. Positive-pressure ventilation causes increased abdominal distention because air is forced through the TEF and may result in gastric perforation and/or respiratory compromise through elevation of the diaphragm.

14. What are the principles of surgical repair of esophageal atresia with TEF?

Surgical repair is done within the first days of life and consists of division of the fistula and establishment of continuity of the esophagus. The esophagus usually is approached through a right retropleural, posterolateral thoracotomy through the fourth intercostal space. Mobilization of the distal esophagus is minimized to protect the blood supply and vagal branches. Proximal pouch mobilization can be more extensive because its cervical blood supply is robust.

15. When was the first successful primary repair of an esophageal atresia performed?

In 1941, at the University of Michigan, Cameron Haight primarily repaired an esophageal atresia in a 12-day-old girl who survived and grew to adulthood. Before this patient, numerous attempts at primary repair by him and other surgeons had been unsuccessful.

16. What is the advantage of an extrapleural approach?

An anastomotic leak results in an esophageal-cutaneous fistula rather than an empyema (if a transpleural approach is used).

17. What is "long-gap" esophageal atresia?

Long-gap esophageal atresia occurs when the proximal and distal ends cannot be joined with a tension-free anastomosis. It generally is defined as a gap of 3 or more vertebral bodies or 5 or more centimeters.

18. What can be done to bridge the gap?

Isolated esophageal atresia is associated with long gaps that shorten by growth if observed for 6–12 weeks. Operative techniques include circular myotomies of the proximal pouch, creation of a tube from an anterior flap of the proximal pouch, and careful mobilization of the distal esophagus and gastroesophageal junction. Replacement of the esophagus with the stomach or colon is used for ultra-long-gap atresia.

19. What are the common complications immediately after repair of esophageal atresia?
Anastomotic leak (10%), esophageal stricture (15%), and recurrent TEF (6–10%) are the most common immediate complications.

20. What long-term problems occur after esophageal atresia repair?
Gastroesophageal reflux is common, occurring in one-half of the children who undergo repair of esophageal atresia. Tracheomalacia occurs in 10–20% of cases. Long-term dysphagia frequently results from disordered motility.

BIBLIOGRAPHY

1. Engum SA, Grosfeld JL, West KW, et al: Analysis of morbidity and mortality in 227 cases of esophageal atresia and/or tracheoesophageal fistula over two decades. Arch Surg 130:502–508, 1995.
2. Harmon CM, Coran AG: Congenital anomalies of the esophagus. In O'Neill JA, Rowe MI, Grosfeld JL, et al (eds): Pediatric Surgery, 5th ed. St. Louis, Mosby, 1998, pp 941–967.
3. Okada A, Usui N, Inoue M, et al: Esophageal atresia in Osaka: A review of 39 years' experience. J Pediatr Surg 32:1570–1574, 1997.
4. Spitz L: Esophageal atresia with and without tracheoesophageal fistula. In Spitz L, Coran AG (eds): Operative Surgery Pediatric Surgery, 5th ed. New York, Chapman & Hall, 1995, pp 111–120.
5. Spitz L: Esophageal atresia: Past, present, and future. J Pediatr Surg 31:19–25, 1996.

10. GASTROESOPHAGEAL REFLUX DISEASE

Jerome M. McDonald, M.D., MAJ, Kenneth S. Azarow, M.D., LTC, and Richard H. Pearl, M.D.

1. What is gastroesophageal reflux?
Gastroesophageal reflux (GER) is uncontrolled vomiting not caused by a noxious stimulus. Virtually all newborns have reflux as demonstrated by "spitting up" while being burped during feeding. Neonatal reflux resolves by 1 year of age and usually is not pathologic.

2. Describe the barriers to GER disease and esophagitis.
Esophageal clearance and mucosal protection are the first factors in prevention of esophagitis. Saliva, which is rich in bicarbonate, coats the esophagus in response to reflux. The production of mucus, prostaglandin, vascularization, and epithelial growth factor helps to prevent damage to the esophageal mucosa. Peristalsis is critical to clear acid from the esophagus and increases in frequency in response to distal esophageal exposure to gastric refluxate. The physiologic high-pressure zone in the distal esophagus (lower esophageal sphincter [LES]) is created by the length of intraabdominal esophagus, intact phrenoesophageal ligaments, pinch-cock action of the diaphragm, mucosal rosette, and increased-amplitude muscular contractions. Additional factors include normal aboral antral contractions, gastric emptying, and a sharp angle of His.

3. Is the lower esophageal high-pressure zone a true sphincter?
No. As described above, this high-pressure zone is created by multiple factors, but it is not a true sphincter like the pylorus.

4. What is the physiologic rationale for the normal neonatal reflux? What is the typical duration?
The distal esophageal high-pressure zone is normally 1 cm in length in infants compared with 2–4 cm in adults. More importantly, a progressive increase in tone of the distal esophageal high-pressure zone is observed from birth to 45 days of age, coincident with improvement in neonatal reflux.

5. True or false: Abdominal wall defects are associated with an increased incidence of GER disease.

True. Both before and after repair, neonates and infants with congenital abdominal wall defects (omphalocele, gastroschisis, and prune-belly syndrome) as well as congenital diaphragmatic hernia are at increased risk of reflux. The highest risk is in patients with large omphaloceles that preclude primary fascial repair (incidence of approximately 70%).

6. List the typical manifestations of GER in neonates, infants, and adolescents.

Neonates	Infants	Adolescents
Apnea	Apnea	Chest pain
Bronchopulmonary dysplasia	Pneumonia	Esophagitis
Recurrent pneumonias	Failure to thrive	Stricture
Poor feeding	Vomiting	Asthma
Coughing	Choking	Barrett's esophagus
Choking	Reactive airways disease	

7. What is Sandifer's syndrome?

This manifestation of esophagitis includes voluntary dystonic contortions of the head, neck, and trunk. Such movements have been shown to improve peristalsis in the lower esophagus.

8. What is the incidence of GER in patients with neurologic impairment?

The incidence of GER is increased in neurologically impaired children; severity and incidence are related directly to the severity of neurologic dysfunction. The rate is as high as 70%, and surgery is required more frequently than in neurologically normal children. The presumed cause is chronic supine positioning, abdominal spasticity, diaphragmatic flaccidity, scoliosis, use of gastrostomy, delayed gastric emptying, retching, and vagal nerve dysfunction.

9. The use of gastrostomy for feeding in neurologically impaired children is associated with GER in what percentage of cases?

The use of gastrostomy, either surgically or by percutaneous endoscopic technique, is associated with an increase in GER due to opening of the angle of His, lowering of the LES pressure, and reduction of LES length. Development of postgastrostomy GER in neurologically impaired children with normal preoperative studies has been reported to be as high as 66%. The Witzel gastrostomy has been associated with a lower incidence of postoperative GER than the Stamm gastrostomy, presumably because the stomach is not tacked to the anterior abdominal wall. Lesser-curvature gastrostomy tubes are associated with less reflux than greater-curvature tubes, possibly because there is no change in the angle of His. However, with the percutaneous technique of insertion, placing the gastrostomy tube specifically in the lesser curvature is not possible.

10. GER complicates repair of esophageal atresia in what percentage of cases?

Symptomatic GER occurs in 30–80% of infants after repair of esophageal atresia; the incidence is related directly to the length of the gap between the ends of the esophagus. Distal esophageal dysmotility and tension on the anastomosis are presumptive causes. GER can be clinically significant, resulting in anastomotic strictures and ultimately necessitating surgical therapy in 15–40% of cases.

11. Does repair or treatment of GER in neurologically impaired children improve life expectancy?

Sometimes. The usual cause of death is recurrent aspiration of saliva, which causes infection regardless of surgical treatment. However, most neurologically impaired children have an improvement in quality of life with better feeding, improved nutrition, decreased or cured gastrointestinal aspiration episodes, and fewer hospital admissions. Although the relentless process caused by the neurologic disorder is not changed, improved nutrition frequently improves overall state of health and well-being.

12. What are the pathologic findings of GER disease on biopsy of the distal esophagus? On bronchoscopy?

Basal cell hyperplasia and increased length of the stromal papilla are typical findings in GER in adolescents but may be normal findings in the distal esophagus of infants. Infiltration of lymphocytes and neutrophils is typical in GER but also may be seen in the normal esophageal mucosa of infants. The finding specific for GER in infants is the presence of eosinophilic infiltration in the esophageal mucosa. On bronchoscopy and lavage, lipid-laden macrophages in the trachea are highly suggestive of GER with aspiration.

13. Describe the evaluation of neonates, infants, and adolescents suspected of having GER disease

Neonates	Infants	Adolescents
Upper gastrointestinal (UGI) series with or without 24-hour pH monitoring	UGI series with or without 24-hour pH study	Esophagogastroduodenoscopy 24-hour pH monitoring
Gastric isotope emptying study (if emptying not visualized on UGI series)	Gastric isotope emptying study (if emptying not visualized on UGI series)	Esophagogastric manometry Gastric isotope emptying study with or without UGI series

14. What are the potential advantages of radionucleotide scintigraphy?

The addition of 99m-technetium to an infant's formula is followed by monitoring with a gamma counter. The test has the advantage of being noninvasive, low in radiation, and widely available. It also can be performed postprandially and used to assess gastric emptying and tracheobronchial aspiration. Limitations include its nonambulatory nature and poor reproducibility.

15. Describe nonsurgical/nonpharmacologic modes of treatment for GER in infants.

The first line of treatment for infants with GER includes positional therapy, thickened feeds, frequent small feedings, and changing the formula to decrease air swallowing. By elevating the head of the bed to 30°, gravitational forces decrease reflux. This mode of therapy is difficult to maintain after the first 60–90 days of life; however, combined with rice cereal thickening of feeds, it allows up to 90% of infants without neurologic deficits to outgrow their reflux. In neurologically normal infants these modes of therapy, not surgery, are the hallmarks of reflux treatment.

16. What pharmacologic treatments for GER disease are presently used?

Until recently, antacids, bethanechol, and metoclopramide were the only pharmacologic treatments available in the United States for treatment of symptomatic GER in children. Although bethanechol and metoclopramide show physiologic improvement of LES pressure and pH monitoring, both have significant side effects with no clinically relevant improvement. Cisapride is now available in the U.S. and has been available in Europe for years. It has become the pharmacologic treatment of choice for neonates and infants after thickening of feeds. Recent reports of the prolonged QT interval with the use of cisapride have generated concern about its safety and have prompted recommendations for limitation of its use. Although controversial, some recommend withholding cisapride in infants with a history of cardiac dysrhythmias, infants receiving drugs known to inhibit its metabolism (e.g., ranitidine, erythromycin), infants with disease or immaturity resulting in reduced cytochrome P450 3A4 activity, and infants with electrolyte abnormalities. Adolescents are treated as adults; omeprazole is the first-line therapy.

17. What other disease processes must be ruled out before operative repair of GER?

Although most patients have no comorbid gastrointestinal disease, the other possibilities include hypertrophic pyloric stenosis before or after repair, intestinal malrotation with Ladd's bands, and H-type tracheoesophageal fistula. Patients with repair of tracheoesophageal fistula or diaphragmatic hernia have a high incidence of postoperative GER. However, before operative repair of GER in such patients, recurrence of the fistula or hernia needs to be excluded.

18. Describe the Nissen fundoplication for control of symptomatic GER. What modifications are common in neurologically impaired infants?

The gastrohepatic ligament is divided as well as the peritoneal covering over the esophagus. The esophagus is mobilized and encircled with a Penrose drain, and the esophageal hiatus and diaphragmatic crura are delineated. The gastrophrenic ligaments are divided to mobilize the posterior aspect of the fundus. Division of the short gastric vessels is then performed as needed. A window is created posterior to the gastroesophageal junction. The right and left leaves of the right crus are approximated over a large bougie (variable depending on esophageal size), and the fundus is passed posteriorly to create at 360° wrap. A 1.0- to 1.5 cm-long wrap is created by approximation of the wrap to the esophagus. Modifications include recreation of the angle of His, pexy of the fundoplication to the esophagus and/or diaphragm, pexy to the crura, addition of an uncut Collis gastroplasty before fundoplication, and reinforcement of the usual closure and wrap sutures with pledgets. A gastrostomy also is frequently placed, particularly in neurologically impaired children.

19. What surgical procedures other than Nissen fundoplication are commonly used for children with symptomatic GER?

The operative choices for repair of reflux include the Toupet, Dor, Thal, Boerema, Boix-Ochoa, and Hill repairs. The two most frequently used are the Toupet and Thal repairs. The Toupet repair is a 180–270° posterior fundoplication with suture approximation to both limbs of the hiatal crura and both anterolateral aspects of the esophagus. This procedure results in four suture lines. The reported advantage is decreased dysphagia and gas bloat. A Thal fundoplication involves anterior approximation of the upper cardia to the anterior two-thirds of the esophagus and the diaphragm at the level of the hiatus. This procedure also permits slightly improved immediate postoperative relief of dysphagia and gas bloat at the expense of increased recurrent GER. The Thal procedure has the advantage of not requiring crural dissection or repair.

20. How effective is the Nissen fundoplication for control of symptomatic pediatric GER?

More than 90% of children have long-term resolution of symptoms with Nissen fundoplication. The cure rate for emesis is nearly 100%. Pulmonary symptoms are relieved in 96% of patients. Weight gain is achieved in nearly all patients, especially those in whom a gastrostomy is placed concurrently. Asthma is improved significantly in approximately 91% of patients.

21. What are the reported complications of surgical therapy for GER disease?

Approximately 15% of patients exhibit surgical complications. The most common include wrap breakdown (with recurrent reflux), dysphagia secondary to a slipped wrap, a wrap that is too tight, torsion of the wrap, and gas bloat (in approximately 10%). Early or late intestinal obstruction occurs in 2–6%. Splenic injury and perforation of the esophagus are rare. Wound infection occurs in approximately 2%. Complications occur more frequently in neurologically impaired children; reported recurrence rates are as high as 30%. With modification of the standard Nissen procedure (see question 18), recurrence rates of < 10% have been reported in neurologically impaired children.

22. What adjunctive measure is often used in reoperative GER surgery?

Because of the higher likelihood of damage to the vagus nerves during dissection at the gastroesophageal junction, many support performing an emptying procedure such as pyloromyotomy or pyloroplasty with the reflux procedure. Clearly, before reoperation a nuclear medicine gastric emptying study should be performed. If the vagus nerves are not clearly identified during the repeat procedure, a gastric emptying study should be considered.

23. What factors are important in deciding for or against the use of gastrostomy in surgical therapy for GER disease?

Three factors need to be considered in the decision to place a gastrostomy at the time of definitive surgical therapy: (1) Is the patient having difficulty with feeding or weight gain? (2) Is gas bloat a concern in the postoperative period? (3) If the patient is neurologically impaired, many surgeons place a gastrostomy because of concerns over air swallowing, ease of feeding, and gas bloat.

Gastrostomy is a relatively simple addition to the procedure and can be temporary; initial placement with subsequent removal, if it proves unnecessary, is a consideration in any patient.

BIBLIOGRAPHY

1. Boix-Ochoa J, Canals J: Maturation of the lower esophagus. J Pediatr Surg 11:749, 1976.
2. Boix-Ochoa J, Rowe MI: Gastroesophageal reflux. In O'Neill JA, Rowe MI, Grosfeld JL, et al (eds): Pediatric Surgery, 5th ed. St. Louis, Mosby, 1998, pp 1007–1028.
3. Carre IJ: Postural treatment of children with partial thoracic stomach. Arch Dis Child 35:569–580, 1960.
4. Foglia RP, Fonkalsrud EW, Ament ME, et al: Gastroesophageal fundoplication for the management of chronic pulmonary disease in children. Am J Surg 140:686–690, 1991.
5. Fonkalsrud EW, Ament ME: Gastroesophageal reflux in childhood. Curr Probl Surg 33:1–80, 1996.
6. Guggenbichler JP, Menard G: Conservative treatment of gastroesophageal reflux hiatus hernia. Prog Pediatr Surg 18:78–83, 1985.
7. Koivusalo A, Rintala R, Lindahl H: Gastroesophageal reflux in children with a congenital abdominal wall defect. J Pediatr Surg 34:1127–1129, 1999.
8. Pearl RH, Robie DK, Ein SH: Complications of gastroesophageal antireflux surgery in neurologically impaired versus neurologically normal children. J Pediatr Surg 25:1169–1173, 1990.
9. Vandenplas Y, Belli DC, Benatar A, et al: The role of cisapride in the treatment of pediatric gastroesophageal reflux. The European Society of Paediatric Gastroenterology, Hepatology, and Nutrition. J Pediatr Gastroenterol Nutr 28:518–528, 1999.

11. CAUSTIC INGESTIONS OF THE ESOPHAGUS

Jennifer I. Lin, Michael G. Caty, M.D., and Kathryn D. Anderson, M.D.

1. What is the most important first step in the evaluation of a child with caustic ingestion?
The first step in the management of children with suspected ingestion injuries is to establish the patency of the airway. Alkaline substances can cause injury to the pharynx and/or larynx. Ongoing swelling can obstruct the airway. Endotracheal intubation or tracheostomy may be necessary in such cases.

2. What substances ingested by children may cause caustic injuries?
Both acids and alkalis are ingested. Strong alkalis in household cleaners are the most commonly ingested substances. Formerly, battery acid was a popular drink with toddlers. Bleach and ammonia usually do not injure children because they take only one swallow and hate the taste.

3. Is there a difference in acid and alkali injuries?
Yes. Strong alkalis tend to be less viscous and injure the proximal pharynx and esophagus. Alkali ingestion causes deeper injury with liquefactive necrosis. Acid ingestion usually results in more distal injury because it is less viscous. Strong acids can cause dramatic injuries of the stomach. Acid ingestion causes coagulation necrosis.

4. What are the complications of caustic injuries?
The severity of complications relates to the depth of the injury. Superficial mucosal injury is painful but resolves without long-term sequelae. Deeper caustic injuries to the esophagus result in healing by fibrosis and subsequent stricture formation. Short-length esophageal strictures may require resection. Greater involvement of the esophagus may mandate esophageal replacement. Full-thickness injury to the esophagus may result in perforation and potential fistula formation to either the trachea or, in extreme cases, the aorta.

5. Does it help to induce vomiting when a child has ingested a caustic substance?

No. In fact, it is contraindicated. Regurgitation of a caustic substance can reinjure the esophagus, pharnyx, or larynx. Regurgitation also places a child at risk for aspiration pneumonitis.

6. What age groups ingest caustic agents?

Ingestion of corrosive substances is seen most commonly in children under 5 years of age. Boys are affected more commonly than girls. Girls are more commonly involved in the adolescent group, when most cases of caustic ingestion are suicide attempts.

7. When is esophagoscopy indicated to assess potential injury to the esophagus?

Endoscopic visualization of the esophagus is indicated whenever a caustic injury is suspected. Esophagoscopy is best done within 24–48 hours after ingestion. It is wise to limit the examination to the first level of injury to avoid perforation.

8. When is esophagoscopy contraindicated?

Endoscopy should not be performed in any patient who lacks a secure airway. For example, in a patient presenting with stridor or evidence of pharyngeal burns, esophagoscopy without first controlling the airway may lead to a complete airway obstruction.

9. When is a contrast study indicated?

A contrast esophagogram with water-soluble contrast should be performed at the initial presentation if perforation is suspected and to assess the length of mucosal injury. An esophagogram usually is done 2–3 weeks after ingestion to determine the presence of strictures.

10. How is an esophageal injury graded endoscopically?

Grade 0	Normal
Grade I	Mucosal edema and hyperemia
Grade IIa	Superficial injury
Grade IIb	Superficial injury with limited areas of deeper or circumferential injury
Grade IIIa	Small scattered necrotic areas
Grade IIIb	Extensive necrosis

11. How does the endoscopic grade of the lesion affect patient management?

For grade I injuries, no specific treatment is indicated. A contrast study may be performed after 2–3 weeks if symptoms of dysphagia are present. More severe injuries involve an increased risk of stricture formation. Patients require close follow-up with endoscopy and esophageal dilatation.

12. What are the indications for immediate surgical exploration?

Free air in the peritoneum or mediastinum, evidence of contrast material extravasating from the esophagus or stomach, or evidence of peritonitis is an indication for emergency exploration. Severe back or retrosternal pain also may indicate the need for exploration after contrast studies.

13. What is the role of antibiotics in managing caustic esophageal injury?

No data support the routine use of antibiotics as prophylaxis. However, antibiotic therapy may be appropriate in patients with evidence of systemic infection or transmural necrosis.

14. How do you manage an esophageal stricture that results from caustic ingestion?

Esophageal dilation should be performed at least once a week with a catheter that is 1–2 French sizes smaller than the stricture. A lumen that remains inadequate after 9–12 months of frequent dilation suggests the presence of irreversible fibrosis, and resection of the stricture or replacement of the esophagus may become necessary.

15. Is caustic injury to the esophagus associated with development of esophageal carcinoma?

Yes. There is a correlation between corrosive esophageal injuries and the development of esophageal carcinoma 15–20 years after the ingestion.

CONTROVERSY

16. Discuss the considerations of steroid therapy in the management of corrosive injuries to the esophagus.

Theoretically, steroids inhibit the inflammatory response and therefore decrease the formation of strictures after caustic ingestion. Although this effect has been shown in animal studies, no statistical benefits were demonstrated in trials with humans. The recent introduction of high-dose dexamethasone in the management of caustic esophageal injuries also requires further studies.

BIBLIOGRAPHY

1. Anderson KD, Rouse TM, Randolph JG: A controlled trial of corticosteroids in children with corrosive injury of the esophagus. N Engl J Med 323:637, 1990.
2. Millar AJW, Cywes S: Caustic strictures of the esophagus. In O'Neill JA, Rowe MI, Grosfeld JL, Coran AG (eds): Pediatric Surgery, 5th ed. St. Louis, Mosby, 1998, pp 969–979.

12. ESOPHAGEAL FOREIGN BODIES

Amanda J. McCabe, M.D., FRCS, Rebeccah L. Brown, M.D.,
Michael G. Caty, M.D., and Philip L. Glick, M.D.

1. Are foreign bodies a public health problem?

Less than a century ago, death and injuries were almost a certainty for all children with persistent foreign bodies lodged in the airway or esophagus. Now there are about 6 deaths per 100,000 ingestions or about 150 deaths per year in the United States. In one survey, parents of children in a suburban pediatric practice reported that 4% of their children had swallowed a coin at some time.

2. What is the most common age for children to present with esophageal foreign bodies?

The peak incidence for ingestion is between 9 and 24 months. More than half of the children are less than 4 years of age. Boys are at greater risk than girls.

3. Where are foreign bodies most commonly trapped in the esophagus?

In the three anatomic narrowings of the esophagus: the cricopharyngeus muscle at the upper esophageal sphincter, the carina and crossover of the aortic arch in the mid esophagus, and the lower esophageal sphincter (LES). In the pediatric population 63–84% are at the cricopharyngeus level, 10–17% at the aortic cross-over, and 5–20% at the LES. In adults most foreign bodies are trapped at the LES.

4. How may a case of foreign body ingestion present?

Adults give a clear history of ingestion and usually localize the level of impaction. In contrast, children may give only a vague history of ingestion, and the parents may have only seen "something in their mouth." Thus the clinician must maintain a high index of suspicion. Often older siblings are unwitting accomplices. Of note, 7–35% of proven pediatric cases of ingestion are asymptomatic. Symptoms may include dysphagia, poor feeding, choking, neck or chest pain, irritability, fever, stridor, cough, and signs of aspiration. Drooling (excessive salivation) is a sign of complete obstruction. Odynophagia may result from esophageal distention secondary to the foreign body, or it may indicate esophageal injury, such as laceration, abrasion, and perforation. Respiratory symptoms, such as cough or wheeze, may result from compression of the trachea by the foreign body.

5. At presentation, what can be done to locate a foreign body accurately?

A chest radiograph (including the cervical spine and soft tissue structures) should be obtained in all cases of suspected foreign body. Both anteroposterior and lateral views are necessary for a full assessment. Abdominal views are needed to screen the rest of the bowel. In cases of nonopaque objects, such as aluminum can tabs, plastic objects, toothpicks, or small bones, plain films have low yield, and unless immediate endoscopy is planned, a contrast esophagogram is indicated. A water-soluble contrast medium is used if esophageal perforation is suspected.

6. What patient populations may be more prone to foreign body ingestion and impaction?

Patients with esophageal strictures secondary to an anastomotic site from repair of esophageal atresia or scarring from ingestion of a caustic substance are at particular risk of impaction. Patients with esophageal atresia seem to be at greatest risk from about 9 months to 5 years of age—the period when they transfer from formulas to solid food—to the period when they can chew and swallow better. During this time certain foods should be avoided (e.g., uncooked carrots, hot dogs, chips, chunks of meat, popcorn). Patients with congenital diverticula also may experience foreign body entrapment. Neurologically impaired and psychiatric patients also are prone to foreign body ingestion and impaction.

7. Where are coins typically trapped?

Coins represent a large proportion of pediatric foreign bodies. Pennies (18 mm in diameter) or dimes (17 mm) usually are seen in the LES or aortic crossover, whereas quarters (24 mm) inevitably are trapped at the upper esophageal sphincter level.

8. How can the location of an ingested coin in the aerodigestive tract be established on plain radiographs?

Coins lodged in the esophagus usually are seen in coronal alignment on anteroposterior (AP) films because the opening of the esophagus is widest in the transverse plane. Coins within the trachea usually are seen in the oblique or sagittal orientation on a plain AP film, because the tracheal cartilage is incomplete posteriorly. The history and symptoms can be misleading with regard to location; therefore, lateral films must be obtained in all cases of foreign body ingestion. Foreign bodies can appear to be in the esophagus on the AP view when actually they are in the pulmonary tree. Because of surface tension, two overlying coins often look like one coin on radiographs, but both need to be detected and removed.

9. Do batteries need to be removed from the esophagus?

Button batteries in the esophagus should be considered an emergency. Prompt removal is essential to prevent complications. Batteries can cause necrosis, esophageal perforation, and, in some cases, death. Three mechanisms explain the tissue damage caused by batteries:
- Electrical burn: an electrical current can be set up between the metal anode and the metallic oxide cathode of the battery in the high-conductive, moist environment of the esophageal mucosa.
- Leakage: potassium hydroxide can leak from an imperfectly sealed battery. This highly corrosive alkali penetrates deeply into tissue layers, causing dissolution of proteins, saponification of lipids, and liquefactive necrosis.
- Pressure necrosis: impaction can result in ischemic, blackened areas of tissue damage from pressure effects alone.

It is likely that a low-voltage electrochemical reaction in tissues contributes to battery corrosion, resulting in further leakage from the battery and subsequent liquefaction necrosis.

10. What follow-up is advised after button battery extraction?

After extraction, the esophagus must be visualized carefully for signs of injury. Repeat esophagograms at 24 hours and again at about 30 days have been recommended to rule out fistula or stricture formation.

11. What underlying condition may be indicated by an ingested toothbrush?

An eating disorder. Bulimia (compulsive binge eating and purging) may affect as many as 20% of adolescent girls. Self-induced vomiting often is achieved by placing a finger or foreign body into the hypopharynx. On occasion, a toothbrush can be swallowed accidentally. Endoscopic removal is preferred, but surgical retrieval may be necessary. Psychiatric consultation is recommended.

12. What complications can arise from esophageal foreign bodies?

Complications are most frequent when foreign bodies have been in situ for more than 24 hours. They range from insignificant to life-threatening. Examples include mucosal scratch/abrasion, esophageal necrosis (button batteries), retropharyngeal abscess, esophageal stricture, esophageal perforation, paraesophageal abscess, mediastinitis, pericarditis, pneumothorax, pneumomediastinum, tracheoesophageal fistula, and vascular injuries including aortic-esophageal fistulas.

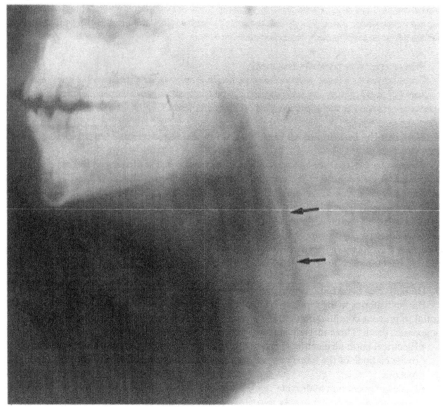

Lateral radiograph of the neck after a history of foreign body ingestion. Note evidence of free air in the neck, with associated esophageal tear.

13. What medical therapies can be used for foreign body dislodgment in the esophagus?

For objects lodged at the LES, the goals of pharmaceutical therapy are to relax the smooth muscle of the LES and to allow the foreign body to pass through the sphincter mechanism into the stomach. From the stomach the vast majority transit the gastrointestinal tract without further problems. The use of glucagon (0.02–0.03 mg/kg; maximal dose of 0.5 mg in children) is reported to have a success rate of 12–50%. More recent reports have used gas-forming solutions with glucagon. Examples include carbonated beverages, sodium bicarbonate, citric acid, and simethicone (E-Z Gas). Success rates approach 75%. The technique is indicated only for smooth objects and in older patients without evidence of a fixed stricture, esophageal diverticulum, or proximal obstruction.

Other medications used for relaxation of the LES include benzodiazepines, calcium channel blockers, anticholinergics, and nitrates, but none of these has been shown to be more effective than glucagon.

In pediatric cases, however, the safest and most efficient way of treating foreign bodies is endoscopic removal by a pediatric surgeon.

14. What techniques can be used to remove foreign bodies from the esophagus?

Endoscopy: the most widely used technique. A rigid esophagoscope combined with general anesthesia is commonly used, although flexible endoscopy under heavy sedation also has been described. When the object is located, it can be grasped with forceps, or, if suitable, a strong sucker can be used. Endoscopy offers the advantage of direct inspection of the esophagus for additional injury or unsuspected additional foreign bodies. Real-time fluoroscopy frequently facilitates removal of radiopaque foreign bodies.

Foley catheter: with the aid of fluoroscopy, ballon extraction has been used for smooth foreign bodies such as coins or buttons. It can be done in the fluoroscopy suite, but the personnel must be prepared to control the airway in all circumstances.

Bougienage: the least commonly used method. It involves the careful passage of a lubricated esophageal dilator into the esophagus. The dilator dislodges the object, allowing it to continue into the stomach, from which it passes without further difficulty. The procedure should be terminated if any resistance is encountered. It is most suitable for objects near the LES or objects not seen on esophagoscopy. In such circumstances, the question arises whether the foreign body was already in the gastric fundus and just appeared at the LES on AP radiograph. A postprocedure chest radiograph is suggested to confirm the passage of radiopaque objects and to rule out esophageal rupture.

Temporization: if the foreign body has lodged in the distal esophagus for less than 24 hours, a trial of passage into the stomach is worthwhile in cases of smooth, innocuous foreign bodies.

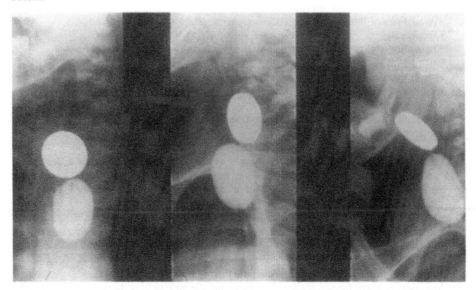

Foley catheter extraction of coin.

15. Which method of extraction is most cost-effective?

In a literature-based comparison of the three methods of pediatric esophageal coin extraction in 1997, the expected cost of endoscopic removal was $2701; of Foley catheter removal, $660; of bougienage removal, $614. Cost-effectiveness, however, cannot be the only consideration in the choice of technique. The availability of trained personnel and suitable facilities both at regular workday times and during on-call evenings and nights must be taken into account. The type of foreign body also is a major determining factor.

16. Who performed the first esophagoscopy?

In 1870 Kussmaul passed a hollow rigid tube through the mouth, pharynx, and esophagus into the stomach of a cooperative professional sword swallower. He used a reflected light source for illumination. With light modifications, the same practice forms a valuable part of the endoscopic management of foreign body retrieval.

17. What is the extraction method of choice for a foreign body just below the cricopharyngeus?

A rigid bronchoscope. Such objects present a particular challenge, because the endoscopic view often is obscured by sphincter closure. With the foreign body against the viewing lens, the scope has to be withdrawn slightly to allow extension of foreign body forceps, and just at this point sphincter closure occurs. A rigid bronchoscope is most effective because the insufflation port helps to keep the field of view open for the grasping action. A portable C-arm fluoroscope also facilitates the removal of difficult-to-visualize foreign bodies.

18. When can balloon extraction be safely used for removal of a foreign body from the esophagus?

This technique has limited use because the esophageal mucosa is not viewed directly. A second foreign body may be missed, and damaged esophageal mucosa may be made worse during blind extraction. Therefore, balloon extraction can be used safely only in the following cases:
- A single, smooth, blunt, radiopaque foreign body
- Ingestion less than 24 hours ago with minimal esophageal inflammation
- No respiratory distress or evidence of perforation
- Availability of fluoroscopy and endoscopy with suitably trained personnel
- Failed cases
- Immediate ability to control the airway if aspiration or laryngeal spasm occurs

19. How is balloon extraction performed?

- Rule out multiple foreign bodies, complete obstruction, and esophageal disease with an esophagogram.
- Have all necessary personnel and equipment for advanced airway management in the fluoroscopy room.
- Place the supine patient in the head-down position.
- Pass a number 12–16 Foley catheter, nasally or orally, past the foreign body under fluoroscopic guidance.
- Inflate the catheter balloon with 5–10 ml of contrast material, taking care not to overinflate the esophagus.
- Using steady traction, remove the catheter and foreign body under fluoroscopic guidance.
- Remove the foreign body from the hypopharynx with MaGill forceps or by cough reflex (see figure in Question 14).

20. What complications should you anticipate during balloon extraction?

Vomiting, epitaxis, foreign body dislodgment into the nose or lung, laryngospasm, hypoxia, and hyperpyrexia. The rate of complication is reported at less than 2%.

21. What are the potential problems of attempting to remove a foreign body from the esophagus in the radiology suite or emergency department?

Neither setting generally is as well equipped as the operating room for airway management if problems arise. During attempts to remove a foreign body with the balloon-tipped catheter technique, the foreign body may be aspirated accidentally into the airway, especially in an inadequately sedated or uncooperative child. Blind bougie insertion in the emergency department to push a foreign body into the stomach is associated with an increased risk of perforation of the esophagus and generally is not recommended.

22. What special considerations are required for the removal of sharp objects from the esophagus?

Sharp objects should be removed upon presentation without a period of conservative waiting. Objects such as open safety pins, razor blades, or bones have a high incidence of esophageal perforation. They are best removed under direct vision with a rigid scope. The rigid scope may allow withdrawal of the object into the sheath for atraumatic removal. Pins or open safety pins may be removed with the sharp end trailing or, if positioned in the opposite direction, pushed into the stomach, turned around, and withdrawn via the blunt end. These procedures must be used with great care, because they may cause diametrically positioned abrasions or linear perforations of the esophageal circumference.

BIBLIOGRAPHY

1. Alvi A, Bereliani A, Zahtz GD: Miniature disc battery in the nose: A dangerous foreign body. Clin Pediatr 36:427–429, 1997.
2. Conners GP: A literature-based comparison of three methods of pediatric esophageal coin removal. Pediatr Emerg Care 13:154–157, 1997.
3. McGahren ED: Esophageal foreign bodies. Pediatr Rev 20:129–133, 1999.
4. O'Neill JA, Rowe MI, Grosfeld JL, et al (eds): Pediatric Surgery, vol. 1. St. Louis, Mosby, 1998.
5. Reilly JS, Cook SP, Stool D, Rider G: Prevention and management of aerodigestive foreign body injuries in childhood. Pediatr Clin North Am 43:1403–1411, 1996.
6. Stack LB, Munter DW: Foreign bodies in the gastrointestinal tract. Emerg Med Clin North Am 14: 493–521, 1996.
7. Wilcox DT, Karamanoukian HL, Glick PL: Toothbrush ingestion by bulimics may require laparotomy. J Pediatr Surg 29:1596, 1994.

13. CONGENITAL LUNG MALFORMATIONS

Drucy Borowitz, M.D., and Bonnie Hudak, M.D.

1. What are the prenatal stages of lung development?
- Embryonic period (0–7 weeks)
- Pseudoglandular period (8–16 weeks)
- Cannalicular period (17–24 weeks)
- Terminal sac period (24 weeks to term)

2. What happens during the embryonic period?
The lung bud branches off from the embryo's primitive foregut.

3. During what stage of prenatal development do the conducting airways form?
Conducting airways form during the pseudoglandular phase. The airway epithelium begins to differentiate, including mucus-secreting cells. All of the airways present in adult life, along with their blood supply, are formed by the 16th week of gestation.

4. During which stages of prenatal development do the gas exchange units form?

Gas exchange units are formed during the cannalicular and terminal sac periods.

5. What happens during the cannalicular period?

Saccules, which consist of terminal bronchioles, alveolar ducts, and alveoli, develop. Blood vessels surrounding the saccules begin to thin out. Supporting tissue is formed, with cartilage in the large airways, collagen in the mid-sized airways, and elastic fibers in the terminal bronchioles. At the end of the cannalicular period, type I and type II cells begin to appear.

6. What happens during the terminal sac period?

More saccules and alveoli form, and the alveolar capillaries increase. This growth is exponential during the last 4 weeks of gestation.

7. What are bronchogenic cysts ? How do they form?

Bronchogenic cysts result from anomalous budding of airways. They are lined with bronchial epithelium, including mucus-secreting cells.

8. Describe the location and attachment of bronchogenic cysts.

Most bronchogenic cysts are located in the mediastinum along the trachea and mainstem bronchi or below the carina. They usually are fixed firmly to the airways but do not communicate with them. If the cysts form at the end of the cannalicular period, they may be located more peripherally in the lungs, usually in the lower lobes, and rarely may communicate with the airways.

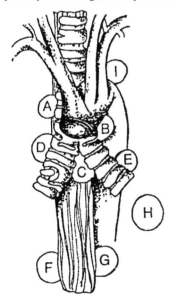

Common locations of bronchogenic cysts: (A) right paratracheal, (B) left paratracheal, (C) subcarinal, (D) above right mainstem bronchus, (E) above left mainstem bronchus, (F) right paraesophageal, (G) left paraesophageal, (H) intraparenchymal, (I) above aortic arch. (From Nobuhara KK, Gorski YC, LaQuaglia MP, Shamberger RC: Bronchogenic cysts and esophageal duplications: Common origins and treatment. J Pediatr Surg 32:1408–1413, 1997, with permission.)

9. True or false: All bronchogenic cysts are located in the chest.

False. Rarely, bronchogenic cysts lose their attachment to the airways and may migrate. They have been reported in the chin, neck, tongue, and abdomen.

10. What are the presenting symptoms of patients with bronchogenic cysts?

Infants may present early in life with respiratory distress due to airway compression and distal pulmonary hyperinflation. Older children and adults may present with chronic cough, wheezing, pneumonia, or hemoptysis. Bronchogenic cysts may be totally asymptomatic and discovered serendipitously on a chest radiograph or at autopsy.

11. What diagnostic tests should be done to delineate bronchogenic cysts?

The diagnosis of a bronchogenic cyst is made most often by abnormal chest radiograph results. Sometimes the presence of a bronchogenic cyst is suggested by noting compression of the esophagus on an upper GI series or compression of the airways during bronchoscopy. Cysts can be further defined by obtaining a computed tomography (CT) scan of the chest with contrast. The wall does not enhance with contrast, but the contrast helps to distinguish the cysts from surrounding mediastinal structures.

12. How are symptomatic bronchogenic cysts treated?

All symptomatic bronchogenic cysts should be removed surgically. Mediastinal lesions can be excised via thoracotomy or sternotomy without resection of lung tissue. Endoscopic resection of tracheal bronchogenic cysts and thoracoscopic removal of small extralobar cysts have been reported. Intrapulmonary cysts are removed with segmental or lobar resection. Occasionally, cysts that are seen on antenatal ultrasound must be drained by a thoracoamniotic shunt to treat fetal distress.

13. What is the treatment of asymptomatic bronchogenic cysts that are found serendipitously?

Controversy surrounds the need for resection of the asymptomatic bronchogenic cyst. There are case reports of malignancies arising in these cysts. However, the true incidence and risk are unknown. An asymptomatic cyst may enlarge and cause airway compression or become infected at a later time.

14. What is a pulmonary sequestration?

A pulmonary sequestration is a mass of nonfunctioning, embryonic lung parenchyma that does not communicate with the tracheobronchial tree and has a systemic arterial blood supply. Pryce first described pulmonary sequestrations in 1946, and there have been many reports since, proving that "the Pryce is right."

15. What types of sequestrations are there?

- **Extrapulmonary sequestrations** have their own separate pleural covering and usually have systemic venous drainage. In 80% of cases the arterial supply comes directly from the aorta.
- **Intrapulmonary sequestrations** do not have their own pleural covering. If intrapulmonary sequestrations are on the left, they drain into the pulmonary veins. If intrapulmonary sequestrations are on the right, they usually drain into the inferior vena cava, creating the "scimitar sign" on chest radiograph. Intrapulmonary sequestrations may have communications with the gastrointestinal tract.

16. How frequently are the different types of sequestrations seen? Where are they located?

Seventy-five percent of sequestrations are intralobar, and the overwhelming majority are found in the lower lobes. Of these, 60–70% are on the left, usually in the left posterior basilar segment. Extrapulmonary sequestrations are found on the left side in 90% of cases, usually between the left lower lobe and the left hemidiaphragm.

17. Are pulmonary sequestrations associated with gender or congenital anomalies?

Intrapulmonary sequestrations usually are not associated with gender or congenital anomalies. Extrapulmonary sequestrations are more common in males (4:1) and may be associated with the following anomalies in up to 50% of cases:

- Right upper lobe bronchial atresia
- Duplication of the colon and/or terminal ileum
- Esophageal communication
- Cervical vertebral anomalies
- Pulmonary vascular lesions, such as pulmonary hypoplasia with absent pulmonary artery
- Congenital diaphragmatic hernia

18. True or false: All pulmonary sequestrations are located in the chest.

False. Very rarely, an extrapulmonary sequestration is found in the retroperitoneum.

19. How do pulmonary sequestrations form?

Pryce proposed that traction by the arterial supply to a segment of fetal lung causes it to separate from the normal lung as it develops. This process may occur either before or after the pleura forms. Other possible mechanisms include:

• An accessory lung bud develops and may or may not be incorporated into lung parenchyma.
• Sequestrations are actually bronchogenic cysts or congenital adenomatous malformations with arterial blood supply.
• Intralobar sequestrations are acquired.

This proves that "Pryce is not the only consideration." The bottom line is that we are not quite sure how sequestrations form.

20. What are the symptoms of pulmonary sequestrations?

Patients with *extrapulmonary* sequestrations are more likely to present in infancy because of the presence of other congenital anomalies. Infants with venous return to the systemic circulation may present with high-output cardiac failure. *Intrapulmonary* sequestration is frequently not diagnosed until childhood or adolescence. Patients may be asymptomatic or have productive cough, chest pain, hemoptysis, or systemic signs of chronic infection such as fever, chills, and weight loss.

21. How are pulmonary sequestrations diagnosed?

Plain chest radiographs may show a solid mass or cystic structure. The diagnosis depends on demonstrating systemic arterial supply. An angiogram demonstrates the aberrant arterial supply and delineates the venous drainage. If a chest CT scan is ordered in a patient in whom sequestration is part of the differential diagnosis, it should be done with contrast in an attempt to delineate the feeding vessels. Magnetic resonance imaging (MRI) is a less invasive way to illustrate blood flow and ultimately may replace angiography.

22. How is pulmonary sequestration treated?

All sequestrations should be removed surgically, including those in asymptomatic patients. Sequestrations may become infected, and fatal hemoptysis has been reported. Because the borders of an intrapulmonary sequestration are not defined by a pleural edge, lobectomy is usually necessary.

23. What are congenital cystic adenomatoid malformations (CCAMs)? How do they form?

CCAMs are cystic masses made up of an overgrowth of terminal bronchioles that resemble fetal lung at 20 weeks gestation (cannnalicular phase). No normal alveoli are present. Because they have conducting airways, they are connected to the tracheobronchial tree. CCAMs probably are caused by a defect in the switch from the cannalicular to the terminal sac periods of development and can be induced in transgenic mice that overexpress keratinocyte growth factor.

24. How are CCAMs classified?

In 1977, Stocker described three types of CCAMs:
• Type I: single or multiple cysts larger than 2 cm in diameter with no adenomatoid areas.
• Type II: a mixture of multiple individual cysts, usually between 0.5 and 1.2 cm in diameter, and adenomatoid areas.
• Type III: entirely adenomatoid, foam-like mass with multiple small (< 0.5 cm) cysts.
(See figure on following page.)

25. How frequently are the different types of CCAMs seen? Where are they located?

Type I lesions account for 70 % of CCAMs. They usually are found on the right side. Type II CCAMs represent 20% of cases and may be found on either side. Less than 10% of CCAMs are type III. Although an entire lung may be affected, usually a single lobe is involved. Lower lobes are involved more frequently than upper lobes.

TYPE I   TYPE II   TYPE III

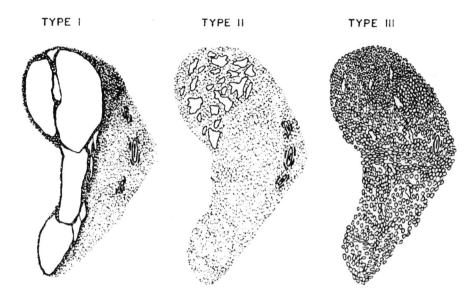

Stocker classification of congenital cystic adenomatoid malformations. Type I, single or multiple large cysts; type II, multiple cysts plus adenomatoid areas; type III, multiple small cysts. (From Stocker JT, Madewell JE, Drake RM: Congenital cystic adenomatoid malformation of the lung. Classification and morphologic spectrum. Hum Pathol 8:155–171, 1977, with permission.)

26. Are CCAMs associated with gender or congenital anomalies?

Type I lesions are not associated with gender or other anomalies. Type II lesions are associated with preterm delivery in 75% of cases, and more than 60–70% of patients have associated anomalies. Type III lesions almost always are seen in males.

27. What is the prognosis for the different types of CCAMs?

Type I lesions usually have a good prognosis. The mortality rate for type II and type III lesions is greater than 50%.

28. True or false: CCAMs are always found in the chest.

Mostly true. There have been case reports of CCAM-sequestration hybrids. The hybrids have been seen with both intrapulmonary and extrapulmonary sequestrations, and at least seven had a retroperitoneal location.

29. How do patients with CCAMs present?

Currently many patients are diagnosed by antenatal ultrasound at some time after 20 weeks gestation. Some patients have associated hydrops or polyhydramnios, which may be fatal if severe. The usual presentation is a newborn with respiratory distress or poor feeding. Initially, the lesions may appear solid until retained fetal lung fluid has cleared. More than 15% of CCAMs are diagnosed in patients over 6 months of age. They usually present with recurrent or persistent infection.

30. What diagnostic tests are used to delineate CCAMs?

When the diagnosis is considered in a neonate, diaphragmatic hernia must be ruled out. The two diagnoses can be difficult to distinguish on plain chest radiograph. A thoracotomy is used for resection of a CCAM, whereas a laparotomy is the usual approach for treatment of diaphragmatic hernia. A chest CT scan or upper GI series should be obtained. The chest CT scan should be ordered with IV contrast to help define blood supply because of the association of CCAMs with pulmonary sequestrations.

31. How are CCAMs treated?

Occasionally, CCAMs have resolved on prenatal ultrasound. In one recent series, however, early postnatal chest CT scans showed residual lesions. CCAMs and CCAM-sequestration hybrids were found at the time of surgery. Whenever CCAMs are seen, the treatment is complete surgical excision. Broncholoalveolar carcinoma, rhabdomyosarcoma, and other malignancies have been reported in children and adults with unresected CCAMs.

Intrauterine thoracoamniotic shunting has been performed on fetuses with cystic masses that have a severe mediastinal shift and are rapidly expanding. Open fetal surgery has been performed, but the type of CCAM may be hard to determine by prenatal ultrasound. Furthermore, because CCAMs may decrease in size during prenatal life, prognostication is difficult. For this reason and because of the risk to the mother as well as the fetus, this option is rarely used.

32. What is congenital lobar emphysema?

Congenital lobar emphysema (CLE) is the overexpansion of a pulmonary lobe. It is also called congenital lobar overinflation. Usually, there is bronchial compression with air-trapping by a ball-valve–like mechanism, which allows air to enter a lobe but not to leave it. Hypoplasia or absence of bronchial cartilage plates is found in up to 79% of cases. Extrinsic compression of a bronchus may be caused by intrathoracic masses such as bronchogenic cysts or teratomas or cardiac or vascular anomalies such as tetralogy of Fallot, patent ductus arteriosus, or vascular rings or slings. Polyalveolar lobes are considered a form of CLE. Such lobes have normal numbers of terminal bronchioles but contain 3–5 times the normal number of alveoli.

33. Which lobes are usually affected?

The left upper lobe is affected most frequently, accounting for about 40% of cases. The second most common sites are the right middle and right upper lobes. About 20% of cases are bilateral. Lower lobes are rarely affected.

34. Is CLE associated with gender or congenital anomalies?

Males are three times more likely to have CLE than females. About 20% of cases are associated with cardiac problems such as ventricular septal defect or patent ductus arteriosus. Another small percentage have rib cage or renal anomalies.

35. How do patients with CLE present?

The overwhelming majority of patients present in the first 6 months of life, and the majority of these present at birth or shortly thereafter. Most present with poor feeding, progressive respiratory distress, and cyanosis. Some patients have a more insidious presentation with tachypnea, dyspnea, wheezing, cough, poor feeding, intermittent cyanosis, or exercise intolerance. Occasionally, CLE is asymptomatic, and the diagnosis is suggested by the chest exam and/or by an abnormal chest radiograph.

36. True or false: Congenital lobar emphysema is always found in the chest.

True.

37. How is CLE diagnosed?

Plain chest radiographs show a hyperlucent, hyperinflated area of the lung, sometimes with shift of the mediastinum or atelectasis of other lobes. If the findings are classic and consistent with the clinical picture, no further work-up is needed. However, in atypical cases or in older patients, additional investigation may be needed. A chest CT scan helps to differentiate the lesion from other lung cysts. A ventilation/perfusion scan demonstrates that both functions are diminished to the affected lobe. Bronchoscopy may demonstrate airway compression, bronchomalacia, or the presence of a foreign body.

38. How is CLE treated?

Newborns presenting with severe respiratory distress require immediate surgical resection. Controversy surrounds the issue of whether patients who have undergone surgical resection have compensatory lung growth, or whether the remaining lobes grow normally but are somewhat hyperinflated. All affected lobes should be removed at the time of surgery, because failure to remove apparently mildly affected areas may result in postoperative hyperinflation of those areas, necessitating a second procedure.

Patients with mild symptoms can be managed medically. Hyperinflation becomes worse during times of intermittent respiratory illnesses but usually resolves with the illness. In such patients, the unresected areas with CLE do not inhibit growth of the remaining lung.

BIBLIOGRAPHY

1. Collin P-P, Desjardins JG, Khan AH: Pulmonary sequestration. J Pediatr Surg 22(8):750–753, 1987.
2. Coran AG, Drongowski R: Congenital cystic disease of the tracheobronchial tree in infants and children. Experience with 44 consecutive cases. Arch Surg 129:521–527, 1994.
3. Eigen H, Lemen RJ, Waring WW: Congenital lobar emphysema: Long-term evaluation of surgically and conservatively treated children. Am Rev Respir Dis 113:823–831, 1976.
4. Holm BA, Kapur P, Irish MS, Glick PL: Physiology and pathophysiology of lung development. J Obstet Gynecol 17(6):519–527, 1997.
5. Hudak BB: Congenital malformations of the lung and airways. In Loughlin GM, Eigen H (eds): Respiratory Disease in Children: Diagnosis and Management. Baltimore, Williams & Wilkins, 1994, pp 501–532.
6. Kravitz RM: Congenital malformations of the lung. Ped Clin North Am Respiratory Medicine II:453–472, 1994.
7. Miller JA, Corteville JE, Langer JC: Congential cystic adenomatoid malformation in the fetus: Natural history and predictors of outcome. J Pediatr Surg 31(6):805–808, 1996.
8. Nobuhara KK, Gorski YC, LaQuaglia MP, Shamberger RC: Bronchogenic cysts and esophageal duplications: Common origins and treatment. J Pediatr Surg 32(10):1408–1413, 1997.
9. Nuchtern JG, Harerg FJ: Congenital lung cysts. Semin Pediatr Surg 3(4):233–243, 1994.
10. Ribet ME, Copin M-C, Gosselin BH: Bronchogenic cysts of the lung. Ann Thorac Surg 61:1636–1640, 1996.
11. Stocker JT, Madewell JE, Drake RM: Congenital cystic adenomatoid malformation of the lung. Classification and morphologic spectrum. Hum Pathol 8(2):155–171, 1977.

14. ACQUIRED LUNG DISEASE

Bradley M. Rodgers, M.D.

EMPYEMA

1. What is empyema?

Empyema is the accumulation of infected fluid within the pleural space. The presence of this fluid may be difficult to differentiate from pulmonary consolidation by plain radiograph (Fig. 1). In such instances the use of transthoracic ultrasound or computerized tomography may help to confirm the presence of pleural fluid.

2. What are the most common causes of empyema in children?

The most common cause of empyema in children is infection of a parapneumonic fluid collection. Other causes include infection of a posttraumatic hemothorax, postoperative infections, and spread from adjacent infections, such as a retropharyngeal or mediastinal abscess.

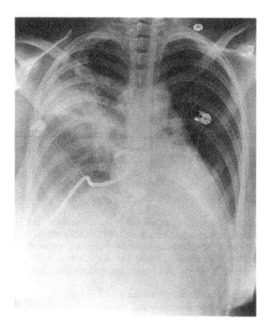

Figure 1.   Frontal chest radiograph of a 17-year-old female with a febrile illness of 7 days duration. A pleural fluid collection has been drained with a pigtail catheter. The radiograph demonstrates patchy infiltrates and atelectasis in the right chest.

3. Describe the typical signs and symptoms of empyema in children.

Children with empyema usually present with respiratory symptoms such as cough and dyspnea. They commonly have significant fever and may complain of dull chest pain. Physical findings include absent breath sounds at the lung bases with dullness to percussion in these regions. Empyema in association with pneumonia may present with rhonchi by auscultation. Laboratory studies usually reveal leukocytosis with a left shift. The diagnosis of empyema is confirmed by thoracentesis. The fluid is usually turbid and contains > 15,000/dl white blood cells. Gram stain may reveal gram-positive or gram-negative organisms.

4. What are the pathologic stages of empyema?

In 1962 the American Thoracic Society described three stages of empyema, which continue to be useful in the classification of the disease. The initial **exudative stage** is characterized by the accumulation of thin pleural fluid with few cellular elements. The Gram stain at this stage is usually negative. Fluid is amenable to drainage by thoracentesis or tube thoracostomy. This stage usually lasts only 24–72 hours and then progresses to the **fibrinopurulent stage**, in which protein and fibrinous material begin to accumulate in the infected pleural fluid with the formation of multiple loculations (Fig. 2). White blood cells are present within the fluid, and the Gram stain is usually positive. The fibrinopurulent stage lasts for 7–10 days and often requires more aggressive treatment to evacuate the fluid. The final stage of empyema is the **organizing stage**. At this point a thick pleural peel forms as a result of fibroblastic proliferation. The lung parenchyma becomes entrapped, forming a fibrothorax. This stage usually occurs within 2–4 weeks after the initial presentation of empyema.

5. What are the most common organisms recovered from empyema fluid?

Bacteria are recovered by culture in only approximately 50% of children with empyema. Many children have been treated with broad-spectrum antibiotics before recovery of fluid, and

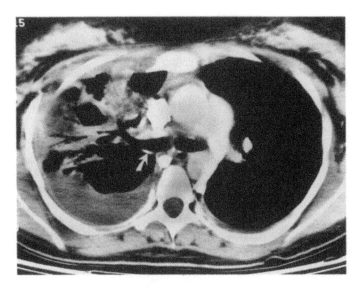

Figure 2. A thoracic CT scan of this patient demonstrates a multi-loculated fluid collection in the right hemithorax in spite of the presence of the pigtail catheter *(arrow)*.

some may be tapped in the exudative stage of the process. Historically, the most commonly cultured organism has been *Streptococcus pneumoniae*, but in recent years, with more routine use of pneumococcal vaccination, *Staphylococcus aureus* has been the most commonly retrieved organism. *Haemophilus influenzae* has been almost completely eliminated as a cause of empyema with widespread immunization. Postoperative and posttraumatic empyemas may contain *Bacteroides* species or *Pseudomonas aeruginosa*.

6. Describe the treatment options for children with empyema.

Successful treatment for empyema requires evacuation of the fluid from the pleural space (Fig. 3). In addition, all patients require antibiotic therapy, tailored to the specific organism cultured or suspected from the clinical course. Evacuation of the hemithorax in the exudative stage may be accomplished by either thoracentesis or tube thoracostomy. Once the empyema has progressed to the fibrinopurulent stage, with intrapleural loculations of infected fluid, either an open pleural debridement or thoracoscopic debridement is required. Recently, thoracoscopic debridement has been shown to be at least as effective as open debridement and results in a shorter hospitalization. Patients presenting in the organizing stage of empyema may require an open pleurectomy to evacuate the fluid and allow the lung to expand to fill the hemithorax. With prompt and effective therapy, such children should do well and should be expected to have clinically normal pulmonary function.

PNEUMOTHORAX

7. What are the causes of pneumothorax in children?

Pneumothoraces can be spontaneous, usually as a result of rupture of a subpleural bleb, or associated with blunt or penetrating trauma. They also may result from disruption of the visceral pleura secondary to increased alveolar pressure, as in patients with asthma, paroxysms of coughing, or mechanical ventilation, or from medical procedures such as central venous catheter insertion or bronchoscopy.

8. What are the presenting signs and symptoms of pneumothorax?

Children with pneumothorax present with the sudden onset of dyspnea and lateralizing chest pain. Physical examination reveals diminished breath sounds on the ipsilateral side. The position of

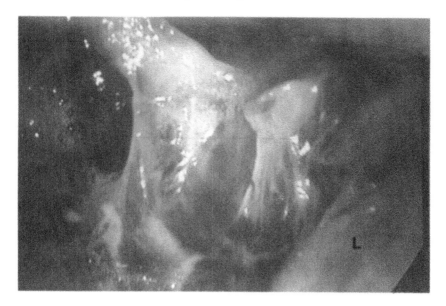

Figure 3. Thoracoscopic view of the pleural space of the patient illustrated in the first figure. Considerable fluid and fibrinous debris is present in the pleural space, with multiple large and small locules. The lung (L) is unable to fully expand until this fluid and material is evacuated.

the trachea should be noted in the suprasternal notch. It usually is in the midline but may be shifted to the contralateral side. Typically, spontaneous pneumothorax occurs in tall, slender adolescent boys.

9. Describe the findings of tension pneumothorax.

Children with a tension pneumothorax may present with severe respiratory compromise. In general, the mediastinum is considerably more mobile in children than in adults, and massive shifts may occur with tension pneumothorax, interfering with contralateral pulmonary ventilation and cardiac function.

The physical examination in children with tension pneumothorax reveals significant respiratory distress, perhaps with cyanosis, and tachycardia. Palpation of the trachea in the suprasternal notch reveals a marked contralateral shift.

The frontal chest radiograph in patients with tension pneumothorax demonstrates shift of the mediastinal structures to the contralateral hemithorax (Fig. 4). The ipsilateral hemithorax is filled with air and lacks lung markings. The ipsilateral diaphragm is depressed, and the intercostal spaces on the ipsilateral side are expanded compared with the opposite side. The collapsed ipsilateral lung may be difficult to identify because it is compressed into the mediastinum.

10. What is the appropriate therapy for a pneumothorax?

Patients presenting with signs and symptoms of a tension pneumothorax require emergent evacuation of the air. A large-bore needle may be placed in the second intercostal space in the midclavicular line to evacuate air rapidly while equipment for insertion of a chest tube is assembled. All symptomatic patients or patients with larger pneumothoraces should be treated with tube thoracostomy. A small chest tube (12–14 French) should be placed in the midaxillary line through the auscultatory triangle. It is not necessary to place a chest tube anteriorly to evacuate a pneumothorax; the anterior tube usually leaves a less cosmetically appealing incision. Asymptomatic patients with small (< 15%) pneumothoraces may be treated with careful observation. Reabsorption of air from the pleural space may be hastened by breathing 100% oxygen to facilitate displacement of nitrogen from the chest.

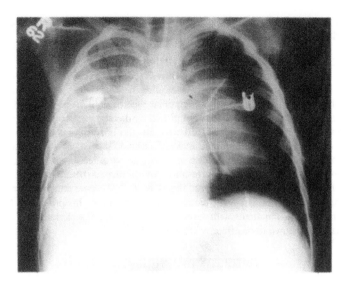

Figure 4. Frontal chest radiograph of a 16-year-old male with metastatic Ewing's sarcoma on intensive chemotherapy. An interstitial pneumonitis developed for which he received intravenous antibiotics. He developed acute worsening of his respiratory condition. The radiograph demonstrates a tension pneumothorax and collapsed lung on the left. The left hemidiaphragm is depressed and the mediastinum is shifted to the right. The entire left hemithorax is larger than the right. The tension pneumothorax was treated with immediate tube thoracostomy.

Patients who have had a single episode of spontaneous pneumothorax have at least a 50% chance of experiencing recurrence in the same hemithorax. Patients who have experienced a second ipsilateral pneumothorax should undergo some form of pleurodesis, either by open pleural abrasion or partial pleurectomy or by thoracoscopic abrasion or talc poudrage. Likewise, patients who have experienced bilateral pneumothoraces should undergo bilateral pleurodesis. Because the development of pneumothorax is associated with a significant mortality rate in patients with cystic fibrosis, most surgeons believe that such children should undergo an ipsilateral pleurodesis with the first episode. This is a difficult decision since most of these patients will become candidates for pulmonary transplantation and a previous pleurodesis complicates that procedure.

CHYLOTHORAX

11. What are the different causes of chylothorax in children?

Chylothorax, the accumulation of lymphatic fluid in the pleural space, may be of various etiologies. Congenital or idiopathic chylothorax is noted in the first few weeks of life and is thought to be secondary to an injury to the thoracic duct or one of its major tributaries during birth. In older children, chylothorax is seen most commonly after cardiac surgery or surgery that involves mediastinal dissection. Posttraumatic chylothorax is uncommon in children, although it may be seen after penetrating thoracic trauma. Chylothorax may result from obstruction of the thoracic duct by mediastinal tumors or by pleural involvement with extensive lymphangiomatosis. In children, thrombosis of the superior vena cava by hyperalimentation catheters may cause chylothorax.

12. How is the diagnosis of chylothorax confirmed?

The diagnosis of chylothorax is confirmed by analysis of fluid obtained by thoracentesis. In a patient who has been eating a normal diet, the fluid appears milky. In patients who must avoid oral ingestion (e.g., after cardiac surgery), the fluid appears serous in color. The specific gravity is greater than 1.012, and a triglyceride level of > 200 mg/dl is usually present. The cell count is > 5000/dl; > 90% of cells are lymphocytes.

13. Describe the treatment of a child with chylothorax.

Treatment of chylothorax begins initially with evacuation of the fluid from the hemithorax, either by thoracentesis or tube thoracostomy. Measures then are undertaken to reduce lymphatic flow through the chest. Elimination of long-chain fatty acids, which are absorbed into the lymphatic system as chylomicrons, may be accomplished by dietary supplementation with medium-chain triglycerides, which are absorbed directly into the portal vein, or by the use of total parenteral nutrition, eliminating all oral fat intake. Continued loss of chyle from the chest results in significant protein depletion and depletion of T lymphocytes, leading to malnutrition and immunologic compromise. If dietary measures have not eliminated the chylothorax within 10–14 days, surgical methods should be considered. Ligation of the thoracic duct by open thoracotomy traditionally has been the mainstay of treatment. In recent years, this procedure has been performed by thoracoscopy. In patients with a more diffuse origin of the chylothorax, a pleural peritoneal shunt has been shown to be effective therapy.

INTERSTITIAL PNEUMONITIS

14. What are the known causes of interstitial pneumonitis in children?

Interstitial pneumonitis is a diffuse interstitial pulmonary process characterized by abnormal gas exchange and restrictive lung disease. It is seen principally in immunocompromised patients. Significant increases in the numbers of children undergoing organ or bone marrow transplantation or receiving chemotherapy for various neoplasms have greatly expanded the population of immunocompromised pediatric hosts. The reservoir of HIV infections in children is also expanding; such patients are susceptible to interstitial pneumonitis.

15. Describe the microbiology of common interstitial pneumonitis infections.

Interstitial pneumonitis in transplant patients is caused most commonly by cytomegalovirus (CMV) infections. CMV-negative recipients who receive tissue from CMV-positive donors are particularly susceptible. Other viruses, such as adenovirus and parainfluenza virus also have been implicated. Other agents responsible for interstitial pneumonitis in this patient population include mycobacteria, protozoan organisms, fungus, and various bacterial organisms. *Pneumocystis carinii* pneumonia, traditionally a common cause of interstitial pneumonitis in immunocompromised patients, is seen less frequently now because of the widespread use of prophylaxis with trimethoprim-sulfamethoxazole (Fig. 5).

16. Describe the diagnostic techniques for interstitial pneumonitis.

Most cases of interstitial pneumonitis require tissue biopsy to establish a diagnosis. Monoclonal antibody stains occasionally allow diagnosis of CMV infections from bronchoalveolar lavage specimens, and occasionally *Pneumocystis carinii* organisms also can be identified in lavage fluid. Transbronchial biopsy performed at the time of bronchoalveolar lavage occasionally provides adequate pulmonary tissue for diagnosis. Often, however, lung biopsy is required by open thoracotomy or thoracoscopic techniques.

BRONCHIECTASIS

17. What is bronchiectasis?

Bronchiectasis is loss of the structural integrity of the conducting airways caused by chronic and recurring pulmonary infections. Destructive loss of the cartilage, elastin, and smooth muscle of these airways leads to dilatation and stasis of secretions. Epithelial metaplasia destroys the ciliated epithelium, replaces it with squamous epithelium, and contributes to inadequate mucus clearance.

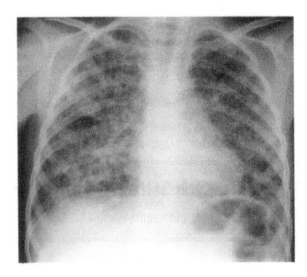

Figure 5.   Frontal chest radiograph of an 8-year-old child one year following a renal transplant. Symptoms of fever and dyspnea developed. Lung biopsy in this patient revealed *Pneumocystitis carinii* infection.

18. What are the common causes of bronchiectasis in children?

Probably the most common cause of bronchiectasis in children is cystic fibrosis. Other causes include bronchial obstruction by retained foreign bodies or endobronchial tumors, congenital disorders (e.g., alpha$_1$ antitrypsin deficiency, Kartagener syndrome), immunodeficiency states (e.g., HIV infection or treatment for transplantation), and chronic aspiration associated with gastroesophageal reflux.

19. What is the treatment for bronchiectasis?

Treatment for early bronchiectasis includes aggressive antibiotic therapy and postural drainage. With recurring infections unresponsive to this therapy, limited surgical resection using segmental pulmonary resection techniques may be quite useful. The major principle of the surgical approach to bronchiectasis is conservation of as much uninvolved lung as possible because many affected children have more diffuse chronic underlying pulmonary disease.

BIBLIOGRAPHY

EMPYEMA
1. Bryant RE, Salmon CJ: Pleural empyema. Clin Infect Dis 22:747–764, 1996.
2. Campbell PW: New developments in pediatric pneumonia and empyema. Curr Opin Pediatr 7:278–282, 1995.
3. Kern JA, Rodgers BM: Thoracoscopy in the management of empyema in children. J Pediatr Surg 28:1128–1132, 1993.
PNEUMOTHORAX
4. Cannon WB, Vierra MA, Cannon A: Thoracoscopy for spontaneous pneumothorax. Ann Thorac Surg 56:686–687, 1993.
5. Davis AM, Wensley DF, Phelan PD: Spontaneous pneumothorax in pediatric patients. Respir Med 87:531–534, 1993.
6. Spector ML, Stern RC: Pneumothorax in cystic fibrosis: A 26-year experience. Ann Thorac Surg 47:204–207, 1989.
CHYLOTHORAX
7. Graham DD, McGahren ED, Tribble CG, et al: Use of video-assisted thoracic surgery in the treatment of chylothorax. Ann Thorac Surg 57:1507–1512, 1994.
8. Valentine VG, Raffin TA: The management of chylothorax. Chest 102:586–591, 1992.

INTERSTITIAL PNEUMONITIS
9. Fan LL, Kozinetz CA, Deterding RR, Brugman SM: Evaluation of a diagnostic approach to pediatric in-
    terstitial lung disease. Pediatrics 101:82–85, 1998.
10. Helman BC: Diagnosis and treatment of interstitial lung disease. Pediatr Pulmonol 23:1–7, 1997.
11. Howenstine MS, Eigen H: Current concepts on interstitial lung disease in children. Curr Opin Pediatr
    11:200–204, 1999.
BRONCHIECTASIS
12. Herman M, Michalkova K, Kopriva F: High resolution CT in the assessment of bronchiectasis in chil-
    dren. Pediatr Radiol 23:376–379, 1993.
13. Lewiston NJ: Bronchiectasis in childhood. Pediatr Clin North Am 31:865–878, 1984.

15. TRACHEOBRONCHIAL FOREIGN BODIES

Rebeccah L. Brown, M.D., and Michael G. Caty, M.D.

1. What age groups usually present with tracheobronchial foreign bodies?
Approximately 80% of children who aspirate foreign bodies are less than 3 years of age.

2. Is there a gender predilection for foreign body aspiration in children?
Yes. Boys outnumber girls by 3:1.

3. What is the most common foreign body identified in the tracheobronchial tree in children?
Nuts, predominantly peanuts, account for about one-half of all foreign body aspirations, followed by vegetable fragments, seeds, popcorn, and a wide array of small plastic and metal objects.

4. What is the most important element in the clinical history?
The history of a choking episode, which may or may not be elicited. About 15% of foreign body aspirations are unwitnessed.

5. What are the symptoms of a foreign body in the airway?
Spasms of coughing, gagging, choking, and wheezing. Stridor may occur with an upper airway foreign body. If the obstruction is complete, the child may become acutely dyspneic and unable to talk, cough, or breathe, then progress rapidly to cyanosis.

6. True or false: If the patient ceases coughing on arrival at the emergency department, the physician can safely assume that the foreign body has probably been coughed out or swallowed.
False. Often the patient ceases coughing because of physiologic adaptation of the sensory receptors of the tracheobronchial tree, giving the false impression to parents and physicians that the foreign body has been cleared from the airway.

7. Where do most foreign bodies become lodged in the tracheobronchial tree?
Classically in the right mainstem bronchus, although a few studies have found the left mainstem bronchus to be slightly more common.

8. What should a parent do if a child experiences a choking episode thought to be due to an aspirated foreign body?
Allow the child to cough it out if possible. If the child is unable to talk, cough, or breathe, perform chest thrusts followed by back blows in children younger than 1 year and abdominal thrusts followed by back blows in children older than 1 year. Seek help.

9. What are the classic physical findings of foreign body aspiration?

Coughing, wheezing, and decreased or absent breath sounds on the affected side. About 75% of patients have at least one component of this classic triad of physical findings.

10. What are the radiographic findings of a tracheobronchial foreign body?

Both inspiratory and expiratory films should be obtained. About 10% of foreign bodies are radiopaque. Otherwise the diagnosis is suspected with hyperinflation of the affected side and mediastinal or tracheal shift away from the side of obstruction. In about 25% of patients, total occlusion of the bronchus results in atelectasis rather than air-trapping. If the foreign body has been present for a prolonged time, pneumonia may be present. Occasionally, the chest radiograph is normal, but this does not exclude the diagnosis in a patient with the appropriate clinical history and symptoms of airway obstruction.

11. What is the treatment for a tracheobronchial foreign body?

Once the diagnosis is suspected, treatment is immediate bronchoscopy with removal of the foreign body. If the foreign body has been present for more than 24 hours, antibiotics usually are administered.

12. Should rigid or flexible bronchoscopy be performed?

Generally, rigid bronchoscopy is performed because of the increased ability to manipulate instruments through the scope and the ability to ventilate through the scope while the procedure is performed. Flexible bronchoscopy may be useful in identifying foreign bodies in the more distal segmental bronchi beyond the reach of the rigid bronchoscope.

13. What is the role of postural drainage in the treatment of tracheobronchial foreign bodies?

Although this therapy may be successful in some cases, generally it is not recommended as a first-line treatment. The longer a foreign body remains in the airway, the more difficult it is to retrieve (especially organic matter) and the higher the risk of pneumonia.

14. What instruments and techniques are available for removal of foreign bodies from the airway?

Grasping forceps (alligator, peanut, or foreign body), Fogarty balloon catheters, and Dormia baskets. If the identity of the foreign body is known, it is useful to practice grasping a similar object ex vivo to ensure that the instrumentation is appropriate for retrieval of the object.

15. What should one do if the foreign body cannot be retrieved endoscopically?

Rarely, thoracotomy, bronchotomy, or lobectomy may be required to extract an aspirated foreign body.

16. How should patients be managed postoperatively?

The patient should be placed on humidified oxygen and observed in a monitored environment. Patients may require racemic epinephrine, bronchodilators, or steroids in the immediate postoperative period because of edema and increased reactivity of the airways. Aggressive pulmonary toilet, including incentive spirometry, chest physiotherapy, and postural drainage, should be provided. A chest radiograph should be obtained postoperatively. Antibiotics may be indicated with long-standing foreign bodies and associated purulent secretions in the airway or pneumonic infiltrate on chest radiograph.

17. What are the indications for repeat bronchoscopy?

Persistent symptoms or radiographic abnormalities on chest radiograph.

BIBLIOGRAPHY

1. Azizkhan RG, Caty MG: Subglottic airway. In Oldham KT, Colombani PM, Foglia RP (eds): Surgery of Infants and Children: Scientific Principles and Practice. Philadelphia, Lippincott-Raven, 1997, pp 901–903.
2. Baharloo F, Veychkemans F, Biettlot MP, et al: Tracheobronchial foreign bodies: Presentation and management in children and adults. Chest 115:1357–1362, 1999.

3. Black RE, Johnson DG, Matlak ME: Bronchoscopic removal of aspirated foreign bodies in children. J Pediatr Surg 29:682–684, 1994.
4. Oguzkaya F, Akcali Y, Kahraman C, et al: Tracheobronchial foreign body aspirations in childhood: A 10-year experience. Eur J Cardiothorac Surg 14:388–392, 1998.

16. LARYNX, TRACHEA, AND MEDIASTINUM

Robert M. Filler, M.D.

1. Why is the neonate primarily a nasal breather?
The pharynx of an infant is short and positioned high, whereas the epiglottis is at the level of the soft palate. This approximation limits air flow through the oral cavity.

2. Why does it matter?
Anything that obstructs the nasal passage or nasopharynx, such as choanal atresia or tubes in the nostrils, adversely affects respiration.

3. What is laryngomalacia?
Laryngomalacia, in which the larynx flops over the glottis, is the most common cause of stridor in infants. It probably results from immaturity of the cartilage, and can be diagnosed by flexible laryngoscopy.

4. Does laryngomalacia require treatment?
The noisy breathing associated with laryngomalacia can be frightening to parents, but cyanosis is rare. Breathing can be improved by placing the child in the prone position. Surgery is rarely required, and it is a self-limiting condition that disappears by 18 months of age.

5. What is epiglottitis?
Epiglottitis is a bacterial infection of the supraglottic structures. In over 90% of cases *Haemophilus influenzae* is the offending organism. The symptoms are rapid onset of severe stridor and airway obstruction, difficulty in swallowing, drooling, and signs of systemic toxicity.

6. What age groups are affected by epiglottitis?
Usually children between 3 and 6 years.

7. Is epiglottitis serious? How is it treated?
Yes, epiglottitis is a serious condition. Treatment, which consists of tracheal intubation to maintain an airway and antibiotic therapy with a third-generation cephalosporin, is needed to prevent mortality and morbidity. If intubation is unsuccessful, tracheostomy is needed.

8. What is acute viral croup (laryngotracheobronchitis)?
Acute viral croup is an infection, usually due to a parainfluenza virus, that affects the tissues below the larynx. Stridor is qualitatively similar to that in epiglottitis, but the course of the illness is not as rapid, airway obstruction is much less severe, and fever and systemic signs are usually less. Viral croup usually affects children under 3 years of age.

9. How is acute viral croup treated?
The vast majority of children have mild airway obstruction and can be managed at home with humidifiers. In more severe cases with cyanosis, however, hospitalization, supplemental oxygen therapy, and racemic epinephrine are needed.

10. When is a tracheostomy needed?

Tracheostomy is used in children only when oral or nasal endotracheal intubation cannot be accomplished. The morbidity and mortality rates of tracheostomy in small children are significant; if it can be avoided by intubation, it should be.

11. What is a laryngeal or laryngotracheal cleft?

If the separation of the embryonic foregut is incomplete, a fissure or cleft may remain between the pharynx and larynx. In more severe cases, the fissure extends caudally to the carina and involves the esophagus and trachea.

12. What symptoms do clefts cause?

Food or saliva gets into the airway, resulting in aspiration pneumonia. The cleft has to be repaired soon after diagnosis to prevent recurrent pulmonary complications. Clefts at the laryngeal level can be repaired through the neck, whereas repair of clefts that extend to the carina may require multiple-staged complicated procedures.

13. What is tracheomalacia?

Tracheomalacia is a condition in which the tracheal wall is especially soft and pliable. It may be due to a developmental defect or follow an injury. In two-thirds of cases tracheomalacia is part of the developmental anomaly that also results in esophageal atresia and tracheoesophageal fistula.

14. Why does tracheomalacia cause respiratory problems?

The diameters of the intrathoracic trachea and bronchi decrease in the expiratory phase of normal respiration, forced expiration, and coughing. In patients with tracheomalacia the abnormally pliable trachea may close completely in such situations. Stridor is expiratory rather than inspiratory (as seen in most fixed airway obstructions).

15. What is the significance of tracheomalacia?

Mild cases involve only a barking cough. In severe cases, however, the cough is ineffective, and retained pulmonary secretions may lead to recurrent pneumonia. The most frightening and life-threatening symptoms are anoxic "dying spells," which are most common in children under 1 year of age. They usually occur during or within 1 or 2 minutes after feeding and may require cardiopulmonary resuscitation. Although reflex apnea has been blamed for such spells, the best data indicate that they are secondary to airway obstruction, which occurs when a full and dilated esophagus compresses the malacic trachea against the aorta.

16. How can one be sure that the dying spells are due to tracheomalacia?

Dying spells may be secondary to neurologic, cardiac, or other causes such as gastroesophageal reflux. In tracheomalacia the narrowing of the tracheal diameter during breathing and swallowing can be appreciated by observing the tracheal air shadow radiographically during breathing and swallowing of radiocontrast material. However, the definitive test is rigid bronchoscopy. The child is anesthetized, but not paralyzed, so that a cough can be stimulated by the scope while the examiner observes the tracheal lumen. In severe tracheomalacia, the anterior and posterior walls of the trachea come together, and the lumen disappears.

17. How is tracheomalacia treated?

The aorta anterior to the trachea can be sutured to the under surface of the sternum (aortopexy). Because of the normal aortic and tracheal adventitial attachments, this maneuver creates more room in the mediastinum and pulls the trachea away from the esophagus so that it cannot be compressed during swallowing. The problem also can be solved by a more recent, relatively noninvasive alternative treatment in which a balloon-inflatable metallic stent is inserted into the trachea to make it more rigid.

18. What about long-term outcomes?

Untreated tracheomalacia tends to improve with growth of the trachea. In mild and moderate cases, symptoms such as noisy respiration usually cease by 1 year of age. Aortopexy is curative without complications or long-term sequelae in more than 95% of patients with severe symptoms. Stenting is equally beneficial because it is less invasive, and the stents can be removed at a later time.

19. At what age does congenital tracheal stenosis become evident?

In patients with the most significant narrowing, symptoms of airway obstruction become evident at about 2–3 months of age. In patients with less severe narrowing, symptoms may not trigger diagnostic studies for 1–5 years.

20. What are the symptoms of tracheal stenosis?

Severe inspiratory stridor is most prominent. The infant with marked obstruction is also tachypneic with labored respirations and cyanosis. Signs of pneumonia also may be present.

21. What is the differential diagnosis of such symptoms?

Congenital tracheal stenosis, vascular ring (double aortic arch), subglottic hemangioma, and, more rarely, unusual tracheal and paratracheal tracheal tumors, cysts, and infections.

22. How is the diagnosis of tracheal stenosis confirmed?

Tracheobronchography with radiocontrast liquid injection into the trachea can be hazardous and further compromise an obstructed airway. Computed tomography (CT) scan with or without three-dimensional reconstruction is a reliable, safe way to obtain definitive information. Magnetic resonance imaging (MRI) is technically difficult to obtain in a critically ill infant. Bronchoscopy can be useful, but when the tracheal lumen is very small, the scope will not pass and it is difficult to evaluate the entire length of narrowing.

23. What is the cause of congenital tracheal stenosis?

In most cases the membranous trachea is totally or almost totally absent, and the trachea is a complete cartilaginous ring. It once was thought that such a ring could not grow in size, but now we have evidence that it can grow, at least to some degree.

24. What are the variations of congenital stenosis?

The length of the narrowed segment is quite variable. It may be quite localized, involving only a few tracheal rings, or it may involve the entire trachea and extend into one or both bronchi. Anomalies in bronchial branching and lung development are often associated with congenital tracheal stenosis.

25. What is the most commonly associated anomaly?

In 50% of cases tracheal stenosis is associated with a pulmonary artery sling, in which the left pulmonary artery arises from the right pulmonary artery and passes between the trachea and esophagus on its way to the left lung. The sling itself usually is not obstructive, but it must be dealt with during repair of the trachea.

26. How is tracheal stenosis treated?

When the narrowing involves less than 50% of the length of the trachea, sleeve resection and end-to-end anastomosis are preferred. For longer lesions tracheoplasty is used. With the aid of cardiopulmonary bypass the narrowed segment is opened longitudinally, and a graft of cartilage or pericardium is sutured to the opening to enlarge the tracheal lumen.

27. How successful is surgery for tracheal stenosis?

Expect excellent results from sleeve resection. Morbidity and mortality from tracheoplasty are significant, depending on the length of tracheal involvement and the degree of inflammation and scarring during the healing process. Insertion of balloon-expandable airway stents may help to deal with such complications, and success can be expected in more than 75% of cases. In some children, however, tracheal stenosis with bronchial involvement is so extensive that surgical correction is not possible.

BIBLIOGRAPHY

1. Backer CL, Mavroudis C, Dunham ME, et al: Repair of congenital tracheal stenosis with a free tracheal autograft. J Thorac Cardiovasc Surg 115:869–874, 1998.
2. Filler RM, Forte V: Lesions of the larynx and trachea. In O'Neill JA, Rowe MI, Grosfeld JL, et al (eds): Pediatric Surgery, 5th ed. St. Louis, Mosby, 1998, pp 863–872.
3. Filler RM, Forte V, Chait P: Tracheobronchial stenting for the treatment of airway obstruction. J Pediatr Surg 33:304–311, 1998.
4. Filler RM, Messineo A, Vinograd J: Severe tracheomalacia associated with esophageal atresia: Results of surgical treatment. J Pediatr Surg 27:1136, 1992.
5. Grillo HC: Slide tracheoplasty for long-segment congenital tracheal stenosis. Ann Thorac Surg 58:613–621, 1994.

17. MEDIASTINAL MASSES

Nicholas C. Saenz, M.D.

1. What is the mediastinum? How is it divided?

There is some debate about the existence of, and therefore the nomenclature for, such an anatomic "compartment." A four-compartment model of the mediastinum separates the superior mediastinum, anteriorly and posteriorly, from the other three compartments. For the purpose of this chapter, the posterior mediastinum refers to Shields' three-compartment model, which consists of an anterior compartment, visceral compartment, and paravertebral sulcus (posterior mediastinum). The posterior mediastinum is the pleural-lined compartment lying posterior to the heart and pericardium, anterior to the vertebral column (but containing the sulci on each side), and between the parietal pleura of the two lungs. The anatomic structures located within the posterior compartment are the thoracic portion of the descending aorta, azygos and hemiazygos veins, esophagus, vagus and splanchnic nerves, thoracic duct, and lymph nodes. Incision of the pleura at the sulcus demonstrates the intercostal lymphatics, nerves, and vessels. The length of the compartment stretches from the apex of the chest cavity to the costodiaphragmatic recess.

2. How do mediastinal masses present?

In infants and children, signs and symptoms related to mediastinal masses are a function of location and/or diagnosis. Masses localized to the anterior mediastinum may present with respiratory distress because the trachea is compressed and deviated. Masses of the middle mediastinum may present in the same fashion. Respiratory distress may be life-threatening. Masses of the posterior mediastinum may present with respiratory distress, neuropathy, or pain. A significant proportion of such masses present incidentally. In addition to mass effect on local structures, the etiology of the tumor may dictate systemic symptoms (i.e., the systemic symptoms of lymphoma). Fetal ultrasound may demonstrate mediastinal masses with significant deviation of the mediastinum into the contralateral hemithorax. Such lesions usually represent simple cysts.

3. Describe the radiographic evaluation of a mass of the mediastinum.

Most lesions are discovered on plain chest radiograph. A lateral view helps to determine in which compartment of the mediastinum the mass is located. Once this is discovered, some form of cross-sectional imaging is necessary. Computed tomography is usually an adequate initial study and is easier to obtain promptly in most institutions. Magnetic resonance imaging is superior at demonstrating foramen encroachment by neurogenic lesions of the posterior mediastinum.

4. What techniques may be used to biopsy mediastinal masses?

Location of the tumor dictates biopsy techniques. Because lymphoma is the most common diagnosis of an anterior mediastinal mass, every effort should be made to make the diagnosis before administration of a general anesthetic. Techniques include bone marrow sampling and superficial node biopsy, when possible. Masses of the anterior mediastinum may be approached percutaneously; in the case of lymphomas, however, cellular markers and immunohistochemistry studies may require a greater bulk of tissue. In this case, a Chamberlain procedure (anterior third interspace) may be useful. If lesions are more superiorly located, an approach posterior to the sternum using mediastinoscopy is another option. Thoracoscopic biopsy may be useful in the evaluation of masses of the middle and posterior mediastinum. Because lesions of the posterior mediastinum usually are resected surgically, formal open thoracotomy may be performed initially if after imaging the lesion appears resectable, as in the case of the neurogenic tumors.

5. What are the most common tumors found in the anterior mediastinum?

Think of the four T's: terrible lymphoma, teratroma, thymoma, and thyroid goiter. Lymphatic malformations (cystic hygromas) must be included in lesions of both the anterior and middle mediastinum.

7. What are the most important considerations of masses of the anterior mediastinum?

To determine whether the lesion is malignant and to ensure that the determination is made safely. Usually such masses are managed in a multidisciplinary fashion.

8. Should all lesions of the anterior mediastinum be initially resected?

No. For example, lymphoma is not treated by resection; it is a systemic disease treated with systemic therapy. Biopsy with careful pathologic evaluation is vital.

BIBLIOGRAPHY

1. Kawashima A, Fishman EK, Kuhlman JE: CT and MR evaluation of posterior mediastinal masses. Crit Rev Diag Imag 33:311–367, 1992.
2. Saenz NC, Schnitzer JJ, Eraklis AE, et al: Posterior mediastinal masses. J Pediatr Surg 28:172–176, 1993.
3. Shields T: Anatomy: Mediastinal Surgery. Philadelphia, Lea & Febiger, 1991.

IV. Cardiovascular

18. CONGENITAL CARDIAC ANOMALIES

Eliot R. Rosenkranz, M.D.

1. You are called to the nursery to evaluate a newborn boy who the pediatrician thinks has a congenital heart defect. How do you proceed?

As in any patient evaluation, review the history, physical exam, and lab work. Write down your findings as you work.

2. What aspects of the history are important?

Although newborns do not have an extensive history, it is important to know what made the pediatrician suspect a heart defect. Was the child breathing hard (tachypneic), "blue" (cyanotic), hypotensive, or in shock? Is he full-term or premature? Are there any other congenital defects (e.g., skeletal, renal, gastrointestinal)? Did the mother have an in-utero ultrasound that was suspicious? Is there any family history of congenital defects?

3. What should you look for during the physical exam?

Is the child dysmorphic or cyanotic? Is he on the ventilator? If the child is breathing on his own, are respiratory rate and effort normal or increased? Focusing on the cardiovascular exam, can you feel pulses in the lower extremities? How do they compare with the right arm (equal or diminished)? Check and compare the blood pressure in the right arm and either leg (equal or decreased in the legs). Listen for murmurs. Note where on the chest or back you hear them, their grade (1–6/6), and when you hear them in the cardiac cycle (systole or diastole). Palpate the liver, and note its size (normal or enlarged) and on which side of the body it is located (right or left). Can you palpate the spleen?

4. What lab tests are important? How are they interpreted?

Look at the pulse oximeter reading or a blood gas analysis to help confirm your assessment of cyanosis. A saturation less than about 88% is consistent with cyanosis. Because the hematocrit in most newborns is elevated, this finding is not too helpful. In older children, a high hematocrit is consistent with cyanotic heart defects. Check the chest radiograph, and look at heart size (normal or enlarged) and position (normal or dextrocardia with the apex pointing toward the right). How do the pulmonary markings look (normal, decreased, or increased)? Look at the liver and stomach bubble below the diaphragm, and determine on which side they are located (normal or situs inversus with the liver on the left and the stomach on the right). At this point, the echocardiogram probably will tell you what the defect is.

5. Echocardiograms are hard to read. What should you look for?

It is best to review the echocardiogram with a pediatric cardiologist. Write down every abnormal finding. The basic anatomic elements to look for include:
- Number of heart chambers (one or two atria and one or two ventricles)
- Location of vena cavae connection to the atria
- Location of pulmonary vein connections to the heart
- Atrium to ventricle connections: correct—right atrium to right ventricle and left atrium to left ventricle; incorrect—right atrium to left ventricle and left atrium to right ventricle. Correct connections are described as concordant, reversed connections as discordant.

- Great artery to ventricle connections: correct—right ventricle to pulmonary artery and left ventricle to aorta; incorrect—right ventricle to aorta and left ventricle to pulmonary artery. Again, correct connections are described as concordant, reversed connections as discordant.
- Holes in the atrial or ventricular septum

Then look at the Doppler, both with the color map and the flow patterns, to determine direction and velocity of blood flow:

- Is the flow in the atria, ventricles, across the valves, or in the great arteries turbulent on the color map? Turbulence should make you think about a hole in the atrial or ventricular septum or obstruction to flow across a heart valve or in an artery.
- If the flow is disturbed, look at the velocity of flow with the Doppler in the turbulent area. By knowing the velocity of the blood flow, you can estimate the difference in blood pressure between the heart chambers or arteries using the following formula:

$$\text{Difference in pressure} = \text{velocity}^2 \times 4$$

6. The infant began to breathe hard when he was fed and could not finish his bottle. He looks normal; he is full-term and pink. He has a systolic heart murmur. What defects should you consider?

Acyanotic or "pink" heart defects can be categorized as:

- Coarctation, patent ductus arteriosus (PDA), vascular rings
- Simple septal defects
- Complex septal defects
- Left-sided valve problems

7. What physiologic changes are caused by these defects?

They cause an increase in the work imposed on the heart due to either (1) a left-to-right intracardiac shunt that causes an increase in volume work on the heart and an increase in the volume of pulmonary blood flow or (2) an obstruction of the flow of blood across a heart valve on the left side of the heart (mitral valve or aortic valve) or in the aorta itself (coarctation of the aorta) that increases the pressure work on the heart. The first physiologic aberration results in pulmonary congestion due to excessive pulmonary blood flow; the second results in pulmonary congestion due to increased pulmonary venous blood pressure.

8. What is a vascular ring?

A vascular ring refers to malformations of the aortic arch or its branches that lead to complete encircling of the esophagus and trachea by blood vessels. The ductus arteriosus completes the ring in most defects.

9. What are the symptoms?

Patients generally present in infancy with symptoms of esophageal obstruction (choking spells) or tracheal stenosis (noisy breathing).

10. Do all vascular rings need surgery?

Patients with symptoms require surgery. Division of the ring usually involves division of the ductus arteriosus. In some rings, such as double aortic arch, the aorta or a branch of the aorta also requires division.

11. How do patients with coarctation present?

It depends on the patient's age. In a newborn, coarctation usually presents with symptoms of heart failure (tachypnea, problems with feeding, acidosis) and even shock when the ductus arteriosus acutely closes. Such patients may or may not have a murmur. Important findings are poor pulses and lower blood pressure in the legs compared with the right arm. The liver and heart are enlarged, and the lungs are congested. In older patients, elevated blood pressure is the most common reason for evaluation of a possible coarctation.

12. What is the best way to treat a newborn with severe coarctation?

The first step is to try to reopen the ductus with an infusion of prostaglandin E1 while simultaneously stabilizing the circulation with fluids, inotropic drugs (e.g., dopamine), and, in some cases, mechanical ventilation. Once the patient is stable, the coarctation should be repaired surgically either by resection and end-to-end anastomosis or by using a subclavian flap. Both techniques have good long-term results. Balloon dilatation and stents are still considered experimental methods and should not be used routinely.

13. What valve problems may be seen in acyanotic patients?

The most common problems are aortic valve stenosis and mitral valve stenosis. Both present with progressive exercise limitation and eventually with congestive heart failure.

14. Do you replace stenotic valves?

The goal is to avoid valve replacement for as long as possible. Aortic stenosis is treated primarily by balloon dilatation with good results. Mitral stenosis is a more difficult problem and generally requires open surgical repair by valve reconstruction.

15. If you have to replace the valves, what procedure is used?

For aortic valve replacement, the preferred procedure is an aortic autograft, which involves transplantation of the pulmonary valve to the aortic position and replacement of the pulmonary valve with a homograft. A homograft is a human valve transplanted from a cadaver donor to the recipient. A homograft aortic valve can be used with good results for isolated aortic valve replacement if an autograft is contraindicated. Replacement of the mitral valve usually requires a mechanical prosthesis, although mitral homograft valve replacement is undergoing clinical evaluation.

16. The autograft operation sounds complicated. Why not just use a mechanical valve replacement?

The autograft is technically more difficult but has two major advantages. First, the valve is viable and has the potential to grow, which is a major advantage for a small child. In addition, anticoagulation is not necessary with the autograft, whereas it is mandatory with the mechanical vale. The need to insert a homograft to replace the pulmonary valve is the Achilles' heel of the procedure. The homograft is likely to require replacement in the future because it does not grow and tends to degenerate.

17. What are the simple septal defects?

They include most atrial septal defects (ASDs) and ventricular septal defects (VSDs) that are not accompanied by other associated heart defects.

18. How and when do you fix simple septal defects?

Most ASDs do not cause significant symptoms during childhood and can be fixed in the first few years of life. The traditional method involves open-heart surgery and closure of the defect either by sewing the edges together or by using a pericardial patch. Closure by a catheter-delivered device is under study at several centers but is not yet widely available. VSDs often present with symptoms of heart failure (poor growth, tachypnea, large heart) in early infancy. The time of presentation depends on the size of the defect and the pulmonary vascular resistance. We recommend closure at the onset of symptoms or elective closure by 1 year of age in asymptomatic patients. VSDs are closed on cardiopulmonary bypass by placement of a prosthetic patch (Dacron, Gore-Tex).

19. How risky is surgical repair of ASDs and VSDs?

Children recover remarkably quickly; most are out of the hospital within 2 or 3 days. All operations carry risk, although the chance of death with this type of heart operation is only 1–2%. Most patients remain well in long-term follow-up.

20. What are complex septal defects?

Complex defects consist of a septal defect or defects with other associated lesions. The more common examples include complete atrioventricular (AV) septal defects (AV canal), double-outlet right ventricle, and combination of VSD with coarctation of the aorta or interrupted aortic arch.

21. How do patients with complex septal defects present? How does their management differ from that of simple defects?

Complex septal defects usually present early in life with symptoms of heart failure and failure to thrive (poor growth in weight and length). The combination of lesions either increases the degree of left-to-right shunt and volume load on the heart or causes a combined volume and pressure load on the heart. It is not uncommon for such patients to come to medical attention in the newborn nursery and to require surgical correction in early infancy.

22. What is a complete AV septal defect (AV canal)?

A complete AV septal defect consists of a VSD located in the inlet portion of the ventricular septum, an ASD located low in the atrial septum in the septum primum, and malformation of the AV (mitral and tricuspid) valves. The VSD and ASD are contiguous defects because they occupy the area of the heart called the AV septum. The AV septum plays a critical role in the development of the AV valves. Although the term *AV canal defect* is deeply rooted in the literature, the term *AV septal defect* is far more descriptive of the lesion.

23. How are patients with complete AV septal defects managed?

Patients generally develop symptoms of heart failure in the first month or two of life as pulmonary vascular resistance falls and left-to-right shunt increases. After the diagnosis is made, such infants should be started on medical therapy, including digoxin and Lasix, and a higher-calorie formula. Surgical repair should be done in the first 6–12 weeks of life.

24. What does the operation entail?

The procedure is done on cardiopulmonary bypass; the heart is stopped with cardioplegia solution. The atrial and ventricular septal defects are closed either by inserting a single patch to close both defects or by inserting separate patches (double-patch technique). Finally, the AV valves are repaired by attaching them to the VSD patch and by closing the "cleft" in the anterior mitral valve leaflet.

25. How successful are such operations? What are the main problems after surgery?

The mortality rate for repair of complete AV septal defect is ~5% at experienced centers. The most common problem in the immediate postoperative period is elevated pulmonary artery blood pressure (pulmonary hypertension), which usually is transient and can be managed with sedation, hyperventilation, vasodilator drugs, and, in some cases, inhaled nitric oxide. Later problems generally involve leakage of the mitral valve, which in some cases requires reoperation.

26. A 2-day-old boy suspected of having congenital heart disease looks blue, and the pulse oximeter indicates a saturation of 78% on 40% oxygen. No murmur is heard, the infant has good pulses, and no other anomalies are present. Is there any difference in your evaluation of the patient?

No. You made a good start by getting some history and doing a physical exam. Infants with blue or cyanotic congenital heart defects are evaluated in the same way as infants with pink or acyanotic heart defects.

27. What defects should be considered in a cyanotic infant?

Simple defects: pulmonic stenosis with right-to-left shunt at the atrial level
Complex defects (often referred to as "T" lesions):
- Tetralogy of Fallot
- Transposition of the great arteries

- Truncus arteriosus
- Tricuspid atresia (an example of single ventricle)
- Total anomalous pulmonary venous return

28. Can you diagnose the specific defect with echocardiography?

Usually. First, of course, you should look at the chest radiograph, which may give important hints. For instance, in tetralogy of Fallot the heart has a configuration like a boot and the pulmonary artery is small. The lungs look black because they have little blood flow. In contrast, children with total anomalous pulmonary venous return may have an obstruction of the connection between the pulmonary veins and the right side of the heart. This obstruction causes the lungs to become highly congested, and on the radiograph the lung fields look white.

29. What should I look for on the echocardiogram?

As in the acyanotic child, first look for the number of heart chambers, the connections of the veins and arteries and the presence of holes between the atria and ventricles. It is important to look for a ductus arteriosus and to determine whether there is flow through it. You want to make special note of whether there is a connection between the right ventricle and pulmonary artery and of the size of the connection (stenotic or normal). Next, you want to determine whether blood is mixed or shunted across any of the septal defects or the ductus. This determination can be made with color Doppler. Finally, piece the anatomy and physiology together to come up with your best diagnosis.

30. Do you ever have to take cyanotic infants to the catheterization lab?

Most often the diagnosis can be made with echocardiography and color Doppler alone. However, you should consider taking the patient to the catheterization lab if the anatomy or physiology is unclear after an adequate echocardiographic exam has been completed or to do a balloon septostomy or balloon valvotomy.

31. What are balloon septostomy and ballon valvotomy?

The cardiologist can do important palliative procedures in the catheterization lab that stabilize patients before surgery and in some instances replace or delay the need for heart surgery. Balloon atrial septostomy involves passing an inflatable balloon across the foramen ovale, inflating the balloon, and pulling it across the foramen. This procedure results in stretching or tearing of the atrial septum, which improves mixing of blue and red blood. A balloon valvotomy is similar. A balloon-tipped catheter is passed across the stenotic aortic or pulmonary valve, and inflation of the balloon stretches the valve open.

32. Why are patients with cyanotic heart defects blue?

There are two basic physiologic problems, which may be present separately or together. First is shunting (mixing) of blue venous blood from the right side into the left side of the heart. This shunt results from a septal defect at either the atrial or ventricular level. Mixing of blue and red blood results in a decrease in the amount of oxygen that is carried in the arterial blood returning to the body. Second is a reduction in the total amount of pulmonary blood flow due to an obstruction of blood flow from the right ventricle to the pulmonary artery. In some cases, the connection between the right ventricle and the pulmonary artery may be absent.

33. How can an infant survive with no connection between the right ventricle and pulmonary artery? How does the blood get to the lungs?

The ductus arteriosus, a blood vessel that connects the aorta and pulmonary artery, is usually patent at birth. Although the blood flows from the pulmonary artery to the aorta via the ductus in utero, the direction of flow typically reverses after birth with blood flowing from the aorta to the pulmonary artery. The ductus then becomes the principal source of pulmonary blood flow in many patients. In patients who depend on the ductus for pulmonary blood flow, prostaglandin E_1 can be given as an continuous infusion to prevent ductal closure.

34. Describe the anatomy of transposition of the great arteries (TGA).

TGA is characterized by discordance in the connection of the ventricles and great arteries. The right ventricle connects to the aorta, and the left ventricle connects to the pulmonary artery.

35. Wait a minute—it sounds like the blood is flowing in two parallel circuits! How do infants with TGA get blood to their lungs? How does oxygenated blood return to the body?

The key defect in TGA is that blood flows in two parallel circuits instead of in series, as in the normal heart. Survival requires mixing of red and blue blood either between the atria (via a patent foramen ovale or ASD), between the ventricles (via a VSD), or between the great arteries (via a PDA). Through any of these sites of mixing, some of the blue blood returning to the right side of the heart crosses the ASD, VSD, or ductus and reaches the left side of the circulation. Then it can go to the pulmonary artery, which in TGA is connected to the left ventricle. Similarly, some of the red blood on the left side of the heart can cross at the atrial, ventricular, or ductal level and reach the right side of the heart, winding up in the aorta.

36. In the echocardiogram of the 2-day-old boy in question 26, the pulmonary artery appears to be connected to the left ventricle and the aorta to the right ventricle. He has no VSD, and the foramen ovale is patent but small. A PDA has bidirectional flow. The diagnosis is TGA. What now?

You need to keep his blood mixing, as discussed earlier, until the defect can be repaired. There are two options: (1) you can continue intravenous prostaglandin to keep the ductus open or (2) a balloon atrial septostomy can be done to improve the mixing of blood at the atrial level. If he has enough mixing of blood via the foramen ovale, it is possible to discontinue the prostaglandin and forego the balloon septostomy.

37. Is one option better than the other?

Not really. It is largely a question of institutional preference. Because prostaglandin has a small risk of causing respiratory depression, some hospitals mechanically ventilate patients receiving prostaglandin infusions. Prostaglandin also may cause fever and fluid retention in higher doses. In many centers, balloon atrial septostomy is done in the catheterization lab, whereas other centers do the procedures at the bedside with echocardiographic guidance. This procedure involves a risk of transient heart block or other arrhythmias. Both strategies can achieve the same goal.

38. What operation does the infant need?

The standard procedure is an **arterial switch** (Jatene) operation, which moves the aorta to the left ventricle, the pulmonary artery to the right ventricle, and the coronary arteries to the aorta. This procedure results in what is often called an anatomic repair because "normal" anatomy is restored. Previously we performed an **atrial switch** (Mustard or Senning) operation. The atrial switch baffled the blue venous blood from the right atrium to the left atrium. From there it went to the left ventricle, which in TGA is connected to the pulmonary artery. Thus, the blue blood reached the lungs. The red pulmonary venous blood was baffled to the right atrium and then to the right ventricle, which is connected to the aorta. Thus, the arterial blood was returned to the body. Atrial switch operations were called physiologic repairs because the anatomy was not normalized but at least the blood reached the correct locations.

39. Why did you "switch your switches"?

Some of the earliest operations in infants with TGA were variants of the arterial switch. However, the surgical mortality rate was quite high. The atrial switch operations, developed independently by William Mustard and Ake Senning, were effective and had much lower mortality rates. They were widely used from the 1960s through the mid 1980s with great success;

however, various problems developed 10–15 years after the operations, including atrial arrhythmia, obstructions of the surgically created atrial baffles, and, in some patients, failure of the right ventricle. For these reasons, surgeons reintroduced the arterial switch operation, which became more successful because of improvements in surgical techniques.

40. Why did the right ventricle fail after atrial switch operations?
The right and left ventricles have different abilities to cope with pressure and volume work. The right ventricle is designed to tolerate variations in the volume of blood that it must pump per minute but is less tolerant of having to work against higher than normal blood pressures for prolonged periods. In patients with TGA who underwent an atrial switch operation, the right ventricle, which is connected to the aorta, must do the work usually done by the left ventricle. Thus, the right ventricle in some patients fails as the patient approaches adulthood.

41. What do you do then?
This problem is very serious. The most common option is to refer the patient for a heart transplant. There is also some experience in converting such patients to an arterial switch, but this procedure is experimental at present.

42. What are the defects in patients with tetralogy of Fallot?
The four abnormalities in tetralogy of Fallot are: (1) ventricular septal defect; (2) right ventricular outflow tract obstruction due to pulmonary stenosis either below, above, or at the pulmonary valve; (3) right ventricular hypertrophy (thickening due to the pulmonary stenosis); and (4) override of the aorta toward the right ventricle. The important parts of the defect in terms of symptoms are the VSD and right ventricular outflow tract obstruction.

43. Who was Fallot?
Fallot was a French pathologist who in 1888 described the four anomalies listed above.

44. Do infants with tetralogy of Fallot present with symptoms like those associated with TGA?
Infants with tetralogy of Fallot are cyanotic, but their clinical presentation varies according the amount of right ventricular outflow tract obstruction. If there is little obstruction, they may be acyanotic and often are referred to as a "pink tetralogy." Such infants usually do not develop problems for several months and may need no immediate care for their heart defect. At the other extreme are infants with tetralogy of Fallot and pulmonary atresia. They have no connection between the right ventricle and pulmonary artery, are usually blue at birth, and need early treatment. Most infants are somewhere between the two extremes and have moderate obstruction.

45. Do all infants with moderate obstruction look blue?
Again, there can be a spectrum of findings. Infants who have right ventricular outflow tract obstruction due to severe stenosis of the pulmonary valve have a "fixed obstruction" that does not vary. They tend to be blue early in life and become bluer as they grow. In contrast, other infants have obstruction of the right ventricular outflow tract due to enlarged muscle bundles in the outflow tract and narrowing of the outflow tract due to malposition of the ventricular septum. The degree of obstruction varies; thus, the condition is called "dynamic obstruction."

46. How do infants with tetralogy of Fallot and pulmonary atresia get blood to their lungs?
The ductus arteriosus is a common source of pulmonary blood flow in such infants. They also may have collateral blood vessels that originate from the aorta or other major arteries. These collateral arteries are often referred to as major aortopulmonary collateral arteries (MAPCAs).

47. Does the source of pulmonary blood supply make a difference?
Infants with pulmonary blood supply from the ductus arteriosus usually have fairly normal pulmonary arteries that distribute blood to all segments of the lung bed. They are

almost always cyanotic at birth. In contrast, infants with MAPCAS often have malformed pulmonary arteries, which may be disconnected from one another. As a result, some segments of the lung may not be connected to the main pulmonary arteries. Although most of these infants are cyanotic at birth, some may be pink and even have congestive heart failure if the MAPCAs are large.

48. A male infant has tetralogy of Fallot with right ventricular outflow tract obstruction both below the valve (due to thickened muscle bundles) and at the pulmonary valve (due to a small annulus). He is cyanotic with an oxygen saturation of 86% on room air. The ductus arteriosus is closed. How should he be managed?

Although the infant is cyanotic, the oxygen level is satisfactory at the moment. The infant may be discharged home and followed for an increase in cyanosis. At that time, surgical intervention will be needed.

49. What if the infant has a patent ductus arteriosus?

Watch the infant in the hospital to see what happens to the oxygen saturation when the ductus closes. If the ductus provides a significant portion of pulmonary blood flow, the infant may become a lot more cyanotic when it closes.

50. If the infant is very cyanotic when the duct closes, what should you do?

The infant can be stabilized by reopening the ductus with a prostaglandin infusion. Then surgical intervention is required.

51. What are the surgical options?

Generally we completely repair the defect as soon as an infant develops symptoms due to tetralogy of Fallot. If the patient remains asymptomatic, we usually repair the defect electively in the first 6 months of life. Currently it is rare for patients with simple tetralogy of Fallot to receive a palliative shunt operation.

52. Why do you prefer complete repair so early in life?

Complete repair early in life leads to less hypertrophy of the right ventricle, which appears to reduce the frequency of late arrhythmias. In addition, early repair reduces the number of surgical procedures that are needed and restores normal oxygen saturation earlier in life, which is important for development.

53. How is the complete repair done?

Surgical repair involves closure of the VSD with a patch and relief of the right ventricular outflow tract obstruction. Generally resection of the obstructing muscle bundles and opening the stenotic pulmonary valve are required. If the valve annulus is well below the normal diameter relative to the child's body size, we may have to put a patch across the outflow tract to enlarge it. Infants with pulmonary atresia often need placement of a conduit between the right ventricle and pulmonary arteries.

54. When do you decide to do a palliative operation?

The modified Blalock-Taussig shunt is the usual palliative operation and involves placing a small polytetrafluoroethylene (PTFE) tube graft between the subclavian artery and a branch pulmonary artery. This procedure is reserved for infants with other medical problems that place them at excessive risk for complete repair. Alternatively, some patients with pulmonary atresia have inadequately large pulmonary arteries to allow complete surgical repair.

55. What is meant by the term "single ventricle"?

The term *single ventricle* (or univentricular heart) refers to a category of cyanotic congenital heart defects that have only one *functional* ventricle. Two ventricles may be physically present, but one or the other is underdeveloped or lacks an inlet or outlet valve and thus cannot participate in the circulation as a functional pumping chamber. In all single-ventricle defects, blue, desaturated blood must mix with the red, fully saturated blood at either the atrial or ventricular level.

56. What specific heart defects are included in the single-ventricle category?
The more common ones are: (1) tricuspid atresia, (2) double-inlet left ventricle, and (3) hypoplastic left-heart syndrome.

57. If only one ventricle is functional, is there also only one atrium? How does blood return to the heart?
Blood returns from the body via the vena cavae and from the lungs via the pulmonary veins to their respective atria in a manner similar to that in the normal biventricular heart. Anatomic malformations of the atria that do not significantly alter their function may be present.

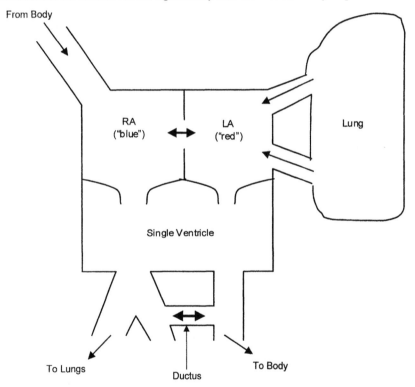

Double-inlet left ventricle. RA = right atrium, LA = left atrium, Ductus = ductus arteriosus.

58. Once the blood returns to the atria, where does it go if there is only one ventricle?
The blood returns to the two atria and then to the single ventricle in two general ways. First, if two AV valves (mitral and tricuspid valves) are present, the blood can traverse the valves into the single ventricle, as in double-inlet left ventricle. Second, in patients with atresia of one of the AV valves (e.g., tricuspid atresia), the affected valve does not form. Instead, a solid plate of muscle prevents the passage of blood from the right atrium to the right ventricle. In this setting an ASD must be present to allow the blood to go into the left atrium and then across the unaffected valve into the ventricle.

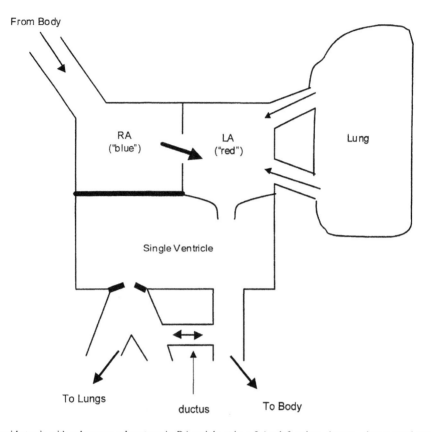

Tricuspid atresia with pulmonary valve stenosis. RA = right atrium, LA = left atrium, ductus = ductus arteriosus.

59. Now that all of the blood is in the ventricle, how does the blue blood get to the lungs and the red blood to the body?

Unfortunately, the blood cannot figure out where to go. Red and blue blood mixes together and then is distributed to the lungs or the body.

60. What determines the relative amounts of blood that go to the body and to the lungs?

The distribution of blood to the lungs and the body is determined by their relative resistances to blood flow. Remember the following equations:

(1) Cardiac output = pressure ÷ resistance
(2) Total cardiac output = cardiac output to lungs + cardiac output to body

In the single ventricle, the blood pressure is equal for blood going to the lungs and blood going to the body. According to equation (1), the amount of blood that goes to the lungs is inversely proportional to the resistance to blood flow to the lungs, and the amount of blood that goes to the body is inversely proportional to the resistance to blood flow in the body. Therefore, an increase in resistance to blood flow to the lungs decreases pulmonary blood flow, and a decrease in resistance to blood flow to the lungs increases pulmonary blood flow. Conversely, an increase in resistance to blood flow to the body decreases systemic blood flow, and a decrease in resistance to blood flow to the body increases systemic blood flow. According to equation (2), if total cardiac output is fixed at a certain amount per minute, an increase in pulmonary blood flow can occur only with a proportionate decrease in systemic blood flow. Conversely, an increase in systemic blood flow can occur only with a decrease in pulmonary blood flow.

61. Can the relative resistances to blood flow to the lungs or body vary from one time to the next?

It is easiest to think of two types of resistances: **fixed resistance** does not vary; **dynamic resistance** varies with time and conditions

A stenotic pulmonary valve and coarctation of the aorta are examples of fixed resistances. In contrast, pulmonary vascular resistance is a dynamic resistance. It can increase or decrease according to changes in the blood gases and maturation of the lung. It is also common to have a combination of fixed and dynamic resistances.

62. This is complicated. How do you keep everything straight so you can predict what is going to happen with the patient?

To determine what an individual patient will do, it is best to draw a diagram based on the figure in question 57. Then modify the diagram, including all of the specific details obtained from the echocardiogram.

63. A cyanotic newborn has an arterial saturation of 78% on room air. The echocardiogram shows tricuspid atresia and severe pulmonary valve stenosis. Blood flows through the ductus arteriosus from the aorta to the pulmonary artery. Do we expect the arterial saturation to change over the next few days?

The figure in question 58 is a diagram for this patient. The blue blood returning from the body mixes with the red blood returning from the lungs, and all of the blood goes into the single ventricle across the mitral valve. If the ductus closes, the total amount of blood going to the lungs decreases. Because of pulmonary valve stenosis (a fixed resistance) more blood cannot flow into the lungs to compensate for the blood that the ductus was supplying. Thus, the infant becomes more cyanotic.

64. Does the infant need a shunt?

A shunt is the best option at this point. Because you predicted this problem from the diagram, you would put the infant on prostaglandin after the diagnosis was made and schedule the shunt electively to prevent a sudden fall in saturation.

65. What if the infant had tricuspid atresia but no pulmonary valve stenosis?

In this case, changes in the pulmonary vascular resistance (a dynamic resistance) are important. The infant is likely to have minimal cyanosis with an arterial saturation in the high 80% range. When the ductus closes, the saturation may fall a bit. However, as infants mature, pulmonary vascular resistance falls; as a result, pulmonary blood flow increases and arterial oxygen saturation rises.

66. Is this bad?

It can be bad, depending on how high the pulmonary blood flow gets. From equation (2) in question 60, we know that if total cardiac output is fixed, an increase in pulmonary blood flow results in a proportional decrease in systemic blood flow. If systemic blood flow decreases too much, organ dysfunction may occur and lactic acidosis develops. On a more chronic basis, the excessive pulmonary blood flow may cause respiratory distress, damage the pulmonary vasculature, cause the heart to dilate and/or hypertrophy, and stunt growth.

67. How do you deal with such problems?

The goal is to balance the relative resistances to ensure adequate amounts of pulmonary and systemic blood flow. In the infant with excessive pulmonary blood flow, the pulmonary artery can be banded to increase pulmonary resistance and thereby decrease pulmonary blood flow.

68. What is the eventual surgical repair for infants with a single-ventricle defect?

The ultimate goal is complete separation of blue and red blood. Complete separation achieves two goals: (1) the arterial saturation approaches a normal level, and (2) the work load on the single ventricle is reduced.

69. What technique is used for surgical repair?

The procedure, called a Fontan operation, involves diverting the systemic venous (blue) blood to the pulmonary arteries, leaving only pulmonary venous (red) blood returning to the single ventricle. The procedure is accomplished in most patients in three staged operations.

The first operation, if necessary, is done in infancy and includes either an aortopulmonary shunt or pulmonary artery band to regulate pulmonary blood flow. Patients with hypoplastic left-heart syndrome and its variants require a more complex procedure that also attacks the underdeveloped aorta.

The second operation, done at approximately 6 months of age, is either a bidirectional Glenn shunt or hemi-Fontan operation. Although the two procedures are different, both divert the superior vena cava to the pulmonary artery and reduce the blood returning to the single ventricle by about 33%.

The final procedure completes the Fontan operation and involves diversion of inferior vena caval blood to the pulmonary artery. This goal can be accomplished by construction of an intracardiac baffle or placement of an extracardiac tube graft between the orifice of the inferior vena cava and pulmonary artery.

70. After the Fontan operation, no ventricle is pumping blood through the pulmonary arteries. How does blood flow in this situation?

The momentum generated when the single ventricle ejects blood into the aorta is the source of energy that powers the blood through the entire circulation. For this situation to exist, systolic and diastolic ventricular function must be normal, pulmonary vascular resistance must be low, and the pulmonary arteries must be well developed.

71. How do such patients do after the Fontan operation?

The surgical mortality rate has decreased to approximately 7–10% for good candidates. Earlier patients with Fontan operations returned to medical attention because of a high incidence of arrhythmias and baffle and conduit obstructions. Changes in surgical techniques have reduced some of these problems. The incidence of late ventricular dysfunction and protein loss in the intestines is still a concern in some patients. However, exercise tolerance is fairly high, and overall the operation is a good palliation for a complex group of patients.

72. What is total anomalous pulmonary venous connection?

The pulmonary veins drain to a structure other than the left atrium.

73. Where do the pulmonary veins connect?

There are four types of total anomalous connection:

Supracardiac: the pulmonary veins drain to a confluence behind the right atrium that empties into the innominate vein via an embryonic residual called an ascending vein.

Infracardiac: the confluence drains to the portal system below the diaphragm via a descending vein.

Cardiac: the confluence drains to the heart directly, usually to the coronary sinus.

Mixed: a combination of the other three types

In partial anomalous venous connection, usually only the right pulmonary veins drain anomalously to the superior vena cava.

74. How does oxygenated blood reach the left ventricle?

An ASD must be present. Red blood and blue blood mix in the right atrium and shunt across the ASD to the left side of the heart.

75. How are these defects repaired?

The goal of the operation is to establish a direct connection between the confluence of pulmonary veins and the back of the left atrium and to close the ASD. Surgery is done on cardiopulmonary bypass.

76. Overall the mortality rate for most congenital heart operations is fairly low. As patients grow, do they need special care and follow-up?

Most if not all patients should be followed for life by a cardiologist familiar with congenital heart defects. Patients with simple defects, such as ASD, VSD, or PDA, are essentially cured and are not expected to develop later problems. In contrast, patients with more complex defects such as single ventricle, operations requiring conduits, and most valve operations, need careful longitudinal follow-up because reintervention is more likely. It also is important to be wary of endocarditis.

BIBLIOGRAPHY

1. Baue AE, Geha AS, Laks H, et al: Glenn's Thoracic and Cardiovascular Surgery, 6th ed. Stamford, CT, Appleton & Lange, 1996.
2. Kirklin JW, Barratt-Boyes BG: Cardiac Surgery, 2nd ed. New York, Churchill Livingstone, 1993.
3. Nichols DG, Cameron DE, Greeley WJ, et al: Critical Heart Disease in Infants and Children. St. Louis, Mosby, 1995.
4. Rosenkranz ER: Caring for the former pediatric cardiac surgery patient. Pediatr Clin North Am 45:907–941, 1998.

19. VASCULAR DISEASE

James A. O'Neill, Jr., M.D.

ARTERIAL DISORDERS

1. What types of arterial disorders affect the renal vessels?

Congenital aneurysms usually involve abdominal visceral vessels. Aneurysms of renal artery branches are among the more common manifestations. When branch vessels of the renal arteries are involved, hypertension is the most common clinical manifestation. Rupture does not tend to occur; thrombosis and embolism are the most common complications. We have encountered renal artery aneurysms in children between the ages of 8 and 18. Undoubtedly, they are present in younger children, but clinical complications usually do not become evident until later in childhood. Disease involving the renal arteries is usually discovered when patients are evaluated for significant hypertension. The etiology of hypertension related to renovascular disease is either congenital or acquired. The various entities are outlined in the table below.

Forms of Renovascular Hypertension

CONGENITAL	ACQUIRED
Arterial aplasia and hypoplasia	Fibromuscular hyperplasia with renal artery stenosis
Neurofibromatosis	Takayasu's disease
Williams' syndrome	Midaortic syndrome
Coarctation of the aorta	Renal artery occlusion after thrombosis or embolism
	Renal artery trauma, anastomotic stenosis
	Pyelonephritis, glomerulonephritis, intrarenal tumor, hemolytic uremic syndrome
	Obstructive uropathy

2. What is the most common cause of renovascular hypertension?

Fibromuscular dysplasia.

3. How are disorders of the renal arteries treated?

Aneurysms of renal artery branches are best treated by excision and reconstruction when the vessels are accessible; when they are intrarenal, partial nephrectomy may be in order. Arterial hypoplasia or aplasia ranges from absence of the kidney to renal hypoplasia associated with significant hypertension. Resection is the only alternative in cases of renal hypoplasia. Arterial reconstruction is an option for patients with renovascular narrowing related to neurofibromatosis, Williams' syndrome, and coarctation of the aorta in either the thoracic or abdominal location. With regard to acquired disorders, obstructive uropathies and tumors usually are associated only with modest elevations in blood pressure and are best treated with renal reconstructive surgery. Nephritis and pyelonephritis may result in malignant hypertension and are best treated pharmacologically.

Renal artery narrowing may result from trauma or primary arterial disease in the form of fibromuscular hyperplasia, which is probably an autoimmune phenomenon and also may involve the aorta and branch vessels. Examples include midaortic syndrome and Takayasu's disease. Patients usually present with significant hypertension; arteriography is diagnostic. It usually is not necessary to determine bilateral renal renins in children when a significant arterial lesion is found in association with hypertension. It is best to defer reconstructive arterial surgery in patients with fibromuscular disease until the sedimentation rate has fallen to normal levels, indicating that the patient does not have active arteritis at the time of surgery. Nephrectomy should be a last resort.

Our preference is arterial reconstruction. Although transluminal balloon dilatation has been successful for branch vessel stenoses, it is not beneficial for lesions located at the aortic orifice. Furthermore, we prefer not to use stents in young children because reconstructive surgery has been so effective. However, all patients who have had treatment of renovascular hypertension require close long-term follow-up because recurrence is a possibility.

When the abdominal aorta is narrowed at its mid portion in association with renovascular narrowing, immediate simultaneous reconstruction of both lesions is preferred. The two approaches are (1) long-patch angioplasty of both the aorta and renal vessels and (2) aortoaortic bypass with bilateral renal artery bypasses when needed. We prefer the second approach. It is usually best to control hypertension before performing surgical correction, but complete control is not always possible for patients with oliguric renal failure or severe malignant hypertension.

4. What percentage of cases of renal hypertension in children are correctable by surgery?

Approximately 80% in the 0- to 5-year-old group, approximately 45% in the 6- to 10-year-old group, and approximately 20% in the 11- to 18-year-old group.

5. What is the cause of mycotic aneurysms? How should they be treated?

Bacterial endocarditis associated with embolism may result in degeneration of the involved arterial wall. *Staphylococcus aureus* is the most common causative organism. Ultrasound may demonstrate the aneurysm, but aortography is useful to delineate the precise anatomic relationships. When mycotic aneurysms result from bacterial endocarditis, both the cardiac lesion and the aneurysm require management if recurrence is to be avoided. Aneurysm resection with either later-staged reconstruction in infants and young children or extraanatomic bypass in older children is indicated. The aortic and mitral valves are the primary valves involved, and the aorta and iliac vessels are the most common sites of mycotic aneurysms. Once an infected aneurysm is recognized, it must be treated immediately to avoid free rupture.

6. What are the major causes of arterial thrombosis and embolism? How are they treated?

First of all, newborn infants may develop spontaneous arterial thromboses, particularly involving the external iliac, various visceral arteries, and proximal upper extremity vessels. Septic infants and infants with severely decreased cardiac output are particularly prone to spontaneous arterial thrombosis. Furthermore, newborn infants are frequently severely polycythemic; infants of diabetic mothers are particularly prone to hyperviscosity associated with thrombosis of various arteries. In addition to manifestations of intestinal ischemia or necrosis, some infants present with gangrene of the extremities. Many such patients can be treated with heparin and urokinase or other lytic agents if urokinase is not available.

Infants with umbilical artery catheters are also prone to thrombotic and embolic complications. They may be treated with intraarterial urokinase and heparin, but occasionally thrombectomy is needed, particularly in the aorta.

7. What are the signs of vascular thrombosis or peripheral embolism?

Absent pulses, coolness, pallor, decreased motor function, decreased tendon reflexes, and pain are the usual manifestations of arterial occlusion. Frequently, iatrogenic events such as placement of intraarterial catheters precede arterial thrombosis and embolism; thus, it is often necessary for the physician to differentiate between arterial spasm and true occlusion. Sequential Doppler and clinical examinations are indicated, but if the process lasts longer than 4–6 hours, spasm is unlikely to be the cause.

8. What is the prognosis for treatment of arterial thrombosis and embolism?

If an arterial thrombosis or embolism is treated before 6 hours with either vascular repair or lytic agent infusion, the results are usually successful. After 8–12 hours the success rate falls markedly. An aggressive approach to arterial occlusion, even in infants, is indicated if amputation is to be avoided.

VENOUS DISEASE

9. How do superficial venous thrombosis and thrombophlebitis present in childhood?

Superficial venous thrombosis usually is associated with superficial venous malformations with tortuous flow patterns or with placement of intravenous catheters for administration of hypertonic solutions. Superficial thrombophlebitis is best categorized as aseptic (frequently traumatic), septic nonsuppurative, and suppurative. Superficial venous thrombosis may or may not be associated with aseptic thrombophlebitis, but the association is common in patients with venous invasions and intravenous infusions. Intravenous catheters that have been in place for 3 days or more may be associated with thrombophlebitis, particularly if hypertonic solutions or solutions at the extremes of pH are administered. In general, discontinuance of the intravenous catheter and solution and application of local heat are sufficient. In septic thrombophlebitis, however, antibiotics are needed. If septic thrombophlebitis is suppurative, venous excision also is indicated.

The signs and symptoms of superficial thrombophlebitis include overlying redness and tenderness as well as low-grade fever, but rarely is the involved extremity swollen. In suppurative thrombophlebitis, these signs are accentuated, and fever is usually prominent. It is often possible to milk pus from the IV entry site.

10. How common is deep venous thrombosis (DVT) in childhood? What causes it?

DVT is recognized with increasing frequency, particularly in tertiary care centers. DVT frequently is associated with the use of long-term indwelling catheters in large veins; it may be associated with trauma, prolonged immobilization, or surgical procedures that are performed on the extremity or that require prolonged periods in the lithotomy position. Upper extremity venous thrombosis in the subclavian and brachial veins ordinarily is categorized as effort thrombosis and frequently is seen in the dominant upper extremity of athletes. DVT also may result from hypercoagulable states, including protein C and S deficiencies, antithrombin III deficiency, and tyrosinemia.

11. How is DVT diagnosed?

Lower extremity edema, calf and thigh pain and tenderness, and a positive Homan's sign (pain with dorsiflexion of the foot) are suggestive. The best noninvasive approaches to diagnosis, in order of preference, are Doppler ultrasound and venous plethysmography. Although venography is also an option, it is no more accurate than the noninvasive methods, is difficult to perform in children, and occasionally results in thrombophlebitis. The best approach in children at present is Duplex scanning or real-time B-mode scanning combined with Doppler ultrasound. With these techniques, actual visualization of the clot, absence of a flow signal, or lack of variance of flow with respiration is diagnostic.

12. How should DVT in childhood be treated?

The basics of treatment are bed rest, elevation, and anticoagulation. Heparin is the best initial approach to treatment with a loading dose of 75 U/kg IV over 10 minutes. The initial maintenance dose is 28 U/kg/hr for infants less than 1 year of age and 20 U/kg/hr for children over 1 year of age. Thereafter heparin dosage is adjusted to maintain the partial thromboplastin time at 60–85 seconds, adjusting the infusion accordingly. An alternate approach is to use enoxaparin. The initial dose is 1.5 mg/kg every 12 hr for infants less than 2 months of age and 1.0 mg/kg every 12 hr for patients older than 2 months of age. The international normalized ratio (INR) should be maintained between 2 and 3 for children. After approximately 5 days of heparin therapy, overlapping on day 1 with oral warfarin, heparin can be discontinued and the patient maintained on warfarin for approximately 3 months.

13. Do children get pulmonary embolism?

Yes, but the exact incidence is unknown. It is assumed to be less frequent than in adults. Of interest, in most instances of pulmonary embolism in childhood the site of DVT is unknown and often is not discovered until autopsy. The extremities usually are not involved.

14. Does DVT result in postthrombotic sequelae?

Yes, but less often than in adults. The sequelae in childhood consist of chronic edema, hyperpigmentation of the skin, eczematous rash, and leg ulcers. They have been noted in approximately 20% of children who sustain DVT but may not become evident for 10–15 years. The same incidence is noted in children who for various reasons have had high venous ligation. Secondary appearance of varicose veins also may occur many years after the episode of venous obstruction.

15. What is the cause of renal vein thrombosis? How does it present?

Renal vein thrombosis is far less common today because most infants who present in shock from sepsis or other causes are resuscitated rapidly. The main cause of renal vein thrombosis is dehydration and hypovolemia, which result in a low flow state. The presence of indwelling catheters in the inferior vena cava also may result in renal vein thrombosis. Acute disease is associated with sudden severe congestion and enlargement of the involved kidney; if both kidneys are involved, oliguric renal failure results. Renal vein thrombosis or occlusion also may result from the presence of tumor thrombus, which usually develops over a lengthy period that permits the establishment of collateral circulation. Some degree of renal function is preserved under these circumstances.

16. What is the best way to treat renal vein thrombosis?

Unilateral renal vein thrombosis in infants is best treated by supportive therapy, which usually results in spontaneous improvement. The same is generally true of bilateral renal vein thrombosis. However, in occasional cases of acute bilateral renal vein and inferior vena caval thrombosis, direct infusion of a lytic agent has been reported to be beneficial.

BIBLIOGRAPHY

1. Andrew M, David M, Adams M, et al: Venous thromboembolic complications (VTE) in children: First analyses of the Canadian Registry of VTE. Blood 83:1251–1257, 1994.
2. Benjamin ME, Hansen KJ, Craven TE, et al: Combined aortic and renal artery surgery: A contemporary experience. Ann Surg 223:255–265, 1996.

3. Berkowitz HD, O'Neill JA: Renovascular hypertension in children. J Vasc Surg 9:46–55, 1989.
4. Blum U, Krumme B, Flugel P, et al: Treatment of ostial renal artery stenoses with vascular endoprostheses after unsuccessful balloon angioplasty. N Engl J Med 336:459–465, 1997.
5. Colburn MD, Gelabert HA, Quinones-Baldrich W: Neonatal aortic thrombosis. Surgery 111:21–28, 1992.
6. Evans DA, Wilmott RW: Pulmonary embolism in children. Pediatr Clin North Am 41:569–584, 1994.
7. Ivarsson SA, Bergqvist D, Lundstrom NR, et al: Takayasu's aortitis with renovascular hypertension. Acta Paediatr 81:1044–1048, 1992.
8. Johannson L, Hedner U, Nillson IM: Familial antithrombin III deficiency as pathogenesis of deep venous thrombosis. Acta Med Scand 204:491–495, 1978.
9. Messina LM, Reilly M, Goldstone J, et al: Middle aortic syndrome: Effectiveness and durability of complex arterial revascularization techniques. Ann Surg 204:331–339, 1978.
10. Nakayama DK, O'Neill JA, Wagner H, et al: Management of vascular complications of bacterial endocarditis. J Pediatr Surg 21:636–639, 1986.
11. O'Neill JA: Long-term outcome with surgical treatment of renovascular hypertension. J Pediatr Surg 33:106–111, 1998.
12. O'Neill JA, Berkowitz H, Fellows KJ, et al: Midaortic syndrome and hypertension in childhood. J Pediatr Surg 30:164–172, 1995.
13. O'Neill JA, Pruitt BA, Moncrief JA: Suppurative thrombophlebitis: A lethal complication of intravenous therapy. J Trauma 8:256–257, 1968.
14. Sarkar R, Coran AG, Cilley RE, et al: Arterial aneurysms in children: Clinicopathologic classification. J Vasc Surg 13:47–56, 1991.

V. Abdominal

20. UMBILICAL PROBLEMS

Mark Stovroff, M.D.

1. How does the umbilicus form?

As the embryo grows, the anterior abdominal wall develops from the infolding of the primitive body wall, narrowing the yolk sac. Part of the yolk sac develops into the mid- and hind-gut; the attenuated connection between the remaining extracolemic yolk sac and mid-gut is the vitelline duct. The vitelline duct fuses with the body stalk containing the umbilical vessels and the allantois (the developing bladder). With time the body wall contracts around this structure and usually closes by birth. This region of closure is the umbilicus.

2. What is the umbilical cord?

It represents the fusion of the yolk sac containing the vitelline duct and body stalk containing the umbilical vessels and allantois. It also contains primitive mesenchymal tissue and an outer layer of amnion.

3. When should the umbilical cord separate?

The normal time sequence is 3 days to 2 months with a mean of 14 days.

4. When should a physician be concerned if separation has not occurred?

Recent reports suggest that the persistence of umbilical cord attachment beyond 3 weeks may be associated with heritable neutrophil mobility defects and widespread infection.

5. What is omphalitis?

An umbilical infection in the newborn period that may progress, if untreated, to necrotizing fasciitis.

6. How is omphalitis managed?

Mild cases generally can be managed by vigorous aseptic drying and application of topical alcohol. However, more severe infection requires hospital admission, administration of parenteral antibiotics, and surgical consultation. Occasionally wide local debridement may be required.

7. How does an umbilical granuloma form?

After cord separation incomplete epithelialization over the ring may lead to formation of a small mass of granulation tissue.

8. How should umbilical granulomas be removed?

Most granulomas resolve with 1 or 2 applications of silver nitrate as a chemical cautery, followed by application of sterile gauze to prevent staining of skin and clothing.

9. If cauterization fails, what should be done next?

An umbilical polyp or sinus tract should be suspected, and referral to a pediatric surgeon for excision should be made.

10. What may cause bilious or prolonged purulent drainage from the umbilicus?

The most likely cause is a vitelline duct anomaly. Anomalies may include a persistent patent vitelline duct with communication to the small intestine or a vitelline cyst or sinus. In such cases the duct has obliterated only partially.

11. What steps should be taken to diagnose a vitelline duct anomaly?

First, a careful examination of the umbilicus may reveal a draining fistula or even the appearance of prolapsed intestinal mucosa. Once the anomaly is found, a contrast study may be obtained to confirm the diagnosis. Occasionally an ultrasound study of the region may reveal an underlying remnant in difficult cases.

12. If an anomaly is found, what surgical approach should be used?

All vitelline duct anomalies require exploration and excision. If they are infected, antibiotics and drainage may be required before umbilical exploration. All remnants must be removed, including the intra-abdominal component.

13. Can urine drain from the umbilicus?

Yes. In a situation analogous to vitelline duct anomalies, the urachus may remain completely or partially patent. A contrast study or ultrasound of the region may be helpful in making the diagnosis. Before operative intervention, the urinary tract should be investigated for a bladder outlet obstruction to explain the persistence of the patent urachus.

Operative intervention is necessary. Through an infraumbilical incision, complete excision of the urachus and/or remnants is performed to the level of the bladder.

14. How does an umbilical hernia develop?

From failure of closure of the umbilical ring after cord separation.

15. Are umbilical hernias common?

An umbilical hernia is the second most common pediatric surgical disorder. The incidence in the general population is 1 of 6 children.

16. What factors predispose to umbilical hernia?

Race and prematurity. Umbilical hernias are 10 times more common in African-American children than in Caucasians. In addition, 75% of infants weighing < 1500 gm have an umbilical hernia at birth. Umbilical hernias also are common in children with trisomy 21, trisomy 13, mucopolysaccharidoses, and congenital hypothyroidism.

17. Do most umbilical hernias close spontaneously?

Spontaneous closure is the rule rather than the exception. The majority of umbilical hernias are closed by age 3 years. The two most important factors in predicting spontaneous closure are the age of the infant and the size of the fascial defect. Spontaneous closure is unlikely after the age of 4 years. In addition, hernias with a diameter greater than 1.5 cm are unlikely to close spontaneously at any age.

18. When should the child with an umbilical hernia be referred for surgical closure?

Timing remains controversial. Any child with symptoms of incarceration or recurrent pain should be referred immediately. For the asymptomatic child with a moderate defect (< 1.5 cm), repair should be done at school age. For the child with a large defect and/or proboscis-like hernia, repair at age 1–2 years allows an easier and more cosmetic repair.

19. How is the repair performed?

Surgical repair is done through an infraumbilical incision, with the sac excised to the level of strong fascia. The defect is closed in a transverse manner with absorbable suture, and the inversion of the umbilical skin is maintained. After skin closure, a small "pressure" dressing is applied.

21. GROIN HERNIAS

Rebeccah L. Brown, M.D., and Philip L. Glick, M.D.

1. What is the processus vaginalis?
The processus vaginalis is a peritoneal diverticulum that extends through the internal ring at approximately 3 months gestation. As the testis descends between the seventh and ninth months of gestation, a portion of the processus vaginalis attaches to the testes and is dragged into the scrotum with the testes.

2. What normally happens to the processus vaginalis after testicular descent?
The portion of the processus vaginalis surrounding the testis becomes the tunica vaginalis. The remainder of the processus vaginalis obliterates, thereby eliminating the communication between the peritoneal cavity and the scrotum.

3. What is the underlying pathophysiology of the development of hernias and hydroceles in infants and children?
Failure of obliteration or incomplete obliteration of the processus vaginalis.

4. In what percentage of patients does the processus vaginalis remain patent?
In approximately 20% of normal adults, the processus vaginalis remains patent throughout life.

5. What is the difference between a hydrocele and a hernia?
A hydrocele occurs with incomplete obliteration of the processus vaginalis so that fluid accumulates around the testicle or the cord structures. This fluid may or may not communicate with the peritoneal cavity. A hernia occurs as a result of distal obliteration of the processus vaginalis with proximal patency or complete failure of obliteration so that both fluid and bowel may be present in the sac.

6. What is the female equivalent of a cord hydrocele?
A hydrocele of the canal of Nuck.

7. What is the pathophysiology of a cord hydrocele?
A cord hydrocele occurs with complete obliteration of the processus vaginalis proximally and distally and patency of the midportion. It may present as a mass in the groin region and may be difficult to differentiate from an incarcerated inguinal hernia.

8. How do hernias in infants and children differ from those in adults?
Almost all inguinal hernias in infants and children are indirect.

9. Anatomically, where should the hernia sac be located in an indirect inguinal hernia?
It should be located anterior and medial to the spermatic cord structures.

10. What is the incidence of groin hernias in infants and children?
Approximately 1–5%.

11. Are groin hernias more common in boys or girls?
Boys outnumber girls 6–10:1.

12. Are groin hernias more common on the right or the left? Why?
Right-sided hernias are more common because the right testis descends later than the left testis; therefore, the right processus vaginalis obliterates at a later date than the left. Consequently, patients who present with a left-sided hernia have a higher incidence of an occult right-sided hernia.

13. What is the anatomic distribution of groin hernias?
60% right, 30% left, and 10% bilateral.

14. What is the incidence of groin hernias in premature infants?
Up to 30%.

15. What is the risk of incarceration of groin hernias in premature infants?
The risk of incarceration exceeds 60% during the first 6 months of life.

16. What other patient populations are more susceptible to groin hernias?
Infants with bladder exstrophy, Ehlers-Danlos syndrome, mucopolysaccaridosis, prune belly syndrome, omphalocele, and gastroschisis; infants and children who have ventriculoperitoneal shunts or who require chronic peritoneal dialysis; and patients with cystic fibrosis.

17. How do most infants with groin hernias present?
Most hernias are found either by parents or during a well-baby or preschool check. Most patients have a history of an intermittent bulge in the groin or scrotum, especially with crying or straining. Often a groin bulge is first noted when the patient is in the bathtub. Most are asymptomatic.

18. What are the symptoms and signs of an incarcerated inguinal hernia?
The patient may be irritable and complain of pain in the groin. Signs of intestinal obstruction, including abdominal distention, vomiting, and obstipation, may follow. Physical examination reveals a tender, sometimes erythematous, irreducible mass in the groin. With strangulation of the bowel, blood may be seen per rectum.

19. What is the silk glove sign?
To demonstrate the silk glove sign, a single finger is laid over and parallel to the inguinal structures, and the finger is lightly rubbed across the cord structures from side to side at the level of the pubic tubercle. A positive silk glove sign imparts a sensation of rubbing two pieces of silk together and indicates thicker-than-normal cord structures, suggesting the presence of a hernia sac.

20. What structures, other than bowel, may become incarcerated in an inguinal hernia sac?
In females, the ovary or fallopian tubes frequently become incarcerated.

21. How does one reduce an incarcerated inguinal hernia?
Standing on the ipsilateral side of the child or at the feet of an infant, the examiner places his or her left index and middle finger on the ipsilateral anterior superior iliac crest and sweeps the fingers down along the inguinal canal toward the ipsilateral scrotum, keeping constant tension on the testicle, hernia mass, or scrotal skin for optimal alignment of the long axis of the hernia with the axis of the inguinal canal. Next, apply pressure with the right index finger and thumb on either side of the hernia neck, which, along with traction on the scrotum, helps to keep the external and internal rings open and prevent the hernia sac from overlapping these structures during reduction. Finally, with the left hand at the apex of the mass and with constant pressure on the inguinal canal from the right index finger and thumb, the fingers are walked slowly up the groin toward the internal ring, keeping constant pressure on the bottom of the hernia contents.

22. What is the differential diagnosis of an inguinal hernia?

Hydrocele, testicular torsion, torsion of the appendix testis, and inguinal lymphadenopathy.

23. Does transillumination reliably distinguish between a hydrocele and a hernia?

No. Bowel may transilluminate as easily as fluid, making it impossible to distinguish reliably between a hydrocele and a hernia.

24. What are the options for management if the parents give a history of an inguinal hernia but it cannot be demonstrated on physical exam?

- Observe the patient with frequent re-examinations.
- Explore the patient based on the clinical history if the parents are thought to be reliable.
- Obtain a herniogram.

25. What is a herniogram?

Water-soluble radiopaque contrast is injected into the peritoneal cavity through a small-bore needle in the infraumbilical region. Radiographs are taken 5, 10, and 45 minutes apart. If a patent processus vaginalis is present, contrast is demonstrated below the inguinal ligament.

26. What are the potential drawbacks and complications of a herniogram?

This relatively invasive procedure may provoke some degree of anxiety in both children and parents. Adverse complications may include intestinal hematoma, intestinal perforation, and contrast reactions.

27. What are the most common indications for a herniogram?

- To confirm a difficult diagnosis
- To check for a suspected femoral hernia
- To rule out recurrent hernia in a postoperative patient with persistent groin symptoms

28. What technique is used to repair pediatric hernias?

High ligation of the sac.

29. When should groin hernias be repaired?

In premature infants, groin hernias should be repaired just before discharge from the neonatal intensive care unit when the infant weighs at least 1800 to 2000 gm and is in optimal medical condition. Other infants should be scheduled electively within about 1 month of making the diagnosis. Incarcerated hernias that can be reduced in the emergency department should be repaired within 24–48 hours. Incarcerated hernias that cannot be reduced in the emergency department should be repaired emergently.

30. What are the complications of groin hernia repair?

- Bleeding
- Infection (< 1%)
- Injury to cord structures (< 2%)
- Recurrence (0.5–1%)
- Iatrogenic cryptorchidism

31. What is the Goldstein test?

Intraoperative diagnostic pneumoperitoneum, also known as the Goldstein test, involves insufflation of air into the peritoneal cavity through a catheter inserted into the hernia sac on the clinically affected side. Crepitance in the contralateral inguinal region or scrotum indicates a patent processus vaginalis on that side. If the test is positive, a contralateral exploration is performed.

32. Describe another technique for assessing the contralateral side.

Laparoscopic exploration of the contralateral side through the open hernia sac on the clinically affected side.

33. What are the relative indications for contralateral exploration?

Premature infants, children less than 1–2 years old (especially girls and children with left-sided hernias), and infants and children with severe, coexisting medical illnesses that significantly increase the anesthetic risk.

BIBLIOGRAPHY

1. Kapur P, Caty MG, Glick PL: Pediatric hernias and hydroceles. Pediatr Clin North Am 45:773–789, 1998.
2. Rescorla FJ: Hernia and umbilicus. In Oldham KT, Colombani PM, Foglia RP (eds): Surgery of Infants and Children: Scientific Principles and Practice. Philadelphia, Lippincott-Raven, 1997, pp 1069–1076.
3. Weber TR, Tracy TF Jr: Groin hernias and hydroceles. In Ashcraft KW, Holder TM (eds): Pediatric Surgery, 2nd ed. Philadelphia, W.B. Saunders, 1993, pp 562–570.

22. GASTROSCHISIS AND OMPHALOCELE

Scott C. Boulanger, M.D., Ph.D., Michael G. Caty, M.D., and Philip L. Glick, M.D.

1. What is the incidence of omphalocele and gastroschisis? Does maternal age matter?

The incidence of gastroschisis and omphalocele is approximately 1 in 2000 live births. Over the past several decades, the incidence of gastroschisis has increased, whereas the incidence of omphalocele has remained unchanged. The incidence of gastroschisis decreases as maternal age increases.

2. Is the incidence related to prematurity?

Yes. The incidence of both gastroschisis and omphalocele is associated with lower gestational age. Birth weight for gestational age is also lower.

3. Define the term cutis navel.

A cutis navel is a small congenital hernia of the umbilicus that has epithelialized. Congenital hernias of the umbilicus differ from omphaloceles in that they are small (< 4 cm) and contain only a few loops of bowel. They are treated with simple primary closure, are not syndrome-related, and have an excellent prognosis.

4. What syndromes are associated with omphalocele?

Several genetic syndromes are associated with omphaloceles: (1) Pentalogy of Cantrell, (2) lower midline syndrome (bladder or cloacal extrophy), (3) Beckwith-Weidemann syndrome, (4) several trisomies (e.g., trisomy 13 and 18), (5) Charge syndrome, (6) prune-belly syndrome, and (7) Meckel-Gruber syndrome. In addition, cardiac anomalies are common in infants with omphalocele, particularly tetralogy of Fallot and atrial septal defects.

5. What syndromes are associated with gastroschisis?

Gastroschisis is not associated with genetic syndromes. However, approximately 10% of cases of gastroschisis are associated with intestinal atresia.

6. What defects comprise pentalogy of Cantrell, lower midline syndrome, and Beckwith-Weidemann syndrome?

Pentalogy of Cantrell consists of an upper midline omphalocele, anterior diaphragmatic hernia, sternal cleft, ectopia cordis, and cardiac anomalies (e.g., ventricular septal defect).

Lower midline syndrome consists of bladder or cloacal exstrophy, imperforate anus, colonic atresia, vesicointestinal fistula, sacral vertebral defects, and meningomyelocele.

Beckwith-Weidemann syndrome consists of gigantism, macroglossia, omphalocele, and pancreatic islet cell hyperplasia. Although both pentalogy of Cantrell and lower midline syndrome are quite rare, approximately 12% of children with omphalocele have Beckwith-Weidemann syndrome.

7. What environmental factors are associated with omphaloceles or gastroschisis?

No specific environmental factors have been associated with formation of either defect. Both omphalocele and gastroschisis have been produced experimentally by various means (i.e., salicylate poisoning, folic acid deficiency, and hypoxia).

8. What genetic factors are associated with omphalocele or gastroschisis?

Familial cases have been reported for both omphalocele and gastroschisis and some have proposed an element of genetic determination.

9. Describe Duhamel's theory about the embryology of omphaloceles.

Duhamel proposed that omphaloceles result from failure of body wall morphogenesis due to a defect in the somatic layer of the cephalic fold. The cephalic fold is one of four folds resulting from the folding over of the lateral parts of the embryonic disc. The cephalic fold eventually forms the thoracic and epigastric walls. The four folds meet to form the umbilical ring. Rapid growth of the midgut during the sixth week causes its herniation through the umbilical ring. A defect in the cephalic fold results in an epigastric omphalocele and other defects associated with pentalogy of Cantrell. In addition, because the midgut remains herniated, affected children usually have malrotation.

Failure of the caudal fold results in lower midline syndrome and a hypogastric omphalocele. If the lateral folds do not meet, a central omphalocele results. In contrast, the embryogenesis of gastroschisis is much less clear. Ultrasound evidence suggests that gastroschisis may arise from in utero rupture of an omphalocele. This evidence may represent the missing link, if one exists, between the embryogenesis and pathogenesis of omphalocele and gastroschisis.

10. Can the diagnosis of an omphalocele or gastroschisis be made prenatally?

Yes. The definitive means of detection is prenatal ultrasound. Because of improvements in method, abdominal wall defects can be detected as early as 10 weeks gestation. Several characteristics allow prenatal differentiation of omphalocele from gastroschisis by ultrasound. Detection of a membranous sac and protrusion of the liver are associated with omphalocele, whereas free-floating bowel is associated with fetuses with gastroschisis.

Other means of detection include measurement of maternal serum alpha fetoprotein (MS-AFP), which is elevated in both gastroschisis and omphalocele. Because elevation of MS-AFP is not specific for ventral wall defects, algorithms for MS-AFP screening have been proposed. A cutoff of two multiples of the mean for screening allows detection of 99% of gastroschisis and 78% of omphaloceles.

11. What is the importance of prenatal diagnosis?

Detection of abdominal wall defects in utero is important for several reasons. In the case of omphaloceles, a search for associated anomalies is made. Results affect prenatal care, timing and mode of delivery, and, in the case of multiple severe anomalies, potential termination of pregnancy. In addition, early parental counseling can be initiated with perinatologists, obstetricians, neonatologists, pediatric surgeons, and ethicists. Such a team approach optimizes prenatal, perinatal, and postnatal care by involving all caregivers who understand the therapeutic options and natural history of the birth defect.

12. What is the best method for delivering a child with an abdominal wall defect?

Most studies show that cesarean section provides no significant advantage over vaginal delivery. One exception is the fetus with a large omphalocele. Several reports have documented dystocia and liver damage during vaginal delivery.

Some experts also recommend early preterm delivery of infants with gastroschisis to avoid excessive exposure to the irritating effects of amniotic fluid. However, most reports do not support this practice. In most cases, therefore, the mode and timing of delivery should be based on obstetric factors—not on the mere presence of an abdominal wall defect.

13. Define the principles of immediate postnatal management in infants with abdominal wall defects.
Infants born with abdominal wall defects are subject to three serious problems at birth. Management is directed at correcting hypovolemia, preventing hypothermia, and monitoring for signs of sepsis. Exposed bowel leads to increased loss of insensible fluid as well as heat loss. Immediate management includes placing the lower half of the infant, including exposed viscera, in a bowel bag ("turkey bag") or wrapping the viscera in sterile gauze; placing the infant in a warmer; initiating intravenous access and fluids; obtaining an airway in cases of respiratory distress; and placement of an orogastric tube to decompress the bowel and decrease the risk of aspiration. Parenteral antibiotics also are initiated soon after delivery to decrease the risk of sepsis.

14. What are the guidelines for fluid resuscitation in newborn infants?
Newborns with abdominal wall defects experience inordinate fluid losses and have been shown to require 2.5–3 times the fluid of normal infants. Fluid resuscitation is begun with a 20 ml/kg fluid bolus with dextrose in 10% lactated Ringer's solution. Additional crystalloid or colloid is continued to achieve a rate of approximately 175 ml/kg/24 hr. A bladder catheter is placed to monitor urine output, and intravenous fluid administration is adjusted to achieve adequate urine output, tissue perfusion, pulse, and blood pressure. The bladder catheter also is used to monitor bladder pressure postoperatively to prevent visceral compartment syndrome if primary closure is performed. Electrolytes, arterial blood gases and serum glucose also should be closely monitored. The subset of infants with Beckwith-Weidemann syndrome are subject to profound hypoglycemia.

15. Some newborns with gastroschisis have evidence of bowel ischemia in the delivery room. How are they managed?
Early bowel ischemia generally results from strangulation due to an abdominal wall defect that is too small. The defect requires prompt enlargement in the delivery room. An emergent upper midline incision should be made in the defect. This incision should relax both skin and fascia. Care should be taken to avoid injury to the bowel, liver, and umbilical vein. The bowel should be inspected to rule out a twist as the cause of vascular compromise. Placing the infant in the left lateral decubitus position optimizes venous return and cardiac output.

16. How is the timing of abdominal wall closure determined?
For infants with gastroschisis or ruptured omphaloceles, surgery is performed as soon as possible after the infant is stabilized because of the higher fluid loss associated with exposed bowel. In some centers, surgery is performed in the delivery room.
Infants with intact omphaloceles do not require urgent surgical intervention. They should undergo evaluation for associated anomalies and closure, if appropriate.

17. What are the options for surgical closure? How do you choose between them?
There are essentially two options: primary closure or staged closure. Most infants with gastroschisis can be closed primarily (80–90%), but primary closure should not be performed if it will significantly compromise ventilation or abdominal viscera. Reduction usually is performed under general anesthesia with careful attention to ventilation. A maximal ventilatory pressure of 25 cm is used as a safe guideline to determine whether primary closure is feasible. If primary closure is not deemed safe, a staged procedure is performed (i.e., silo formation).

18. How is primary closure performed?
The steps for primary closure are straightforward. The abdominal wall defect is extended 1–2 cm superiorly and inferiorly. The abdominal wall cavity is stretched manually. The meconium in

the colon is reduced by manual compression through the anus. The viscera then are carefully reduced into the abdominal cavity as long as acceptable intraabdominal pressure is maintained (see questions 19 and 20). The abdominal wall fascia is closed in a single layer. Skin can be closed using a subcuticular running suture. Whenever possible, an umbilicus is reconstructed.

19. What methods are available to measure intraabdominal pressure?

Several methods are available to quantitate intraabdominal pressure and have proved useful in determining whether primary closure is possible. Examples include CVP measurement, intravesicular pressure, and intragastric pressure.

20. Describe staged closure.

Staged closure involves placing a reinforced silastic silo over the exposed viscera and attaching it to the fascia. Silos come in prefabricated versions or can be custom fabricated using sheets of reinforced silastic (0.03-inch thickness). Slowly the silo contents are reduced into the abdominal cavity. Most infants can be closed within 7–10 days using this method. The silo protects the herniated bowel and redirects the pressure in the abdomen to promote enlargement of the abdominal cavity.

21. When is staged closure appropriate?

Currently the decision to use a silo is based primarily on clinical criteria. High-risk infants or those with large defects generally are not closed primarily. Studies have shown that intragastric pressure greater than 20 mmHg or a rise in central venous pressure greater than 4 mmHg is associated with intolerance of primary closure. Lacey et al. have shown that intraabdominal pressure less than 20 mmHg, as measured indirectly by intravesicular pressure monitoring, is associated with safe primary closure.

22. Describe the construction of a silo.

After reduction of as much bowel as the child will tolerate, silastic sheets are sutured to the fascia. The silastic sheets then are sutured together with walls perpendicular to the abdominal cavity to avoid a funnel shape. Nonabsorbable suture is used throughout. Betadine ointment is placed at the base of the silo, which then is wrapped in sterile gauze for support. Under sterile conditions, the silo is reduced over the next several days. A special roller clamp has been manufactured for this purpose, but various other methods are available.

23. What is the role of nonoperative management of omphaloceles?

Nonoperative management is reserved for infants with extremely large defects or small abdominal cavities or high-risk infants such as those with severe congenital heart defects, pentalogy of Cantrell, or trisomy 13 or 18.

24. What methods are available for nonoperative management?

One method uses topical application of an agent to promote eschar formation. Several agents have been used, such as mercurochrome, silver sulfadiazine, 70% alcohol, and silver nitrate. An alternative method for large omphaloceles involves placement of an elastic wrap, such as op-site, that allows gradual reduction of viscera into the abdominal cavity and epithelialization.

25. What must be monitored if mercurochrome or betadine is used?

With mercurochrome, serum levels of mercury must be monitored to prevent mercury toxicity, which can lead to death. With betadine, iodine levels should be monitored because iodine toxicity has been described. Therefore, both techniques should be avoided.

26. What are the alternatives for closure of the abdomen if prosthetic material for a silo is not available?

Alternatives to prosthetic material include dura, an intact omphalocele sac, amnion, mesh, an empty plastic IV bag, or tissue expanders to create a skin flap.

27. What disadvantage do these methods have in common?
They leave a ventral hernia unless the fascia is closed at a later date.

28. Name a theoretical risk specific to the use of dura for closure.
There is a slight risk of transmission of Jacob-Creuzfeldt disease.

29. What is the mortality rate in infants with omphaloceles?
Mortality rates range from 30% to 60%.

30. Survival of infants with omphaloceles depends on which four factors?
- Size of the defect
- Prematurity
- Sac rupture
- Associated anomalies (most important)

31. What two factors primarily contributed to improved survival in the 1970s?
Parenteral nutrition and staged closure.

32. What is the expected mortality rate for infants with gastroschisis?
10%.

33. Identify five ways to clinically distinguish an omphalocele from a gastroschisis.
- **Location of defect**. A gastroschisis is located lateral to the cord (usually on the right), whereas omphaloceles are defects of the umbilical ring.
- **Cord**. The cord inserts into the sac in an omphalocele and is inserted normally in a gastroschisis.
- **Sac**. A gastroschisis has no sac. An omphalocele usually has a sac or, if it ruptures in utero, a remnant of a sac.
- **Defect size**. Omphaloceles normally have larger defects.
- **Content of defect**. Gastroschisis contains hollow viscera and occasionally tubes and ovaries, but never liver. Omphaloceles, on the other hand, commonly contain liver as well as all of the above.

34. What is the most common postoperative complication after repair of gastroschisis?
Prolonged adynamic ileus is common in the postoperative period. Most children can take all of their calories enterally by 1 month. Because intestinal atresia is present in 10% of cases, it must be ruled out in children with signs of obstruction.

35. What is the long-term outlook for children with abdominal wall defects?
Studies have shown that such children are prone to growth delay and lower IQ, even with normal bowel function.

36. Should an appendectomy be performed at the time of the original operation?
Because all children with abdominal wall defects have malrotation, appendicitis may present atypically in the future. Many pediatric surgeons recommend removal of the appendix if it is available at the time of the original operation. Appendectomy should not be performed in tight primary closure or delayed closure involving prostatic material.

37. Define amniotic band syndrome. How is it related to abdominal wall defects?
Amniotic bands are ringlike constrictions of the skin apparently due to premature separation of the amnion from the chorion, which gives rise to strands of amnion that can disrupt normal morphogenesis. Multiple defects may arise, including abdominal wall defects, limb amputations, and craniofacial defects.

38. Describe three options for managing an associated intestinal atresia in infants with gastroschisis.

The three options are primary resection with reanastomosis, creation of a stoma, and delayed resection after resolution of inflammation. The best option is controversial and usually is determined by surgeon preference and condition of the bowel.

39. Describe the appearance of bowel in children with gastroschisis.

The bowel appears inflamed, thickened, matted, and foreshortened.

40. What organs are most commonly herniated in gastroschisis? In omphalocele?

Stomach, small bowel, and large bowel are most commonly eviscerated in a gastroschisis. The liver is rarely herniated. In omphaloceles, the stomach and intestines are herniated. The liver also is herniated in about 50% of cases of omphalocele.

41. What is the male-to-female ratio for gastroschisis and omphalocele?

Omphalocele, 1.5:1; gastroschisis, 1:1.

42. Describe the potential complications when the liver is reduced into the abdominal cavity.

Reduction of the liver can be complicated by adherence to the sac. Therefore, when reducing the liver, one must take care not to cause torsion of the hepatic veins and portal vein or tear the liver capsule. The former can lead to chronic decrease in venous return and cardiac output, and the latter can cause life-threatening exsanguination.

BIBLIOGRAPHY

1. Bethel C, Seashore J, Touloukian R: Caeserean section does not improve outcome in gastroschisis. J Pediatr Surg 24:1, 1989.
2. Cooney DR: Defects in the abdominal wall. In O'Neill JA Jr, Rowe MI, Grosfeld JL, et al (eds): Pediatric Surgery. St. Louis, Mosby, 1998.
3. Duhamel B: Embryology of exomphalos and allied malformations. Arch Dis Child 38:142, 1963.
4. Glick PL, et al: The missing link in the pathogenesis of gastroschisis. J Pediatr Surg 20:406, 1985.
5. Glick PL, et al: Maternal serum alpha-fetoprotein is a marker for fetal anomalies in pediatric surgery. J Pediatr Surg 23:16, 1988.
6. Ingalls TM, et al: Genetic determinants of hypoxia-induced congenital anomalies. J Hered 44:185, 1953.
7. Jones KL: Smith's Recognizable Patterns of Human Malformations, 4th ed. Philadelphia, W.B. Saunders, 1988.
8. Kirk EP, Wah RM: Obstetric management of the fetus with omphalocele or gastroschisis: A review and report of one hundred twelve cases. Am J Obstet Gynecol 146:512, 1983.
9. Klein P, et al: Short-term and long-term problems after Duraplastic enlargement of the anterior abdominal wall. Eur J Pediatr Surg 1:88, 1991.
10. Lacey SR, et al: Bladder pressure monitoring significantly enhances care of the infant with abdominal wall defects: A prospective clinical study. J Pediatr Surg 28:1370, 1993.
11. Lacey SR, et al: Relative merits of various methods of indirect measurement of intraabdominal pressure as a guide to closure of abdominal wall defects. J Pediatr Surg 22:1207, 1987.
12. Langer JC: Gastroschisis and omphalocele. Semin Pediatr Surg 5:124, 1996.
13. Nakayama DK, et al: Management of the fetus with an abdominal wall defect. J Pediatr Surg 19:408, 1984.
14. Nelson MM, et al: Multiple congenital abnormalities resulting from transitory deficiency of pteroylglutamic acid during gestation in the rat. J Nutr 56:349, 1955.
15. Palomaki GE, et al: Second trimester maternal serum alpha-fetoprotein levels in pregnancies associated with gastroschisis and omphalocele. Obstet Gynecol 71:906, 1988.
16. Phillipart AI, Canty TG, Filler RM: Acute fluid volume requirements in infants with anterior abdominal wall defects. J Pediatr Surg 7:553, 1972.
17. Rowe MI, O'Neill JA, Grosfeld JL, et al (eds): Essentials of Pediatric Surgery. St. Louis, Mosby, 1995.
18. Schuster SR: A new method for staged repair of large omphaloceles. Surg Gynecol Obstet 125:837, 1967.
19. Sermer M, et al: Prenatal diagnosis and management of congenital defects of the anterior abdominal wall. Am J Obstet Gynecol 156:308, 1987.

20. Stanley-Brown EG, Frank J: Mercury poisoning from application to omphalocele. JAMA 216:2144, 1971.
21. Sawin R, et al: Gastroschisis Wringer clamp: A safe, simplified method for delayed primary closure. J Pediatr Surg 27:1346, 1992.
22. Thompson DJ: Obstructed labour with complicated presentation and exomphalos. BMJ 2:45, 1944.
23. Warkany J, Takacs E: Experimental production of congenital malformations in rats by salicylate poisoning. Am J Pathol 35:315, 1959.

23. PRUNE-BELLY SYNDROME, BLADDER EXSTROPHY, AND CLOACAL EXSTROPHY

Scott C. Boulanger, M.D., Ph.D., Michael G. Caty, M.D., and Philip L. Glick, M.D.

PRUNE-BELLY SYNDROME

1. Who coined the term prune-belly syndrome? By what other names is the syndrome known?

The term *prune-belly syndrome* was coined in 1901 by William Osler because of the wrinkled appearance of the abdominal wall in affected patients. Prune-belly syndrome also is known as the triad syndrome, because it has three major manifestations (see Question 4), and Eagle-Barrett syndrome.

2. What is the incidence of prune-belly syndrome?

The incidence is approximately 1 in 50,000 live births. It is much more common in males than females.

3. Describe the three major theories for the development of prune-belly syndrome.

One theory postulates that the yolk sac does not resorb. The abdomen closes around it, leaving the abdominal musculature highly redundant. Another theory suggests that the dilated urinary tract causes redundancy in the abdominal wall. The mesodermal defect theory suggests that abnormal migration of the thoracic somites is responsible.

4. What are the three major manifestations of prune-belly syndrome?

Urinary tract malformations, cryptorchidism, and absent or deficient abdominal wall musculature are present in fully expressed prune-belly syndrome. The term *pseudo–prune-belly syndrome* has been coined to describe males who do not fully manifest all three abnormalities and females with abnormalities in abdominal wall musculature.

5. What percentage of patients with prune-belly syndrome have normal kidneys?

Approximately 50% have normal kidneys. The other 50% display a range of renal dysplasia, up to and including renal agenesis (Potter's syndrome). The two kidneys may have differing degrees of dysplasia.

6. Describe the most common genitourinary manifestation in prune-belly syndrome.

Ureteral dilatation is the most common genitourinary abnormality. The ureters typically are long and tortuous, but the degree of abnormality varies between the two ureters and from patient to patient. Moreover, the distal third of the ureters generally is more dilated than the proximal two-thirds. The dilatation usually does not result from obstruction. Histologic examination confirms some deficiency in the smooth muscle of the ureters.

7. Is ureteral obstruction present?

Hardly ever. The dilatation of the ureters and the ureteropelvic junction is the result of decreased smooth muscle and increased collagen. Moreover, the degree of dilatation and tortuosity is much greater than in patients with obstruction due to urethral valves.

8. Vesicoureteral reflux is present in what percentage of patients?

About 80%.

9. Vesicoureteral reflux and urine stasis often result in what complication?

Reflux and stasis can lead to infection. The resulting inflammation and fibrosis can lead to a deterioration of renal function if not treated appropriately. All tests that involve intubation of the urinary tract should be covered with antibiotics.

10. Describe the appearance of the bladder in patients with prune-belly syndrome.

The bladder usually is quite enlarged and sometimes contains a diverticular-shaped dome. The muscle wall is thick and highly vascular without trabeculations. Muscle usually is deficient, but collagen and fibrous tissue are abundant. The ureteral orifices are displaced laterally and dilated. The urachus may remain patent, especially if urethral atresia is present.

11. Do most patients have normal urodynamics?

Surprisingly, the answer is yes. Patients often are able to empty their bladder completely. Those who cannot are at significant risk of urinary infection.

12. Where are the testes usually located in prune-belly syndrome?

The testes, whicy usually are smaller than normal, typically lie intra-abdominally above the ureters at the level of the iliac arteries, but they may lie as high as the inferior pole of the kidney.

13. Why are male patients sterile but not impotent?

Although the testes of infants appear normal, cell maturation over time is insufficient. The defect in spermatogenesis, along with deficiencies in production of prostatic fluid, results in sterility. Such patients are not impotent, but they are subject to retrograde ejaculation.

14. Do patients have an increased risk of testicular malignancy?

Yes. The risk of malignancy appears to be increased, but it is no higher than that of normal patients with cryptorchidism.

15. What area of the abdominal wall is primarily deficient?

The main deficiency is found in the lower portion of the abdominal wall. The rectus muscles and internal and external obliques are less well developed than in the upper abdomen.

16. Why does the wrinkled appearance of the abdominal wall diminish over time?

Over time adipose tissues deposit in the subcutaneous tissue of the abdominal wall. This process tends to decrease the wrinkled appearance after the first year of life.

17. The deficiency of abdominal wall musculature places patients at greater anesthetic risk. Why?

The deficiency in abdominal wall musculature can lead to retention of pulmonary secretions and subsequent pneumonia.

18. What skeletal, gastrotintestinal, and cardiac anomalies are common?

The most common skeletal abnormality is dislocation or dysplasia of the hip. Polydactyly, limb absence, and pectus excavatum, among others, also have been reported. Malrotation is common, but midgut volvulus is rare. Imperforate anus may been seen in severe forms of the syndrome. A large variety of cardiac malformations have been reported. Up to 10% of patients have some cardiac ab-normalities, most commonly patent ductus ateriosum and atrial and ventricular septal defects.

19. What radiographic tests should be obtained in newborns with prune-belly syndrome?
Ultrasound of the kidneys and urinary tract should be obtained. A voiding cystourethrogram is obtained at 4 months of age to evaluate for reflux. Diethylenetriamine penta-acetic acid (DPTA) scans also are obtained around this time to assess renal function. In addition, ultrasound of the heart and abdominal and chest radiographs should be obtained.

20. What factor limits survival in patients with prune-belly syndrome?
The limiting factor in survival is most often the degree of severity of the genitourinary mal-formation. If prune-belly syndrome is associated with Potter's syndrome, pulmonary develop-ment often limits survival.

21. Is urinary diversion indicated in newborns?
Usually not. It is indicated for infants with a documented site of obstruction, which is rare in prune-belly syndrome. The simplest method of diversion is percutaneous nephrostomy, es-pecially in the presence of a dilated renal pelvis. If the renal pelvis is not dilated, cutaneous ureterostomy may be a better option, although it may lead to more difficult reconstruction later.

22. When should surgical reconstruction be considered?
Timing is quite controversial. Some experts advocate immediate reconstruction, believing that it reduces the risk of infection and progressive renal failure. However, results of reconstruc-tion have not been uniformly positive. Other experts recommend nonoperative management be-cause urinary tract function often improves with age. Indications for reconstruction include recurrent infection and worsening renal function.

23. By what age should orchidopexy be performed? Abdominoplasty?
It generally is recommended that orchidopexy be performed by age 2 years. The purpose of orchidopexy is psychologial, not functional. Abdominoplasty may be performed at any time, but often it is done at the time of other surgery.

BLADDER EXSTROPHY

24. Describe the anatomic abnormality in bladder exstrophy.
Bladder exstrophy is a defect of the anterior bladder wall and abdominal wall. It results in ex-posure of the bladder and urethra. In addition, the pubic bones are splayed open to varying degrees.

25. How common is bladder exstrophy?
The incidence is between 1 in 10,000 and 1 in 40,000 live births. The male-to-female ratio is approximately 4:1.

26. Describe the most likely embryogenesis of bladder exstrophy.
Most experts believe that bladder exstrophy is a result of overdevelopment of the cloacal membrane. Rupture of the membrane after the cloaca has been divided into the urogenital sinus and the rectum results in exstrophy.

27. Describe the range of anatomic variants of bladder exstrophy. What percentage is made up of classic bladder exstrophy?
The exstrophy complex is a spectrum of malformations. The range includes pubic diastasis, female epispadias, male epispadias, classic bladder exstrophy, superior vesical fistula, duplex

exstrophy, bladder exstrophy with imperforate anus, and cloacal exstrophy. Classic bladder exstrophy is present in 50% of cases.

28. How should the umbilical cord and exposed bladder mucosa be managed at birth?
The umbilical stump should be sutured closed instead of clamped, and moist, nonadherent dressings should cover the exposed bladder mucosa. These steps should prevent damage to the bladder plate.

29. When should bladder reconstruction begin?
Bladder reconstruction is performed in a staged fashion. The first step is performed in the immediate neonatal period. The pliability of the pelvic ring in neonates allows pelvic and often bladder closure.

30. What are the steps for staged bladder reconstruction?
The first step is primary closure of the bladder and pelvis, which involves iliac osteotomies to close the pelvic ring and creation of paraexstrophy flaps to close the bladder. Epispadias repair in males usually is performed at 1 year of age. In males and females continent reconstruction is performed at 4 years of age. Before this stage the kidneys and urinary tract should be evaluated thoroughly with ultrasound, voiding cystourethrography, and urodynamics. At this time bladder augmentation may be performed for patients with inadequate capacity.

31. When should urinary diversion be performed instead of reconstruction?
Most patients should undergo staged reconstruction. Urinary diversion is reserved for patients with inadequate bladder plates and the 10–20% who remain incontinent after reconstruction.

CLOACAL EXSTROPHY

32. What is cloacal exstrophy? How common is it?
Cloacal exstrophy involves an anterior abdominal wall defect in which the two hemibladders are visible and separated by a midline intestinal plate, an omphalocele, and an imperforate anus. This anomaly is seen in only 1 in 100,000 to 200,000 live births. The male-to-female ratio is roughly 1:1. With current management techniques, survival rates have increased from 50% to 90%.

33. How common are associated anomalies?
Gastrointestinal, skeletal, and renal abnormalities are quite common.

34. Why are most patients assigned a female gender?
Patients often are assigned a female gender because the phallic structures usually are inadequate to perform a male reconstruction. This topic, however, is quite controversial. Every case must be considered individually by a multispecialty team, including pediatric surgeons, pediatric urologists, pediatric orthopedists, neonatologists, psychologists, endocrinologists, geneticists, ethicists, and the child's family.

35. Is the embryogenesis similar in cloacal and bladder esxtrophy?
Yes. In the case of cloacal exstrophy, the cloacal membrane is believed to rupture before the cloaca divides into the urogenital sinus and rectum.

36. What is generally the first step in surgical repair?
Closure of the omphalocele is performed first; bladder closure may be performed at the same time. Intestinal reconstruction with end colostomy is the third step. These procedures are performed in the neonatal period. Epispadias repair is performed at 1 year of age in males and continent reconstruction at 4 years of age, as in patients with exstrophy of the bladder. On some occasions, anal reconstruction can be performed if the pelvic floor is adequate.

BIBLIOGRAPHY

1. Brock JW III, O'Neill JA Jr: Bladder exstrophy. In O'Neill JA Jr, Rowe MI, Grosfeld JL, et al (eds): Pediatric Surgery. St. Louis, Mosby, 1998, pp 1709–1725.
2. Geskovich FJ III, Nyberg LM Jr: The prune belly syndrome: Review of its etiology, defects, treatment and prognosis. J Urol 140:707–712, 1988.
3. Hendren WH, Carr MC, Adams MC: Megaureter and prune belly syndrome. In O'Neill JA Jr, Rowe MI, Grosfeld JL, et al (eds): Pediatric Surgery. St. Louis, Mosby, 1998, pp 1631–1652.
4. O'Neill JA: Cloacal exstrophy. In O'Neill JA Jr, Rowe MI, Grosfeld JL, et al (eds): Pediatric Surgery. St. Louis, Mosby, 1998, pp 1725–1731.
5. Rowe MI, O'Neill JA, Grosfeld JL, et al (eds): Essentials of Pediatric Surgery. St. Louis, Mosby, 1995.

VI. Gastroenterology

24. NORMAL EMBRYOLOGY, ANATOMY, AND PHYSIOLOGY OF THE GASTROINTESTINAL TRACT

Charles N. Paidas, M.D.

1. What is gastrulation?

Gastrulation is the process of transformation from a bilaminar (endoderm and ectoderm) to a trilaminar germ disc (endoderm, ectoderm, and mesoderm). The mesoderm is derived from epiblasts as are the ecto- and endoderm. The ectoderm lines the amnion, the endoderm lines the yolk sac, and the mesoderm migrates between the two other layers. Gastrulation occurs during the third week of embryogenesis.

2. Why is gastrulation important?

Transformation to a three-layer germ disc facilitates the formation of all germ cell derivatives. In addition, it establishes bilateral symmetry and the craniocaudal axis of the embryo. Without all three germ cell layers, the embryo is doomed to death or teratology.

3. From which areas of the developing gut is mesoderm excluded?

The buccopharyngeal membrane and the cloacal membrane. The buccopharyngeal membrane gives rise to the oral cavity. The cloacal membrane disintegrates and gives rise to openings for the anus and urinary tract.

4. What are the major derivatives of ectoderm, endoderm, and mesoderm?

Ectoderm: epidermis, central and peripheral nervous systems, mammary glands, pituitary gland, adrenal medulla, distal rectum, and anus.

Mesoderm: connective tissue, muscle, bone, cartilage, blood, lymphocytes, lymphatics, heart, adrenal cortex, kidneys, gonads, and spleen.

Endoderm: endothelium, epithelium of the gastrointestinal tract up to the proximal rectum, lungs and bronchi, urinary tract, thyroid, parathyroid, liver, gallbladder, common bile duct, and pancreas.

5. When is organogenesis complete within the embryo?

In general, all organs are formed by the eighth week of gestation.

6. What is the definition of embryonic period? Fetal period?

The embryonic period is defined as the time between gastrulation and organogenesis (weeks 4–8). The Carnegie Collection of Human Embryos consists of 23 development stages based on the morphologic states of development of the human embryo and corresponds to weeks 1–8 of gestation. Bone marrow formation in the humerus begins in the fetal period, usually the at the eighth to ninth week of gestation. It is a time of growth and maturation that culminates at 38 weeks gestation.

7. When is intestinal rotation completed in the embryo?

Intestinal rotation is completed at the tenth week of gestation. At the same time the abdominal coelomic cavity closes.

8. What is the omphalomesenteric duct? What is its clinical significance?
Also called the vitelline duct or yolk stalk, the omphalomesenteric duct connects the yolk sac to the intestinal tract to provide nutrients for the embryo. As the embryo grows and no longer requires the yolk sac, the omphalomesenteric duct fuses with both the body stalk and umbilical vessels to form the umbilical cord. Vestigial remnants of the omphalomesenteric duct or failure to obliterate completely may result in a polyp, sinus, cyst, fibrous cord, and fistula. The best-known omphalomesenteric remnant is the Meckel diverticulum.

9. What is normal rotation of the intestinal tract?
The intestinal tract normally rotates 270° counterclockwise along the axis of the superior mesenteric artery.

10. What is the normal relationship of the duodenum and superior mesenteric artery?
The duodenum normally lies beneath the artery.

11. Which abdominal structures are considered retroperitoneal?
The duodenum, ascending and descending colon, inferior vena cava, aorta, kidneys, ureters, pancreas, and adrenal glands.

12. What are the derivatives of the foregut, midgut, and hindgut?
Foregut: pharynx, entire esophagus, lungs, pharyngeal pouches, stomach and duodenum (up to the ampulla), liver, gallbladder, biliary tree, and pancreas.
Midgut: duodenum below the ampulla, jejunum, ileum, ascending colon, and proximal two-thirds of the transverse colon.
Hindgut: distal one-third of the transverse colon, descending and sigmoid colon, and rectum.

13. What structures hold the stomach in place and prevent gastric volvulus?
The stomach is held in place by the esophageal hiatus, phrenoesophageal ligament, fixation of the duodenum in the retroperitoneum, short gastric vessels, and gastrocolic ligament. Gastric volvulus, which probably results from abnormal fixation of the these structures, is classified as either organoaxial or mesenteroaxial. Organoaxial volvulus is rotation of the stomach along its long axis; the greater curvature rotates anteriorly or posteriorly. Mesenteroaxial volvulus is rotation on an axis drawn from the greater to the lesser curvature.

14. Is omphalocele associated with failure of rotation?
Yes. In fact, the failure of the midgut to return into the abdominal coelomic cavity by the tenth week of gestation is a probable cause for the development of an omphalocele.

15. What are the sources of intrauterine and postnatal hematopoiesis?
Blood-forming organs during intrauterine life include the liver, spleen, and thymus. The spleen continues to be a source of red blood cells until 5 months of age; afterward the bone marrow is the sole source of hematopoiesis.

16. Does the position of the cecum in a barium enema help to diagnose malrotation?
No. The cecum can be positioned anywhere on the right side of the abdominal cavity. Its free-floating position makes it a poor indicator of the rotational status of the gut.

17. What is the osmolarity of full-strength gastrograffin?
1900 mOsm/L. However, we usually use half strength or quarter strength for any diagnostic or therapeutic enema.

18. What are the normal constituents of chyle?
B lymphocytes, triglycerides, white blood cells, and protein (> 3 gm/dl). Its specific gravity is greater than 1.015.

19. **In what percentage of the population is asymptomatic malrotation discovered at autopsy?**
20%.

20. **What are typical caloric and electrolyte requirements for a healthy, full-term newborn?**
- Total calories = 120 kcal/kg/day
- Sodium = 2–3 mEq/kg/day
- Protein = 2–3 gm/kg/day
- Potassium = 1–2 mEq/kg/day

21. **What is the caloric concentration of protein, fat, and carbohydrate in kcal/gm?**
- Protein = 4.0 kcal/gm
- Fat = 9.0 kcal/gm
- Carbohydrate = 3.4 kcal/gm

22. **What is the relationship of total body, extracellular, and intracellular water to body weight from birth to adulthood?**
A classic analysis of body water compartments was done by Friis-Hansen. Total body water is approximately 75% of body weight at birth and slowly falls to 60% by 1 year of life, where it remains through adulthood. Extracellular water is 45% of body weight at term and, like total body water, continues to fall postnatally. Adult levels of 20–25% are reached by 1–2 years of age. In contrast, intracellular water is 30% at term and rises to adult levels of 45% by 3–4 months of age. In summary, there is a shift from extracellular to intracellular water from fetal to neonatal life; relative total body water and extracellular water decrease with gestational age and adulthood.

23. **The terminal ileum is necessary for absorption of which nutrients?**
Vitamins A, D, E, and K (fat-soluble vitamins), vitamin B_{12}/intrinsic factor complex, and bile salts.

24. **The umbilical cord normally is composed of which structures? Where do they communicate?**
The umbilical cord normally is composed of two arteries and one vein. The right umbilical vein disintegrates, but the left umbilical vein traverses the liver and becomes the ductus venosus, providing venous flow to the suprahepatic cava. The left umbilical vein is not part of the portal circulation. However, a catheter in the umbilical vein may obstruct flow in the portal circulation by causing thrombosis and stasis of the tributaries of the ductus venosus.

25. **What is the normal epithelium of the intestinal wall from mouth to anus?**
Squamous mucosa lines the oropharynx, and columnar epithelium lines the esophagus, stomach, and intestinal tract to the anus. At the anus the mucosa again becomes squamous. The junction of the columnar and squamous cells of the rectum and anus is called the dentate or pectinate line.

26. **Describe the innervation of the bowel.**
Intestinal innervation can be divided into an intrinsic (relaxation) and extrinsic (contraction) system. The intrinsic system consists of neurotransmitters located in Meissner, Auerbach, and Henle ganglia within the muscularis mucosa and between the circular and longitudinal muscle layers of the bowel wall. Common neurotransmitters located within these ganglia include nitric oxide and gamma-aminobutyric acid. The extrinsic system is composed of the vagus nerve, sacral plexus, and sympathetic chain. The two systems communicate in the wall of the intestine to coordinate a balance of contraction and relaxation.

27. **What happens to the circular and longitudinal muscle of the rectum as it becomes the anus?**
The outer longitudinal smooth muscle interdigitates as connective tissue with the striated muscle of the external sphincter. The inner circular smooth muscle of the bowel wall thickens to become the internal sphincter.

28. What is the normal quantity of gastric output in newborns?
15–20 ml/kg/day of a secretion virtually identical to normal saline.

29. Why should soy-based formulas be avoided in preterm infants?
Soy-based formulas, such as Isomil and Prosobee, contain phytates that bind calcium and phosphorus, resulting in hypocalcemia and osteopenia, respectively. Breast milk can be fortified for use in preterm infants.

30. Why is the sodium requirement of a preterm newborn higher than that of a full-term newborn?
In preterm infants the fractional excretion of sodium is much higher because renal absorption of sodium is much less efficient; therefore, sodium requirements approach 10 mEq/kg/day.

31. What is the role of glutamine in the intestinal tract?
The amino acid glutamine generally is regarded as the principal fuel source for gut mucosa. Lack of glutamine supplementation causes reduced levels of immunoglobulin A and increased bacterial translocation. Parenteral nutrition supplemented with glutamine has been shown to reverse the depression of gut-associated lymphoid tissue.

32. What is the action of omeprazole on the gastric musoca?
Omeprazole stops gastric acid secretion by inhibition of the hydrogen-potassium-adenosine triphosphatase enzyme system of the parietal cell. This enzyme system is the acid or proton pump within the gastric mucosa; its inhibition shuts down acid production. Omeprazole is not an anticholinergic or an H_2 antagonist. Serum gastrin levels usually increase during the first two weeks of administration but then plateau.

33. What is the action of metaclopramide on the gastrointestinal tract? Where does it have its greatest effect?
Metaclopramide stimulates contraction of the gastric antrum, relaxes the pylorus and duodenal bulb, and increases peristalsis of the duodenum and jejunum. Thus, metaclopramide preferentially stimulates motility of the upper gastrointestinal tract. It has no effect on either the gallbladder or colon. Although its mechanism of action is unknown, it is used to treat gastroesophageal reflux as well as delayed gastric emptying. Effects of metaclopramide do not depend on vagal stimulation, but anticholinergic medications may abolish its actions.

34. How long does it take for intestinal flora to colonize the gut after birth?
2–3 days.

35. What is the role of gastrin in the intestinal tract?
Gastrin belongs to a family of gastrointestinal peptides produced by G cells of the antrum and duodenum. Gastrin stimulates gastric acid and promotes cell proliferation in the stomach, small bowel, and colon. The most important stimulus for gastrointestinal peptide secretion is food. For gastrin, polypeptides and amino acids in the antrum are the most important food stimuli. Neither carbohydrates nor fats stimulate the release of gastrin. In addition, gastrin is stimulated by vagal discharge through gastrin-releasing peptide from nerve terminals. Gastric distention, alkalinization of the gastric antrum, short bowel syndrome, and hypercalcemia also cause release of gastrin. Antral acidification inhibits gastrin release through release of the inhibitory peptide somatostatin (from D cells of the antrum). Along with histamine and acetylcholine gastrin stimulates the parietal cell to make hydrochloric acid.

36. When is meconium aspiration a problem?
Meconium begins to accumulate in the gastrointestinal tract of a 3–4-month-old fetus. When an infant is asphyxiated or stressed in utero or at delivery, it usually passes meconium. However,

this response is rarely present before 34 weeks gestation. Thus, we rarely see meconium aspiration in a preterm newborn less than 34 weeks old.

37. What is the mechanism of action for cisapride?
Cisapride is a serotonin receptor agonist and promotes gastric motility by enhancing the release of acetylcholine at the myenteric plexus. It does not induce muscarinic or nicotinic receptor stimulation, nor does it inhibit acetylcholinesterase activity. Gastric acid is not affected by cisapride.

38. What electrocardiographic abnormality is associated with the use of cisapride?
Prolonged QT interval. The mechanism by which cisapride alters ventricular depolarization is unclear. However, QT prolongation causes ventricular arrhythmias and is associated with sudden infant death syndrome. An EKG is recommended for premature infants and newborns receiving cisapride.

39. What intestinal enzyme deficiency most commonly causes osmotic diarrhea?
Lactase deficiency. In contrast to a continuous watery stool output (secretory diarrhea), children with lactase deficiency have a significant postprandial increase in diarrhea (the hallmark of osmotic diarrhea). Lactose is a disaccharide composed of glucose and galactose. Normally, lactase breaks down the lactose, and the two products are absorbed. If malabsorption occurs, the carbohydrates remaining in the intestinal lumen increase the osmotic pressure. In addition, bacteria ferment the undigested carbohydrate (lactose) in both the terminal ileum and the colon, exacerbating the osmotic gradient and subsequent diarrhea. Extensive jejunal resection often leads to significant carbohydrate malabsorption due to the loss of the primary site of disaccharidase activity. Undigested and malabsorbed carbohydrate contributes to osmotic diarrhea.

40. Does an infant who has gastric residuals when fed a dilute formula benefit from undiluted formula?
Yes. Gastric emptying and intestinal motility are slowed with nutrients that are either hyposmolar or hyperosmolar compared with breast milk. Thus, breast is best!

41. What are the major components of bile?
Bile acids in the form of salts (cholic and chenodeoxycholic acids), bile pigment (bilirubin diglucuronide), cholesterol, phospholipids, proteins, electrolytes, and, of course, water. Secret tip: whenever you have electrolytes, you have water, but the converse is not necessarily true.

42. What is the role of bile acids in absorption of nutrients?
The bile acids, cholic and chenodeoxycholic acid, are made in the liver from cholesterol. Deoxycholic and lithocholic acid are formed by anaerobic bacteria in the intestine. All of these acids are conjugated with either glycine or taurine in the liver and then secreted into the bile salt pool as detergents for the storage and breakdown of fats. Unconjugated bile acids are reabsorbed in the terminal ileum and recirculated as a component of the enterohepatic circulation. Bile salt malabsorption following ileal resection may contribute to watery diarrhea and malabsorption of fat- and lipid-soluble vitamins.

43. How are proteins broken down in the intestinal tract?
Proteins undergo initial degradation into oligopeptides and amino acids in the stomach by the action of pepsin. When these degradation products enter the intestine, cholecystokinin and secretin stimulate the pancreas to secrete proteases (trypsin, chymotrypsin, carboxypeptidase, and elastase) and bicarbonate. Protein breakdown culminates with the absorption of individual amino acids and small peptides (dipeptides and tripeptides), using distinct transport systems. Amino acids generally are absorbed in the proximal gut (jejunum) and peptides throughout the intestinal tract (jejunum and ileum).

44. What is bethanecol?
Bethanecol stimulates the muscarinic parasympathetic nerves of the stomach and thus increases gastric tone. It also increases the tone and contraction of the bladder detrussor muscle. Nicotinic effects of cholinergic stimulation are not affected because of the selective action of bethanecol.

45. How long does it take for the newborn to develop intestinal flora similar to the adult?
3–5 days.

46. Human breast milk contains which carbohydrate? What is its caloric equivalent in kcal/oz?
Human breast milk contains lactose, a glucose/galactose disaccharide. Breast milk is 20 kcal/oz (two-thirds of a calorie per ml) and has an osmolarity of 300 mOsm/kg water.

47. Describe bowel lengthening from the antenatal period to adulthood.
Total intestinal length during 19–27 weeks is approximately 142 cm; it nearly doubles during the last trimester. Small intestine length at term ranges from 250 to 300 cm. The colon measures approximately 30–40 cm at term. Postnatal small bowel length increases to a maximum of 2.5–3.5 meters in adulthood, and the colon grows to 1.5–2 meters.

CONTROVERSIES

48. What is the optimal management of a child with gastroesophageal reflux and evidence of malrotation on upper gastrointestinal studies?
Fix the malrotation with a Ladd procedure, and hope that the reflux can be treated medically. Some surgeons include an antireflux procedure with the Ladd procedure.

49. What is the difference between nonrotation and malrotation?
Three letters! These terms frequently are used interchangeably—and incorrectly—in the literature. Nonrotation occurs when the intestine fails to undergo additional rotation after the duodenum makes its normal counterclockwise rotation. As a result, the cecum and ascending and descending colon are not retroperitoneal. Nonrotation occurs in children with congenital diaphragmatic hernia, omphalocele, or gastroschisis and occasionally in otherwise normal children. Malrotation is total or partial failure of fixation of the duodenum and remaining midgut.

50. What is the single best radiologic test for the diagnosis of the normal rotation of the intestinal tract?
Some physicians say barium enema, but the best test is the upper gastrointestinal series to look for the position of the duodenum with the ligament of Treitz across the midline to the left of the spine.

BIBLIOGRAPHY

1. Broussart DL: Gastrointestinal motility in the neonate. Clin Perinatol 22:37–59, 1995.
2. El-Dahr SS, Chevalier RL: Special needs of the newborn infant in fluid therapy. Pediatr Clin North Am 37:323–336, 1990,
3. Friis-Hansen B: Body water compartments in children. Changes during growth and related changes in body composition. Pediatrics 28:169–181, 1961.
4. Koenig WJ, Amarnath RP, Hench V, Berseth CL: Manometries for pre-term and term infants: A new tool for old questions. Pediatrics 95:203, 1995.
5. Larsen W: Human Embryology. New York, Churchill Livingstone, 1993.
6. Lewin MB, Bryant RM, Fenrich AL, Grifka RG: Cisapride-induced long QT interval. J Pediatr 128:279–281, 1996.
7. O'Rahilly R, Muller F: Developmental Stages in Human Embryos. Washington, DC, Carnegie Institution, 1989.
8. Schwartz PJ, Stramba-Badiale M, Segantini A, et al: Prolongation of the QT interval and the sudden infant death syndrome. N Engl J Med 338:1709–1714, 1998.

9. Souba WW, Herskowitz K, Salloum R, et al: Gut glutamine metabolism. J Parent Ent Nutr 14(Suppl): 40S–67S, 1990.
10. Touloukian RJ, Walker Smith GJ: Normal intestinal length in preterm infants. J Ped Surg 18:720–723, 1983.
11. Walker WA, Durie PR, Hamilton JR, et al: Anatomy and embryology. In Pediatric Gastrointestinal Disease: Pathophysiology, Diagnosis, Management, vol. 1, 2nd ed. St. Louis, Mosby, 1996, pp 9–30.

25. SMALL INTESTINAL OBSTRUCTION

Alfred A. de Lorimier, M.D.

1. What are the major causes of intestinal obstruction?
- Intussusception
- Adhesions
- Hernia
- Inflammation
- Volvulus
- Neoplasm
- Fecal impaction
- Enterocolitis of Hirschsprung's disease
- Meconium ileus equivalent
- Trauma
- Ileus

Each of these entities is discussed in detail in other chapters. This chapter focuses on the diagnosis and management of small bowel obstruction due to adhesions, but the general principles apply to bowel obstruction of any etiology.

2. What are adhesions? How do they cause intestinal obstruction?
Adhesions are collagenous bands of scar tissue that most commonly follow the trauma of a laparotomy. Adhesions may obstruct the intestine in several ways. The seromuscular layer of one loop of bowel may become densely adherent to another loop and in the process kink the intestine, much like bending a garden hose. Another form of adhesion may have the configuration of a single violin string or involve multiple bands of scar (similar to crabgrass) that entrap the intestine and block the bowel lumen.

Congenital adhesive bands are associated with malrotation of the midgut, remnants of the omphalomesenteric duct that bridge the ileum and umbilicus, or a persistent vitelline vein or artery remnant between the mesentery and umbilicus.

3. How frequently do adhesions cause intestinal obstruction?
Adhesions frequently develop after open abdominal operations. The incidence of adhesion formation may be less frequent with laparoscopic procedures. The risk of intestinal obstruction after a laparotomy may be as high as 10% over the lifetime of the patient. The risk of obstruction is higher after pelvic operations than after upper abdominal procedures.

4. What are the various kinds of bowel obstruction?
A **simple** intestinal obstruction occurs when one end of the bowel lumen is obstructed. A simple obstruction may be **complete** or **incomplete**.

In **closed-loop obstruction** both proximal and distal ends of a segment of intestine are obstructed. Closed-loop obstruction usually occurs when a loop of bowel has herniated through a narrow orifice, such as an indirect inguinal hernia or mesenteric defect, or when adhesive bands have formed. A volvulus may produce a closed-loop obstruction in the absence of compromised blood supply. Closed-loop obstruction also may occur in the large intestine when distal obstruction with an intact ileocecal valve that prevents decompression of colonic contents into the small bowel. The isolated loop becomes progressively distended with enteric fluid, because it cannot decompress through the intestine proximally.

5. What is the significance of a closed-loop obstruction?

In a closed-loop obstruction the bowel grows progressively dilated from the accumulated se-cretions. Over time the increasing pressure within the lumen is transmitted to the bowel wall and eventually exceeds the perfusion pressure of the circulation, resulting in gangrene. The bowel above the proximal point of obstruction accumulates swallowed air and enteric secretions, which are evi-dent on radiographs. However, the closed loop of bowel tends to be a gasless, fluid-filled mass.

6. What is a strangulating obstruction?

A strangulating obstruction occurs when the circulation to a segment of intestine is impaired. The ischemia progresses to gangrene without prompt operative repair. Volvulus, in which the mesenteric blood supply to the bowel becomes twisted, is the obvious example of strangulating obstruction. The other example is closed-loop obstruction (see Question 5). In the usual se-quence, the first step is venous compression; because arterial pressure is not yet compromised, the bowel wall and lumen become suffused (hemorrhagic) with blood. Subsequent cessation of all blood flow produces infarction.

7. Why is a strangulating obstruction more lethal than a simple obstruction?

The unique combination of bacteria and their toxins, blood, and necrotic tissue is particu-larly lethal. As these products are absorbed from the lymphatics and peritoneum, the result is septic shock with a high mortality rate.

8. What are the symptoms and signs of intestinal obstruction?

The three prominent symptoms are **pain, vomiting,** and **abdominal distention**.

9. Describe the pain of intestinal obstruction.

An obstruction in the proximal intestine produces a dull, constantly painful sense of epigas-tric fullness. More distal obstruction in the small bowel causes recurring, intermittent episodes of cramping pain or colic, located periumbilically. Typically the cramping begins abruptly with crescendo intensity, lasting for 1–3 minutes, and then subsides in decrescendo fashion. There may be a pain-free interval for a varying period, but colic recurs. Initially the waves of cramping occur at short intervals, but as the obstruction progresses, the bowel fatigues, and cramping be-comes more like a steady dull pain. The patient finds some relief by drawing the legs up and as-suming a fetal position.

10. What are borborygmi?

Borborygmi are the loud rumbling and gurgling sounds due to the movement of air and fluid that has puddled in the widely dilated bowel lumen. They are said to coincide with the waves of colic, but in reality the coincidence of colicky pain and the borborygmi is unusual.

11. What is the character of the vomiting?

Initially vomiting may be a reflex response, and the emesis consists only of gastric contents. The intestine responds to obstruction with increased peristaltic activity. In addition, the mucosa no longer absorbs luminal fluids, and fluid secretion into the lumen increases. As the volume of fluid backs up to the stomach, the emesis becomes greenish-brown and develops a fecalent odor. The fecalent odor does not imply a colonic obstruction; it is due to the overgrowth of enteric or-ganisms in the luminal fluid. *Bilious vomiting must be considered a sign of intestinal obstruction until proved otherwise.* A distal ileal obstruction may not produce bilious vomiting for a pro-longed period after the onset of obstruction because of the distance that enteric contents must travel back to the stomach.

12. Is the presence of abdominal distention necessary for a diagnosis of bowel obstruction?

No. The abdomen is not distended with proximal bowel obstruction. Because it takes time for the accumulation of swallowed air and fluid to fill the obstructed intestine, the abdomen is not distended in the early stages of the obstruction.

13. How do you assess the clinical status of patients with bowel obstruction?

The physical examination is helpful to a limited degree. Vital signs of pulse, respiratory rate, blood pressure, and temperature usually are normal initially. As the patient loses fluid into the bowel and with vomiting, diminished plasma volume is reflected in tachycardia, narrowing of pulse pressure, and low-grade fever. At the onset of the obstruction the patient appears relatively normal between bouts of colic. Over time, however, the patient develops an anxious expression with sunken eyes, dry skin and mucous membranes, and prolonged capillary refilling time.

The presence of an abdominal scar from a previous laparotomy almost ensures that the bowel obstruction is due to adhesions. Distended bowel loops may be visible and palpable through the abdominal wall. The presence of a mass may indicate an inflammatory process (such as an appendicele abscess), infarcted bowel, or matted intestinal loops due to Crohn's disease. If peritonitis has developed, the abdomen is rigid and diffusely tender with signs of rebound tenderness.

14. What physical signs suggest a gangrenous obstruction?

In patients with a strangulating obstruction, blood and bacteria eventually ooze into the peritoneal cavity, resulting in parietal peritoneal irritation. The patient tends to be highly agitated and moves about, attempting to find a position of comfort. There is no period of pain relief between bouts of colic. The pain becomes constant, with tenderness and guarding localized to the area of infarction. Subsequently, a generalized peritonitis develops. Frequently, however, the surrounding normal and obstructed intestine tends to cover the gangrenous bowel, therefore obscuring the findings of peritonitis.

15. Is a rectal examination helpful?

A rectal examination usually reveals an empty rectum with obstruction in the small bowel because, with the onset of hyperperistalsis from the obstruction, stool usually is evacuated from the colon. A rectum impacted with stool implies constipation. Children with Hirschsprung's disease have a rectum full of liquid stool. When you withdraw the examining finger, stand back—typically there is an explosive discharge of stool and gas. The rectal examination also may reveal a mass in the cul de sac due to infarcted bowel, abscess, or tumor.

16. Is auscultation of the abdomen helpful?

Auscultation of the abdomen reveals high-pitched tinkles at irregular and random intervals, with occasional periods of hyperactive bowel sounds that last for seconds or minutes. If there is little air in the bowel, however, the abdomen is silent. Contrary to common lore, correlation between episodes of hyperperistaltic rushes and expression of pain is not very high.

17. Which laboratory studies are useful?

Blood count may reveal a high hematocrit secondary to hemoconcentration due to reduced plasma and extracellular fluid volume. Reductions in plasma and extracellular fluid volume result from large fluid losses from the serosa of the bowel into the peritoneal cavity and bowel lumen as well as from vomitus and perspiration. Anemia occurs if blood has suffused into the obstructed bowel because of prominent mesenteric venous compression. The white blood count may be normal or elevated in either simple or strangulating obstruction.

18. Why is assessment of serum electrolytes helpful?

A proximal small bowel obstruction results in loss of fluids that resemble gastric juice and thus produces hypokalemic and hyperchloremic metabolic alkalosis. For more distal small bowel obstruction, fluid losses are usually isotonic. Serum electrolytes are normal until sufficient dehydration results in metabolic acidosis, as demonstrated by low serum bicarbonate and elevated serum chloride.

19. What radiologic studies should be obtained?

Plain radiographs of the abdomen, supine and upright, are necessary. If the patient has difficulty in maintaining an upright position, the study can be obtained with the patient lying on the side—the so-called lateral decubitus position. It may require about 6 hours for sufficient swallowed air and fluid to fill the obstructed intestine and thus produce the radiographs typical of obstruction. Over time the bowel loops become dilated and contain air/fluid levels.

20. What radiologic findings define a small bowel obstruction?

Sometimes it is difficult to determine whether the dilated bowel is colon or small intestine. Typically, the obstructed and dilated small bowel is located centrally in the abdomen, and the bowel loops are oriented in a transverse direction. A dilated colon is located at the flanks and oriented vertically, except for the transverse colon. Obstructed small bowel is characterized by the presence of valvulae conniventes, which traverse the entire diameter of the small intestine at short intervals, like a stack of coins. In contrast, the colon is recognized by haustra, which do not extend across the entire lumen. In the case of complete bowel obstruction, the colon usually contains little or no gas, because during the course of obstruction the entire intestine tends to develop hyperperistalsis and the colon empties of gas and stool. The presence of gas in the colon suggests a partial intestinal obstruction if the symptoms have been present for many hours.

21. How do abdominal radiographs suggest a gangrenous obstruction?

A distinct loop of gas-containing, dilated bowel that is bent on itself and looks like a coffee bean suggests a closed-loop, gangrenous obstruction. However, a closed-loop obstruction or a gangrenous loop of bowel may appear as a gasless mass with the density of water. Sometimes a gangrenous obstruction is associated with an absolutely gasless abdomen and no dilated intestine is discernible.

22. What is the role of contrast studies?

In certain settings plain abdominal x-ray studies may be supplemented with contrast studies. In patients with a partial small bowel obstruction or paralytic ileus, the distention and distinguishing radiologic features of obstruction may be absent. Therefore, contrast material may be given by mouth or through a nasogastric tube, and the transit through the bowel can be followed with fluoroscopy and periodic abdominal radiographs.

23. What is the preferred contrast material?

Barium is preferred because Gastrografin and nonionic water-soluble contrast become diluted in the fluid-filled intestine and define the intestine poorly. Barium has been maligned as a contrast medium because of concern that it may become inspissated in the colon as water is resorbed from the lumen and thus contribute to obstruction. In cases of delayed evacuation, the barium must be expelled by either motility agents, such as Dulcolax, or saline enemas.

24. What other imaging studies may be helpful?

Abdominal ultrasound is a superb, noninvasive technique for diagnosing masses such as a closed-loop or gangrenous obstruction, intussusception, abscesses, and tumors. Computerized tomography and magnetic resonance scans are expensive studies that are rarely used in children with intestinal obstruction.

25. How do you distinguish a simple small bowel obstruction from a strangulating obstruction?

The short answer: there is no sure way with current diagnostic measures. Essentially every patient with a complete intestinal obstruction should be considered to have a gangrenous obstruction. Eventually gangrenous bowel provokes signs of peritonitis with fever, localized or generalized abdominal rigidity, rebound tenderness, and elevated white blood count. However, it takes time for strangulated intestine to exude the toxic products of necrosis that irritate the parietal peritoneum. Thus, patients must be reevaluated carefully at frequent intervals. Clearly concern should be greater when these signs are present and when symptoms have changed from episodic cramping to constant and intense pain with radiation to the back and increasing abdominal tenderness. Nevertheless, experience has shown that such features may not be present when frank gangrene has occurred, and not infrequently, they may be present with simple obstruction. Occasionally a mass that is palpable through the abdominal wall or in the cul de sac indicates the presence of a gangrenous loop of bowel. Because of the great difficulty in identifying strangulating obstruction, an old surgical doctrine advises, "Never let the sun rise or set on a bowel obstruction." A laparotomy is indicated as soon as possible. This principle applies for complete intestinal obstruction.

26. How do you care for a patient with small bowel obstruction?

Volume replacement is the first priority. One or two large-bore intravenous cannulas should be placed, and blood should be obtained for complete blood count and type and cross-match in case a transfusion is necessary. Sometimes the mobilization of adhesions results in an extremely bloody operation. Ringer's lactate solution should be infused rapidly, providing a bolus of 10–20 ml/kg or a quantity equivalent to 15% of estimated normal blood volume. In children the normal blood volume is about 85 ml/kg. The objective is to return tissue perfusion to normal.

27. How do you know how much fluid replacement to give?

End-points to determine adequate tissue perfusion are limited: skin turgor, capillary refilling time, pulse, blood pressure (pulse pressure), and urine output. After blood volume has been restored, a right atrial catheter may be placed to monitor central venous pressures as an additional measure of proper volume replacement. Skin capillary perfusion tends to reflect intestinal perfusion and can be assessed by the rate of return of capillary flow in the nailbeds if the extremity is warm. The fingertips are compressed, thereby expressing blood from the nailbed capillaries. With release of the compression color should return within 1 second. Tachycardia due to hypovolemia slows toward a normal rate with volume replacement. The pulse pressure may be quite narrow, and as blood volume is corrected, the pulse pressure widens with a rise in the systolic pressure.

28. What is considered adequate urinary output?

Adequate kidney perfusion occurs when urine output is greater than 1–2 ml/kg/hour.

29. What is the significance of central venous catheter pressures?

It is possible to have a normal central venous pressure in the presence of hypovolemia because of venous vasoconstriction. During the course of intravenous fluid replacement, restoration of normal blood volume is recognized by a progressive rise in central venous pressure toward an upper normal level of about 12–15 cm H_2O.

30. What other measures are necessary to proper treatment of patients with intestinal obstruction?

A nasogastric tube should be passed into the stomach and a vacuum applied. A large-bore tube with a sump double lumen should be used so that, as the stomach collapses around the tube, a small side lumen will draw air to prevent the wall of the stomach from occluding the tube. The tube evacuates fluid and air from the bowel and minimizes further distention from swallowed air. The air that accumulates in obstructed intestine is due almost exclusively to swallowing, not to fermentation by bowel organisms. Usually gastric decompression helps to relieve some of the pain, and the lack of pain relief should raise concern for gangrenous bowel. The attempt to pass a long tube into the distal small bowel, as sometimes advocated in adults, is time-consuming and ineffective.

31. What is the role of nonoperative management?

Clearly conservative, nonoperative management should not be attempted for patients with fever (temperature > 37.5°C), localized abdominal tenderness or palpable mass, leukocytosis, or radiologic evidence of complete obstruction of the colon. Such patients require emergency laparotomy.

Patients with a partial bowel obstruction due to adhesions and patients with a history of repeated adhesive bowel obstruction may be treated nonoperatively for a certain period to see whether the obstruction will resolve. Nasogastric decompression, intravenous fluid, and electrolyte resuscitation should be continued, and patients must be observed carefully for symptoms and signs indicative of possible intestinal vascular compromise. They should be reexamined repeatedly for changing abdominal findings that suggest strangulation and for development of fever or leukocytosis. Abdominal radiographs should be repeated at least once daily to detect progression or resolution of the obstruction. Resolution of the obstruction is suggested when the symptoms of colic diminish, the volume of nasogastric output decreases, and its color changes, assuming that the tip of the tube is not in the duodenum. In addition, there should be evidence of evacuation of gas and stool.

32. How long should conservative care be continued?
Nonoperative management may be continued for up to 4 days, with the expectation that about 75% of obstructions will resolve. During the observation period about 20–30% of patients develop criteria requiring laparotomy. Of patients whose initial obstruction resolves with conservative treatment, about 35% later develop a recurrent obstruction. A repeated conservative approach results in resolution of about 40% of recurrent obstruction, whereas 60% require surgery.

33. Describe surgical treatment of intestinal obstruction.
Preoperatively, the patient should receive intravenous antibiotics to control intestinal flora. At present, ampicillin, gentamicin, and flagyl or clindamycin are combined to provide a relatively inexpensive regimen that is effective against aerobic and anaerobic enteric organisms. When close-to-normal blood volume has been restored, anesthesia may be started with a reduced risk of inducing hypotension.

In patients with previous surgery, the same incision may be used for cosmetic reasons, but bowel may be densely adherent to the incision site. Perforation of the intestine during the course of entering the abdomen is a major risk. Therefore, the incision usually is started in an area beyond the original incision and extended into the peritoneal cavity. Then the surgeon can detect the presence of adherent bowel and extend the original incision line while mobilizing the adherent intestine from the abdominal wall. To prevent further adhesion formation, the bowel should be manipulated in a way that avoids abrasion of serosal surfaces; saline-soaked, soft sponges can be helpful in this endeavor. Glove powder of various sorts may be highly inflammatory, and it should be removed thoroughly by washing in a basin of sterile saline solution before the abdomen is entered.

Abdominal exploration may reveal only one bowel-entrapping band, which is readily excised. If adhesions are extensive and dense, the surgeon is in for a long day of tedious attempts to find normal planes to dissect between the wall of one bowel loop plastered to another. On some occasions bowel segments are so densely adherent that the lumen is entered in numerous places and it becomes necessary to resect the entire area. The extremely dilated bowel near the point of obstruction must be handled carefully because the wall may be so thin and edematous that it is easy to perforate.

34. What do you do about fluid-filled, dilated bowel?
What to do about the large amount of intraluminal gas and fluid before closing the abdomen is still debated. Many surgeons advocate milking the contents of the intestine either into the colon or retrograde into the stomach, where it can be aspirated by the nasogastric tube. However, the manipulation of the intestine required to empty its contents contributes to abrasion of the serosal surfaces and may contribute to further adhesion formation. Another technique is to insert a large-bore needle obliquely through the bowel wall into the lumen and to connect it to a vacuum. This approach involves the risk of peritonitis due to spillage of enteric contents or a subsequent leak from the needle hole. Decompression is necessary when the intestine is so distended that closure of the abdomen is difficult. Otherwise, there may be good reason to leave the intestine somewhat

distended in an attempt to minimize kinking and future obstruction. With resolution of ileus the fluid in the lumen is absorbed and evacuated rectally.

35. What is the chance that bowel obstruction will recur?

About 15% of operated patients develop recurrent small bowel obstruction. Of these, two-thirds respond to conservative treatment and one-third require another operation.

36. How do you avoid adhesions in the future?

Currently there is no way to prevent adhesion formation. Numerous substances have been instilled into the abdominal cavity or given systemically without benefit. However, adhesions readily form with abrasion of serosal surfaces of the parietal peritoneum and intestine. In addition, foreign bodies such as glove powder, nonabsorbable sutures, bits of sponges, and necrotic tissue at the end of ligated mesenteric or omental vessels become a nidus for adhesions.

37. How do you manage the patient with intestinal obstruction due to recurrent and extensive adhesions?

Unfortunately, some children develop such extensive adhesions that the abdominal cavity is totally obliterated with no planes between bowel loops or between the intestine and abdominal wall. An ongoing inflammatory reaction, possibly a reaction to glove powder, latex, or other components used in the manufacture of gloves, involves all serosal surfaces. Once the bowel has been mobilized completely, it is worthwhile to pass a long silicone catheter via a gastrostomy or jejunostomy through the entire small bowel in an effort to prevent sharp angles of curvature as the intestine is folded back into the abdominal cavity. With this approach, recurrent adhesions have little chance of kinking the bowel. The tube should have an adequate diameter so that it cannot be kinked. It probably should be left in place for 1 month or more to allow time for the adhesive reaction to subside. This approach involves several risks. A very rigid tube may erode through the intestine. In addition, subsequent attempts to remove the tube can be difficult. Clearly, a long-standing indwelling tube should be used only in desperate circumstances.

38. Describe the approach to strangulating obstruction.

When necrotic bowel is encountered, it must be removed. At times it may be difficult to determine whether apparent ischemic infarction is reversible after the obstruction is relieved. Viability is determined by noting the return of normal color and motility, vigorous mesenteric pulsations, and brisk bleeding when a nick is made in the bowel wall. These signs are not entirely reliable, however, because they are qualitative: how close to normal is the color of the bowel wall, how vigorous are the pulsations, and how brisk is the bleeding cut?

If an extensive length of intestine is affected, it is prudent to delay resection and allow time to ensure that blood perfusion does not resume. It is important to ensure restoration of a normal blood volume and establishment of excellent mesenteric arterial and venous blood flow in normal areas of gut. Occasionally, a Doppler probe is used to confirm blood flow. Sometimes the intravenous injection of fluorescein dye is used to observe perfusion of the bowel wall; an ultraviolet light source identifies the presence or absence of the typical chartreuse, fluorescent color change in the suspect area.

When the area of possibly necrotic bowel is extensive and resection may result in short bowel syndrome, it is prudent to leave the intestine in place and close the abdomen for a short period. The intestine should be replaced in the abdomen in a way that maintains optimal mesenteric blood flow. About 1 day later, the abdomen should be reexplored to assess the viability of the intestine and to determine whether resection is indicated.

39. What is the differential diagnosis of intestinal obstruction?

The greatest concern is to ensure that the symptoms of pain and vomiting are not due to a **surgical emergency**. In addition to the various causes of intestinal obstruction, other surgical problems to consider in childhood include acute appendicitis, Meckel's diverticulitis, biliary colic, and pancreatitis. The pain of appendicitis and Meckel's diverticulitis is not characterized as cramping and usually is localized to the right lower abdomen. Biliary disease produces pain in the right upper quadrant. The pain of pancreatitis may be predominantly in either the right or left upper quadrant, but in most cases it is in the deep epigastrium. Vomiting is usually nonbilious. In contrast, the pain of small bowel obstruction is mid-abdominal, periumbilical in location and decidedly cramping.

The symptoms of colicky abdominal pain and vomiting may occur with a wide assortment of nonsurgical problems. Children are particularly prone to develop such symptoms within the broad umbrella of **indigestion**. Some cases are due to overindulgence of certain foods, and others are related to food intolerance, such as true allergies or lactase deficiency.

Bacterial enteritis due to *Shigella, Salmonella, Yersinia,* and *Campylobacter* species also presents as cramping abdominal pain. **Urinary tract infections** may produce prominent symptoms of abdominal pain. **Viral enteritis** due to enteric adenovirus and rotavirus also produces symptoms of cramping abdominal pain and vomiting. Usually the infectious causes are associated with systemic symptoms of malaise, weakness, and prominent fever. In each of the nonsurgical problems, diarrhea develops in the course of the illness. Fever and headache commonly precede the onset of abdominal pain due to infection.

Recurrent abdominal pain of childhood or "functional abdominal pain" may be a challenging problem. This entity is probably a variant of irritable bowel syndrome in adults. The pain varies from a dull ache to rather intense cramping. The pain is poorly localized and commonly described as involving the whole abdomen, but it may be periumbilical in location. Vomiting is uncommon, but in some cases nonbilious vomiting develops. Diarrhea is unusual. Generally, there is a discrepancy in the overall demeanor of the patient and the expressed intensity of the pain. Patients lack the facial expressions and autonomic responses (increased pulse rate, pallor, and sweating) that are typical of small bowel obstruction. Some children (usually adolescents) complain bitterly. Crying out during episodes of cramping may be an emotional overreaction in response to discomfort. Usually such highly expressive children flail about during the pain, whereas patients with a true bowel obstruction tend to draw up the legs and become somewhat withdrawn and quiet with obvious anguish.

40. Why is the diagnosis of abdominal pain so important?

Even with the magnificent imaging studies currently available, the abdomen can be a "black box," and assessment of the causes of abdominal pain may be an enormous challenge. The clinician must be concerned at all times that the patient with abdominal pain does not have a surgical problem. Delay in treating the various sources of intestinal obstruction can be disastrous. Infarction and gangrene must be avoided to prevent significant morbidity and mortality.

BIBLIOGRAPHY

1. Akgur FM, Tanyel FC, Buyukpamukcu N, et al: Adhesive small bowel obstruction in children: The place and predictors of success for conservative treatment. J Pediatr Surg 26:37–41, 1991.
2. Janik JS, Ein SH, Filler RM, et al: An assessment of the surgical treatment of adhesive small bowel obstruction in infants and children. J Pediatr Surg 16:225–229, 1981.
3. Silen W, Hein MF, Goldman L: Strangulation obstruction of the small intestine. Arch Surg 85:121, 1962.
4. Sarr M, Bulkley GB, Zuidema GD: Preoperative recognition of intestinal strangulation obstruction. Am J Surg 145:176, 1983.

26. PANCREAS

Joel Shilyansky, M.D.

1. How does the pancreas develop?

The dorsal pancreatic primordium, derived from the duodenum and giving rise to the body and tail of the pancreas, and the ventral pancreatic primordium, derived from the hepatic diverticulum and giving rise to the head and uncinate process of the pancreas, fuse by the seventh week of gestation. The main pancreatic duct of Wirsung, which is formed by the fusion of the ventral duct and distal dorsal duct, drains into the duodenum at the ampulla of Vater. The proximal duct may persist as the duct of Santorini, draining through an accessory papilla cephalad and posterior to the ampulla of Vater. The islets of Langerhans are recognizable by the end of the third month.

2. Where is the pancreas located?

The pancreas is a retroperitoneal organ located at the level of L1. The head is intimately associated with the duodenal C loop, whereas the tail lies in the hilum of the spleen. The blood supply of the pancreas is from the celiac axis via the splenic artery, gastroduodenal artery, and superior pancreaticoduodenal arteries. The latter vessels join with the inferior pancreaticoduodenal arteries arising from the superior mesenteric artery. Pancreatic veins drain into the splenic and superior mesenteric veins, which join to form the portal vein. To assess the integrity of the pancreatic head, an extensive Kocher maneuver is required. The body and tail of pancreas are examined through the lesser sac.

3. What is the function of the pancreas?

The pancreas has two main functions: production of digestive enzymes and regulation of metabolism and glucose homeostasis. Lipase and amylase are secreted as active enzymes, whereas proteolytic enzymes are secreted as proenzymes by acinar cells and activated by duodenal enterokinases. Cholinergic vagal stimulation during the cephalic phase and cholecystokinin (released from intestinal mucosa) during the intestinal phase of digestion stimulate pancreatic secretions. Somatostatin release inhibits pancreatic secretions. Pancreatic ductal cells secrete bicarbonate and water in response to secretin released by duodenal mucosa exposed to acid. Proteolytic activity is nearly normal in neonates, but amylase and lipase levels increase over the first year of life.

The pancreas contains 1–2 million islets of Langerhans (1–2% of pancreas), containing glucagon (α cells), insulin (β cells), somatostatin (δ cells), and pancreatic polypeptide (PP cells). Insulin secretion is affected primarily by serum glucose concentration, leading to glyconeogenesis and lipogenesis. Somatostatin and glucagon decrease insulin secretion. Sympathetic stimulation, glucocorticoids, and sepsis may blunt the response to insulin.

4. What are the most common congenital pancreatic anomalies?

Annular pancreas arises from incomplete migration of the ventral pancreatic anlage. The annular portion drains independently into the duodenum or into Wirsung's duct. It may be associated with trisomy 21 (15%), malrotation, or intrinsic duodenal obstruction (40%). Other midline anomalies are also seen (e.g., tracheoesophageal fistula with esophageal atresia and congenital heart lesions).

Pancreatic divisum, defined as separate and distinct drainage of the dorsal and ventral pancreatic ducts into the duodenum, occurs in 5–10% of patients. Most children with this anatomic arrangement are asymptomatic. However, stenosis of the minor or accessory papilla may lead to recurrent acute pancreatitis.

Cystic fibrosis (CF) is the most frequent lethal genetic disease in North America (1 in 2500 live births, 5% carrier rate). CF is transmitted in an autosomal recessive fashion. The disease presents with bronchiolar obstructions that lead to frequent pulmonary infections and pulmonary insufficiency. Children suffer from pancreatic insufficiency, as manifested by malabsorption, weight loss, steatorrhea, and gallstones. The diagnosis can be made by a sweat test demonstrating excessive chloride concentration (> 60 mEq/L). Genetic analysis is diagnostic in 75–85% of children. Pancreatic insufficiency can be corrected in most children with pancreatic enzyme replacement.

Persistent hyperinsulinemic hypoglycemia of the neonate (nesidioblastosis) presents at birth or in early infancy with poor feeding, perioral cyanosis, lethargy, hypotonia, irritability, and seizures. Children may appear well until they suffer a minor viral illness. The hallmark of the disease is elevated insulin levels despite persistent hypoglycemia. Severe neurologic injury and death can result, because cerebral glucose concentration approaches zero when plasma glucose concentration is below 40 mg/dl (2.2 mmol/L).

5. How do children with annular pancreas present?

The malformation often is associated with duodenal atresia or stenosis and presents during the neonatal period with feeding intolerance, bilious vomiting, and a "double-bubble" sign on radiographic examination of the abdomen. In the absence of associated anomalies, annular pancreas may be asymptomatic.

6. How is annular pancreas treated?

The pancreatic tissue should not be divided because injury to pancreatic and biliary ducts results. Furthermore, the associated duodenal obstruct is not corrected. The duodenal obstruction should be bypassed by performing duodenoduodenostomy or duodenojejunostomy.

7. How does pancreatic divisum present?

Most children with this anatomic arrangement are asymptomatic. However, stenosis of the minor or accessory papilla may lead to recurrent acute pancreatitis. Diagnosis is suspected when endoscopic pancreaticogram fails to demonstrate the main pancreatic duct. The minor (accessory) papilla may be visualized during the endoscopic study.

8. What are the therapeutic options for pancreatic divisum?

Pancreatic divisum is usually asymptomatic; however, when associated with recurrent episodes of pancreatitis it may be treated with surgical sphincteroplasty. The role of endoscopic treatment of pancreatic divisum has not been defined.

9. What is the differential diagnosis of newborns with hypoglycemia?

- Sepsis
- Prematurity
- Small size for gestational age
- Gestational diabetes
- Hormone deficiencies (adrenal insufficiency, growth hormone insufficiency, hypopituitarism)
- Metabolic deficiency (hepatic insufficiency, galactosemia, glucose-6-phosphate dehydrogenase [G6PD] deficiency, glycogen storage disease)
- Persistent hyperinsulinemic hypoglycemia of the neonate (PHHN), islet-cell adenoma

10. What syndrome is associated with PHHN?

Beckwith-Wiedemann syndrome, which consists of hemihypertrophy, organomegaly, macroglossia, gigantism, hypoglycemia, and Wilms' tumors.

11. What are the diagnostic criteria for PHHN?

- Hypoglycemia: persistent serum glucose levels < 40 mg/dl (2.2 mmol/L)
- Hyperinsulinemia: detectable serum insulin despite serum glucose levels < 40 mg/dl (2.2 mmol/L)
- Requirement for glucose infusion at a rate greater than maximal hepatic production (> 8–10 mg/kg/min)
- Low serum ketones and fatty acid levels

12. What are the goals of PHHN treatment?

The primary goal of treatment is to limit episodes of hypoglycemia and the resulting neurologic injury. The secondary goal is to minimize the development of diabetes mellitus.

13. What strategies are used for the medical treatment of PHHN?
- Glucose infusion (via central line)
- Diazoxide
- Glucagon
- Octreotide (somatostatin analog)
- Continuous or frequent enteral feedings (via gastrostomy)

14. Describe the surgical treatment of PHHN.
- Enucleate nodules, which may be found in the minority of children.
- Perform a 75–85% or 95% distal pancreatectomy. In some children (45% and 30%, respectively) a subsequent near-total (99%) pancreatectomy is required to control hypoglycemia. Diabetes rarely occurs after an 85% pancreatectomy, is delayed by 3–10 years after 95% pancreatectomy, and rapidly develops after 99% pancreatectomy.

15. What are the presenting signs and symptoms of pancreatitis in children?

Complaints: abdominal pain, back pain, feeding intolerance, anorexia, vomiting

Physical findings: epigastric tenderness, distention, mass

Laboratory findings: elevated amylase and lipase are commonly found, but normal values do not rule out pancreatitis. Multiorgan dysfunction is infrequent in children with pancreatitis but bodes a poor prognosis.

Radiographic findings: intestinal gas pattern is consistent with paralytic ileus, including a distended duodenal sweep. Chest radiographs may be consistent with respiratory distress syndrome in children with severe pancreatitis. Ultrasound or computed tomography (CT) may demonstrate pancreatic enlargement and peripancreatic fluid accumulation and can estimate pancreatic necrosis.

16. What are the Ranson criteria?

Ranson criteria, which are markers of organ dysfunction, help to predict survival of patients with severe pancreatitis.

On admission:
- Associated diseases (age > 55 years in the original description)
- White blood cell count > 16,000
- Glucose level > 200 mg/dl
- Lactate dehydrogenase > 350 IU/L
- Aspartate aminotransferase > 250 IU/L

After 48 hours:
- 10% decrease in hematocrit
- 5-mg/dl increase in blood urea nitrogen
- Calcium < 8 mg/dl
- Partial pressure of oxygen in arterial blood < 60 mmHg
- Base deficit > 4 mEq/L
- Fluid sequestration > 100 ml/kg

17. What are the most common causes of pancreatitis in children?
- Trauma
- Idiopathic (cause unknown)
- Biliary disease, gallstones
- Chemotherapeutic agents, corticosteroids (other medications)
- Viral and bacterial infections
- Familial pancreatitis

18. How is pancreatitis treated in children?

Medical treatment of acute pancreatitis is supportive. The goals are to correct pulmonary dysfunction, replace fluids, and provide parenteral nutrition. Enteral nutrition is withheld initially.

Long-term nutritional support with elemental formula via a nasojejunal tube is controversial. Prophylactic antibiotic administration and treatment with octreotide failed to demonstrate improved outcome in clinical trials.

Surgical debridement is required for necrotizing pancreatitis, especially when it is associated with infection of the necrotic peripancreatic fat and deteriorating clinical status. The presence of infection may be ascertained by needle aspiration of peripancreatic fluid during CT or ultrasound imaging. The procedures entail a generous abdominal incision, debridement of necrotic material, and extensive drainage. The abdomen is packed open, explored repeatedly, or lavaged through large drains.

Other surgical procedures are performed after pancreatitis subsides and aimed at preventing recurrences, including treatment of gallstones, choledochal cysts, pancreas divisum, and pancreatic ductal anomalies.

19. List the complications of pancreatitis.
  • Pancreatic necrosis and hemorrhage
  • Pseudocyst formation
  • Abscess formation
  • Pancreatic fistulas, ascites, and pleural or pericardial effusions
  • Chronic pancreatitis
  • Biliary obstruction
  • Pancreatic insufficiency
  • Diabetes (rare in children)

20. What are the indications for drainage of pseudocysts?
Most pancreatic pseudocysts in children resolve with expectant management. The indications for drainage are increasing size (usually > 5 cm), infection, gastrointestinal obstruction, bleeding, rupture, and symptomatic persistence (> 6 weeks).

21. What are the options for drainage of pseudocysts?
Percutaneous, radiographically guided aspiration of the cyst fluid is a good initial treatment option in the absence of bleeding or cyst rupture. Contrast injection into the pseudocyst helps to define pancreatic ductal anatomy and to determine the presence of infection and aids in surgical planning. All infected cysts and all cysts with immature capsule should be drained externally, whether by percutaneous or open route. External drainage may be complicated by fistula formation and recurrences (~25% of cases). Internal drainage into the stomach, cystgastrostomy, duodenum, cystduodenotomy or a roux-en-Y loop, and cystjejunostomy are safe and associated with a low recurrence rate (~5%). Distal pancreatectomy for cysts in the tail or body of the pancreas results in the lowest recurrence rate.

22. How does chronic pancreatitis present in children?
Chronic pancreatitis manifests with recurrent or persistent abdominal pain, associated with decreased enteral intake and hyperamylasemia.

23. How is chronic pancreatitis treated?
Medical management consists of analgesia and exocrine enzyme replacement.

Surgical management is directed toward eliminating focal aberrant pancreatic tissue and drainage of obstructed pancreatic ducts. Resection of the tail (distal pancreatectomy) or head (Whipple procedure) of the pancreas is appropriate in children with focal pancreatic changes, normal remaining gland, and small pancreatic duct. Children with dilated pancreatic duct (> 6 mm) should be treated with drainage into a roux-en-Y loop. An end-to-end drainage of the tail of the pancreas is appropriate in cases of a single ductal stricture in the head of the pancreas. To treat multiple ductal strictures, a side-to-side longitudinal pancreaticojejunostomy (Puestow procedure) should be considered.

24. What are the most common masses of the pancreas in children?
Cystic masses
- Duplication   • Pseudocyst
- Retention   • Multicystic disease

Solid masses
- Solid and cystic tumor of the pancreas (papillary-cystic neoplasm of the pancreas)
- Pancreaticoblastoma
- Mucinous cystadenoma and cystadenocarcinoma
- Ductal carcinoma
- Lymphoma
- Endocrine tumors, which may secrete gastrin, insulin, somatostatin, glucagon, vasoactive intestinal peptide, and other hormones
- Sarcomas (rhabdomyosarcoma)

25. How are tumors of the pancreas treated in children?
Since tumors of the pancreas are rare in children, treatment is individualized. In general, operative exploration is mandated to obtain tissue diagnosis and determine resectability.

Benign lesions of the exocrine pancreas should be resected when feasible; alternatively cystic epithelialized lesions should be drained with a roux-en-Y loop, and large simple cysts can be marsupialized.

Malignant tumors of the pancreas should be resected even in the presence of local invasion. Long-term survival is expected for solid and cystic tumors of the pancreas, which metastasize infrequently and represent the most common histologic variant in children.

Endocrine tumors of the pancreas, malignant or benign, can lead to significant morbidity due to secretion of biologically active polypeptide hormones. Functional lesions should be treated by enucleation from the pancreatic head and body or distal pancreatic resection of the tail. The peripancreatic lymph nodes must be examined carefully and removed because small deposits of tumor cells can continue to produce active hormones. The presence of hormonally active lesions in the submucosa of the duodenum should be sought, especially when preoperatively localized to the head of the pancreas. Because the lesions are frequently small, a duodenotomy should be performed.

26. What syndromes are associated with endocrine tumors of the pancreas?
- Zollinger-Ellison syndrome   • Von Hippel-Lindau syndrome
- Multiple endocrine neoplasia type I • Neurofibromatosis

27. How do patients with endocrine tumors of the pancreas present?

SYNDROME	PRESENTATION	HORMONE SECRETED	DIAGNOSTIC TESTS
Insulinoma	Hypoglycemia, confusion, fainting, altered behavior, weight gain	Insulin	Elevated insulin/glucose ratio, elevated C peptide in serum
Gastrinoma	Severe peptic ulcer disease, diarrhea, acid hypersecretion, hypercalcemia	Gastrin	Fasting gastrin > 150 pg/ml Positive secretin test
Somatostatinoma	Steatorrhea, diabetes, cholelithiasis, neurofibromatosis	Somatostatin	Elevated serum somato-statin
VIPoma	Watery diarrhea, hypochlorhydria, achlorhydria, diarrhea resistant to nasogastric suction, flushing	VIP	Elevated serum VIP, hypo-kalemia
Glucoganoma	Necrolytic migratory erythema, stomatitis, glossitis, diabetes, normochromic anemia	Glucagon	Elevated glucagon level, hypoaminoacidemia

VIP = vasoactive intestinal peptide.

BIBLIOGRAPHY

1. Guice KS: Acute pancreatitis. In Greenfield LJ, Mulholland MW, Oldham KT, Zelenock GB (eds): Essentials of Surgery: Scientific Principles and Practice. Philadelphia: Lippincott-Raven, 1997.
2. Lillehei C. Pancreas. In Oldham KT, Colombani PM, Foglia RP (eds): Surgery of Infants and Children: Scientific Principles and Practice. Philadelphia, Lippincott Raven, 1997.
3. Shilyansky J, Cutz E, Filler RM: Endogenous hyperinsulinism: Diagnosis, management and long term follow-up. Semin Pediatr Surg 6:115, 1997.
4. Vane DW. Lesions of the pancreas. In Ashcraft KW, Holder TM (eds): Pediatric Surgery. Philadelphia. W.B. Saunders, 1993

27. INTESTINAL ATRESIA AND WEBS

Anthony Sandler, M.D.

DUODENAL ATRESIA AND STENOSIS

1. What is the proposed theory for development of duodenal atresia?
Failure of epithelial apoptosis (programmed cell death) results in incomplete canalization of the duodenal lumen. Normally, the solid cord stage of the distal foregut canalizes at the end of the eighth-to-tenth week of gestation.

2. What are the three types of duodenal atresia?
Type I involves a mucosal diaphragmatic membrane.
Type II involves a short fibrous cord that connects the two ends of atretic duodenum.
Type III involves complete separation of the two atretic duodenal ends.

3. Is the windsock anomaly a sign of foul intestinal air traffic?
No. It is a form of type I duodenal atresia in which an intact membrane takes the shape of a windsock web. The site of the origin of the windsock is proximal to the distal level of obstruction.

4. Is vomiting most often bilious or nonbilious with duodenal atresia?
Vomiting is most often bilious because 85% of obstructions are distal to the entry of the bile duct into the duodenum.

5. What other gastrointestinal conditions are associated with duodenal atresia and stenosis?
Approximately one-third of patients have either annular pancreas or malrotation associated with duodenal atresia. An anterior portal vein, second distal web, and biliary atresia are rarely associated (2–4%).

6. What is the most common genetic anomaly associated with duodenal atresia?
Approximately one-third of infants born with duodenal atresia and stenosis have trisomy 21 (Down syndrome).

7. Can duodenal atresia be diagnosed prenatally?
Polyhydramnios is present in about 50% of fetuses with duodenal atresia. Prenatal ultrasound demonstrating a dilated, fluid-filled stomach and proximal duodenum in the presence of polyhydramnios is highly suggestive of duodenal atresia.

8. If an abdominal radiograph reveals the classic double-bubble sign of duodenal atresia and small, scattered amounts of air distal to the second bubble, is duodenal obstruction excluded?
Not necessarily. The presence of distal air suggests a partial obstruction that may be consistent with duodenal stenosis, perforate web, annular pancreas, duodenal duplications, preduodenal

portal vein, or malrotation with Ladd's bands. Alternatively, a duodenal atresia associated with a duplicated bile duct may result in distal intestinal air. An upper gastrointestinal contrast study is helpful in defining the anomaly.

9. Is duodenoduodenostomy preferred to duodenojejunostomy for treatment of duodenal atresia?

Yes. The Kimura diamond-shaped anastomosis is preferred. A proximal transverse duodenal incision is anastomosed to a distal longitudinal duodenal incision. Kimura refers to the anastomosis as "somebody's procedure." While he was conducting clinical rounds as a visiting professor, a resident described the procedure performed on a child with duodenal atresia but could not remember the surgeon for whom the procedure was named. The resident coined the term, "somebody's procedure."

10. Is complete excision the ideal management of a windsock web variant?

No. The web should be opened along its lateral side after duodenotomy. The papilla usually is located in the medial portion of the web. Thus, partial excision of the lateral aspect is performed, followed by simple closure of the duodenotomy.

11. What is the overall survival rate for patients with duodenal anomalies?

Over the past 25 years, the survival rate has improved from about 65% to greater than 90%.

12. What is the most common long-term complication in patients with congenital duodenal anomalies?

A megaduodenum with duodenal dysmotility is seen most commonly in long-term follow-up. Clinically, the child may present with recurrent episodes of malodorous vomiting. Successful treatment consists of reoperation and a tapering duodenoplasty or duodenal plication.

NEONATAL SMALL INTESTINAL OBSTRUCTION

13. Is polyhydramnios always associated with jejunal atresia?

No. Only 24% of cases of jejunal atresia are associated with maternal polyhydramnios. About 25–40% of amniotic fluid is swallowed by the fetus in the fourth or fifth month, and the fluid is reabsorbed in the first 25–30 cm of jejunum. Thus, more distal atresias may not be associated with polyhydramnios.

14. What are the five major causes of bilious vomiting in the newborn?

- Intestinal atresia
- Malrotation with or without volvulus
- Meconeum ileus
- Hirschsprung's disease
- Imperforate anus

Bilious vomiting in a neonate is pathologic and must be carefully investigated. Obstruction of the intestine distal to the ampulla of Vater results in bilious emesis.

15. What is considered the most likely cause of intestinal atresia?

Mechanical in utero intestinal accidents, including vascular occlusions, are most likely responsible for intestinal atresia. Animal models of mesenteric vascular occlusion cause intestinal atresia, and multiple clinical examples demonstrate the development of atresia from in utero vascular insults such as volvulus, internal hernia, intussusception, and constriction of bowel via a tight gastroschisis defect.

16. What is the most common site of intestinal atresia?

Atresias occur most commonly in the jejunum. Duodenal atresias occur more commonly than ileal atresias, whereas ileal atresias are more common than colonic atresias. Most atresias are single (90%), but 10% of patients may have multiple atresias.

17. How is intestinal atresia classified?
Type I consists of a mucosal web with an intact muscularis.
Type II atretic segments are separated by a fibrous band.
Type IIIa consists of an atresia with a V-shaped mesenteric gap defect.
Type IIIb is the "apple-peel" deformity, in which the distal atretic segment receives retrograde blood supply from the ileocolic or right colic artery.
Type IV takes the form of multiple atresias with a "string of sausage" effect.

18. When an atresia is suspected, what study is preferred to make the diagnosis?
A contrast enema study identifies a microcolon (or unused colon) and therefore indicates the level of obstruction. It also helps to differentiate meconium ileus, malrotation, and Hirschsprung's disease from intestinal atresia. If malrotation is suspected, an upper gastrointestinal contrast study is preferred as the initial study.

19. Is a sweat-chloride test helpful in diagnosing intestinal atresia?
The sweat-chloride test is not helpful for diagnosing atresia; it is used for diagnosing cystic fibrosis. However, about 10% of jejunoileal atresia occurs in infants with cystic fibrosis, suggesting that a sweat-chloride test may be useful to identify cases of atresia associated with cystic fibrosis and complicated meconium ileus.

20. What is the surgical management of intestinal atresia?
An end-to-end or end-to-oblique anastomosis is performed when possible. In patients with near-normal bowel length, part of the proximal dilated, abnormal atretic segment can be resected. The distal bowel should be evaluated for additional atresias or stenosis by passage of injected air or saline or a soft, appropriately sized catheter.

21. Is the initial management of atresia complicated by possible short bowel syndrome different from the initial management of pure intestinal atresia?
Yes. The remaining proximal atretic segment in such patients must be preserved. The bowel must not be excised, nor should a tapering enteroplasty be performed. It is reasonable to imbricate the dilated bowel; this approach effectively reduces the caliber of the bowel and allows function to resume. If indeed short gut syndrome is present, the bowel can be lengthened with the Bianchi procedure in the future.

COLONIC OBSTRUCTION

22. What other anomalies are associated with colonic atresia?
The incidence of colonic atresia as an isolated defect is low. Colonic atresia may be associated with cloacal extrophy, vesicointestinal fissure, and abdominal wall defects.

23. Is the management of colonic atresia different from the management of small intestinal atresia?
Most authors recommend treating such patients with a preliminary colostomy and subsequent ileocolic or colocolic anastomosis. Some authors recommend primary anastomosis for colonic atresias in the right-sided or transverse colon, with temporary colostomy for atresias affecting the sigmoid colon.

BIBLIOGRAPHY

1. Dalla Vecchia LK, Grosfeld JL, West KW, et al: Intestinal atresia and stenosis: A 25-year experience with 277 cases. Arch Surg 133:490–496, 1998.
2. Grosfeld JL, Rescoria FJ: Duodenal atresia and stenosis: Reassessment of treatment and outcome based on antenatal diagnosis, pathologic variance, and long-term follow-up. World J Surg 17:301, 1993.
3. Kimura K, et al: Diamond-shaped anastomosis for duodenal atresia: An experience with 44 patients over 15 years. J Pediatr Surg 25:977, 1990.

4. Kimble RM, Harding JE, Kolbe A: Does gut atresia cause polyhydramnios? Pediatr Surg 13:115–117, 1998.
5. Roberts HE, Cragan JD, Cono J, et al: Increased frequency of cystic fibrosis among infants with jejunoileal atresia. Am J Med Genet 78:446–449, 1998.
6. Weber TR, Vane DW, Grosfeld JL: Tapering enteroplasty in infants with bowel atresia and short gut. Arch Surg 117:684, 1982.

28. MALROTATION AND MIDGUT VOLVULUS

Richard H. Pearl, M.D.

1. What is normal rotation?

During the fourth week of embryonic life the intestine moves outside the abdominal wall into the base of the umbilical cord. As the bowel matures and enlarges, the intestine returns to the abdominal cavity during the tenth week of gestation; rotation and fixation are complete by the end of the eleventh week. The direction of rotation during this process is 270° counterclockwise; proper placement is evidenced when the ligament of Treitz is fixed left of the spine and the cecum is located in the right lower quadrant (RLQ).

2. What are malrotation and nonrotation?

Normal rotation is 270°; any rotation that is less than complete has some element of malrotation. Nonrotation, or return of the gut to the abdomen without rotation, is reported in 0.5–2.0% of patients at autopsy or during contrast gastrointestinal (GI) studies. Rarely is nonrotation pathologic. Because malrotation can occur with varying degrees of rotation, the exact placement of the GI tract as found during surgery is variable. However, the most common findings are a duodenum that does not cross the midline on upper GI studies and a cecum that is high-riding or superior to the transverse colon in the right upper quadrant.

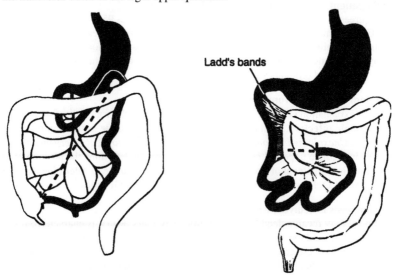

Left, The cecum descends into the right lower quadrant. Note the normal broadness of the small bowel mesentery *(dashed line)*. **Right,** In malrotation, the duodenal loop typically lacks 90° of its normal 270° rotation, and the cecocolic loop lacks 180° of its normal rotation.

3. Do all patients with malrotation become symptomatic?
No, but most do so at a very young age.

4. What causes the symptoms?
A midgut volvulus (MGV) is the most common (and catastrophic) cause of symptoms in patients with malrotation; 30% occur in the first week of life and 50% occur before 1 month of age. MGV results from the narrow mesenteric base (see previous figure, right image). The small bowel hangs down in the abdomen like a bell clapper. This position allows the bowel to twist, become obstructed, and cause symptoms.

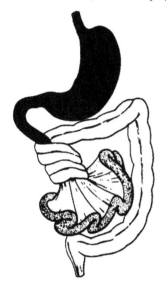

In midgut volvulus, the small bowel becomes supported only by a narrow pedicle containing the superior mesenteric artery. As a result, the small bowel may twist in a clockwise direction about this narrow axis.

5. How do patients with malrotation and MGV present?
Bilious (green) vomiting is the sentinel event, occurring in > 95% of patients with malrotation and MGV. The most common scenario is green vomiting for no reason in an infant who has a flat abdomen (initially), is afebrile, and has not been previously ill. Soon the infant may become jittery, tachycardic, pale, and diaphoretic. Abdominal distress and rectal bleeding may occur, although they are late and ominous signs.

6. If an infant has bilious vomiting, what should be done?
If no other explanation is apparent (e.g., bilious vomiting with profuse diarrhea and fever may identify a systemic infection, such as gastroenteritis), an immediate evaluation for malrotation should be done. *Unexplained bilious vomiting in an infant is a surgical emergency until proved otherwise.* An immediate upper GI contrast study is ordered to determine the position of the duodenojejunal junction (ligament of Treitz), or a contrast enema is done to determine the position of the cecum in the RLQ. Most pediatric surgeons prefer the upper GI series.

7. If the diagnosis is delayed, what may occur?
Dead bowel may mean a dead baby in as little as 6 hours. MGV is characterized by a 720° twist of the bowel around the axis of the superior mesenteric artery (SMA). This twist, caused by the narrow mesenteric base created by the malrotation, occludes first venous outflow, then arterial inflow to the gut. Ischemia, bleeding, necrosis, and perforation relentlessly and quickly ensue.

8. How can this worst-case scenario be prevented?
By quick and effective diagnosis (upper GI or contrast enema), stabilization and resuscitation, and expeditious operative intervention. As the operating room is prepared, a large-bore

intravenous line should be placed, normal saline should be given rapidly, broad-spectrum antibiotics should be infused, and a nasogastric tube should be positioned and placed on suction. However, the operation should not be delayed for resuscitation, which continues during surgery. The mortality rate of MGV ranges from 2% to 24%; the presence of necrotic bowel at surgery, associated anomalies, and the patient's age (young) are predictive of worse outcomes.

9. How is the surgery performed?

The operation usually is conducted through an upper abdominal transverse incision (although a midline incision also can be used). Upon entering the abdomen, the ischemic small bowel is immediately visible in the surgical field. The bowel varies from normal in appearance to purple or black and frankly necrotic. It is derotated counterclockwise, because volvulus is always a clockwise twisting of the bowel around the SMA axis. The bowel is observed for reperfusion, and warm saline packs are placed around the intestines for several minutes. After the bowel has recovered, Ladd's procedure is performed.

10. What is Ladd's procedure?

1. Identify abnormal peritoneal attachments of the right colon, cecum, and duodenum (Ladd's bands) that cause the narrow mesenteric base between the duodenum and cecum.

2. Complete division of these abnormal attachments allows maximal separation between the duodenum and cecum and thereby widens the base of the small bowel mesentery.

3. The bowel then is returned to the abdomen in the nonrotated position by placing the entire small bowel on the right, the large bowel on the left, and the cecum in the left upper quadrant.

4. The operation is concluded with an incidental appendectomy.

11. Why is the operation called Ladd's procedure?

William Ladd, the first surgeon-in-chief of Boston Children's Hospital, described malrotation with MGV and its surgical correction in a landmark paper in the *New England Journal of Medicine* in 1932. He described 10 cases treated by derotation and division of the abnormal peritoneal bands. Subsequently, others have called them Ladd's bands to honor his contribution.

12. For history buffs: How many chiefs of surgery have there been at Boston Children's Hospital since its inception? Name them.

1. William Ladd, M.D.   4. Hardy Hendren, M.D.
2. Robert Gross, M.D.   5. Moritz Ziegler, M.D.
3. Judah Folkman, M.D.

13. Why is this historical information important?

Ladd and Gross are considered the fathers of pediatric surgery. Ladd was the first surgeon in the United States to dedicate his practice to surgical problems in infants and children. He subsequently trained Gross, who was his successor. Gross' trainees (and their trainees) have trained two-thirds of practicing pediatric surgeons (directly or indirectly by tracing surgical lineage).

14. Besides upper GI and contrast enema, what other studies help to diagnose malrotation and MGV?

Ultrasound may suggest malrotation by picking up the relationship of the SMA, superior mesenteric vein (SMV), and duodenum. Normally the SMV lies to the right of the SMA. If their relationship is different (left or anterior), malrotation may be the cause. However, this test is not as specific or accurate as GI contrast studies.

15. If a plain abdominal radiograph is ordered for an infant with bilious vomiting in the emergency department, what findings may suggest malrotation?

• Gastric outlet obstruction
• Large gastric air bubble
• Relatively gasless abdomen (except for air in the stomach)

• Duodenal obstruction with a "double-bubble" sign
• Multiple air-fluid levels and dilated loops of bowel (a late and ominous finding)

16. Does a normal abdominal radiograph exclude the diagnosis of malrotation?
No. If unexplained green vomiting is present, refer to question 6. Malrotation must be ruled out by contrast study.

17. After a successful Ladd's procedure, can volvulus recur?
Yes. Recurrent volvulus is reported in 2–6% of cases. It is due to the narrow mesenteric base and lack of fixation after surgery. However, after postoperative adhesions have developed, recurrent volvulus is highly unlikely.

18. How does recurrent MGV present?
Green vomiting, crampy abdominal pain, no gas, no stool.

19. To prevent recurrence, should we "pex" the cecum in the RLQ?
No. The mesentery is not wide enough to locate the cecum in the RLQ. In addition, cecopexy to the abdominal wall was performed in the past and did not improve results.

20. What other diagnoses can be confused with malrotation?
Any anomaly or disease that causes obstruction of the upper GI tract can be confused with malrotation, including:
• Duodenal atresia
• Gastric or duodenal web (windsock deformity)
• Proximal jejunal atresia
• Duplication of the duodenum and proximal jejunum with compression and obstruction
• Mesenteric cyst with obstruction
• Necrotizing enterocolitis

21. Can pyloric stenosis be confused with malrotation?
Not if you know anatomy! When the pylorus is obstructed, the vomiting is white (formula), not green (bile), because the obstruction is proximal to the ampulla of Vater.

22. If you encounter necrotic bowel at surgery, is the length of necrosis a predictor of survival?
Yes. Patients with 10% necrosis have a survival rate of virtually 100%; patients with 50% necrosis have a 90% survival rate; and patients with 75% necrosis have only a 35% survival rate.

CONTROVERSY

23. If you encounter complete necrosis of the midgut, what should you do?
This finding means necrotic bowel from the ligament of Treitz to the mid-transverse colon. To survive with short gut requires 20 cm of bowel with an intact ileocecal valve and 40 cm of bowel without it. In this scenario, less than 10 cc of small bowel is represented by the duodenum and proximal jejunum. Some surgeons resect the bowel, create stomas, place a central line, and start total parenteral nutrition (TPN). Others close without resection and allow the infant to die. Currently I prefer the second option because bowel transplantation is far from perfected and usually is not performed until infants weigh 10 kg. In addition, the long-term results are far worse than for liver, kidney, and heart transplantation. As results from intestinal transplantation improve and as morbidity associated with TPN for newborns decreases, surgery will be a more viable option. Clearly, however, prevention of complete necrosis with early diagnosis and surgery obviates the need for this draconian decision.

BIBLIOGRAPHY

1. Gross RC: Malrotation of the intestines. In Gross RE (ed): The Surgery of Infancy and Childhood. Philadelphia, W.B. Saunders, 1953, pp 192–203.
2. Ladd WE: Congenital obstruction of the duodenum in children. N Engl J Med 215:705, 1932.

3. Messineo A, MacMillan JH, Pauder SB, Filler RM: Clinical factors affecting mortality in children with malrotation of the intestines. J Pediatr Surg 27:1343–1345, 1992.
4. Rescorla EJ, Shedd F, Grosfeld JL, et al: Anomalies of intestinal rotation in childhood: Analysis of 447 cases. Surgery 108:710–716, 1990.
5. Warner BW: Malrotation. In Oldham KT, Colombani PM, Foglia RP (eds): Surgery of Infants and Children: Scientific Principles and Practice. Philadelphia, Lippincott-Raven, 1997, pp 1229–1240.

29. GASTROINTESTINAL SURGICAL ASPECTS OF CYSTIC FIBROSIS

Michael S. Irish, M.D., Michael G. Caty, M.D., Philip L. Glick, M.D., and Drucy Borowitz

1. What is cystic fibrosis?

Cystic fibrosis (CF) is an inherited disease resulting from mutations in the gene that codes for a cell membrane protein termed the *cystic fibrosis transmembrane (conductance) regulator* (CFTR). This protein is an adenosine 3'-5' cyclic phosphate (cAMP)-induced chloride channel, which also regulates the flow of other ions across the apical surface of epithelial cells. The alteration in CFTR results in an abnormal electrolyte content in the environment external to the apical surface of epithelial membranes. The abnormal electrolyte content leads to desiccation and reduced clearance of secretions from tubular structures lined by affected epithelia.

2. What organ systems are affected by CF?

Clinically CF is characterized by the triad of chronic obstruction and infection of the respiratory tract, insufficiency of the exocrine pancreas, and elevated sweat chloride levels. The disease is insidious and variable and affects the lungs, digestive system, reproductive system, and sinuses; it can cause degeneration of several organs of the body, including the kidneys, liver, and heart.

3. How does CF affect the lungs?

Thick mucus in the lungs reduces the ability to clear bacteria and leads to cycles of infection and inflammation that ultimately damage lung tissues. Lung function is progressively lost; respiratory failure is the major cause of death in patients with CF.

4. How does CF affect the pancreas and intestinal tract?

Development of both the pancreas and intestinal tract in fetuses with CF is abnormal. Abnormal pancreatic secretions obstruct the duct system, leading to autodigestion of the acinar cells, fatty replacement, and ultimately fibrosis. Beginning in utero, this progressive process occurs variably over time. Approximately two-thirds of infants found to have CF by neonatal screening have pancreatic insufficiency at birth. Approximately 10% of patients with CF retain pancreatic sufficiency and tend to have a milder course. The production of insulin usually is unaffected by CF in early life, but diabetes becomes an increasingly common complication in older patients. Liver damage may be another late-onset complication of CF.

5. How does CF affect the reproductive system? What other complications may occur?

CF also affects the male reproductive system, causing infertility. Clinical variants, such as adult men with bilateral absence of the vas deferens and little other clinical involvement, have recently been described. Fertility in women is reduced only slightly, if at all. Other potential complications of CF include sinusitis, nasal polyps, and arthritis.

6. How is CF inherited?

Cystic fibrosis is an autosomal recessive disease with a heterozygote frequency estimated at 1 in 29 in the Caucasian population. A single correctly encoded allele is adequate for normal CFTR production. Thus, only people with two defective CFTR alleles have CF; people with a single defective allele are carriers. Each offspring of two heterozygote parents has a 1 in 4 chance of developing the illness. A family history of CF has been noted in 10–40% of new patients with meconium ileus.

7. What is the ΔF508 mutation?

In 1989, the CF locus was localized through linkage analysis to the long arm of human chromosome 7, band q31. The most common mutation of the CFTR gene is a three base pair deletion that results in the removal of a phenylalanine residue at amino acid position 508 of CFTR. This is called the *ΔF508* mutation. Over 600 CFTR mutations have been reported to the CF Genetic Consortium as of October 1995. Approximately 50% of patients with CF are homozygous for ΔF508, and another 25–30% have one copy of ΔF508 along with another mutation. Certain alleles cluster with increased frequency in specific populations. For example W1282X is common in Ashkenazi Jews, and A455E is common in both the Dutch and people from northern Quebec. Genotype-phenotype correlation demonstrates that homozygosity of ΔF508 nearly always confers pancreatic exocrine insufficiency.

8. What is the incidence of CF?

Approximately 40,000 people in the United States have CF. About 1 in 23 people in the United States carry at least one defective gene; it is the most common genetic defect of its severity in the United States.

9. Can the CF status of a high-risk fetus be predicted?

Yes. Noninvasive CFTR analysis can be done using a technique for recovering DNA from cells obtained by buccal brushing. Although these tests are highly specific, commercial tests screen, at most, for only 70 of the over 600 CF mutations. Thus, negative tests must be interpreted with some caution.

10. How is CF diagnosed?

CF must be suspected in all cases of fetal or neonatal bowel obstruction, and diagnostic tests should be performed as soon as possible.The diagnosis of CF should be confirmed or refuted by a sweat test performed with a technique that meets all standards of the NCCLS. Sweat tests may be performed at any time after the first 48 hours of life, provided that the patient is not edematous. The minimal amount of sweat needed is 75 mg or 15 µl. This quantity may be difficult to obtain in young infants. Sweat should not be pooled from multiple sites to obtain the required quantity, because the rate of sweating determines its electrolyte content. Mutation analysis, performed on buccal or blood cells, is useful in diagnosis if it yields two known CF mutations.

11. What is the survival outlook for patients with CF?

In the 1960s the life expectancy of people with CF was about 8 years. Today the median life expectancy is just under 30 years and increasing. Advances in the perinatal diagnosis and management of CF and its complications, as well as understanding of the CFTR protein, have vastly improved the outlook.

MECONIUM ILEUS

12. What is meconium ileus?

Meconium ileus (MI) is a bowel obstruction caused by inspissated meconium in the newborn with CF. Meconium ileus is the earliest clinical manifestation of CF, occurring in approximately 16% of patients. Meconium ileus is either *simple* or *complicated*. Each form occurs with a frequency of approximately 50%. In the simple form, thickened meconium begins to form in utero;

as it obstructs the mid-ileum, proximal dilatation, bowel wall thickening, and congestion occur. Complicated MI is associated with volvulus, atresia, necrosis, perforation, meconium peritonitis, and pseudocyst formation.

13. What causes MI?

Meconium in patients with MI has a higher protein and lower carbohydrate concentration than meconium in controls. However, the lack of concordance between MI and severity of pancreatic disease suggests that intraluminal intestinal factors contribute to its development. Postnatal intestinal disease is characterized by a glandular abnormality in which hyperviscous mucus is produced. It is speculated that the CFTR ion channel defect leads to dehydration of intraluminal contents. In fetuses with CF and MI, the meconium has increased viscosity and decreased water content compared with meconium in normal controls.

Abnormal intestinal motility also may contribute to the development of MI. Some patients with CF have prolonged small intestinal transit times. Other diseases associated with abnormal gut motility, such as Hirschsprung's disease and chronic intestinal pseudo-obstruction, have been associated with MI-like disease, suggesting that decreased peristalsis may allow increased resorption of water and thus favors the development of MI.

14. Can meconium ileus be diagnosed prenatally?

Yes, by ultrasound.

15. What sonographic characteristics are associated with MI?

Sonographic characteristics associated with MI include hyperechoic masses (inspissated meconium in the terminal ileum), dilated bowel, and nonvisualization of the gallbladder. Fetal meconium, when visualized in the second and third trimesters on ultrasound, is usually hypoechoic or isoechoic to adjacent abdominal structures. The sensitivity of intraabdominal echogenic masses in the detection of CF is reported to be between 30% and 70%. The importance of hyperechoic fetal bowel is related to gestational age at detection, ascites, calcification, volume of amniotic fluid, and the presence of other fetal anomalies. Furthermore, prenatal diagnosis of MI using the sonographic features of hyperechoic bowel must take into account the a priori risk of the parents.

The finding of dilated bowel on prenatal ultrasound has been reported less frequently than that of hyperechoic bowel. Bowel dilation in MI is caused by meconium obstruction but mimics similar findings with midgut volvulus, congenital bands, bowel atresia, intestinal duplication, internal hernia, meconium plug syndrome, or Hirschsprung's disease. However, studies suggest that dilated fetal bowel warrants parental testing for CF and continued sonographic surveillance of the fetus.

Inability to visualize the gallbladder on fetal ultrasound also has been associated with CF. Combined with other sonographic features, nonvisualization of the gallbladder can be useful in prenatal detection. However, it should be interpreted with caution because the differential diagnosis includes biliary atresia, omphalocele, and diaphragmatic hernia. Interpretation of sonographic findings must include consideration of the risk of the fetus of having CF. In the low-risk group, the diagnosis is suspected when the sonographic appearances of MI are found on routine prenatal ultrasound. All pregnancies subsequent to the birth of a CF-affected child are considered at high-risk. Parents of a child with CF are obligate carriers of a CF mutation.

16. How accurate is prenatal ultrasound in detecting MI?

The positive predictive value of hyperechoic masses in a high-risk fetus is estimated at 52%, whereas in a low-risk fetus the estimate is only 6.4%.

17. How do you evaluate the fetus suspected of having MI or CF?

We have established an algorithm which may be used in decision making and management of the fetus suspected of having MI based on prenatal ultrasound findings (see Figure below). If both parents have identified CF mutations, subsequent evaluation of the fetus can be made by amniocentesis. If only one parent or neither parent has an identified CF mutation, but the couple already have a child with CF, the status of the fetus can be predicted by analysis of restriction fragment length polymorphisms (RFLPs). Genetic material from both parents, the affected sibling, and the fetus must be available for RFLP testing. If the results predict CF in the fetus, the mother should be followed at a tertiary care facility for further management. Alternatively, the parents may consider termination. If either DNA analysis or amniocentesis is refused or is nondiagnostic, we recommend close sonographic follow-up at 6-week intervals.

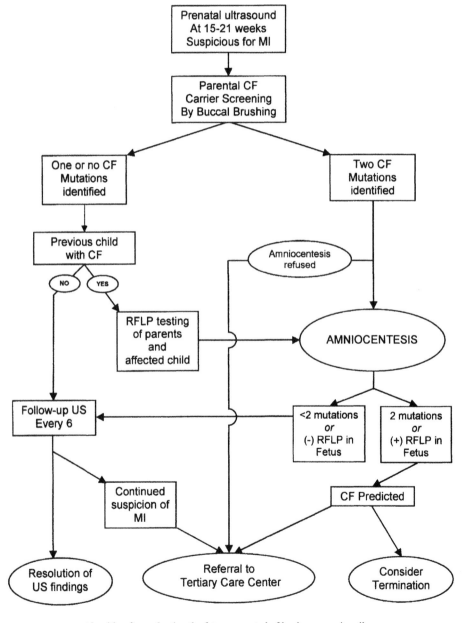

Algorithm for evaluating the fetus suspected of having meconium ileus.

18. Describe the clinical and radiographic features of *simple* MI.

Simple MI usually presents with abdominal distention at birth. Failure to pass meconium, bilious vomiting, and progressive abdominal distention eventually occur. Often dilated loops of bowel become visible on exam and have a doughy character that indents on palpation. Typically, the rectum and anus are narrow, a finding that may be misinterpreted as anal stenosis.

Uncomplicated MI is characterized by a pattern of unevenly dilated loops of bowel on abdominal radiograph with variable presence of air-fluid levels. As air mixes with the tenacious meconium, bubbles of gas may be seen. This soap-bubble appearance depends on the viscosity of the meconium and is not a constant feature. However, its presence is pathognomonic and distinguishes MI from other causes of newborn intestinal obstruction. Although none of these features alone is diagnostic of MI, collectively and in patients with a family history of CF, they strongly suggest the diagnosis.

19. Describe the clinical and radiographic features of *complicated* MI.

Complicated MI presents more dramatically. At birth severe abdominal distention with abdominal wall erythema and edema may be present. Abdominal distention may be sufficiently severe to cause respiratory distress. Signs of peritonitis include tenderness, abdominal wall edema, distention, and clinical evidence of sepsis. A palpable mass may indicate pseudocyst formation. Often the neonate is in extremis and needs urgent resuscitation and surgical exploration.

Radiologic findings in complicated MI vary with the complication. Speckled calcifications on abdominal plain films are highly suggestive of intrauterine intestinal perforation and meconium peritonitis. A pseudocyst is suggested by radiographic findings of obstruction and a large dense mass with a rim of calcification. In utero perforation (CF- or non–CF-related) can lead to meconium peritonitis or meconium pseudocyst formation; therefore, only intraoperative inspection can differentiate CF- and non–CF-related meconium peritonitis or pseudocyst formation.

20. How is the diagnosis of MI confirmed in the newborn?

If MI is clinically and radiographically suspected, a contrast enema of barium may be performed for diagnosis, followed by a therapeutic Gastrograffin enema, if MI is likely. Some advocate water-soluble contrast initially for both diagnosis and treatment. Contrast instillation is followed fluoroscopically and demonstrates a colon of small caliber (microcolon of disuse), often containing small rabbit pellets (scybala) of meconium. Progression of the contrast proximally also may outline pellets of inspissated meconium. If contrast is successfully refluxed proximal to the obstruction, dilated loops of small bowel are seen.

21. How is MI managed nonoperatively?

After birth both simple and complicated MI should be managed as a newborn intestinal obstruction. Resuscitative measures, including mechanical respiratory support, if necessary, and intravenous hydration, are initiated along with gastric decompression, evaluation and correction of coagulation disorders, and empiric antibiotic coverage. When MI is suspected or diagnosed, immediate surgical evaluation should be obtained and a Gastrograffin enema should be performed.

22. What are the criteria for attempting a Gastrograffin enema in a newborn with MI?

- An initial diagnostic contrast enema must exclude other causes of neonatal distal intestinal obstruction.
- The infant must show signs of uncomplicated MI with no clinical or radiologic evidence of complicating factors, such as volvulus, gangrene, perforation, peritonitis, or atresia of the small bowel.
- The infant should be well prepared for the enema, with adequate fluid and electrolyte replacement and correction of hypothermia.
- The enema must be done under fluoroscopic control.
- Intravenous antibiotics should be administered.
- Close surgical supervision is imperative.

23. What is Gastrograffin? Describe its therapeutic effect.

Gastrograffin (Bristol-Meyers Squibb, Princeton, NJ) is meglumine diatrizoate, a hyperosmolar, water-soluble, radiopaque solution containing 0.1% polysorbate 80 (Tween 80) and 37% organically bound iodine. The osmolarity of the solution is 1900 mOsm/L. Upon instillation, fluid is drawn into the intestinal lumen osmotically, hydrating and softening the meconium mass. Both transient osmotic diarrhea and diuresis follow. Thus, adequate resuscitation and hydration in anticipation of fluid losses is paramount.

24. Describe the technique of performing a Gastrograffin enema in a newborn.

Under fluoroscopic control, a 25–50% solution of Gastrograffin is infused slowly at low hydrostatic pressure through a catheter inserted into the rectum. To minimize the risk of rectal perforation, balloon inflation is avoided. Upon completion, the catheter is withdrawn and an abdominal radiograph is obtained to rule out perforation. The infant then is returned to the neonatal care unit for intensive monitoring and fluid resuscitation. Warm saline enemas containing 1% N-acetylcysteine may be given to help complete the evacuation. Usually rapid passage of semiliquid meconium continues in the ensuing 24–48 hours. Radiographs should be taken in 8–12 hours, or as clinically indicated, to conform evacuation of the obstruction and to exclude late perforation. In the nonoperative management of MI, if evacuation is incomplete or if the first attempt at Gastrograffin evacuation does not reflux contrast into dilated bowel, a second enema may be necessary. Serial Gastrograffin enemas can be performed at 6- to 24-hour intervals if necessary. However, if progressive distention, signs of peritonitis, or clinical deterioration occurs, surgical exploration is indicated. The success rate of Gastrograffin enemas in patients with uncomplicated MI ranges from 63% to 83%.

After successful evacuation and resuscitation, 5 ml of a 10% N-acetylcysteine solution is administered every 6 hours through a nasogastric tube to liquefy upper gastrointestinal secretions. Feedings with supplemental pancreatic enzymes for infants with confirmed CF may be initiated when signs of obstruction have subsided, usually within 48 hours.

25. What is the major complication of Gastrograffin enemas?

The major complication is rectal perforation, which can be avoided with careful placement of the catheter under fluoroscopic guidance and avoidance of inflating balloon-tipped catheters. Early perforation during administration of the enema is usually readily apparent under fluoroscopy. The risk of perforation increases with repeated enemas. Potential causes of late perforation, between 12 and 48 hours after the initial enema, include severe bowel distention by fluid osmotically drawn into the intestine or direct injury to the bowel mucosa by the contrast medium.

26. What is the goal of operative management of uncomplicated MI?

Over the years various surgical approaches to the treatment of uncomplicated MI have been proposed, and success rates with each method have been variable. The approach to each infant should be individualized. The goal of operative management in simple, uncomplicated MI is evacuation of meconium from the intestine with preservation of maximal intestinal length.

27. Describe the technique of Hiatt and Wilson and its variations.

In 1948, Hiatt and Wilson of Babies Hospital in New York reported the first successful surgical management of five infants with MI through intraoperative disimpaction of meconium with saline instilled into the bowel via a tube enterostomy. In 1989, Fitzgerald proposed a similar technique in which an appendectomy is performed and a cecostomy catheter is placed through the appendiceal stump for insertion of irrigant and evacuation of impacted meconium.

Variations on the theme of Hiatt and Wilson's technique involve placement of indwelling ostomy tubes for postoperative bowel irrigation decompression and/or feeding. In 1970, O'Neill reported success with tube enterostomy with and without resection. Harberg described a similar procedure in which a T-tube enterostomy is used. In either situation, irrigations are begun on the first postoperative day. After successful clearance of the obstruction (7–14 days), the tube can be removed and the enterocutaneous fistula allowed to close spontaneously.

28. What are the advantages and disadvantages of the Mikulicz double-barreled enterostomy?

The Mikulicz double-barreled enterostomy, first reported by Gross, has three distinct advantages. First, because complete evacuation of inspissated meconium is not necessary, operating and anesthetic times are reduced. Second, an intraabdominal anastomosis is avoided, preventing the risk of anastomotic leakage. Third, the bowel can be opened after complete closure of the abdominal wound, thereby reducing the risk of intraperitoneal contamination. After surgery solubilizing agents can be given through both the proximal and distal limbs of the stoma as well as per rectum or via nasogastric tube. As classically described, a crushing clamp may be applied to the two limbs to create continuity for distal flow of intestinal fluids.

Disadvantages of this and other procedures employing resection and stoma(s) are potential postoperative fluid losses through high-volume stomas, bowel shortening by resection, and the need for a second procedure to reestablish intestinal continuity.

29. Describe the Bishop-Koop enterostomy.

The distal chimney enterostomy, described by Bishop and Koop, involves resection with anastomosis between the end of the proximal segment and the side of the distal segment of bowel approximately 4 cm from the opening of the distal segment. The open end is brought out as the ileostomy. This technique allows normal gastrointestinal transit while providing a means for managing distal obstruction through the ileostomy.

30. Describe the proximal enterostomy developed by Santulli.

The reverse of the Bishop-Koop enterostomy is the proximal enterostomy described by Santulli in 1961. After resection the end of the distal limb is anastomosed to the side of the proximal limb. The end of the proximal limb is brought out as the enterostomy. This arrangement enhances proximal irrigation and decompression, and it is not necessary to evacuate the proximal small bowel at the time of surgery. As with the distal chimney enterostomy, catheter access to the distal limb, with the catheter exiting through the stoma, provides means of irrigating the distal bowel. The apparent disadvantage of this technique is the presence of a high-output stoma and the inherent risk of dehydration. Care must be taken to replenish fluids, electrolytes, and nutrients in accordance with stomal output. Reinstillation of stomal output from the proximal to the distal limb often is performed via the indwelling catheter.

31. Describe the technique of resection with primary anastomosis.

Resection with primary anastomosis, first suggested by Swenson in 1962, met with initial difficulty and the complication of leakage from the anastomosis. Improved results have been noted with adequate resection of compromised bowel, complete proximal and distal evacuation of meconium, and preservation of adequate blood supply to the anastomosis.

We prefer a modification of the technique, originally described by Gross in 1953. Celiotomy is performed through a muscle-sparing, horizontal incision just above the umbilicus. Upon exploration, the decision to create an enterostomy for irrigation and evacuation of meconium or to resect the segment of impacted intestine, is based on the viability and length of involved bowel. We then create side-by-side, separate enterostomies without a common wall. Stomas are placed within the abdominal incision and may be covered with a single ostomy collecting device. Postoperatively each stoma may be irrigated to remove residual meconium. Dilute enteral feedings high in glutamine may be instilled via the distal stoma to stimulate growth of the unused distal bowel. Intestinal continuity generally is restored within 6–8 weeks if bowel function has resumed and the infant tolerates oral feedings.

32. What are the options for operative management of complicated MI?

Surgery is always indicated in cases of complicated MI. Complications necessitating surgical management include persistent or worsening abdominal distention, persistent bowel obstruction, enlarging abdominal mass, intestinal atresia, volvulus, perforation, meconium cyst formation with peritonitis, and bowel necrosis. Resection is more often necessary in cases of complicated MI than in cases of simple MI. Temporary stomas are always required.

33. Discuss the postoperative feeding of patients with MI.

Infants with uncomplicated MI and CF may be given breast milk or routine infant formula, enzymes, and vitamins. Caution must be used in prescribing enteric enzyme medication to patients with MI and CF. Treatment failures and complications, such as fibrosing colonopathy due to excessive enzyme doses, distal intestinal obstruction syndrome, and problems related to generic substitutions for proprietary medications, have been reported. Patients with a complicated surgical course require either continuous enteral feedings or total parenteral nutrition (TPN). We recommend the use of predigested infant formula (Alimentum or Pregestimil) for enterally fed infants.

Prestenotic dilation of the small bowel caused by the obstructing meconium theoretically may lead to mucosal damage that contributes to poor peristalsis or malabsorption. Patients with complicated MI and/or sizeable bowel resection who are fed enterally may tolerate continuous feedings better than bolus feedings. Because the bowel mucosa may or may not be damaged by stasis, feedings are begun with predigested, diluted, formula, usually at one-half strength and low volume. If this formula is well tolerated, the strength may be increased first and then the volume, while observing for signs of feeding intolerance (abdominal distention, heme-positive stools, and/or increasing emesis).

Once oral feedings are begun, pancreatic enzymes must be given orally (even with predigested formula), starting at 2,000–4,000 lipase units per 120 ml of full-strength formula. For example, a 2.5-kg infant receiving 4 ml/kg/hr of formula, should receive one-half of a Pancrease capsule (4000 lipase units per capsule) orally every 12 hours. Capsules containing enteric-coated microspheres can be opened and the contents mixed with applesauce. The combination is given orally. The microspheres should not be crushed, because crushing exposes the enzymes to the acid of the stomach, where they will be destroyed. Uncrushed pancreatic enzymes should be given even with MCT-oil containing formulas. Destin ointment (zinc oxide) can be applied to perianal skin if pancreatic enzymes cause skin breakdown.

34. What complications affect the postoperative feeding of patients with MI?

Infants with MI are at risk for cholestasis, particularly if they receive TPN. Alkaline phosphatase, alanine aminotransferase, aspartate aminotransferase, and bilirubin should be monitored weekly. Infants with significant bowel resection (greater than one-third) may be difficult to manage, especially if the ileocecal valve has been resected. In addition, the presence of an ileostomy may lead to excessive loss of fluid and sodium. Ostomies should be taken down as soon as possible. In the interim, if access to the distal, defunctionalized bowel is feasible, ostomy-drip feeds of glutamine-enriched formula should be given at low volumes to enhance bowel growth and help prevent bacterial translocation.

Gastric acid hypersecretion is seen in patients with short-bowel syndrome. An acid intestinal environment inactivates pancreatic enzymes and prevents dissolution of enteric-coated microcapsules. H_2 blockers may be used as an adjunct to pancreatic enzyme therapy in patients with significant bowel resections. Patients with the double burden of excessive sweat and intestinal sodium losses may have compensation for total body sodium deficit. Urine sodium should be measured in infants with ileostomies, especially in cases with failure to grow, even if serum sodium levels are normal. Patients with urine sodium less than 10 mEq/L need sodium (and possibly bicarbonate) supplementation.

35. What is the prognosis of infants with MI?

Early series, subsequent to Hiatt and Wilson's report of the first survivors with MI in 1948, showed mortality rates of 50–67%. With the advent of improved nonoperative and operative treatments, good nutritional support, and better treatment of bacterial infection, the prognosis for infants with both complicated and simple MI has improved dramatically. Survival rates of

85–100% have been reported. On the whole, once infants are discharged from the hospital, they do well. Long-term follow-up of patients with MI shows pulmonary function at age 13 years to be no different between those born with MI and those without MI.

GASTROESOPHAGEAL REFLUX

36. What percentage of patients with CF experience significant gastroesophageal reflux disease?

Gastroesophageal reflux (GER) occurs with increased prevalence in patients with CF and may exacerbate their respiratory status. Pathologic reflux (i.e., endoscopic and histologic esophagitis) is present in over 50% of patients with CF. Most patients with CF also have an abnormal quantity of reflux, as defined by pH probe, that may be associated with prominent respiratory symptoms. Thus early diagnosis and treatment are of prime importance to curtail the complications of pathologic reflux and to maximize respiratory function.

37. Why are patients with CF prone to GER?

The particular mechanism of GER in CF is unclear, but a number of factors may contribute to the increased susceptibility to the development of pathologic GER. First, it has been shown that most reflux episodes in CF occur during transient lower esophageal sphincter relaxations. These transient relaxations are increased during distention of the gastric fundus, a feature that can predispose these patients to reflux especially when receiving large supplemental bolus feeds. This cycle of events may be further exacerbated in the event of poor gastric emptying. Gastric emptying of liquids was initially thought to be delayed in patients with CF. Second, the head-down posture adopted during chest physiotherapy places gastric liquid content in an optimum position at the LES for reflux in the event of a transient period of relaxation. Associated coughing and forced expiration, which both increase the abdominothoracic pressure gradient, will also facilitate reflux action. Last, medications such as theophylline and alpha-adrenergic drugs, used in the treatment of respiratory disease in the CF patient, are known to decrease the resting tone in the LES and could conceivably facilitate reflux activity.

BILIARY TRACT DISEASE

38. What are the biliary manifestations of CF?

Gallbladder disease is prevalent in patients with CF. Abnormal oral cholecystograms are found in 46% and cholelithiasis in 12%. Abnormalities include a microgallbladder containing thick, colorless "white bile" with occlusion of the cystic duct; gallstones; biliary dyskinesia; and sclerosing cholangitis. Bile acid metabolism is disturbed in patients with pancreatic insufficiency who do not receive adequate pancreate enzyme supplementation. Bile acids probably are bound to malabsorbed fat and as a result are lost in feces, which in turn depletes the bile acid pool and supersaturates cholesterol in the gallbladder. This condition promotes stone formation.

Many patients with CF and gallbladder sludge or stones are asymptomatic, but approximately 4% have the classic symptoms of cholecystitis. Laparoscopic cholecystectomy is the treatment of choice in such cases, because it involves less postoperative pain and therefore less pulmonary compromise compared with the open technique. The role of cholecystectomy in patients with asymptomatic gallstones remains unclear.

DISTAL INTESTINAL OBSTRUCTION

39. What is distal intestinal obstruction syndrome?

Distal intestinal obstruction (DIOS), formerly called meconium ileus equivalent, is a recurrent postneonatal partial or complete intestinal obstruction unique to patients with CF. Most cases occur in adolescents and adults, but all age groups can be affected. The overall incidence is approximately 15%.

40. What causes DIOS?

The exact cause is unknown, but patients are more likely to have a history of steatorrhea due to pancreatic exocrine insufficiency despite adequate enzyme therapy. Various aspects peculiar to the gastrointestinal function of patients with CF may help, in part, to explain this syndrome. Examples include abnormal intestinal mucins, abnormal intraluminal water and electrolyte content, and inherently slow intestinal motility. Neurotensin, a gastrointestinal hormone that delays motility, is secreted from the distal ileum in the presence of unabsorbed fat. Additional precipitating factors may include relative dehydration, especially in a postoperative period; inadequate enzyme supplementation; and changes in diet.

41. What are the clinical features of DIOS?

The cardinal features of the syndrome are cramping abdominal pain, often localized to the right lower quadrant (RLQ), a palpable mass in the RLQ, and decreased frequency of defecation. Degrees of obstruction range from partial, which is most common, to complete, which is characterized by vomiting, distention, and absolute constipation. Colicky pain may be provoked by meals, resulting in anorexia as a method to avoid further pain. Physical examination in uncomplicated DIOS usually reveals a tender mass in the RLQ with no evidence of peritonitis. Rectal examination shows no fecal impaction or dehydrated stool, and the stool is heme-negative.

42. How is DIOS diagnosed?

Because of the nonspecific nature of DIOS, which has no pathognomonic radiologic features, an accurate diagnosis of abdominal pain in patients with CF is not easy. Plain supine and erect abdominal radiographs are still the most helpful initial investigation when the diagnosis is suspected. They show bubbly granular material in the right iliac fossa and variable degrees of small bowel obstruction (i.e., air-fluid levels with proximal small bowel dilatation). Plain films support, but do not prove, the diagnosis. Inspissated material in the right iliac fossa also can be demonstrated with a water-soluble contrast enema. Intussusception can be excluded, and the investigation may prove therapeutic in some cases of DIOS.

Particularly difficult is the differentiation from partial small bowel obstruction caused by adhesions from previous abdominal surgery or appendiceal disease, which occurs in 1.5–2% of patients with CF. Abdominal pain is a common complaint of patients with CF, and because they often are treated with antibiotics and steroids, the classic clinical signs and symptoms of appendicitis may be masked and the critical diagnosis missed. The result is a high incidence of perforation and substantial morbidity. Despite the blunting of clinical signs, evidence of pyrexia and leukocytosis may be present. Depending on the appendix location, a contrast enema may show deformity of the cecum with an associated mass effect rather than the inspissated material typical of DIOS. An abdominal ultrasound scan, or if necessary a computed tomography scan, shows free fluid or an abscess collection in the region of the cecum. In such cases treatment should proceed with appendectomy. If the diagnosis is still in doubt, the surgeon may choose laparoscopic investigation and then proceed appropriately in light of the findings.

43. How is DIOS treated?

In the absence of partial small bowel obstruction due to adhesions, appendiceal disease, or complete obstruction, DIOS is suitable for a trial of medical management. After adequate rehydration a balanced polyethylene glycol-electrolyte solution, such as XXX GoLytely or Colyte, can be given orally or by nasogastric tube. The dose is 20–40 ml/kg/hr with a maximum of 1200 ml/hr. Prokinetic agents such as metoclopramide can be used to limit the amount of nausea and bloating. Successful treatment is judged by the passage of stool, resolution of symptoms, and disappearance of a previously palpable right iliac fossa mass. Sequential plain abdominal radiographs help to document the resolution of DIOS, but if symptoms persist the differential diagnosis outlined above must be reconsidered.

Contrast enemas should be used for patients with emesis due to DIOS after placement of a nasogastric tube for gastric suction. As long as the patient remains clinically stable, contrast enemas may be repeated at intervals of several hours over several days. But careful monitoring must be initiated before, during, and after the procedure because large fluid and electrolyte shifts can be induced by the contrast material.

With complete obstruction or evidence of peritonitis, surgical intervention is necessary and all oral or rectal therapies are contraindicated. A nasogastric tube should be passed to help with decompression, and adequate resuscitative measures should be initiated. At laparotomy the bowel wall feels thickened and filled with tenacious material. It can be decompressed and irrigated with Gastrograffin, usually via a small catheter placed through the appendix stump, as described for meconium ileus. It is also possible to leave an irrigating tube in situ to irrigate the bowel postoperatively.

GUT NEOPLASMS

44. Do patients with CF have an increased risk of malignancy?
The overall risk of cancer in patients with CF is similar to that of the general population, but the risk of digestive tract cancers is increased. Examples include tumors of the esophagus, stomach, small intestine, large intestine, liver or biliary tract, and pancreas.

The differential localization and expression of the CFTR gene may play a role in the neoplastic disease process. Furthermore, increased cellular turnover in response to the persistent irritation of GER, gallstones, or steatorrhea in digestive tract organs also may offer an explanation for these findings.

FIBROSING COLONOPATHY

45. What is fibrosing colonopathy?
Fibrosing colonopathy is a newly described entity in children with CF. Findings at laparotomy in children with CF who presented with presumed DIOS that failed to respond to medical therapy include colonic strictures with histopathologic changes of postischemic ulceration repair, mucosal and submucosal fibrosis, destruction of the muscularis mucosa, and eosinophilia. In some patients a change from conventional enteric-coated pancreatic enzymes to high-strength products 12–15 months before presentation has been described. In the largest case-control study reported, the absolute dose of pancreatic enzymes rather than the type of enzyme was the strongest predictor of fibrosing colonopathy.

46. How is fibrosing colonopathy diagnosed?
The diagnosis of fibrosing colonopathy should be considered in patients with CF who have been exposed to high doses of pancreatic enzymes and present with symptoms of abdominal pain, distention, chylous ascites, change in bowel habit, or failure to thrive. Continued diarrhea also may be a prominent feature; unfortunately, it may prompt the family to increase supplemental enzymes. On occasion the diarrhea may be bloody. A barium enema may reveal mucosal irregularity, loss of haustral markings, and a foreshortened colon with varying degrees of stricture formation. In some cases, the whole colon is involved. Colonoscopy may show an erythematous mucosa and areas of narrowing, from which it is advisable to take multiple forcep-pinch biopsies.

47. How is fibrosing colonopathy managed?
Initial management should reduce enzyme dosage to the recommended levels of 500–2500 lipase units/kg per meal. This reduction should be accompanied with adequate nutritional supplementations, which may be enteral elemental feeding or even TPN for a time. Patients who show signs of unrelenting failure to thrive, obstruction, uncontrollable diarrhea, or chylous acites need surgical intervention.

48. What are the surgical options for fibrosing colonopathy?

When surgery is planned electively for patients with intractable symptoms, gentle bowel preparation can be given preoperatively. The goals of surgical intervention are to resect the affected bowel and to make a primary anastomosis. Unfortunately, these goals are not possible in the event of pancolonic or rectal involvement. As a result, the patient requires an ostomy, which often is the safest option. Patients and parents must be fully aware of and prepared for this possibility preoperatively. Because it is also not clear whether fibrosing colonopathy completely resolves with a reduction in enzyme dosage and surgical resection, patients require regular follow-up for any signs of deterioration.

RECTAL PROLAPSE

49. What is the incidence of rectal prolapse in patients with CF?

Rectal prolapse occurs in approximately 20% of patients with CF. The initial prolapse occurs most commonly between 1 and 3 years of age and may be recurrent. It also may be the sole presenting feature of a CF in about 3% of cases.

50. What are the risk factors for rectal prolapse?

Factors that directly predispose patients with CF to prolapse include constipation, diarrhea with increased frequency and volume of movement, malabsorption, and colonic distention. Indirect contributors related to increased intraabdominal pressure caused by coughing or pulmonary hyperinflation.

51. How do you manage the patient with CF and rectal prolapse?

Initial management involves manual reduction of the prolapse. Medical management to maximize fat absorption aids overall control. Reassure parents that the number of prolapse episodes is likely to decrease with age. However, further intervention is warranted in patients who have persistent pain or incontinence with each episode of prolapse.

The **acute prolapse** is easily reduced if action is taken promptly before edema formation. Parents can be taught to grasp the herniated bowel with the fingertips of a gloved hand and apply circumferential pressure with an inward push. Sustained pressure may be required to achieve full reduction. If prolapse immediately recurs, the buttocks can be strapped together with adhesive tape for 7–14 days.

Recurrent prolapse can be treated by rectal submucosal injection. The procedure is performed under general anesthesia after the rectum has been emptied with a suppository. With the patient in the lithotomy position the needle is inserted through the skin just outside the mucocutaneous junction and guided into position by a finger placed in the rectum. As the needle is slowly withdrawn, 2–3 milliliters of 5% phenol in almond oil or hypertonic saline (30%) are injected in a linear track into four different quadrants. A single treatment controls approximately 90% of patients. Linear electrocauterization in the four quadrants also has been described to produce perirectal inflammation. This technique requires a longer hospital stay and may be complicated by rectal bleeding and/or rectal stenosis.

When all conservative options are exhausted, a surgical approach may be considered. However, many different operations have been described to control rectal prolapse. Through a transabdominal approach the rectum can be fixed to the hollow of the sacrum by a prosthetic or fascia lata graft sutured to the bowel and the presacral fascia, thus creating a new pelvic floor. Other operations include rectal suspension and levator ani muscle repair through a posterior sagittal approach. The diversity of options highlights the unsatisfactory results often achieved in these difficult cases.

BIBLIOGRAPHY

1. Bishop H, et al: Management of meconium ileus: Resection, roux-en-Y anastomosis and ileostomy irrigation with pancreatic enzymes. Ann Surg 145:410–414, 1957.
2. Borowitz D, et al: Preventive care for patients with chronic illness: Multivitamin use in patients with cystic fibrosis. Clin Pediatr 33:720–725, 1994.

3. Borowitz D: Pathophysiology of gastrointestinal complications of cystic fibrosis. Semin Resp Crit Care Med 15:391–401, 1994.
4. Borowitz DS, et al: Use of pancreatic enzyme supplements for patients with cystic fibrosis in the context of fibrosing colonopathy. Consensus Committee. J Pediatr 127:681–684, 1995.
5. Boue A, et al: Prenatal diagnosis in 200 pregnancies with a 1-in-4 risk of cystic fibrosis. Hum Genet 74:288–297, 1986.
6. Colledge WH, et al: Generation and characterization of a delta F508 cystic fibrosis mouse model. Nature Genet 10:445–452, 1995.
7. Collins FS, et al: The cystic fibrosis gene: Isolation and significance. Hosp Pract 25:47–57, 1990.
8. Fitzgerald R, et al: Use of the appendix stump in the treatment of meconium ileus. J Pediatr Surg 24:899–900, 1989.
9. Foulkes AG, et al: Localization of expression of the cystic fibrosis gene in human pancreatic development. Pancreas 8:3–6, 1993.
10. Hardy JD, et al: Sweat tests in the newborn period. Arch Dis Child 48:316–318, 1973.
11. Hiatt R, et al: Therapy of meconium ileus: Report of 8 cases with review of the literature. Surg Gynecol Obstet 87:317–327, 1948.
12. Irish MS, et al: Meconium ileus: Antenatal diagnosis and perinatal care. Fetal Matern Med Rev 8:79–83, 1996.
13. Irish MS, et al: Prenatal diagnosis of the fetus with cystic fibrosis and meconium ileus. Pediatr Surg Int 12:434–436, 1997.
14. Gross R: The Surgery of Infants and Childhood. Philadelphia, W.B. Saunders, 1953.
15. Harberg FJ, et al: Treatment of uncomplicated meconium ileus via T-tube ileostomy. J Pediatr Surg 16:61–63, 1981.
16. Oppenheimer EH, et al: Hepatic changes in young infants with cystic fibrosis: Possible relation to focal biliary cirrhosis. J Pediatr 86:683–689, 1975.
17. Raffensperger J: Surgical problems in cystic fibrosis. In Lloyd-Still J (ed): Textbook of Cystic Fibrosis. Boston, John Wright PSG, 1983, pp 371–382.
18. Santulli T: Meconium ileus. In Holder T, Ashcraft K (eds): Pediatric Surgery. Philadelphia, W.B. Saunders, 1980.
19. Swenson O: Pediatric Surgery, 2nd ed. New York, Appleton-Century-Crofts, 1962.
20. Tsui LC: Genetic markers on chromosome 7. J Med Genet 25:294–306, 1988.
21. Tsui LC, et al: Molecular genetics of cystic fibrosis. Adv Exp Med Biol 290:9–17; discussion 17–18, 1991.
22. O'Neill JAJ, et al: Surgical treatment of meconium ileus. Am J Surg 119:99–105, 1970.
23. Noblett HR: Treatment of uncomplicated meconium ileus by Gastrograffin enema: A preliminary report. J Pediatr Surg 4:190–197, 1969.
24. Noblett H: Meconium ileus. In Ravtch M, Welch K, Benson C, et al (eds): Pediatric Surgery. Chicago, Year Book, 1979, pp 943–951.

30. NECROTIZING ENTEROCOLITIS

Jeffrey S. Upperman, M.D., Evan P. Nadler, M.D., and Henri R. Ford, M.D.

1. What is the overall incidence of necrotizing enterocolitis?

The incidence of necrotizing enterocolitis (NEC) is approximately 1–3 cases per 1000 live births in the United States, or about 25,000 new cases of NEC worldwide per year.

2. What is the mortality rate associated with NEC?

Reported mortality rates range from 10% to 70%. Over the past three decades, the overall survival rate has improved steadily.

3. Which infants are at the greatest risk for developing NEC?

NEC is a disease of prematurity, especially in low-birth-weight infants. Small-for-gestational-age infants have less of a risk. Infants weighing less than 1500 gm have significantly increased rates of morbidity and mortality.

4. With what event is the onset of NEC often associated?

The onset of NEC is associated strongly with the initiation of feeding. The age at which feeding is initiated and the osmolarity of the feeding may be important factors in development of the disease.

5. What are the most common sites of intestinal involvement in NEC?

The most common site is the terminal ileum, followed by the colon. NEC can involve single (50%) or multiple segments of the intestine. In some cases, nearly the entire intestine (75%) can be involved; this finding is called pannecrosis.

6. What gross pathologic changes of the intestine are commonly seen in NEC?

The bowel often is distended, with fibrous exudate covering the serosal surface. Patchy necrosis also may result. The diseased bowel wall may be thinned and contain subserosal gas collections. Mucosal ulcerations with associated epithelial sloughing may be extensive.

7. What is the most common microscopic lesion in NEC?

Coagulation necrosis (bland necrosis) of the superficial mucosa resulting in cell "ghosts."

8. In which layer does pneumatosis first appear?

Pneumatosis begins in the submucosa and then progresses to the muscularis and subserosal layers.

9. What causes NEC?

The cause of NEC is not clear. Compromised intestinal immune function has been implictaed as necessary but not sufficient for the development of NEC. In addition, some have suggested that inflammatory cytokines and nitric oxide play a role in disease development.

10. How do neonates with NEC usually present?

Infants with NEC usually have abdominal distention, but they may present solely with signs of sepsis (i.e., apnea, bradycardia, unstable temperature, hypotension, or hypoglycemia). In progressive cases, the abdomen may feel firm, with a mass-like effect due to abdominal wall edema. The abdominal wall also may be erythematous. Emesis, hematemesis, and rectal bleeding (gross or occult) also are common.

11. What changes in the complete blood count are typically associated with NEC?

Leukopenia and thrombocytopenia. Both may be profound.

12. What other laboratory abnormalities are associated with active NEC?

Metabolic acidosis, positive Clinitest stool, and guaiac-positive stool are common findings. Others include elevated urinary lactate excretion and elevated hydrogen breath excretion (less common).

13. What does the Clinitest detect?

If carbohydrates are malabsorbed in the small intestine because of mucosal damage, they pass into the colon and are fermented. Clinitest tablets detect reducing substances in the stool, a byproduct of fermentation.

14. What plain-film findings are commonly associated with NEC?

Bowel distention, pneumatosis intestinalis, dilated intestinal loops, portal venous air, pneumoperitoneum, and ascites.

15. What is the fixed-loop sign? What does it suggest?

The fixed-loop sign is a single loop or multiple loops of bowel that remain in the same position or shape on plain film for 24–36 hours. The sign suggests full-thickness bowel necrosis and is an indication for operation. Routine abdominal films should be obtained every 6–8 hours in patients with NEC.

16. How does air get into the portal venous system?

Portal venous air or gas is gas dispersed in the fine radicals of the portal venous system. There are two potential mechanisms: (1) gas tracks up the venous sysem from the intestinal wall into the portal veins, and (2) gas-forming bacteria enter the portal system and produce gas. Some believe that portal venous air is an absolute indication for surgical exploration, but others think that it is merely a secondary indicator.

17. Are barium studies useful in making the diagnosis of NEC?

No. If a bowel perforation is present, barium, which is nonabsorbable, can exacerbate the peritonitis. It is best to use a water-soluble ionic contrast agent, but contrast studies are not the first-line diagnostic tools.

18. What is the Bell staging system for NEC?

Stage I	Infants with features suggestive of NEC
Stage II	Infants with definitive NEC
Stage III	Infants with evidence of bowel necrosis and clinical deterioration

19. What are the principal components of nonoperative management of NEC?

Nonoperative management consists of nasogastric decompression, total parenteral nutrition, and broad-spectrum antibiotics.

20. What are the indications for surgery?

The major indications for going to the operating room include free air in the abdomen, deteriorating clinical course, erythema of the abdominal wall, the fixed-loop sign, an abdominal mass, and positive paracentesis.

21. How does one decide the extent of intestine to resect?

The optimal operative approach is to resect perforated or clearly diseased bowel, while preserving as much viable intestine as possible.

22. What do you do if multiple segments of the bowel are diseased?

One approach is to resect the necrotic segments, create a proximal stoma, and, if possible, anastomose the distal defunctionalized segments. Others advocate the creation of multiple stomas. Stoma closure usually can follow in 4–6 weeks after a contrast study.

23. Is it safe to perform a primary anastomosis if there is a single diseased segment?

It depends. In selected cases, the surgeon may perform a primary anastomosis, but the standard approach is to construct a stoma proximal to the resected segment and bring out the distal intestine as a mucous fistula. In some cases, the distal intestine can remain in the abdomen (Hartman's pouch).

24. What do you do if the entire intestine is involved (pannecrosis)?

Some surgeons simply close if the disease appears to involve the intestine just distal to the ligament of Treitz. In some instances, however, the surgeon may create a very high jejunostomy and save a significant length of bowel.

25. Can you bring the stoma or mucous fistula out through the incision?

Yes. There is no increase in wound infection rates.

26. What are the most common long-term complications of the nonoperative and operative management of NEC?

Strictures and short-gut syndrome, respectively.

BIBLIOGRAPHY

1. Albanese C, Rowe M: Necrotizing enterocolitis. In O'Neill J, Rowe M, Grosfeld J, et al (eds): Pediatric Surgery. St. Louis, Mosby, 1998, pp 1297–1320.
2. Ford H, Watkins S, Reblock K, et al: The role of inflammatory cytokines and nitric oxide in the pathogenesis of necrotizing enterocolitis. J Pediatr Surg 32:275–282, 1997.
3. Rowe M, O'Neill J, Grosfeld J, et al: Essentials of Pediatric Surgery. St. Louis, Mosby, 1995.

31. MECKEL'S DIVERTICULUM

William Tisol, M.D., and Richard H. Pearl, M.D.

1. Who first described Meckel's diverticulum?

Meckel's diverticulum was first reported in 1598 by Fabricus Hildanus. Alexis Littre described the presence of the diverticulum in a hernia in 1745 (hence the term Littre's hernia). In 1809, Johann Friederich Meckel was the first to describe the embryologic relationship between the diverticulum and the omphalomesenteric duct.

2. Who described Meckel's diverticulum as "frequently suspected, often looked for, and seldom found"?

Charles Mayo in 1933.

3. Is Meckel's diverticulum a true diverticulum?

Yes. The diverticulum contains all intestinal layers.

4. Describe the embryology of Meckel's diverticulum.

The omphalomesenteric (vitelline) duct connects the primitive gut to the yolk sac. In normal fetal development, the omphalomesenteric duct regresses between the fifth and seventh weeks of fetal life. Failed regression results in various anomalies, including Meckel's diverticulum.

5. What other anomalies arise from failed regression of the omphalomesenteric duct?

Although Meckel's diverticulum is the most common anomaly, failed regression also may lead to an umbilical polyp, omphalomesenteric fistula, umbilical sinus, umbilical cyst, and persistent fibrous band.

6. What congenital anomalies are associated with Meckel's diverticulum?

Associated congenital anomalies include cardiac defects, congenital diaphragmatic hernia, duodenal atresia, esophageal atresia, imperforate anus, gastroschisis, malrotation, omphalocele, Hirschsprung's disease, and Down's syndrome.

7. Describe the blood supply to a Meckel's diverticulum.

The blood supply is derived from the embryonic right and left vitelline arteries, which originate from the aorta. The left vitelline artery usually involutes. The proximal portion of the right vitelline artery persists as the superior mesenteric artery, and the distal portion supplies blood to the diverticulum as an end artery.

8. Does a Meckel's diverticulum arise from the mesenteric or antimesenteric side of the small bowel?

The diverticulum arises from the antimesenteric side of the bowel wall.

9. What is the "rule of 2's"?

In general, Meckel's diverticulum occurs in 2% of the population, usually is located within 2 feet of the ileocecal valve, is 2 inches in length and 2 centimeters in diameter, becomes symptomatic before age 2, contains 2 types of heterotopic tissue (gastric and pancreatic), and is 2 times more common in males.

10. Are most patients with Meckel's diverticulum symptomatic or asymptomatic?

Most patients are asymptomatic. Only 4–35% of patients have related symptoms. Children are more likely to be symptomatic than adults; infants and young children are the most likely to present with symptoms.

11. What is the lifetime risk of developing symptoms of a Meckel's diverticulum?

The lifetime risk is between 4% and 6% and decreases with age.

12. Describe the common symptoms associated with Meckel's diverticulum.

Abdominal pain, nausea, emesis, rectal bleeding, and abdominal distention are the most common symptoms. However, some symptoms are associated with specific age groups. Intestinal obstruction, usually due to volvulus or intussusception, is the most typical presentation in newborns. In older infants and younger children, painless lower gastrointestinal bleeding is most common. Older children usually present with inflammation, as in appendicitis.

13. How is a Meckel's diverticulum diagnosed?

Diagnosis depends on presentation. The test of choice for a bleeding Meckel's diverticulum is a technetium-99m pertechnetate isotope scan (Meckel scan) which preferentially concentrates the isotope in ectopic gastric mucosa. The Meckel scan has a sensitivity of 85% and a specificity of 95%. If obstruction from either intussusception or volvulus is suspected, a pneumatic or barium enema or upper gastrointestinal study with small bowel follow-through is suggestive; however, the diagnostic yield is low. Inflammatory symptoms are similar to those of appendicitis and are diagnosed clinically.

14. How is a symptomatic Meckel's diverticulum treated?

The treatment of choice is diverticulectomy through a right lower quadrant incision with transverse closure of the ileum to maintain luminal patency. Closure may be hand-sewn or stapled. Small bowel resection with end-to-end anastomosis is an alternative method, especially if hemorrhage has occurred. Incidental appendectomy is also performed.

CONTROVERSY

15. How is an asymptomatic Meckel's diverticulum treated?

Treatment of the asymptomatic Meckel's diverticulum is controversial. In general, resection of the incidental Meckel's diverticulum is indicated in children less than 8 years old because infants and young children are at the greatest risk for symptomatic complications. In older children, resection of the incidental Meckel's diverticulum is not indicated. Asymptomatic resection also is indicated in patients of any age who have a Meckel's diverticulum containing heterotopic tissue.

BIBLIOGRAPHY

1. Ashcraft KW, Holder TM: Pediatric Surgery, 2nd ed. Philadelphia, W.B. Saunders, 1993.
2. O'Neil JA, Rowe MI, Grosfeld JL, et al: Pediatric Surgery, 5th ed. St. Louis, Mosby, 1998.
3. Rowe MI, Fonkalsrud EW, O'Neil JA, et al: Essentials of Pediatric Surgery. St. Louis, Mosby, 1995.
4. St-Vil D, Brandt ML, Panic S, et al: Meckel's diverticulum in children: A 20-year review. J Pediatr Surg 26:1289–1292, 1991.

32. APPENDICITIS

Richard Pearl, M.D., Michael Caty, M.D., and Philip Glick, M.D.

1. Is knowledge of appendicitis important in the surgical care of children?

Yes. Appendicitis is the most common reason for both consultation in the emergency department for abdominal pain and emergency abdominal surgery in children.

2. What causes appendicitis?

Luminal obstruction causes appendicitis, as demonstrated in animal experiments in the 1930s by Wangensteen. Causes of obstruction include proliferation of submucosal lymph tissue, which coincides with the peak incidences of appendicitis in the second and third decades of life; fecaliths coincident with appendicitis, suggesting that fecal matter can be a nidus of obstruction; tumors (colon cancer and carcinoids); parasites; and foreign bodies (e.g., nails, bones, seeds, barium).

3. True or false: The most common reason for appendicitis is a fecalith.

False. The incidence of fecaliths in pathologic specimens is as follows: negative appendectomy, 1.2%; acute appendicitis, 7.0%; and perforated appendicitis, 12%. Most cases of appendicitis are not associated with fecaliths.

4. How frequently does cancer cause acute appendicitis?

Cancer was observed in 0.5% of specimens reviewed in a series of almost 5000 patients who underwent surgery for appendicitis.

5. Describe the usual presentation of a child with appendicitis.

The typical child presents with gradual onset of generalized, periumbilical pain. The pain gradually becomes located to the right lower quadrant. Once the pain is located in the right lower quadrant, anterior abdominal tenderness usually occurs. Pain continues to become worse. At this time medical attention usually is sought. However, the presentation is often atypical, and the astute clinician must be watchful for any clues that may help to arrive at the correct diagnosis.

6. Why does the type of pain change in appendicitis?

The initial, periumbilical pain results from distention of the appendix. This typical visceral pain is vague and located at the T10 dermatome, which includes the umbilicus. The localized right lower quadrant pain and tenderness result from full-thickness ischemia and inflammation of the appendix. When the inflamed appendix touches the adjacent peritoneum, localized parietal pain results from the ensuing peritonitis. Atypical anatomic locations of the appendix cause confusing physical findings, such as pelvic, right flank, or right upper quadrant tenderness from appendices located near the right ovary, behind the right colon, or near the gall bladder, respectively. An inflamed appendix touching the bladder may cause painful micturition, mimicking a urinary tract infection; in such cases, however, although the urine may contain white cells, it should show no bacteria on Gram stain or culture.

7. How do you diagnose appendicitis?

The key to successful diagnosis of appendicitis is a careful history, thorough physical exam, and analysis of selected laboratory studies. If two of these three criteria are suggestive of appendicitis, further evaluation is usually unnecessary. Only in confusing cases or atypical presentations should ancillary diagnostic studies be ordered. Plain abdominal radiographs usually contribute little to the diagnosis of appendicitis and are not recommended. However, if they are ordered, findings consistent with appendicitis include the presence of fecaliths, an atypical right lower quadrant gas pattern ("sentinel loops" thought to be due to localized ileus), and lordosis away from the right side. Chest radiographs can be particularly helpful to evaluate for occult pneumonic processes, which can mimic appendicitis. In experienced hands, ultrasound is quite helpful, especially in adolescent girls. The finding of an enlarged, noncompressible appendix is virtually diagnostic. Other findings, such as tubo-ovarian pathology, help to rule out the diagnosis. Computed tomography (CT) scanning also has proved effective in adults and is now selectively used in children.

8. What other problems can be confused with appendicitis?

Disease entities that may mimic appendicitis include Crohn's disease, viral gastroenteritis, mesenteric adenitis, pneumonia, Meckel's diverticulitis, ovarian pathology, psoas abscess, and typhlitis.

9. How is uncomplicated, nonperforated acute appendicitis treated?

Most cases of acute appendicitis are treated with immediate appendectomy, which can be done with either an open technique or the laparoscope. Alternative approaches appropriate for the delayed diagnosis of appendicitis include a combination of intravenous antibiotics, percutaneous abscess drainage, and interval appendectomy.

10. What is an interval appendectomy? When is it appropriate?

Interval appendectomy refers to a delay in the performance of an appendectomy until a certain interval of time has passed. This strategy usually is applied to the patient who presents with complicated appendicitis that is minimally symptomatic and not associated with diffuse peritonitis. A CT scan or ultrasound demonstrates a loculated right lower quadrant collection of fluid or phlegmon. After the patient is admitted, intravenous antibiotics are administered. If an abscess is present, it is drained percutaneously. Antibiotics are continued until the patient is afebrile, intestinal function is normal, and the white blood cell count is less than 10,000. Much of this intravenous antibiotic therapy can be done as home care. After patients recover from acute illness, they return in 8–12 weeks for appendectomy. In selected patients the advantage of this approach is much greater ease and safety of appendectomy due to resolution of periappendiceal infection and inflammation.

11. How is perforated appendicitis treated?

The appendix is removed, and any interloop adhesions of the bowel are taken down. Irrigation of the peritoneal cavity is performed. The value of antibiotics in irrigation fluids is controversial and often depends on the science of individual preference. We recommend postoperative antibiotics to continue until the fever resolves, intestinal function is normalized, and the white blood cell count is less than 10,000 (although this policy is not universally accepted). Compared with adults, wounds are rarely left open postoperatively in children with ruptured appendicitis. Intraoperative placement of drains in the abdomen in perforated appendicitis seems to have little value and in fact has increased the length of stay in several studies with no decrease in infectious complications.

12. How long should patients be treated with antibiotics for appendicitis?

In uncomplicated cases of acute appendicitis, a single preoperative and postoperative dose of a broad-spectrum antibiotic is sufficient. In a series of 1366 children so treated, cefoxitin was the choice in 65% of cases, with few infectious complications. In cases of perforation, triple regimens were chosen more frequently (ampicillin, gentamicin, and clindamycin or flagyl). Therapy is continued until the patients are afebrile for 24 hours and the white blood cell count has returned to normal (< 10,000). With this regimen the average length of stay was 3 days and 7 days for acute and perforated appendicitis, respectively.

13. What are the complications of perforated appendicitis?

Common complications of perforated appendicitis include wound infection, intraabdominal abscess, and small bowel obstruction. Less common complications include pneumonia, pyelephlebitis, and fascial dehiscence. Several series have demonstrated reduced fertility in women after perforated appendicitis, although this finding has been refuted in a large report from Great Britain.

14. What is an acceptable infectious complication rate in properly treated perforated appendicitis?

This question is highly controversial. Posttreatment abscess rates from 0% to upward of 15% are reported. However, with early diagnosis and treatment followed by appropriate antibiotic therapy, the goal should be wound infections in < 2% and abscesses in < 2.5% of treated patients. Unfortunately, lack of early referral causes infectious complications beyond the control of the treating surgeon. Infectious complications are proportional to the appendiceal rupture rate.

15. How common are delayed referrals in children suffering from appendicitis?

Fifty-two percent of children with appendicitis perforate before seeing a doctor, and 70% are perforated before they are first seen by a surgeon. Parental education and a high index of suspicion by the primary care doctor are needed to decrease these embarrassing statistics.

16. Why are delayed referrals for surgical consultation so common?

As with any disease, 85% of early diagnosis depends on an accurate history. Therefore, the ability to diagnose appendicitis is related inversely to the patient's age. In children less than 3 years old, appendicitis is virtually never diagnosed before perforation. Perforation rates approach those seen in adolescents and young adults (20%) only after children reach 8 years of age. The dilemma is communication. By the time a toddler can give sufficient information about abdominal discomfort to achieve the level of suspicion necessary for parents or caregivers to seek medical attention, it is almost always too late. In fact, in evaluating a 3- or 4-year-old child with appendicitis in the emergency department, the most common scenario is several days of high fever, abdominal distention, and small bowel obstruction on acute abdominal radiographs. Clearly this is a late presentation.

17. What is the time frame from the first symptom to perforation in children with appendicitis?

Scientific data are difficult to provide; in our experience the interval from first symptom to perforation is usually 24–36 hours. This time frame is important, because in evaluating a child with suspected appendicitis with a brief history and equivocal findings, the correct approach is to admit, observe, and reexamine. If the child has appendicitis, the serial physical examination is critical in the accurate, timely, and correct diagnosis. This is the key to improving our results and thereby decreasing the perforation rates. Perforation rates as high as 55% have been reported in children entirely because of late presentation. However, rarely do children perforate after they have been evaluated by a surgeon (< 2%), proving that early presentation and evaluation are critical if we are to improve results and decrease the complication rates.

18. What is McBurney's point? Who was McBurney?

McBurney's point is located between an inch-and-a-half to two inches from the anterior spinous process of the ilium on a straight line drawn from the process to the umbilicus. Another useful description of McBurney's point is one-third the distance from the anterior superior iliac crest in a direct line to the umbilicus. This anatomic landmark was attributed to McBurney because his detailed report of the removal of the appendix in 1889 used this measurement in the operative description.

19. Where does the term "appendicitis" come from?

In 1886, the pathologist Reginald Fitz demonstrated that the clinical entity known then as "perityphlitis" was due to inflammation of the appendix; therefore, he described the disease process as appendicitis. He also predicted that its treatment would be surgical.

20. Are the terms "peritoneal signs," "acute abdomen," and "surgical abdomen" synonyms?

Yes. For the most part, surgeons use these terms interchangeably. With few exceptions, when a patient is determined to have peritoneal signs, acute abdomen, or surgical abdomen, an operation is indicated.

21. How are peritoneal signs detected?

The experienced pediatric diagnostician looks for subtle or obvious signs of parietal peritoneal irritation. In the case of appendicitis, when parietal peritoneal irritation begins to occur, localized signs develop. These signs can be elicited by gentle finger palpation of the child's abdominal wall, looking for evidence of rectus or oblique muscle rigidity. As parietal peritoneal irritation develops, these findings become less subtle; hence, the "board-like" abdomen associated with diffuse peritonitis. If the tip of the appendix is located retrocecally or in the pelvis, peritoneal findings in the anterior abdominal wall may be replaced by psoas muscle or obturator muscle irritation. For this reason, check for the "psoas sign" and "obturator sign" in doing a thorough exam of children suspected of having an abdominal process.

22. What is guarding?

There are two types of guarding: voluntary and involuntary. **Voluntary guarding** occurs in any child who voluntarily contracts the abdominal muscles. It may occur from laughing or crying or as a protective mechanism. It has no pathologic significance.

On the other hand, **involuntary guarding** is a sign of peritoneal irritation and usually suggests the need for a surgical procedure. Patients have no control over involuntary guarding; it is a spinal cord reflex, initiated when peritoneal irritation develops. It can be elicited with gentle finger or hand palpation of the anterior abdominal wall, looking for localized or diffuse rigidity of the rectus or oblique muscles. The examining physician must specify in the record whether patients have voluntary or involuntary guarding; writing "+ guarding" in the chart is of no value in the medical record.

23. What is rebound tenderness?

Rebound tenderness is abdominal pain or tenderness elicited by the examiner with deep palpation, followed by abrupt removal of the examining fingers. It may be positive not only in illness requiring surgery, but also in illnesses not requiring surgical intervention. In addition, it is extremely painful and cruel to test for rebound tenderness. Therefore, testing for rebound tenderness should not be performed in children.

24. What is Rovsing's sign?

Gentle palpation or percussion of the left side of the abdomen elicits pain at McBurney's point in cases of appendicitis. It is a valuable part of the physical exam in children suspected of having appendicitis.

BIBLIOGRAPHY

1. Anderson KD, Parry RL: Appendicitis. In O'Neill JA, Rowe MI, Grosfeld JL, et al (eds): Pediatric Surgery. St. Louis, Mosby, 1998, pp 1369–1377.
2. Hale DA, Malloy M, Pearl RH, et al: Appendectomy: A contemporary appraisal. Ann Surg 225:252–261, 1997.
3. Hale DA, Molloy M, Pearl RH, et al: Appendectomy: Improving care through quality improvement. Arch Surg 132:153–157, 1997.
4. Irish MS, Pearl RH, Caty MG, Glick PL: The approach to common abdominal diagnosis in infants and children. Pediatr Clin North Am 54:725–772, 1990.
5. Pearl RH, Hale DA, Molloy M, et al: Pediatric appendectomy. J Pediatr Surg 30:173–181, 1995.

33. INTUSSUSCEPTION

Jeff C. Hoehner, M.D., Ph.D.

1. What is intussusception?
Full-thickness invagination of the proximal bowel into the distal contiguous intestine.

2. What names are ascribed to the proximal and distal bowel components of an intussusception?
The proximal invaginating intestine is termed the **intussusceptum,** the distal receiving bowel (outer part) is the **intussuscipiens.**

3. What age group is most commonly affected?
80–90% of intussusceptions occur in children between 3 months and 3 years of age.

4. What are "red currant jelly" stools?
Red currant jelly stools are a frequent finding in patients with intussusception. Intussusception results in intestinal edema, lymphatic obstruction, local venous hypertension, vascular stasis, and subsequent mucosal sloughing. This combination of intraluminal fluid, blood, and mucosal tissue fragments results in stools with the appearance, color, and consistency of red currant jelly.

5. What are classic clinical findings of intussusception?
Crampy abdominal pain, vomiting, rectal bleeding, and abdominal mass. Although each finding alone is quite common, this constellation is identified in only 10% of patients. Profound lethargy, dehydration, and abdominal distention are also frequent findings.

6. What is the most common finding on abdominal plain film?
A normal radiograph, although partial or complete bowel obstruction occasionally is seen. Infrequently the intussuscipiens is visualized as an opacity within a radiolucent, gas-filled distal bowel.

7. What segment of the bowel is most frequently affected?
The most common intussusception is ileocolic—the ileum invaginates into the cecum or right colon. Ileoileal or colocolic intussusceptions are less frequent and associated more often with a "pathologic lead point."

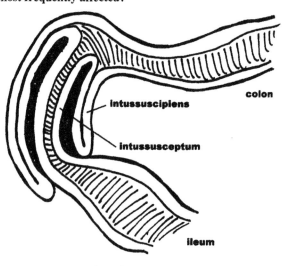

Ileocolic intussusception

8. What is meant by a "pathologic lead point" in intussusception?

The pathologic lead point is a recognizable intraperitoneal anomaly or abnormality that tethers or obstructs the bowel, initiating the process of intussusception. Meckel's diverticulum, intestinal polyps, intestinal duplications, B-cell lymphoma, and indwelling enteral feeding tubes are among the more frequent pathologic lead points.

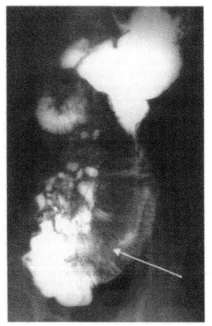

Upper gastrointestinal contrast study shows an uncommon jejunojejunal intussusception just distal to the ligament of Treitz. An arrow indicates the intussuscepted intestine. A jejunal polyp acted as the pathologic lead point in this patient with Peutz-Jeghers syndrome.

9. What is the usual cause of intussusception?

The best answer is that the cause is unknown. However, an unproven theory suggests that, because intussusception frequently follows a viral illness (gastroenteritis, respiratory infection), the resultant hyperplasia of distal ileal lymphoid tissue is to blame. Hyperplastic tissues, called Peyer's patches, involve the entire circumference of the distal ileum, thus causing luminal narrowing and tethering that encourages intussusception.

10. What is the sign of Dance?

The sign of Dance is the absence of the cecum in the right iliac fossa during palpation, as first described by Dance, a New York pediatrician.

11. How is intussusception diagnosed?

Usually suspected clinically, the diagnosis is confirmed by either ultrasonography (target or bullet sign) or contrast enema (fist or coiled-spring sign).

12. When the diagnosis is suspected or confirmed, is the patient emergently referred for reduction?

No. Dependable IV access, rehydration, and surgical consultation are essential. Insertion of a nasogastric tube and intestinal decompression are recommended before reduction is attempted.

13. Is urgent operative treatment required in all patients with intussusception?

No. Most centers have the capability of performing either hydrostatic or pneumatic reduction of the intussusception. Reduction is accomplished by inserting and securing a catheter into the rectum, taping the buttocks together to obtain an occlusive seal, and instilling either radio-opaque fluid or air into the colon. Under fluoroscopic guidance, pressure within the distal bowel pushes the intussuscipiens proximally. Complete reduction is confirmed only when air or contrast freely fills more proximal loops of bowel with reflux into the terminal ileum.

14. What kind of pneumatic or hydrostatic reduction pressures are safe?

Despite some debate, elevation of a barium column higher than 1 meter or insufflation of air at pressures > 150 mmHg is not recommended.

15. What is the next step if initial attempts at pneumatic or hydrostatic reduction fail?

You may try again, especially if the patient remains stable and partial reduction was achieved at the first attempt. However, more than two unsuccessful attempts at nonoperative reduction usually are associated with an increased incidence of perforation.

16. When is operative treatment indicated?

Irreducibility by pneumatic or hydrostatic means, perforation, shock, and hemodynamic instability are indications for urgent operative treatment. Reported relative indications include clinical peritonitis, age > 6 years, and duration of symptoms > 24 hours.

17. Do all patients treated operatively require intestinal resection?

No. Gentle manipulation by pushing the intussusceptum out of the intussuscipiens (rather than by pulling with traction) frequently results in reduction. If reduction is accomplished, no further intervention is required. If attempts at reduction cause undue injury to the bowel wall, if bowel necrosis or perforation is present, or if a pathologic lead point is identified or suspected, resection and primary anastomosis are indicated.

18. Does reduction prevent subsequent recurrences?

No. Recurrences may occur in 5–11% of children. Some children may experience multiple recurrences. Operative reduction, even with resection, maintains a 1–4% incidence of recurrence.

19. What medical processes are associated with intussusception?

Two classic examples are cystic fibrosis and Henoch-Schonlein purpura (HSP). Intussusception in cystic fibrosis is probably a result of the thick, putty-like material adherent to the intestinal mucosa, which acts as a partial obstruction or lead point equivalent to meconium ileus. In HSP, a submucosal hematoma acting as a lead point is the most common cause.

20. How should you evaluate a 2-year-old child presenting with a mid-small bowel obstruction 10 days after a fundoplication/gastrostomy?

With an abdominal ultrasound and/or contrast enema and upper gastrointestinal study. The incidence of intussusception after laparotomy in children is 0.1–0.5%. Postoperative intussusception occurs most typically 8–11 days after a laparotomy. Abdominal distention with bilious vomiting is a more frequent feature than abdominal pain. Neurologically impaired children are at highest risk. The intussusception usually involves the small bowel, and operative reduction is typically required.

BIBLIOGRAPHY

1. Daneman A, Alton DJ, Lobo E, et al: Patterns of recurrence of intussusception in children: A 17-year review. Pediatr Radiol 28:913–919, 1998.
2. Doody DP: Intussusception. In Oldham KT, Colombani PM, Foglia RP (eds): Surgery of Infants and Children. Philadelphia, Lippincott-Raven, 1997, pp 1241–1249.
3. Ein SH, Alton D, Palder SB, et al: Intussusception in the 1990s: Has 25 years made a difference? Pediatr Surg Int 12:374–376, 1997.
4. Fecteau A, Flageole H, Nguyen LT, et al: Recurrent intussusception: Safe use of hydrostatic enema. J Pediatr Surg 31:859–861, 1996.
5. Grant HW, Buccimaza I, Hadley GP: A comparison of colo-colic and ileo-colic intussusception. J Pediatr Surg 31:1067–1610, 1996.

6. Hoehner JC, Kimura K, Soper RT: Postoperative intussusception as a consequence of inversion appendectomy. Pediatr Surg Int 10:51–53, 1995.
7. Palder SB, Ein SH, Stringer DA, et al: Intussusception: Barium on air. J Pediatr Surg 26:271–275, 1991.
8. Reymond RD: The mechanism of intussusception: A theoretical analysis of the phenomenon. Br J Radiol 45:1–7, 1972.
9. West KW, Stephens B, Rescorla FJ, et al: Postoperative intussusception: Experience with 36 cases in children. Surgery 104:781–785, 1988.
10. Young DG: Intussusception. In O'Neill JA Jr, Rowe MI, Grosfeld JL, et al (eds): Pediatric Surgery, 5th ed. St. Louis, Mosby, 1998, pp 1185–1195.

34. SMALL LEFT COLON SYNDROME

J. Stephen Marshall, M.D., FACS

1. What is small left colon syndrome?

Small left colon syndrome (SLCS) results in clinical and radiologic evidence of a low colon obstruction without an anatomic defect to explain the microcolon.

2. What congenital defects can result in congenital microcolon?

• Atresias
• Partial or total colonic Hirschsprung's disease
• Cystic fibrosis
• Colonic meconium plug

3. What studies should be used for the diagnosis of SLCS?

Contrast enemas should be used for the diagnosis of SLCS. Positive studies demonstrate a narrowed colon from the rectum to the splenic flexure. Gastrogaffin enemas may stimulate the colon, resulting in resolutin of SLCS. Contrast enemas also should be used in cases of atresia to rule out multiple atresias and may be therapeutic in cases of meconium plugs. Contrast studies also suggest the diagnosis of Hirschsprung's disease when a radiologic transition zone is seen.

4. What common prenatal factors do children with SLCS share?

Most are children of diabetic mothers. In fact, approximately 40% of children of diabetic mothers show some manifestation of SLCS.

5. How does maternal diabetes cause SLCS?

Infants of diabetic mothers are believed to have postnatal hypoglycemia, which may have two effects on the gastrointestinal tract that result in SLCS. Elevated levels of glucagon can cause decreased intestinal motility in the left colon, and hypoglycemia can produce vagal stimulation that increases intestinal motility in the area of distribution of the vagus nerve, which ends at the splenic flexure. The combination of these two events explains the characteristic radiologic findings in SLCS.

It is believed that the high production of glucagon in children exposed to high maternal levels of insulin causes a narrowing of the left colon, which may be more sensitive to the effects of glucagon. This also may explain why the syndrome may resolve after a contrast enema as the glucagon level normalizes.

6. What is the natural history of SLCS?

SLCS produces a funtional colon obstruction with a significant risk of cecal perforation if not treated promptly.

7. What is the best surgical approach to SLCS?

Observation. The treatment of SLCS is nonsurgical. Water-soluble contrast enemas are diagnostic and, in most cases, therapeutic, although more than one enema may be necessary. Involvement of the surgical service is mandatory, however, because cecal perforation may occur early in the disease process, and other surgical diseases may be the source of the obstruction.

8. What is the megacystitis-microcolon syndrome?

The more accurate name for this entity is the megacystitis-microcolon-intestinal hypoperistalsis syndrome. Affected children have a large, distended bladder, microcolon, and shortened, nonrotated midgut. Clinical presentation includes abdominal distention and bilious vomiting in the newborn period. Ganglion cells and acetylcholinesterase activity are normal, but smooth muscle cells of the bladder and ileum demonstrate vacuolar degeneration with increased connective tissue between cells. The absence of motility in the ileum yields a microcolon without stool. This disease is associated with a high mortality rate despite pharmacologic and surgical intervention.

BIBLIOGRAPHY

1. Davis WS, Allen RP, Favara BE, Slovis TL: Neonatal small left colon syndrome. Am J Roentgenol Radium Ther Nuclear Med 120(2):322–329, 1974.
2. Davis WS, Campbell JB: Neonatal small left colon syndrome. Occurrence in asymptomatic patients of diabetic mothers. Am J Dis Children 129:1024, 1975.
3. Oldham KT: Atresia, stenosis, and other obstructions of the colon. In O'Neill JA, et al (eds): Pediatric Surgery, 5th ed. St. Louis, Mosby, 1998.
4. Stewart DR, Nixon GW, Johnson DG, Condon VR: Neonatal small left colon syndromes. Ann Surg 186(6):741–745, 1977.

35. DISORDERS OF COLONIC MOTILITY

David J. Hackam, M.D., Ph.D., and Richard H. Pearl, M.D.

HIRSCHSPRUNG'S DISEASE

1. What is Hirschsprung's disease?

Congenital aganglionosis of the intestine.

2. Define the incidence of Hirschsprung's disease and associated risk factors.

Hirschsprung's disease occurs in 1 in 1000 live births. The male-to-female ratio is 4:1. Most cases are sporadic, but long-segment aganglionosis and total colonic aganglionosis are associated strongly with familial disease (15% and 50%, respectively). The incidence of trisomy 21 is 5–15%.

3. Is there a genetic basis for Hirschsprung's disease?

Yes. A dominant gene for Hirschsprung's disease maps to the proximal region of the long arm of chromosome 10, which was identified as the *RET* protooncogene. Mutations in *RET* occur in approximately 25% of familial cases and 15% of sporadic cases.

4. From what are enteric ganglion cells derived?

Vagal neural crest cells.

5. Describe the normal embryogenesis of the myenteric nervous system.

Neural crest-derived neuroblasts appear in the esophagus at 5 weeks, then migrate to the anal canal during weeks 5–12. These cells form immediately outside the circular layer and then become sandwiched between the longitudinal muscle layers. The submucous plexus is formed by the neuroblasts, which migrate from the myenteric plexus across the circular muscle layer and into the submucosa and mucosa.

6. True or false: The internal sphincter is aganglionic.

True. Affected children truly have a tight sphincter.

7. Is the location of the aganglionosis variable?

Yes. The aganglionosis is rectosigmoid in 75% of patients. It is located in the sigmoid, splenic flexure, or transverse colon in 17% of cases, and 5–8% of cases involve the total colon with a short segment of terminal ileum.

8. Describe the gross pathologic features of Hirschsprung's disease.

Dilation and hypertrophy of the proximal colon with transition to normal-sized or narrow distal (i.e., aganglionic) bowel. The abnormally dilated bowel actually has ganglionic cells (which really stumped early pathologists and surgeons).

9. What are the histologic features of Hirschsprung's disease?

Absence of ganglion cells in the myenteric and submucous plexuses and presence of hypertrophied, nonmyelinated nerve trunks in the space normally occupied by the ganglion cells.

10. How does Hirschsprung's disease present?

Delayed passage of meconium in the first 24 hours (over 90% of patients) is associated with constipation, abdominal distention, and bilious vomiting in the first few days of life. Rectal examination may cause explosive passage of meconium and gas, causing acute relief of the obstruction.

11. True or false: Hirschsprung's disease is never fatal.

False. Never say never in surgery. About 10–30% of children develop enterocolitis, which may be the initial presentation and is an important potential cause of mortality.

12. What is the differential diagnosis of Hirschsprung's disease in the neonatal period?

Malrotation with volvulus, intestinal atresias or stenosis, duodenal obstruction, meconium ileus, and imperforate anus. Virtually any congenital obstruction of the gastrointestinal tract may be considered initially because the length of aganglionosis is so variable.

13. How is Hirschsprung's disease diagnosed?
- Plain abdominal radiographs. Distended bowel occupies the entire abdomen with air/fluid levels, often with no or a small amount of air in the undilated rectum.
- Contrast enema identifies the transition zone and also is helpful if barium is retained in the colon for over 24 hours. The post-evacuation film can be particularly helpful.
- Anorectal manometry reveals absence of internal sphincter relaxation in response to rectal distention.
- Rectal biopsy, the gold standard, is performed 2–3 cm proximal to the dentate line. Biopsy identifies the absence of ganglion cells and the increase in immunohistochemical staining for acetylcholinesterase activity in the lamina propria and muscularis. It can be done via rectal suction biopsy (preferred) or transanal full-thickness biopsy.

14. What are the major principles in treating Hirschsprung's disease?

The historical standard is to obtain diversion proximal to the aganglionic segment in the neonatal period, then to perform a definitive pull-through operation at 9–12 months of age when the bowel is at normal caliber. This procedure is followed by stoma closure if it was not performed at the time of the pull-through. However, most pediatric surgeons now use a one-stage approach. A definitive pull-through procedure is performed at the time of diagnosis without proximal diversion. This strategy has been applied to neonates and older infants with results equivalent to the multiple-staged approach. The one-stage approach requires a shorter total hospital stay and can be done as an open procedure, laparoscopically, transanally, or as a combination of these methods.

15. Define the pull-through operations performed for Hirschsprung's disease.
   - Duhamel procedure. The aganglionic colon is resected to the rectum, which is left in place. Normally innervated proximal colon is pulled through behind the rectum, and side-to-side colorectal anastomosis is performed with a transanal GIA stapler.
   - Soave procedure. Aganglionic bowel is resected, and an endorectal dissection in the submucosal plane is performed from the proximal rectum to the anus. Ganglionic proximal bowel is then pulled through the rectal muscular cuff and anastomosed to the distal rectum.
   - Swenson procedure. Aganglionic colon is resected, followed by extramural rectal dissection with pull-through of ganglionic proximal bowel and anastomosis of colon to distal rectum just above the dentate line.

16. What are the major complications of pull-through procedures?
   - Anastomotic leak (1–5%)
   - Stricture (3–5%)
   - Intestinal obstruction (5%)
   - Wound infection (1–10%)
   - Enterocolitis (2–27%)

17. What are the principles for treating Hirschsprung's enterocolitis?
   - Correction of dehydration and electrolyte imbalance
   - Rectal irrigation
   - Broad-spectrum antibiotics (consider vancomycin because of 30% association with *Clostridium difficile*)
   - Decompression of intestine

18. What important principles apply to long-segment Hirschsprung's disease?
   Total colonic aganglionosis, which may extend to the small intestine, is a severe form of Hirschsprung's disease. The male predominance is less evident than with other forms of Hirschsprung's disease (1.5:1 to 2:1), and the familial incidence is approximately 20%. Such cases account for 2–14% of all forms of aganglionosis. Most patients present with neonatal obstruction. Radiography may show a colon of normal transition or caliber. Treatment involves ileostomy, followed by a pull-through operation, although one-stage pull-through can be performed in selected stable patients.

INTESTINAL NEURONAL DYSPLASIA

19. What is intestinal neuronal dysplasia?
   Intestinal neuronal dysplasia (IND) is a condition that clinically resembles Hirschsprung's disease; however, ganglion cells are present but abnormal. The characteristic features include hyperganglionosis of the submucous and myenteric plexus, giant ganglia, ectopic ganglia, increased acetylcholinesterase (AChE)-positive nerve fibers around submucosal vessels, and increased AChE-positive nerve fibers in the lamina propria.

20. How is IND managed?
   Laxatives and enemas, followed by internal sphincter myectomy if symptoms persist. Resection and pull-through may be indicated for extensive IND.

FUNCTIONAL CONSTIPATION

21. Define functional constipation.

Functional constipation refers to a disorder of delayed colonic motility in which no organic or anatomic cause can be found. Diagnosis depends on history and physical examination as well as the selective use of barium enema, anorectal manometry, transit studies, and rectal biopsy to exclude neurologic, mechanical, or systemic causes.

22. How do the history and physical examination assist with the diagnosis?

Acute constipation suggests an organic cause, whereas chronic constipation is usually functional. Failure to thrive and abdominal distention suggest Hirschsprung's disease. In functional constipation the rectum is distended and full of stool, whereas in Hirschsprung's disease it is empty and tight.

23. How does functional constipation present?

Constipation, encopresis, and fecal incontinence.

24. How is functional constipation treated?

Through the combined, multidisciplinary implementation of defecation trials, dietary modification, and laxatives. Psychosocial counseling is often beneficial as part of multimodality management. The selective use of biofeedback training may be of benefit—use whatever works.

25. What percentage of neurologically normal children with fecal incontinence have functional constipation as an underlying disorder?

Approximately 95%.

BIBLIOGRAPHY

1. Banani AS, Forootan HR, Kumar PV: Intestinal neuronal dysplasia as a cause of surgical failure in Hirschsprung's disease: A new modality for surgical management. J Pediatr Surg 31:572–574, 1996.
2. Berger S, Ziebell P, Offsler M, Hofmann-von Kap-herr S: Congenital malformations and perinatal morbidity associated with intestinal neuronal dysplasia. Pediatr Surg Int 13:474–479, 1998.
3. Cord-Udy CL, Smith VV, Ahmed S, et al: An evaluation of the role of suction rectal biopsy in the diagnosis of intestinal neuronal dysplasia. J Pediatr Gastroenterol Nutr 24:1–6, 1997.
4. Hackam DJ, Filler RM, Pearl RH: Enterocolitis after the surgical treatment of Hirschsprung's disease: Risk factors and financial impact. J Pediatr Surg 33:830–833, 1998.
5. Hackam DJ, Superina RA, Pearl RH: Single-stage repair of Hirschsprung's disease: A comparison of 109 patients over 5 years. J Pediatr Surg 32:1028–1032, 1997.
6. Kleinhaus S, Boley SJ, Sheran M, et al: Hirschsprung's disease: A survey of the surgical section of the American Academy of Pediatrics. J Pediatr Surg 14:588–597, 1979.
7. Kobayashi H, Hirakawa H, Surana R, et al: Intestinal neuronal dysplasia is a possible cause of persistent bowel symptoms after pull-through operation for Hirschsprung's disease. J Pediatr Surg 30:253–257, 1995.
8. Lyonnet S, Bolino A, Pelet A, et al: A gene of Hirschsprung's disease maps to the proximal long arm of chromosome 10. Nature Genet 4:346–350, 1993.
9. Oldham KT, Coran AG, Wesley JR: Pediatric abdomen. In Greenfield LJ, Mulholland M, Oldham KT, et al (eds): Surgery: Scientific Principles and Practice, 2nd ed. Philadelphia, Lippincott-Raven, 1997, pp 2028–2101.
10. Polley TZ, Coran AG, Heidelberger KP, et al: Suction rectal biopsy in the diagnosis of Hirschsprung's disease and chronic constipation. Pediatr Surg Int 1:84–87, 1986.
11. Puri P: Hirschsprung's disease. In Puri P (ed): Newborn Surgery. Oxford, Butterworth Heinemann, 1996, pp 363–379.
12. Puri P, Wester T: Intestinal neuronal dysplasia. Semin Pediatr Surg 7:181–186, 1998.
13. So HB, Schwartz DL, Becker JM, et al: Endorectal "pull-through" without preliminary colostomy in neonates with Hirschsprung's disease. J Pediatr Surg 15:470–471, 1980.

36. INFLAMMATORY BOWEL DISEASE

Steven W. Bruch, M.D., and Peter C. W. Kim, M.D.

1. Name the two most common types of inflammatory bowel disease in children.
Ulcerative colitis and Crohn's disease.

2. What are the predisposing risk factors for Crohn's disease?
Crohn's disease is more common in Jewish people, especially those of middle European origin. A genetic predisposition may exist. At the time of diagnosis, there is a 5–25% chance that a first-degree relative of the patient will have an inflammatory bowel disease, and siblings of a patient with Crohn's disease are 17–35 times more likely to develop the disease compared with the general population. Human leukocyte antigen (HLA) studies suggest an association with Crohn's disease and the HLA-DR4 allele.

3. What are the predisposing risk factors for ulcerative colitis?
Again, people of Jewish descent are more likely to develop ulcerative colitis than the general population. A family history is the most consistent risk factor for children. HLA studies show that patients with ulcerative colitis are more likely to have the HLA-DR2 allele. Nonsmokers are more likely to develop ulcerative colitis, and smoking may improve symptoms in patients with ulcerative colitis. (This is *not* a recommendation to start smoking, however.)

4. When does inflammatory bowel disease most commonly affect children?
The most common age of onset for newly diagnosed cases of Crohn's disease in the pediatric population is the mid-to-late teens. Approximately 15% of all cases of Crohn's disease occur during childhood. Children with ulcerative colitis are most commonly diagnosed between the ages of 5–16; onset during infancy accounts for < 1% of reported cases.

5. What are common presenting symptoms of inflammatory bowel disease?
The most common symptoms are crampy abdominal pain and diarrhea, which may contain mucus and/or blood. In Crohn's disease, the pain is usually right-sided and may be associated with a mass in the right lower abdomen that mimics acute appendicitis. Perirectal disease manifested as fistulas, fissures, and tags is present in about 15–30% of patients. In ulcerative colitis, the pain is usually lower abdominal, crampy pain that is most intense during defecation.

6. What are the extraintestinal symptoms of inflammatory bowel disease?
In most patients with Crohn's disease extraintestinal manifestations include fever, fatigue, and weight loss. The other common target organs are the skin, joints, liver, eyes, and bone. Ulcerative colitis may be associated with weight loss, delayed growth and sexual maturation, mucocutaneous lesions, renal calculi, primary sclerosing cholagangitis, and ocular disease.

7. Describe the common laboratory findings in patients with inflammatory bowel disease.
The most common laboratory findings in patients with Crohn's disease are anemia (70%), elevated erythrocyte sedimentation rate (80%), hypoalbuminemia (60%), and thrombocytosis (60%). Patients with ulcerative colitis present with similar laboratory findings, but up to 36% of pediatric patients with ulcerative colitis have no abnormal blood tests. The stool of patients suspected of having ulcerative colitis should be cultured to exclude enteric pathogens as a cause of the symptoms.

8. Describe the radiologic findings in patients with inflammatory bowel disease.
In Crohn's disease radiologic studies are used to diagnose and stage the disease. Because the small bowel is involved in over 80% of cases, an upper gastrointestinal series with small bowel

follow-through is essential. Common findings with Crohn's disease are irregular, nodular or "cobblestoned," and thickened bowel loops with deep ulcers, fistulas, and stenotic areas depicted as a "string sign."

Contrast studies of the colon typically are not obtained in patients with ulcerative colitis, as endoscopy is now used to diagnose and stage this disease. In fulminant cases of ulcerative colitis and Crohn's disease plain films should be obtained to look for a toxic megacolon.

9. Describe the endoscopic findings in patients with inflammatory bowel disease.

Endoscopically, Crohn's disease and ulcerative colitis have distinct characteristics that some-times overlap and thus make the two difficult to distinguish. Crohn's disease commonly presents with rectal sparing, which is unusual in ulcerative colitis. Crohn's disease is also characterized by aphthous ulcers and patchy inflammation interspersed with grossly normal–appearing colon. Deep-fissuring ulcers, heaped-up edematous mucosa or pseudopolyps, and a granular, friable, edematous ileocecal valve also may be present in the colon of patients with Crohn's disease. Ulcerative colitis produces a continuous inflammation from the rectum to various levels of the proximal colon. Biopsy is essential to diagnose inflammatory bowel disease and to distinguish Crohn's disease from ulcerative colitis.

10. What are the clinical differences between Crohn's colitis and ulcerative colitis?

Comparison of Clinical Manifestations of Crohn's Colitis and Ulcerative Colitis

	CROHN'S COLITIS	ULCERATIVE COLITIS
Rectal involvement	Often absent (50%)	Always present
Colonic pattern of involvement	Skip areas, focal and discontinuous involvement	Continuous involvement from rectum proximally
Anal lesions	Multiple fistulas frequent (75%)	Infrequent and less severe (< 25%)
Mucosal appearance	Cobblestone pattern with multiple ulcerations	Inflamed mucosa: red, granular, and friable
Serosal involvement	Serositis characteristic with creeping fat	Serositis occurs only with fulminant disease
Small bowel involvement	Frequent; terminal ileitis most common (30%)	Infrequent; "backwash ileitis" in 10%

11. What pathologic features differentiate Crohn's colitis from ulcerative colitis?

Comparison of Pathologic Features in Crohn's Colitis and Ulcerative Colitis

	CROHN'S COLITIS	ULCERATIVE COLITIS
Bowel wall involvement	Transmural	Limited to mucosa and submucosa
Ulcerations	May be deep and fissured	Erosive and superficial
Granulomas	Frequently present (> 50%)	Absent
Crypt disease	Epithelial erosions next to uninvolved crypts	All crypts are involved with cryptitis
Goblet cells	Depleted in affected crypts only	Generalized goblet cell depletion
Vasculitis	May be present	Absent

12. Describe the medical management of a pediatric patient with inflammatory bowel disease.

The goals of treatment are to control symptoms, avoid complications, and prevent recurrence. Corticosteroids are used to improve symptoms in the acute phase of both small bowel and colonic disease and as maintenance therapy to prevent recurrence. The most significant side effects of chronic steroid use are bone demineralization and restriction of growth. These side effects can be minimized by the addition of 5-aminosalicylate agents, which also are used to induce remission and to prevent recurrence. Sulfasalazine, which is activated in the colon, is used for both Crohn's disease and ulcerative colitis, whereas Crohn's disease in the small bowel is treated with mesalamine, which is activated in the small bowel. Immunosuppressive agents are used in cases refractory to steroids or cases that require high doses of steroids to control symptoms. Azathioprine and 6-mercaptopurine have been used extensively in pediatric patients, and other agents, such as methotrexate and cyclosporine, are now used more frequently. Antibiotics are used to treat complications of Crohn's disease, especially intraabdominal abscesses. Metronidazole is useful in perianal disease and in severe cases of Crohn's colitis. Adequate nutrition is important in the management of inflammatory bowel disease to eliminate malnutrition as a cause of growth failure.

13. What are the indications for surgery in patients with Crohn's disease?
About 50–70% of children with Crohn's disease require surgery within 10–15 years of diagnosis. The complications of Crohn's disease lead to operative intervention; the disease itself is not cured surgically. Examples include perforation, bleeding, obstruction, toxic megacolon, abscess formation, fistula formation, and intractability.

14. What are the indications for surgery in patients with ulcerative colitis?
Surgery for ulcerative colitis is curative in both adults and children. The main indications in children are intractable disease (64%), refractory growth failure (14%), toxic megacolon (6%), hemorrhage (4%), perforation (3%), and cancer prophylaxis (2%).

15. What are the goals of surgical therapy for Crohn's disease?
Surgery for the complications of Crohn's disease should remove enough bowel to relieve the complication while attempting to maintain the maximal amount of intestine possible. The resected specimen should include all bowel involved grossly with induration and creeping fat, along with a short segment (< 10 cm) of grossly normal–appearing bowel. In children with multiple stenotic areas, strictureplasty without resection allows preservation of the maximal amount of intestine. In patients with severe colonic involvement, surgical options include segmental colectomy, subtotal colectomy with ileoanal anastomosis, or a proctocolectomy and Brooke ileostomy. An endorectal pull-through with ileal pouch–anal anastomosis should not be attempted in patients with Crohn's disease because of the risk of recurrence in the J-pouch and rectal muscular sleeve. Children with severe perianal disease and nonhealing fistulas often require a proctocolectomy with ileostomy. Proximal diversion alone often does not allow healing of the excluded portion of bowel.

16. What are the goals of surgical therapy for ulcerative colitis?
To cure ulcerative colitis the entire colonic mucosa down to the dentate line must be removed. This goal is best accomplished with total abdominal colectomy, mucosal proctectomy, and endorectal pull-through using a J-pouch ileoanal anastomosis. In emergency situations (toxic megacolon, extensive rectal bleeding) colectomy and ileostomy are initially performed, followed by a pull-through procedure as a second elective procedure.

BIBLIOGRAPHY

1. Ament ME, Vargas JH: Medical therapy for ulcerative colitis in childhood. Semin Pediatr Surg 3:28–32, 1994.
2. Coulson WF: Pathologic features of inflammatory bowel disease in childhood. Semin Pediatr Surg 3:8–14, 1994.
3. Dudgeon DL: Ulcerative colitis. In Oldham KT, Colonbani PM, Foglia RP (eds): Surgery of Infants and Children: Scientific Principles and Practice. Philadelphia, Lippincott-Raven, 1997, pp 1301–1312.
4. Fonkalsrud EW: Inflammatory bowel disease. In Ashcraft KW, Holder TM (ed): Pediatric Surgery, 2nd ed. Philadelphia, W.B. Saunders, 1993, pp 440–452.
5. Fonkalsrud EW: Surgery for pediatric ulcerative colitis. Curr Opin Pediatr 7:323–327, 1995.
6. Fonkalsrud EW: Surgical management of ulcerative colitis in childhood. Semin Pediatr Surg 3:33–38, 1994.

7. Gitnick G: Current views of the etiology of inflammatory bowel disease. Semin Pediatr Surg 3:2–7, 1994.
8. Griffiths AM: Inflammatory bowel disease. Nutrition 14:788–791, 1998.
9. Hyams JS: Crohn's disease in children. Pediatr Clin North Am 43:255–277, 1996.
10. Kirschner BS: Ulcerative colitis in children. Pediatr Clin North Am 43:235–253, 1996.
11. Langer JC: Crohn disease. In Oldham KT, Colonbani PM, Foglia RP (eds): Surgery of Infants and Children: Scientific Principles and Practice. Philadelphia, Lippincott-Raven, 1997, pp 1253–1264.
12. Mack DR: Ongoing advances in inflammatory bowel disease, including maintenance therapies, biologic agents, and biology of disease. Curr Opin Pediatr 10:499–506, 1998.
13. Telander RL, Schmeling DJ: Current surgical management of Crohn's disease in childhood. Semin Pediatr Surg 3:19–27, 1994.
14. Telander RL: Surgical management of Crohn's disease in children. Curr Opin Pediatr 7:328–334, 1995.
15. Vargas JH: Medical management of Crohn's disease in childhood. Semin Pediatr Surg 3:15–18, 1994.
16. Van Allmen D, Goretsky MJ, Ziegler MM: Inflammatory bowel disease in children. Curr Opin Pediatr 7:547–552, 1995.
17. Wyllie R, Sarigol S: The treatment of inflammatory bowel disease in children. Clin Pediatr 37:421–426, 1998.

37. GASTROINTESTINAL BLEEDING

T. A. Brown, M.D., MAJ, and Kenneth Azarow, M.D., LTC

1. A child with lower gastrointestinal bleeding requires blood replacement. At what point is surgery absolutely indicated?

Children tolerate a low hematocrit better than adults for various reasons, including lack of artherosclerotic disease. However, replacement of one-half of blood volume in a 24-hour period is an absolute indication for surgical intervention. Rebleeding during the same hospitalization is also considered an absolute indication by many physicians. The blood volume of an infant is approximately 80 ml/kg.

2. List the most common causes of upper and lower gastrointestinal bleeding in infants and children.

	NEWBORN	1 MO TO 1 YR	1–2 YR	> 2 YR
Upper GI tract	Hemorrhagic disease Swallowed maternal blood	Esophagitis Gastritis	Peptic ulcer disease	Varices
Lower GI tract	Anal fissure	Anal fissure (constipation)	Polyps	Polyps
	Necrotizing enterocolitis	Intussusception	Meckel's diverticulum	Inflammatory bowel disease Intussusception

3. In the 1- to 2-year-old toddler, what is the number-one cause of painless, massive gastrointestinal bleeding requiring a transfusion?

Meckel's diverticulum.

4. What is Meckel's diverticulum?

Meckel's diverticulum is a remnant of the embryonic vitelline or omphalomesenteric duct caused by failure of normal regression of the duct. It is a true diverticulum that occurs in the ileum, typically within 2 feet of the cecum (see Chapter 31).

5. What percentage of Meckel's diverticula contain heterotopic tissue? What type of heterotopic tissue is present?

The two common types of heterotopic tissue are gastric and pancreatic. Gastric mucosa is more common and is found in 10% of asymptomatic patients and 50% of symptomatic patients.

6. What is the most common presentation of symptomatic Meckel's diverticulum?

The most common symptom is bleeding. However, most Meckel's diverticula are discovered incidentally during surgery for some other disorder.

7. Describe the management of a bleeding Meckel's diverticulum.

Bleeding is typically episodic, and most patients can be stabilized to undergo elective surgery. The diverticulum can be amputated with a stapler, or a wedge resection can be completed with a transverse closure to avoid narrowing of the ileum. Occasionally, the bleeding vessel may be found on the mesenteric wall opposite the diverticulum; if noted, the vessel should be oversewn. Segmental bowel resection is an option; however, the bleeding (from an ulcer in the adjacent ileum) will stop regardless of how the Meckel's diverticulum is removed.

8. List the three most frequent types of polyps in the pediatric population.

Juvenile (80%), lymphoid (15%), and adenomatous (3%) polyps.

9. Differentiate juvenile polyps from adenomatous polyps.

Juvenile polyps are hamartomas—malformed colonic mucosa arranged in a bizarre or random fashion. They are not considered to be premalignant unless they are part of a polyposis syndrome. Adenomatous polyps represent dysplastic growth of colonic epithelial cells in an organized progression. Adenomatous polyps are premalignant and eventually lead to invasive adenocarcinoma.

10. What is the most common presentation of juvenile polyps?

Bleeding is seen in 93% of symptomatic patients, typically in the form of blood-streaked feces.

11. What number of polyps in a child constitutes a polyposis syndrome?

More than 5 polyps without a family history of polyposis syndrome or any number of polyps with a family history of polyposis syndrome.

12. What is the treatment of Peutz-Jeghers syndrome?

The cumulative risk of cancer in patients with Peutz-Jeghers syndrome approaches 70% by age 60. Therefore, an aggressive screening and biopsy program should be undertaken, including annual exam with complete blood count, breast and pelvic exams with cervical smears and pelvic ultrasound in females, mammography at age 25, testicular exam in males, pancreatic ultrasound, and biennial upper and lower endoscopy. Early surgery should certainly be undertaken for dysplastic changes, rapid growth, and persistent bleeding.

13. What is the most common cause of bright red blood per rectum in 1- to 10-year-old children?

Anal fissure secondary to constipation.

14. Which of the following are treatments for anal fissures:

A. Botulinum toxin (Botox)   D. Metronidazole
B. Stool softeners and sitz baths E. Sphincterotomy
C. Topical nitroglycerin   F. All of the above

Most patients with acute fissures respond well to gentle dilation, stool softeners, and sitz baths. Chronic or nonhealing ulcers may respond to metronidazole or measures to reduce sphincter tone, such as botulinum toxin, nitroglycerine, and sphincterotomy. Thus, the correct answer is "F."

15. Describe a Sengstaken-Blakemore tube and how it is used.

A Sengstaken-Blakemore tube is a triple-lumen tube with a separate gastric and esophageal balloon and a manometer to control pressure in the balloons. In acute, uncontrollable upper GI bleeding, the tube is passed into the stomach, the gastric balloon is inflated, and the tube is pulled back, effectively causing tamponade of upper gastric bleeding. Persistent bleeding indicates an esophageal source. The esophageal balloon is then inflated to control esophageal hemorrhage (see Chapter 42).

16. List the treatment options for bleeding varices.

- Sclerotherapy
- Local epinephrine injection
- Intravenous vasopressin
  with systemic nitroglycerin
- Octreotide
- Thermal coagulation
- Laser coagulation
- Sengstaken-Blakemore tube
- Variceal banding
- Transjugular intrahepatic
  portosystemic shunt
- Surgery

17. Describe the various portosystemic shunts used for portal decompression in the treatment of bleeding esophageal varices.

Portosystemic shunting can be achieved with excellent results in children. The various central shunt procedures include the portacaval shunt in an end-to-side or side-to-side manner in which the portal outflow is diverted into the inferior vena cava. The mesocaval and portacaval interposition shunts with autogenous vein or polytetrafluoroethylene (PTFE) successfully divert flow from the portal system to the inferior vena cava. Small-diameter grafts are used to maintain prograde portal hepatic perfusion.

The distal shunts include the splenorenal shunt, either central or distal, which diverts flow from the portal system into the systemic system via an anastomosis between the divided splenic vein and renal vein. These shunts are not indicated for acute bleeding, but rather for prophylaxis in patients with recurrent bleeding. They are contraindicated in the presence of ascites but exhibit less encephalopathy than to central shunts.

18. How is bleeding from a swollen rosette of rectal mucosa with circular folds best treated?

The description suggests rectal prolapse. Treatment with conservative measures, including stool softeners and fiber supplements, is successful in most cases. In the acute phase, the herniated bowel is reduced with gentle manual pressure. A rectal exam rules out other causes. The underlying cause should be treated. Constipation is most common, followed by diarrhea, parasites, and cystic fibrosis.

19. How should persistently bleeding hemorrhoids be controlled in patients with portal hypertension?

Primary hemorrhoids are extremely rare in children, but they are found in 4–5% of children with portal hypertension representing a portosystemic anastomosis. Exam under anesthesia with simple oversewing of the bleeding hemorrhoid is the treatment of choice. Hemorrhoidectomy should be avoided because it may exacerbate the underlying portal hypertension. The underlying portal hypertension can be treated with beta blockers and vasopressin, if necessary.

20. What drug is the leading cause of gastritis and peptic ulcer disease in children?

Aspirin. However, the incidence of gastritis secondary to ibuprofen is on the rise.

21. What is the diagnostic modality of choice for an upper GI bleed?

Endoscopy is the gold standard. Both diagnostic and therapeutic interventions are available.

22. What is hemorrhagic disease of the newborn?

Hemorrhagic disease of the newborn is a bleeding diathesis resulting from vitamin K_1 deficiency. It presents as bruising, gastrointestinal and umbilical bleeding, and persistent oozing. Most newborns are vitamin K_1-deficient, and this deficiency can result in failure to produce clotting factors II, VII, IX, and X. As a result, prothrombin time and activated partial thromboplastin time are prolonged, even when platelet count and fibrinogen level are normal. The mother's milk does not have a sufficient quantity of vitamin K_1; intramuscular administration of vitamin K after birth is preventative.

23. What percentage of patients with Crohn's disease present with a GI bleed?
14%.

24. What is the likely cause of duodenal ulcer bleeding in a 1-week-old infant with no other apparent illness or stress? What is the treatment of choice?
Typically, duodenal ulcers result from hypersecretion caused by maternal gastrin production. They often respond to nasogastric decompression, saline lavage to clear clots, volume replacement, and a 2- to 4-week course of H_2 blockers. If surgery is necessary, suture ligation of the ulcer bed is sufficient.

25. How is acute bleeding from ulcerative colitis best managed?
Acute bleeding associated with exacerbation of ulcerative colitis is managed initially with sulfasalzine and corticosteroids. Rarely are other treatments necessary. Cyclosporine, methotrexate, azathioprine, and other drugs also have been shown to be beneficial in refractory cases, but their use is questionable because of side effects and poor long-term remission rates. However, to convert emergent surgery in an immunocompromised patient to elective surgery, cyclosporine has been shown to be effective. Progressive bleeding despite maximal medical management is best treated by colectomy.

26. What is blue rubber bleb nevus syndrome?
This rare condition, found primarily in children, is manifested by cutaneous and gastrointestinal cavernous hemangiomas. Bleeding may be severe, leading to anemia and consumptive coagulopathies. Blue rubber bleb nevus syndrome should be considered in cases of unexplained gastrointestinal bleeding. Therapy is symptomatic.

27. What is the "split notochord" theory? In what percentage of patients does it relate to GI bleeding?
The "split notochord" theory is one explanation of duplication cysts. Affected patients have an adhesion between the endoderm and ectoderm of the neural crest early in development. As the notochord grows, it splits because of persistent adherence, resulting in diverticula of the endoderm and ultimately a duplication cyst. Presenting symptoms vary widely, depending on the location of the cyst. Gastric, duodenal, small intestine, and colonic duplication cysts may present with gastrointestinal hemorrhage.

BIBLIOGRAPHY

1. Arensman RM: Gastrointestinal bleeding. In O'Neill JA, Rowe MI, Grosfeld JL, et al (eds): Pediatric Surgery, 5th ed. St. Louis, Mosby, 1998, pp 1253–1255.
2. Besson I, Ingrand P, Person B, et al: Sclerotherapy with or without octreotide for acute variceal bleeding. N Engl J Med 333:555–560, 1995.
3. Brynskov J, Freund L, Rasmussen SN, et al: A placebo-controlled, double-blind, randomized trial of cyclosporine therapy in active chronic Crohn's disease. N Engl J Med 2321:845–850, 1989.
4. Evans S, Stovroff M, Heiss K, Ricketts R: Selective distal splenorenal shunts for intractable variceal bleeding in pediatric portal hypertension. J Pediatr Surg 30:1115–1118, 1995.
5. Grand RJ, Ramakrishna J, Calenda KA: Inflammatory bowel disease in the pediatric patient. Gastroenterol Clin North Am 24:613–632, 1995.
6. Gui D, Cassetta E, Anastasio G, et al: Botulinum toxin for chronic anal fissure. Lancet 344:1127–1128, 1994.
7. Maksoud JG, Goncalves ME: Treatment of portal hypertension in children. World J Surg 18:251–258, 1994.
8. Mestre J: The changing pattern of juvenile polyps. Am J Gastroenterol 81:312–315, 1986.

9. Oranje AP: Blue rubber bleb nevus syndrome. Pediatr Dermatol 3:304–310, 1986.
10. Panes J, Teres J, Bosch J, Rodes J: Efficacy of balloon tamponade in treatment of bleeding gastric and esophageal varices. Digest Dis Sci 33:454–459, 1988.
11. Phillips RKS, Spigelman AD: Peutz-Jeghers syndrome. In Phillips RKS, et al (eds): Familial adenomatous polyposis and other polyposis syndromes. Boston, Little, Brown, 1994, pp 188–202.
12. St-Vil D, Brandt ML, Panic S, et al: Meckel's diverticulum in children: A 20-year review. J Pediatr Surg 26:1289–1292, 1991.

38. ANORECTAL DISORDERS

Steve C. Chen, M.D., and Tom Jaksic, M.D., Ph.D.

CONGENITAL ANORECTAL DISORDERS

1. What is imperforate anus?

Imperforate anus is an abnormal termination of the anorectum. It has a wide spectrum of clinical presentations, ranging from a fistula in the perineum to a blind-ending rectum without a fistula.

2. What is the incidence of imperforate anus? What is the male-to-female ratio?

The overall incidence is 1 in 5,000 live births; it is slightly higher in males (55% to 65% of cases).

3. How is imperforate anus classified?

In the past malformations were classified according to gender and as low, intermediate, or high, depending on the termination of the rectum relative to the puborectalis muscle complex. The defect can be further characterized by the accompanying fistula to the urogenital system or perineum.

4. What is the most common high variant of imperforate anus in males? In females?

In males, it is imperforate anus with a rectourethral fistula; in females, it is imperforate anus with a rectovaginal fistula.

5. What is the most common low defect in males? In females?

In males, it is imperforate anus with a perineal fistula to the median raphe of the scrotum or base of the penis; in females, it is imperforate anus with a rectovestibular fistula (i.e., to the vestibule of the vagina).

6. What is the incidence of associated malformations?

The incidence of associated malformation varies from 50% to 60% of cases.

7. What are common associated anomalies?

The VACTERL association (vertebral, anal, cardiac, tracheoesophageal, renal, and limb defects), Down's syndrome, Hirschsprung's disease, and duodenal atresia.

8. Name the key steps in managing an infant with imperforate anus.

- Perineal examination for fistula and urinalysis with observation up to 24 hours
- Imaging studies to differentiate high vs. low malformations
- Further investigations to detect associated anomalies (i.e., VACTERL)
- Perineal anoplasty for low defects and colostomy followed by posterior sagittal anorectoplasty (PSARP) for high defects. Recently primary repair of high defects in one stage without colostomy has been successfully performed in selected neonates.

9. What is PSARP?

PSARP (posterior sagittal anorectoplasty), also known as the Peña procedure, is a posterior sagittal pull-through procedure with anorectal anastomosis.

10. What are the key steps of PSARP?
- Place the patient in a prone position with pelvic elevation.
- Identify the center of sphincter complex with an electrical stimulator.
- Make an incision in the sacral midline.
- Separate muscle layers with care to preserve the muscle complex.
- Identify the rectum and associated fistula.
- Divide the fistula.
- Taper the rectum.
- Pull the rectum through the puborectalis sling.
- Approximate midline structures.
- Perform an anorectal anastomosis, and recreate the external sphincter around the anal pull-through.
- Initiate a postoperative anal dilatation program starting 2–3 weeks after surgery.

11. Name the common surgical complications of high lesions.

The mortality rate is low; death generally is secondary to associated cardiac and renal anomalies. Urologic investigations are mandatory in high defects. Other complications include anal stenosis, constipation, rectal mucosal prolapse, and incontinence.

12. What is cloaca?

The word *cloaca* in Latin means sewer. In anorectal malformations, cloaca is defined as the rectum, vagina, and urinary tract emptying into a single common channel.

13. What is the incidence of a cloacal anomaly?

1 in 50,000 births.

14. Name the key steps in management of cloacal malformations.
- Identify the perineal opening.
- Perform cystoscopy, vaginoscopy, and retrograde contrast studies to visualize the anatomy.
- Do a colostomy.
- Use the posterior sagittal approach for complete reconstruction, usually at about 1 year of age.

15. What is cloacal exstrophy?

Cloacal exstrophy is the most severe form of anorectal and ventral abdominal wall defects. The features of classic cloacal exstrophy include imperforate anus, omphalocele, blind-ending microcolon, and two exstrophic hemibladders with an everted cecum between them. Boys also have a rudimentary hemipenis on each side.

16. What is the incidence of cloacal exstrophy?

The incidence is 1 in 400,000 births with a male predominance.

17. Name the key steps in managing infants with cloacal exstrophy.
- Careful preoperative investigation
- Omphalocele closure
- Separation of gastrointestinal tract from hemibladders with construction of gastrointestinal stoma
- Closure of hemibladders, if possible
- Approximation of widely separated pubis
- Usually delayed additional urogenital reconstruction, depending on sex assignment

ACQUIRED ANORECTAL DISORDERS

18. Where do anal fissures occur?
In the mucosa and skin lining the anal canal, often in the posterior midline.

19. What differential diagnosis is associated with laterally located anal fissures?
Crohn's disease and immunodeficiency states.

20. What are the presenting symptoms of anal fissures?
Perianal pain and a small amount of hematochezia with bowel movements.

21. Describe the characteristics of chronic fissures.
Anal sphincter hypertrophy, chronic ulceration, sentinel skin tag, and anal papilla.

22. What are the main therapeutic options for anal fissures?
Acute fissures are treated conservatively with stool softeners and sitz baths. Inflammatory bowel disease and immunodeficiency states should be ruled out in patients with persistent lateral anal fissures.

23. What are the common causes of perianal abscess?
Usually anal crypt gland infections and occasionally infected diaper rash.

24. What are the common organisms?
Staphylococcal and gram-negative enteric organisms.

25. How is perianal abscess treated?
Incision and drainage followed by sitz baths. Antibiotics are useful only for associated cellulitis.

26. What is fistula in ano?
Fistula in ano is a communication between an anal crypt and the perianal skin. Crohn's disease must be considered in older children, particularly if multiple fistulas are seen.

27. What percent of perianal abscesses progress to fistula in ano?
30–50%.

28. What is the main therapeutic option for fistula in ano?
The main therapy is fistulectomy (removal of the entire sleeve of granulation tissue). Supralevator and other complex fistulas are rare in children. Goodsall's rule, which predicts the location of the internal opening of anal fistulas in adults, does not usually apply in infants with anal fistula. In infants the internal opening generally is located radially opposite the external opening.

29. What are the most common causes of rectal prolapse in children? What is the peak age for prolapse?
Constipation and idiopathic disease are the most common causes. The incidence peaks at ages 1–3 years.

30. Who is at risk for developing rectal prolapse?
Children with cystic fibrosis, neuromuscular disorders, and tenesmus.

31. What are the main therapeutic options for rectal prolapse?
Manual reduction is usually successful but may be required on more than one occasion. Nonreducible prolapse may require surgical rectopexy or rarely resection.

32. What is the causative agent in perianal condyloma acuminatum?
Human papilloma virus (HPV). Subtypes 6, 11, 16, and 18 are most common in the pediatric population.

33. How is HPV transmitted?
Under 1 year of age, vertical transmission from the mother is likely. Sexual abuse is highly associated with condyloma acuminatum in older children.

34. What are the main therapeutic options for condyloma acuminatum?
• Medical therapy with topical agents such as podophylline or bichloroacetic acid
• Surgical fulguration with electrocautery or laser

BIBLIOGRAPHY

1. Abercrombie JF, George BD: Perianal abscess in children. Ann R Coll Surg Engl 74:385–386, 1992.
2. Ashcraft KW, Garred JL, Holder TM: Rectal prolapse: 17-year experience with the posterior repair and suspension. J Pediatr Surg 25:992–994, 1990.
3. Ashcraft KW, Holder TM: Acquired anorectal disorders. In Ashcraft KW, Holder TM (eds): Pediatric Surgery, 2nd ed. Philadelphia, W.B. Saunders, 1993, pp 410–415.
4. Cohen BA, Honig P, Androphy E: Anogenital warts in children: Clinical and virologic evaluation for sexual abuse. Arch Dermatol 126:1575–1580, 1990.
5. de Vries PA, Pena A: Posterior sagittal anorectoplast. J Pediatr Surg 17:638–643, 1982.
6. Hendren WH: Cloaca, the most severe degree of imperforate anus: Experience with 195 cases. Ann Surg 228:331–346, 1998.
7. Palder SB, et al: Perianal complications of pediatric Crohn's disease. J Pediatr Surg 26:513–515, 1991.
8. Pena A: Imperforate anus and cloacal malformations. In Ashcraft KW, Holder TM (eds): Pediatric Surgery, 2nd ed. Philadelphia, W.B. Saunders, 1993, pp 372–392.
9. Pena A: Anorectal malformations. Semin Pediatr Surg 6:35–47, 1995.
10. Poenaru D, Yazbeck S: Anal fistula in infants: Etiology, features, management. J Pediatr Surg 28:1194–1195, 1993.
11. Shaul DB, Harrison EA: Classification of anorectal malformations: Initial approach, diagnostic tests, and colostomy. Semin Pediatr Surg 6:187–195, 1997.
12. Smith EA, et al: Current urologic management of cloacal exstrophy: Experience with 11 patients. J Pediatr Surg 32:256–261, 1997.

VII. Hepatobiliary and Spleen

39. BILIARY ATRESIA

Frederick M. Karrer, M.D., and Denis D. Bensard, M.D.

1. What is biliary atresia?

Unlike other atresias, which are characterized by a point obstruction with proximal dilatation, biliary atresia is a panductular obliterative process. Recent evidence implicates a progressive, sclerosing, inflammatory process that begins in utero or just after birth. The incidence of biliary atresia is about 1 of 10,000–15,000 live births.

2. How do infants with biliary atresia present?

Physiologic jaundice should resolve by about 2 weeks of life. Persistence of hyperbilirubinemia should prompt evaluation. Most infants with biliary atresia are of normal birth weight and initially have good weight gain. Mild hepatomegaly is common. Stools may be pigmented initially but become acholic by presentation.

3. Describe the work-up of a jaundiced infant.

Bilirubin analysis reveals increased direct-reacting fractions. Alanine aminotransferase, aspartate aminotransferase, alkaline phosphatase, and glutamyl transpeptidase are modestly elevated. If infections and metabolic and endocrine causes of cholestasis are ruled out, further work-up to identify mechanical causes of obstruction is necessary. Ultrasound of the liver and gallbladder is helpful mainly to rule out other causes of extrahepatic biliary obstruction (e.g., choledochal cyst, spontaneous perforation of the bile ducts). The gallbladder in biliary atresia is usually tiny or not seen at all. Hepatobiliary imaging (hepato-iminodiacetic acid scan) shows good uptake by the liver but no enteric excretion in infants with biliary atresia. If these studies support the diagnosis of biliary atresia, exploratory laparotomy with intraoperative cholangiogram should be done. A Kasai procedure should follow, if indicated.

4. What is a Kasai procedure?

A Kasai operation (hepatic portoenterostomy) takes advantage of the fact that tiny hepatic ducts remain patent in the upper end of the fibrous biliary remnant. The biliary remnant is dissected up to the liver hilum and amputated. A roux-en-Y is constructed, and the jejunal limb is anastomosed to the hepatic hilum. Numerous modifications to the original technique of enteric drainage have been designed to reduce the incidence of cholangitis.

5. What are the most common postoperative complications?

Cholangitis, caused by the combination of enteric bacteria and partial biliary obstruction, is almost universal. The modifications to Kasai's original procedure were intended to reduce the incidence of cholangitis; however, none has fully achieved that goal. Portal hypertension develops in over 50% of long-term survivors (see Chapter 43). Manifestations of portal hypertension include esophageal variceal bleeding, hypersplenism, and ascites.

6. What is the prognosis of infants with biliary atresia?

Without the Kasai operation all infants develop progressive liver failure and die within 2 years, most before their first birthday. Even with the Kasai portoenterostomy, only about one-third survive 10 years without liver transplantation. Another third either fail to drain bile altogether or have only temporary drainage and are considered early failures. The remaining third have bile drainage but develop complications of cirrhosis and/or liver failure and require liver transplantation by age 10.

7. What are the major prognostic factors?

The major prognostic factor is age prior to surgery. Many reports have demonstrated better results in infants who have earlier surgery. The long-term (10-year) survival rate for patients having surgery before age 60 days is 68%, whereas for patients having surgery after 90 days the survival rate is only 15%. Other important positive prognostic factors include clearing of jaundice after the Kasai procedure, absence of fibrosis and cirrhosis, on liver biopsy larger-sized ducts at the porta hepatis (> 200 μm), and absence of portal hypertension.

CONTROVERSY

8. Should infants with biliary atresia initially undergo a Kasai portoenterostomy or a liver transplant?

Infants who have timely diagnosis and achieve bile drainage have a chance for long-term survival without the need for immunosuppression. Beyond the increased risks of immunosuppression (infectious and neoplastic), the number of donors is inadequate to supply the needed organs if all patients with biliary atresia went first to transplantation. Innovative techniques such as reduced-sized, split, and living-related liver donors have partially addressed the organ shortage, but liver transplantation is still a formidable undertaking. We favor an initial Kasai procedure, followed by liver transplantation for failures. Failure is indicated by recurrent cholangitis, progressive jaundice, portal hypertension complications, poor hepatic synthetic function, and growth failure.

BIBLIOGRAPHY

1. Bates MD, Buchvalas JC, Alonson MH, et al: Biliary atresia: Pathogenesis and treatment. Semin Liver Dis 18:281–293, 1998.
2. Karrer FM, Price MR, Bensard D, et al: Long-term results with the Kasai operation for biliary atresia. Arch Surg 131:493–496, 1996.
3. Ohi R, Nio M: The jaundiced infant: Biliary atresia and other obstructions. In O'Neill JA, Rowe MI, Grosfeld JL, et al (eds): Pediatric Surgery, 5th ed. Mosby, St. Louis, 1998, pp 1465–1481.

40. CHOLEDOCHAL CYST

Samuel M. Alaish, M.D., and Eric L. Lazar, M.D.

1. What are the five types of choledochal cyst? Which type is most common?

Type I: saccular or diffuse fusiform dilatation of the common bile duct, usually inferior to the confluence of the left and right hepatic ducts

Type II: diverticulum of the common bile duct

Type III: intraduodenal dilatation of the common bile duct; choledochocele

Type IV: multiple cysts of the intra- or extrahepatic bile ducts (or both)

Type V: single or multiple intrahepatic cysts

Type I is the most common type.

2. What is Caroli's disease?

Single or multiple intrahepatic biliary cysts classified as type V are referred to as Caroli's disease when they are associated with hepatic fibrosis.

3. What are the two main types of choledochocele?
In the more common type, the common bile duct and pancreatic duct enter the intraduodenal choledochocele separately. In the less common type, the choledochocele is a diverticulum off the common duct at the level of the ampulla of Vater; the pancreatic duct enters the end of the common bile duct in the usual location.

4. What is the incidence of choledochal cyst?
The worldwide incidence is approximately 1 in 100,000.

5. In what part of the world is choledochal cyst more common?
Choledochal cyst is more common in Asia, with an incidence of 1 in 1000 in Japan.

6. Is choledochal cyst more common in males or females?
Choledochal cyst is three times more common in females than males.

7. What is thought to be the cause of congenital biliary dilatation?
The cause of biliary dilatation is unproved. The two most commonly accepted theories are (1) reflux of trypsin and other pancreatic enzymes into the proximal biliary ductal system because of a congenitally abnormal insertion of the pancreatic duct into the common duct and (2) obstruction of the distal duct.

8. What is the classic triad associated with choledochal cyst?
Jaundice, pain, and an abdominal mass. But at most 15% of children present with the classic triad.

9. What laboratory abnormalities are associated with choledochal cyst in infants?
Conjugated hyperbilirubinemia, increased alkaline phosphatase, and other serum indicators of obstructive jaundice. If biliary obstruction has been present for a substantial period, patients may have a mildly abnormal coagulation profile.

10. With regard to clinical course and prognosis, what disease process does choledochal cyst mimic in infants?
Biliary atresia.

11. What is the treatment of choice for types I, II, and IV?
Cyst excision, cholecystectomy, and roux-en-Y hepaticoportoenterostomy.

12. What is the treatment for choledochocele (type III)?
A longitudinal duodenotomy is used to expose the intraduodenal choledochocele. The cystic space is unroofed, and the mucosa is reapproximated with multiple interrupted absorbable sutures. The entry points of the common bile duct and pancreatic duct must be carefully identified and calibrated to determine whether sphincteroplasty of the ducts is necessary. Sphincteroplasty of the duct openings is necessary in most cases, usually because the duct openings are narrowed by chronic inflammation. On rare occasions, choledochoceles are located in the head of the pancreas and are not amenable to internal drainage into the duodenum. If alternate internal drainage procedures cannot be accomplished, pancreaticoduodenectomy may be required.

13. What, if any, is the surgical treatment for Caroli's disease?
Partial hepatic lobectomy should be done when the disease is localized and amenable to resection, but unroofing with drainage into a roux limb of the jejunum may be needed when proximal ductal obstruction is encountered. Bilobar disease is treatable only by liver transplantation.

14. What are the complications of cyst excision and hepaticojejunostomy?
Complications include cholangitis, pancreatitis, lithiasis, and anastomotic stricture.

15. Is it possible to diagnose choledochal cyst in utero? If so, how?
Prenatal ultrasound has demonstrated choledochal cysts at various intervals ranging from 15 to 37 weeks gestation. The size of the cyst increases steadily as gestational age advances.

16. In cases diagnosed prenatally, what is the optimal timing for surgery?
Because of the frequency of hepatic fibrosis, known to be reversible with surgical repair, as well as the potential complications of cyst enlargement, hepatic dysfunction, and perforation, optimal timing appears to be 1–2 weeks of age. At this time the infant is usually stable.

17. How often do patients present with cyst rupture and bile peritonitis? What is the treatment of choice?
One to two percent of patients present with cyst rupture and bile peritonitis. In cases of spontaneous rupture, the treatment of choice consists of cystectomy, cholecystectomy, and roux-en-Y hepaticoportoenterostomy.

18. Does choledochal cyst carry a risk of malignant degeneration?
Carcinomas arising in choledochal cyst walls are well recognized and are believed to be the result of chronic inflammation. Carcinoma rarely has been reported in childhood and affects primarily adults. The typical form of malignancy is adenosquamous carcinoma; occasional patients have small cell carcinoma.

19. Should cholecystectomy be included as part of the treatment for choledochal cyst? What if the cystic duct is not dilated?
Cholecystectomy always should be performed.

20. What is the treatment of choice in older patients who have had recurrent bouts of cholangitis and who have a substantial amount of pericystic inflammation and adherence to adjacent hepatic vessels?
As originally reported by Lilly, cyst excision is performed using a plane of dissection between the inner and outer layers of the cyst wall. The portion of the cyst wall adherent to the portal vein and hepatic artery is left undisturbed. Cholecystectomy is performed, and reconstruction is achieved using a roux-en-Y hepaticojejunostomy.

21. What complications are associated with a choledochal cyst left untreated?
- Cholangitis
- Lithiasis
- Pancreatitis
- Biliary cirrhosis
- Rupture
- Carcinoma
- Portal hypertension

BIBLIOGRAPHY

1. Altman RP, Lilly JR, Greenfield J, et al: A multivariate risk factor analysis of the portoenterostomy (Kasai) procedure for biliary atresia: Twenty-five years experience from two centers. Ann Surg 226:348–353, 1997.
2. Ando K, Suda K: Histopathological study of the liver in congenital biliary dilatation and abnormal pancreatico-choledochal duct junction. J Jpn Soc Pediatr Surg 28:10, 1992.
3. Babbitt DP: Congenital choledochal cyst: New etiological concept based on anomalous relationships of common bile duct and pancreatic bulb. Ann Radiol 12:231, 1969.
4. Fieber SS, Nance FC: Choledochal cyst and neoplasm: A comprehensive review of 106 cases and presentation of two original cases. Am Surg 63:982–987, 1997.
5. Howard ER: Choledochal cysts. In Howard ER (ed): Surgery of Liver Disease in Children. Oxford, Butterworth-Heinemann, 1991, p 94.
6. Howell CG, et al: Antenatal diagnosis and early surgery for choledochal cyst. J Pediatr Surg 18:387, 1983.

7. Karnak I, Cahit Tanyel F, Buyukpamukcu N, Hicsonmez A: Spontaneous rupture of choledochal cyst: An unusual cause of acute abdomen in children. J Pediatr Surg 32:736–738, 1997.
8. Kasai M, Kimura S, Asakura Y, Suzuki H: Surgical treatment of biliary atresia. J Pediatr Surg 3:665–675, 1968.
9. Lazar EL, Altman RP: Surgical disease of the biliary tract. In Morris PJ, Wood WC (eds): Oxford Textbook of Surgery. Oxford, Oxford University Press, 1999.
10. Lilly JR: Total excision of choledochal cyst. Surg Gynecol Obstet 146:254, 1978.
11. Lilly JR: The surgical treatment of choledochal cyst. Surg Gynecol Obstet 149:36, 1979.
12. Matsubara H, et al: Is it possible to differentiate between choledochal cyst and congenital biliary atresia (type 1 cyst) by antenatal ultrasonography? Fetal Diagn Ther 12:306–308, 1997.
13. Miyano T, et al: Hepaticoenterostomy after excision of choledochal cyst in children: A 30-year experience with 180 cases. J Pediatr Surg 31:1417, 1996.
14. Moss RL, Musemeche CA: Successful management of ruptured choledochal cyst by primary cyst excision and biliary reconstruction. J Pediatric Surg 32:1490–1491, 1997.
15. Nakamura T, Okada A, Higaki J, et al: Pancreaticobiliary maljunction-associated pancreatitis: An experimental study on the activation of pancreatic phospholipase A2. World J Surg 20:543–550, 1996.
16. Ohi R, et al: Surgical treatment of congenital dilatation of the bile duct with special reference to late complications after total excisional operation. J Pediatr Surg 25:613, 1990.
17. O'Neill JA: Choledochal cyst. Curr Probl Surg 29:365, 1992.
18. O'Neill JA: Choledochal cyst. In O'Neill JA, Rowe MI, Grosfeld JL, et al: Pediatric Surgery, Vol II. St. Louis, Mosby, 1998, pp 1483–1493.
19. Rha SY, Stovroff MC, Glick PL, et al: Choledochal cysts: A ten-year experience. Am Surg 62:30–34, 1996.
20. Rossi RL, et al: Carcinomas arising in cystic conditions of the bile ducts. A clinical and pathological study. Ann Surg 205:377, 1987.
21. Samuel M, Spitz L: Choledochal cyst: Varied clinical presentations and long-term results of surgery. Eur J Pediatr Surg 6:78–81, 1996.
22. Stinger MD, Dhawan A, Davenport M, et al: Choledochal cysts: Lessons learned from a 20 year experience. Arch Dis Child 73:528–531, 1995.
23. Todani T, et al: Congenital bile duct cysts. Classification, operative procedures, and review of 37 cases including cancer arising from choledochal cyst. Am J Surg 134:263, 1977.
24. Tsuchija R, et al: Malignant tumors in choledochal cysts. Ann Surg 186:22, 1978.
25. Tugo-Vicente HL: Prenatally diagnosed choledochal cysts: Observation or early surgery. J Pediatr Surg 30:1288, 1995.
26. Yeong ML, Nicholson GI, Lee SP: Regression of biliary cirrhosis following choledochal cyst drainage. Gastroenterology 82:332, 1982.

41. GALLBLADDER DISEASE

Steven Rothenberg, M.D.

1. What is the presentation of the acute cholecystitis?

Children often present with signs of dehydration, fever, nausea, and right upper quadrant pain with abdominal wall tenderness and guarding. Some patients may have a tender, palpable mass (Murphy's sign).

2. What laboratory tests are helpful?

Patients usually have an elevated white blood cell count with a left shift. Liver function studies may be elevated (alkaline phosphatase more than serum transaminases), although not to the same degree as with hepatitis. Serum bilirubin is usually not elevated unless stones obstruct the bile duct (which is uncommon).

3. What are the types of gallstones?

Cholesterol, pigment, and mixed. Pigment stones are associated with conditions that cause hemolysis, ileal resection, or treatment with hyperalimentation. They are also more common in Asians.

4. Why do ileal resection and diseases of the terminal ileum cause stone formation?
Bile salts are absorbed in the terminal ileum.

5. Which conditions may cause hemolysis in childhood?
- Sickle cell anemia
- Spherocytosis
- Thalassemia major
- Pyruvate kinase deficiency
- Hexose kinase deficiency
- Autoimmune hemolytic anemia

6. What neonatal conditions may be associated with cholelithiasis?
- Prematurity
- Ileal resection
- Cystic fibrosis
- Hyperalimentation
- Prolonged fasting

7. What conditions are associated with gallstones in older children?
- Obesity
- Family history
- Use of oral contraceptives
- Native American or
  Hispanic descent
- Pregnancy
- Chronic illness from other diseases
- (e.g., cystic fibrosis, spinal cord diseases)
  or chemotherapy

8. Who described the first case of cholecystitis in a child?
Gibson in 1737.

9. Why do cholesterol stones form?
Cholesterol stones are a combination of cholesterol, bile, and lecithin. A change in the percentage of these three components results in conditions that cause supersaturation of cholesterol and thus a nidus for stone formation (increasing percentage of cholesterol, decreasing percentage of bile salts and lecithin). Remember the stupid triangular-phase diagram: it is a frequent question on board exams.

10. What is acalculous cholecystitis? Who gets it?
Acalculous cholecystitis is the presence of acute or chronic inflammation of the gallbladder without the presence of stones. The exact cause is not known, but it is usually associated with recent stress or trauma resulting in dehydration, ileus, and gallbladder stasis. The signs and symptoms are the same as those of acute cholecystitis except that the ultrasound fails to show stones. Biliary scintigraphy (hepato-iminodiacetic acid [HIDA] scan) shows normal liver uptake but no visualization of the gallbladder. Treatment consists of intravenous hydration, antibiotics, and, if necessary, cholecystectomy.

11. What is biliary dyskinesia?
Biliary dyskinesia is a poorly understood condition characterized by inadequate contraction and clearance of the gallbladder with stimulation. It may present as colicky or chronic right upper quadrant pain but without the signs and symptoms of acute infection. Diagnosis is made by obtaining a cholecystokinin-stimulated HIDA scan that shows poor biliary excretion (decreased ejection fraction), usually less than 20%. The incidence in children is not known, but it is diagnosed with increasing frequency.

12. What is the differential diagnosis of right upper quadrant pain?
In addition to the entities already discussed, acute appendicitis, peptic ulcer disease, inflammatory bowel disease, hepatitis, pancreatitis, and (in infants) intussusception.

13. What is the treatment for acute cholecystitis and cholelithiasis?
Initial treatment consists of intravenous hydration and antibiotics. Nonsurgical treatment for stones includes dissolution therapy (with primary bile acids) and extracorporeal shock-wave

lithotripsy. Both therapies have low success and high recurrence rates and are rarely used in children. In neonates on total parenteral nutrition (TPN), resumption of oral feeds and discontinuance of TPN often result in dissolution of sludge and small stones. Stones diagnosed in utero frequently resolve after birth and therefore should be followed with ultrasound.

14. What is the appropriate surgical therapy?
Although cholecystotomy and drainage of the gallbladder occasionally have been advocated, especially in critically ill patients, cholecystectomy is the standard of care. The vast majority of these procedures, even in children, are performed laparoscopically.

15. When should an intraoperative cholangiogram be performed?
This issue is relatively controversial. If you want to survive surgical rotation, find out your attending's bias and swear to it. Most surgeons agree that evidence of bile duct obstruction is an absolute indication. Signs of obstruction include jaundice, elevated bilirubin, dilated common bile duct, and gallstone pancreatitis. Other indications include multiple small stones in the gallbladder, elevated liver function tests, and a need to identify anatomy during surgery. Some surgeons believe that a cholangiogram should be performed in every case, especially if the procedure is done laparoscopically.

16. What are the surgical options in patients with common duct stones?
Preoperative endoscopic retrograde pancreatography with stone extraction and sphincterotomy, followed by laparoscopic cholecystectomy a few days later; laparoscopic common bile duct exploration; or open duct exploration.

17. What are the boundaries of the foramen of Winslow?
The gallbladder above; the duodenum below; the portal vein, common hepatic duct, and hepatic artery anteriorly; and the vena cava inferiorly.

18. What structures comprise the triangle of Calot?
The cystic duct, common hepatic duct, and cystic artery.

BIBLIOGRAPHY
1. Holcomb GW III, Pietsch JB: Gallbladder disease and hepatic infections. In Ravitch MM, Randolph JG, Welch KJ, et al (eds): Pediatric Surgery, 4th ed. Chicago, Year Book, 1986.
2. Gilger MA: Cholelithiasis and cholecystitis. In Wyllie R, Hymans JS (eds): Pediatric Gastrointestinal Disease. Philadelphia, W.B. Saunders, 1993, pp 931–944.
3. Rowe MI, O'Neill JA Jr, Grosteld JL, et al: Gallbladder disease. In Essentials of Pediatric Surgery. St. Louis, Mosby, 1995, pp 656–662.
4. Holcomb GW III: Laparoscopic cholecystectomy. Semin Laparosc Surg 5:2–8, 1998.

42. PORTAL HYPERTENSION

Frederick M. Karrer, M.D., and Denis D. Bensard, M.D.

1. List the various types of varices and the routes for collateral flow between the portal and systemic venous systems.
- Esophageal varices: portal vein → left gastric (coronary vein) → esophageal veins → azygous/hemiazygous veins → superior vena cava.
- Hemorrhoids: portal vein → inferior mesenteric vein → superior hemorrhoidal (rectal) veins → middle and inferior hemorrhoidal (rectal) veins → internal iliac veins → inferior vena cava.

- Caput medusae: portal vein → umbilical vein (ligamentum teres) → superficial veins of the abdominal wall → superior and inferior epigastric veins → superior and inferior vena cava.
- Retroperitoneal varices: portal vein → duodenal, pancreatic, and colonic veins → retroperitoneal (veins of Retzius) → inferior vena cava.
- Diaphragmatic varices: portal vein → hepatic ligaments/bare area (veins of Sappey) → phrenic veins → inferior vena cava.

2. What is the initial management of upper gastrointestinal hemorrhage due to variceal bleeding?

Volume resuscitation and stabilization are givens. Blood should be obtained for determination of hemoglobin and hematocrit, platelet count, coagulation studies, and immediate type and cross-matching. Fortunately, variceal bleeding in children usually stops spontaneously, especially in children with portal vein thrombosis. If bleeding persists, the next step is initiation of an intravenous drip of octreotide. Octreotide reduces splanchnic blood flow and portal venous pressure.

3. What is a Sengstaken-Blakemore tube?

Sengstaken-Blakemore (SB) tubes or modifications thereof are like huge Foley catheters. The balloon is placed into the stomach, and the position is confirmed radiographically before balloon inflation. When the gastric balloon is inflated, it is placed on traction, compressing venous inflow to the esophageal varices. Persistent massive hemorrhage is now rare, but if a SB tube is used, endotracheal intubation is recommended to prevent aspiration. Traction on the SB tube can be maintained by having the child wear a football helmet with the SB tube tied securely to the face mask.

4. What endoscopic techniques are used?

Endoscopy should be performed as soon as the patient is hemodynamically stable to diagnose the cause of the hemorrhage and to initiate treatment. Two main endoscopic treatments are widely used, sclerotherapy and endoscopic band ligation. For endosclerosis, sclerosant solutions such as sodium morrhuate, ethanolamine, or tetradecyl sodium are injected in or near the varix. Endoscopic band ligation is accomplished by placing a small elastic band around the varix. Both achieve thrombosis and scarring of the varices in the distal esophagus and control acute hemorrhage in 90–95% of children. Continued endoscopic treatment and surveillance are necessary because recurrence of varices is common.

5. Are portosystemic shunts still used?

Shunts are designed to divert blood from the portal to the systemic venous system and were the mainstay of treatment for portal hypertension for 25 years. Largely replaced with endoscopic treatments and liver transplantation, shunts still have a role in children who are not candidates for liver transplantation, children in whom endoscopic techniques fail, or children who live in remote areas.

6. What shunts are used most often in children?

For children with portal vein thrombosis, standard portacaval shunting is not an option. The most often used shunts are mesocaval (superior mesenteric vein to inferior vena cava) and splenorenal shunts (splenic vein to left renal vein). The distal splenorenal shunt (Warren's shunt) is a selective shunt that decompresses only the esophageal varices, maintaining perfusion pressure to the liver.

BIBLIOGRAPHY

1. Karrer FM: Portal hypertension. Semin Pediatr Surg 1:134–144, 1992.
2. Orloff MJ, Orloff MS, Rambotti M: Treatment of bleeding esophagogastric varices due to extrahepatic portal hypertension: Results of portal-systemic shunts during 35 years. J Pediatr Surg 29:142–154, 1994.

43. SPLEEN

J. B. Joo, M.D., and Richard H. Pearl, M.D.

1. When can the spleen be identified during fetal development?

The splenic precursor is recognized by 5 weeks gestation. The spleen appears on the left side of the dorsal mesogastrium near the dorsal pancreas.

2. Does the spleen serve a function during gestation?

Yes. The spleen is a major site of fetal hematopoiesis during mid-gestation.

3. When does the spleen stop growing in normal development?

The spleen enlarges from about 11 gm at birth to an average of about 135 gm by puberty before diminishing in size during adulthood.

4. What are the major functions of the spleen?

- Blood homeostasis. The spleen is capable of hemoatopoietic functions throughout life, although with age its relative contribution declines reciprocally to the increase in bone marrow hematopoiesis. The spleen also serves as the principal graveyard for senescent or damaged blood cells.
- Resistance to infection. The spleen provides an important defense against infection by acting as a phagocytic filter for infectious organisms and by producing specific antibodies.

5. Describe the splenic blood flow.

After entering the spleen, blood passes through the small central arteries of the white pulp, where perpendicular branches skim off plasma, particulate material, and some lymphocytes. The remaining blood in the central arteries flows into the red pulp, where it drains into the splenic sinuses directly or indirectly via the splenic cords.

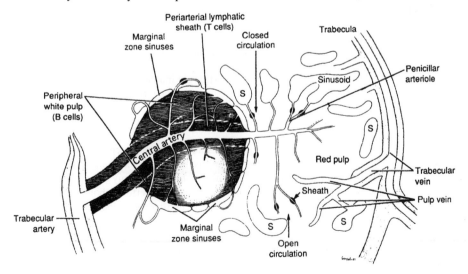

Blood circulation of the spleen. Theories of open and closed circulation are represented. Splenic sinuses (S) are indicated. (Redrawn and reproduced from Greep RO, Weiss L: Histology, 3rd ed. New York, McGraw-Hill, 1973; with permission.)

6. Why is the splenic blood flow system important?
Sluggish flow of blood through the red pulp facilitates phagocytosis by fixed macrophages of nondeformable or antibody-coated blood cells as well as particulate matter such as bacteria.

7. What types of red blood cells predominate after a splenectomy?
Howell-Jolly bodies, which are red cells with inclusions (fragments of nuclear material).

8. What percentage of infants with congenital asplenia survive the first year of life?
Only 10%. Death usually is due to associated cardiac anomalies.

9. Where are the two most common locations for an accessory spleen?
• Splenic hilum
• Tail of pancreas
Accessory spleens also have been located in small and large bowel mesentery, pelvis, and scrotum.

10. What is the most common hereditary anemia in the white population?
Hereditary spherocytosis.

11. What is the abnormality in hereditary spherocytosis?
A deficiency or dysfunction of spectrin (a structural protein) in the red blood cell membrane. This deficiency allows the red cells to deform.

12. Describe the classic laboratory test for hereditary spherocytosis.
In the osmotic fragility test, normal red blood cells remain intact in lower saline concentrations, whereas spherocytes hemolyze in decreased osmolar solutions.

13. Why does splenomegaly occur in spherocytosis?
The less deformable spherocytes become trapped in the splenic microcirculation, causing localized increase in blood pressure in the splenic microcirculation with gradual splenic enlargement.

14. In patients with hereditary spherocytosis, when should a splenectomy be performed?
Splenectomy is the only treatment for hereditary spherocytosis and should be done even when the child is asymptomatic. A splenectomy is strongly indicated when frequent hemolytic crises, as manifested by profound drops in hematocrit, necessitate transfusion.

15. What preoperative examination is essential before a splenectomy for any chronic hemolytic condition?
Ultrasound of the gallbladder should be performed to assess the presence of bilirubin stones. The more severe and the longer the duration of hemolysis, the greater the likelihood of gallstones. Gallstones occur in 85% of cases. Hence, a concomitant cholecystectomy should be performed. However, in the absence of chronic inflammation, some surgeons perform cholecystostomy with extraction of stones because stone formation should not occur after the splenectomy.

16. What is the mode of transmission for beta-thalassemia? Where is the highest incidence?
The mode of transmission is autosomal dominant. The highest incidence is in the Mediterranean countries and parts of Africa and Southeast Asia.

17. What are the two causes of anemia in beta-thalassemia?
• Ineffective erythropoiesis. Impaired beta-globin synthesis leaves unstable alpha-globin aggregates, which cause cell membrane damage and ultimately lead to apoptosis of red cell precursors.

- The red cells that survive are at increased risk for sequestration and destruction in the spleen. The result is hypersplenism.

18. True or false: Splenectomy is curative for beta-thalassemia.

False. Splenectomy is palliative. It reduces the number of required transfusions by half but does not alter the metabolic defect.

19. Describe the signs and symptoms of acute splenic sequestration in sickle cell anemia.

Fever, cough, diarrhea, vomiting, drowsiness, and bone pain. When the spleen becomes rapidly engorged and painful, a clinical shock-like picture may develop because of sequestration and decreased effective hemoglobin.

20. What is the role of splenectomy in sickle cell anemia?

Patients with recurrent acute splenic sequestration, which causes sickle cell crisis, or hypersplenism with splenomegaly sometimes require splenectomy. Otherwise, the spleen infarcts, resulting in an autosplenectomy.

21. What is the best test to diagnose idiopathic thrombocytic purpura?

None. Idiopathic thrombocytic purpura (ITP) is a diagnosis of exclusion.

22. What causes ITP?

Circulating antiplatelet autoantibodies attach to platelets, making them susceptible to destruction.

23. Do patients with ITP have splenomegaly?

No. The spleen is seldom enlarged unless there is an underlying disease process.

24. When is a splenectomy indicated for ITP?
- Acute bleeding episode
- Persistent thrombocytopenia
- Lack of response to steroids
- Relapse after steroids
- Steroid complications
- Chronic disease

25. What is the cure rate of splenectomy for ITP?

90%.

26. What is overwhelming postsplenectomy infection?

Overwhelming postsplenctomy infection (OPSI) manifests as sudden onset of fever, nausea, vomiting, confusion leading to seizures, shock, disseminated intravascular coagulation with Waterhouse-Friderichsen syndrome, coma, and death within hours. OPSI is due to the lack of clearing bacteremia of encapsulated organisms: *Pneumococcus* species, *Meningogoccus* species, *Escherichia coli*, *Haemophilus influenzae*, *Staphylococcus* species, and *Streptococcus* species.

27. What preoperative prophylactic measures are suggested with asplenic patients?

The 1994 recommendations of the American Academy of Pediatrics include vaccinations for *Haemophilus influenzae* type B, 23-valent *Streptococcus pneumoniae* before 2 years of age, and *Neisseria meningitidis* after 2 years of age.

CONTROVERSY

28. What is the value of antibiotic prophylaxis in asplenic children?

Children less than 15 years of age have a greater overall risk (0.13–8.1%) for OPSI compared with adults (0.28–1.9%).

Prophylactic antibiotics have been studied extensively in asplenic children with sickle cell disease. Oral penicillin, 125 mg given twice daily, was highly efficacious in patients younger than 5 years. Many pediatricians, however, prescribe penicillin prophylaxis in other high-risk patients, such as those with thalassemia, immunodeficiency states, and malignancy. Another consideration is to use penicillin prophylaxis for only 2 years after splenectomy, the period of highest risk for fatal OPSI. Because patient compliance is an issue, some physicians use intramuscular bicillin shots once a month to obviate the need for daily oral medication. Others provide a supply of penicillin to be started immediately at the onset of febrile illness.

BIBLIOGRAPHY

1. Committee on Infectious Diseases: 1994 Red Book: Report of the Committee on Infectious Diseases, 23rd ed. Elk Grove, IL, American Academy of Pediatrics, 1994, pp 57–58.
2. Coon WC: Surgical aspects of splenic disease and lymphoma. Curr Probl Surg 35:548–646, 1998.
3. Cotran RS, Kumar V, Collins T: Red Cells and Bleeding Disorders: Robbins Pathologic Basis of Disease, 6th ed. Philadelphia, W.B. Saunders, 1999, pp 601–643.
4. Ein SE: Splenic lesions. In Ashcraft KW, Holder TM: Pediatric Surgery, 2nd ed. Philadelphia, W.B. Saunders, 1993, pp 535–545.
5. Eraklis AJ, Filler RM: Splenectomy in childhood: A review of 1413 cases. J Peditr Surg 7:382–388, 1972.
6. French J, Camitta BM: The spleen. In Nelson WE, Behrman RE, Kleigman RM, Arvin AM: Nelson Textbook of Pediatrics, 15th ed. Philadelphia, W.B. Saunders, 1996, pp 1438–1440.
7. Junqueira LC, Carneiro J, Kelley RO: The Immune (Lymphoid) System: Basic Histology, 7th ed. East Norwalk, CT, Appleton & Lange, 1992, pp 261–280.
8. Lane PA: The spleen. In Rudolph AM, Hoffman JIE, Rudolph CD: Rudolph's Pediatrics, 20th ed. Stamford, CT, 1996, pp 1233–1235.
9. Lane PA: The spleen in children. Curr Opin Pediatr 7:36–41, 1995.
10. Lynch AM, Kapila R: Overwhelming postsplenectomy infection. Infect Dis Clin North Am 10:693–707, 1996.

VIII. Head and Neck

44. CERVICAL LYMPHADENOPATHY

Robert E. Kelly, Jr., M.D.

1. Describe the distribution of lymph nodes in the neck.

Lymph nodes of the head and neck may be divided into horizontal and vertical groups. The **horizontal nodes** are positioned at the junction of the head with the neck and include the submental, submandibular, superficial parotid (preauricular), mastoid, and suboccipital nodes, all of which drain the superficial tissues of the head.

The **vertical nodes** drain the deep structures of the head and neck. The internal jugular nodes follow the course of the internal jugular vein to drain via the thoracic duct or right lymphatic duct. The external jugular or superficial cervical nodes lie along the course of the external jugular vein and drain the parotid and lower part of the ear. The infrahyoid, prelaryngeal, and pretracheal nodes drain the thyroid, larynx, trachea, and part of the pharynx. The retropharyngeal nodes drain the nose, pharynx, and eustachian tube. All of the cervical nodes ultimately drain to the deep cervical group. At the base of the neck, just posterior to the clavicles, are the supraclavicular nodes.

2. What size is too large for a cervical lymph node?

Most normal children have palpable cervical lymph nodes. In general, a cervical lymph node is considered enlarged if it measures more than 10 mm at its longest diameter. Palpable supraclavicular nodes are always considered abnormal.

3. Which historical features are important in evaluating a patient with cervical lymphadenopathy?

Evaluation of a child with lymphadenopathy requires a thorough history and physical examination. Onset and duration of symptoms as well as rate of lymph node enlargement should be sought. Exposure to animal bites or scratches, presence of risk factors for HIV infection, contact with tuberculosis, and recent travel outside the geographic region of residence should be noted. Weight loss, protracted fever, rash, and other symptoms of systemic disease should be queried. Parents should be asked whether the child has received any antibiotics and, if so, how the symptoms and lymphadenopathy responded. Tuberculin skin test status also should be ascertained.

4. On physical examination, what distinguishes hyperplastic lymph nodes from pyogenic nodes?

Hyperplastic lymph nodes that develop in response to viral infections are small, discrete, mobile, nontender, and bilateral; usually they are not accompanied by cellulitis or periadenitis. **Pyogenic nodes** tend to be unilateral, large, warm, and tender with surrounding erythema and edema.

5. On physical examination, what features should raise suspicion of malignancy?

Nodes associated with malignancy are generally firm or hard, discrete, and nontender. They tend to be rubbery in texture without surrounding inflammation. Over time, they become matted together and fixed to the skin or underlying structures. Suppuration is not a characteristic of nodes with a neoplastic origin. It may be impossible to distinguish on examination a lymph node affected by chronic infection from one involved with malignancy.

6. Which viral illnesses are commonly associated with cervical lymphadenopathy?

Lymph nodes associated with viral upper respiratory infections are usually small, soft, and bilateral, without warmth or erythema of the overlying skin. Cervical adenopathy is a prominent feature of both Epstein-Barr virus and cytomegalovirus infections. Less commonly, adenovirus-associated upper respiratory infection, herpes simplex gingivostomatitis, rubeola, roseola, and coxsackievirus infections.

7. Name the most common causes of bacterial cervical lymphadenitis.

Acute, unilateral, cervical lymphadenitis in children is caused by *Staphylococcus aureus* or *Streptococcus pyogenes* in 40–80% of cases. Staphylococcal infections are commonly seen in children between 1 and 4 years of age.

8. What cervical lymph nodes are most commonly affected by purulent infection?

The primary sites of bacterial cervical lymph node infection are submandibular (50–60%), upper cervical (25–30%), submental (5–8%), occipital (3–5%), and lower cervical (2–5%). Fluctuation occurs in 25% of patients with acute bacterial cervical adenitis and is seen more commonly in lymphadenitis secondary to *S. aureus.*

9. How may suppurated cervical nodes be managed?

Suppurative cervical adenopathy is managed by administration of antibiotics and drainage of purulence when fluctuation is present. Repeated needle aspiration may be effective and may be attempted in cosmetically important areas (i.e., submental or preauricular nodes) but often is difficult in an uncooperative toddler or child. Many surgeons advocate incision and drainage under anesthesia; this approach provides the best chance to break up and drain all loculations of the abscess.

10. How is atypical mycobacterial infection of cervical nodes managed?

In the United States, nontuberculous or atypical mycobacteria account for most cases of cervical adenitis due to mycobacteria. Constitutional signs are rare. Onset of adenopathy may be quite sudden, with a gradual increase in size over a 2- to 3-week period. Infection of lymph nodes with atypical mycobacteria is managed by surgical excision of the affected nodes, which is curative. Affected children do not need to undergo the prolonged systemic antibiotic treatment necessary for *Mycobacterium tuberculosis* infection. If complete excision is impractical because of the extent of disease, debulking should be attempted.

11. Do cats really cause cat scratch disease?

Cat scratch disease results from the scratch of a cat or kitten in 95% of cases. Constitutional symptoms, including fever, malaise, and fatigue, are usually mild and present in fewer than 50% of patients. Nodes suppurate in 10–35% of patients. The causative agent for most cases of cat scratch disease is *Bartonella henselae*, a gram-negative, rickettsial organism. Management is symptomatic because the disease is usually self-limited. Painful, suppurative nodes can be treated with needle aspiration for relief of symptoms. Surgical excision is generally unnecessary.

12. Describe the approach to the patient with a cervical node suspected of harboring malignancy.

Lymphoma (Hodgkin's and non-Hodgkin's), leukemia, and metastatic solid tumors may present with cervical lymphadenopathy. An enlarging, painless, nontender lymph node, which is larger than the expected size, should raise concern. Other factors to take into account are the absence of an inflammatory focus in the drainage area, a suspicious mass or radiographic finding in the drainage area, and systemic symptoms, especially the B symptoms of Hodgkin's disease (fever, night sweats, weight loss, and malaise). Histologic evaluation may be necessary to make a distinction.

13. Explain the controversy about the use of fine-needle aspiration to diagnose malignancy in children.
Recent reports advocate the use of needle biopsy techniques in evaluation of possible malignancy. Success in diagnosis of conditions as varied as sarcoidosis and cat scratch disease has been reported. However, pathologists in many pediatric centers remain uncomfortable with assigning the diagnosis of lymphoma based on cytopathology or a small core of a lymph node. Success rates of diagnostic techniques in studies with adults and children are improved by high rates of metastatic carcinoma or melanoma, which are histologically much easier to diagnose. Thus, before committing a patient to chemotherapy with its potentially significant morbidity, most centers favor an open biopsy so that the diagnosis can be as secure as possible.

14. How should a biopsy specimen suspected of lymphoma be handled?
At biopsy, the surgeon should bring the specimen in saline to the pathologist immediately after removal. Evaluation for lymphoma includes a number of studies that are compromised or made impossible by formalin fixation, including chromosome translocation studies, flow cytometry, in situ hybridization, and immunoperoxidase staining.

15. How frequently are biopsied lymph nodes malignant?
Peripheral lymph node biopsies in 239 children resulted in a specific diagnosis in only 41% of cases. In this series, reactive hyperplasia was diagnosed in 52% of the nodes, granulomatous disease in 32%, and neoplasia in 13%. Hodgkin's and non-Hodgkin's lymphoma accounted for 24 of the 31 cases; neuroblastoma was diagnosed in 4 cases and rhabdomyosarcoma in 3 cases.

BIBLIOGRAPHY

1. Chernoff WG, Lampe HB, Cramer H, et al: The potential clinical impact of the fine needle aspiration/ flow cytometric diagnosis of malignant lymphoma. J Otolaryngol 1(Suppl 21):1–15, 1992.
2. Chesney PJ: Cervical lymphadenitis and neck infections. In Long SS, Pickering LK, Prober CF (eds): Principles and Practice of Pediatric Infectious Diseases. New York, Churchill Livingstone, 1997, p 188.
3. Ellis H: Clinical Anatomy. Oxford, Blackwell Scientific, 1983, pp 289–366.
4. Grossman M, Shiramiuzu B: Evaluation of lymphadenopathy in children. Curr Opin Pediatr 6:68–76, 1994.
5. Kelly CS, Kelly RE Jr: Lymphadenopathy in children. Pediatr Clin North Am 45:875–888, 1998.
6. Knight PJ, Mulne AF, Vassy LE: When is lymph node biopsy indicated in children with enlarged peripheral nodes? Pediatrics 69:391–396, 1982.
7. Pappa VI, Hussain HK, Reznek RH, et al: Role of image-guided core-needle biopsy in the management of patients with lymphoma. J Clin Oncol 14:2427–2430, 1996.
8. Schuit KE, Powell DA: Mycobacterial lymphadenitis in childhood. Am J Dis Child 132:675–677, 1978.
9. Steel BL, Schwartz MR, Ramzy I: Fine needle aspiration biopsy in the diagnosis of lymphadenopathy in 1103 patients: Role, limitations and analysis of diagnostic pitfalls. Acta Cytol 39:76–81, 1995.
10. Szelc Kelly CM, Goral S, Perez Perez GI, et al: Serologic response to *Bartonella* and *Afipia* antigens in patients with cat scratch disease. Pediatrics 96:1137–1142, 1995.

45. THYROGLOSSAL DUCT CYSTS AND SINUSES

Rebeccah L. Brown, M.D., and Philip L. Glick, M.D.

1. What is the embryologic origin of thyroglossal duct cysts/sinuses?
Thyroglossal duct cysts are ectodermal remnants that develop along the line of descent of the thyroid gland in the neck.

2. Describe the embryologic descent of the thyroid gland and its relationship to the hyoid bone.
During the fourth to seventh week of gestation, the foramen cecum at the base of the tongue is the site of development of the thyroid diverticulum, which descends in the anterior midline of the neck. It maintains its connection to the foramen cecum via the thyroglossal duct. Simultaneously, the hyoid bone forms from the second branchial arch; as a result, the thyroglossal duct passes either anterior or posterior or dissects directly through the central portion of the hyoid bone. Normally, the thyroglossal duct is obliterated once the thyroid gland reaches its final destination in the anterior neck.

3. Why do thyroglossal duct cysts and sinuses develop?
They develop because of failure of obliteration of the thyroglossal duct.

4. What is the typical location of thyroglossal duct cysts and sinuses?
Thyroglossal duct cysts and sinuses are located in the anterior midline of the neck at any point along the line of descent of the thyroid gland. Most are located at or immediately adjacent to the hyoid bone; however, about 3% are sublingual and up to 7% are substernal.

5. How often is ectopic thyroid tissue identified within the thyroglossal duct remnant?
In about 25–35% of cases.

6. What happens with complete failure of descent of the thyroid gland?
Complete failure of descent results in a lingual thyroid, which may present as a mass at the base of the tongue.

7. At what age do thyroglossal duct cysts and sinuses usually present?
Although thyroglossal duct cysts and sinuses are congenital, they rarely present in the newborn period. More commonly, they are noted in children 2–10 years old. Of interest, up to one-third of lesions are not identified until after the age of 20.

8. During the physical examination, what maneuver(s) may help to diagnose a thyroglossal duct cyst or sinus? Why?
Because of the embryologic attachments to the foramen cecum at the base of the tongue and to the hyoid bone, thyroglossal duct cysts and sinuses may rise in the neck when the patient is asked to swallow or stick out his tongue. However, this is not a consistent finding.

9. What is the major complication associated with thyroglossal duct cysts and sinuses as well as the primary indication for excision?
The major complication seen with thyroglossal duct cysts and sinuses is infection with oral bacterial flora due to communication with the base of the tongue at the foramen cecum. The risk of infection also represents the primary indication for excision. Infection makes excision more difficult and increases the risk of recurrence.

10. What is the differential diagnosis of a midline anterior neck mass?
Ectopic thyroid tissue, thyroid neoplasm, dermoid cyst, sebaceous cyst, lipoma, and submental lymphadenitis.

11. Should the clinician obtain a preoperative radioisotope thyroid scan to ascertain that the lesion does not contain all of the patient's thyroid tissue?
Although this issue is somewhat controversial, a preoperative radioisotope thyroid scan is not generally recommended because excision is indicated regardless of the findings. If the surgical specimen contains significant thyroid tissue on pathologic examination, postoperative thyroid function tests identify patients who have no remaining thyroid tissue. Replacement therapy then can be initiated.

12. Describe the Sistrunk procedure.
The Sistrunk procedure, described in 1920, is the complete excision of the thyroglossal duct cyst and its sinus tract up to the base of the tongue, including the central portion of the hyoid bone with the specimen.

13. How does one manage an infected thyroglossal duct cyst or sinus?
Management includes warm soaks, antibiotics, and, if necessary, incision and drainage. Complete excision should follow resolution of the infection.

14. What are the predisposing factors for recurrence after excision of a thyroglossal duct cyst or sinus?
Recurrence is most common in patients who have had a previously infected cyst or incomplete excision of the sinus tract with failure to include the central portion of the hyoid bone.

15. What is the risk of recurrence?
The risk of recurrence should be less than 10%.

16. Is malignancy associated with thyroglossal duct cysts and sinuses?
Papillary adenocarcinoma has been described in up to 10% of patients undergoing thyroglossal duct excision in adulthood.

BIBLIOGRAPHY

1. Brown RL, Azizkhan RG: Pediatric head and neck lesions. Pediatr Clin North Am 45:889–905, 1998.
2. Fallat ME: Neck. In Oldham KT, Colombani PM, Foglia RP (eds): Surgery of Infants and Children: Scientific Principles and Practice. Philadelphia, Lippincott-Raven, 1997, pp 847–848.
3. Rowe MI: Neck lesions. In O'Neill JA, Grosfeld, Fonkalsrud EW, et al (eds): Essentials of Pediatric Surgery. St. Louis, Mosby, 1995.
4. Tapper D: Head and neck sinuses and masses. In Ashcraft KW, Holder TM (eds): Pediatric Surgery, 2nd ed. Philadelphia, W.B. Saunders, 1993, pp 927–929.
5. Telander RL, Deane SA: Thyroglossal and branchial cleft cysts and sinuses. Surg Clin North Am 57:779–791, 1977.
6. Telander RL, Filston HC: Review of head and neck lesions in infancy and childhood. Surg Clin North Am 72:1429–1447, 1992.

46. BRANCHIAL CLEFT AND ARCH ANOMALIES

Rebeccah L. Brown, M.D., and Philip L. Glick, M.D.

1. How many branchial clefts and arches are there? Why are they important in development?
During the fourth to eighth week of gestation, the human embryo develops four pairs of branchial arches with intervening clefts that give rise to the mature structures of the head and neck.

2. What is the function of the first branchial arch?
The first branchial arch forms the mandible and maxillary process of the upper jaw. Abnormal development results in anomalies such as cleft lip and palate, abnormal shape and contour of the external ear, and malformation of the internal ossicles.

3. What is the function of the first branchial cleft?
The first branchial cleft forms the eustachian tube, tympanic cavity, and mastoid air cells. Failure of development results in microtia and aural atresia.

4. What is the function of the second branchial arch?
The second branchial arch forms the palantine tonsil, tonsillar fossa, and hyoid bone.

5. What is the function of the third branchial arch?
The third branchial arch gives rise to the inferior parathyroid glands and thymus.

6. What is the function of the fourth branchial arch?
The fourth branchial arch gives rise to the superior parathyroid glands and ultimobranchial body, which is responsible for the development of the thyrocalcitonin-producing parafollicular cells of thyroid gland.

7. Describe the characteristic location and tract of first branchial cleft anomalies.
First branchial cleft anomalies are rare. A draining sinus lying anterior to the ear may be identified in infancy, whereas a small cyst overlying the parotid gland may be seen in children and adults. The sinus tract typically extends to the external auditory canal in close association with the branches of the facial nerve.

8. Are preauricular pits, sinuses, and cysts the same as first branchial cleft anomalies?
No. Although sometimes they are classified with first branchial cleft anomalies, preauricular pits, sinuses, and cysts are not of true branchial cleft origin. Instead, they represent ectodermal inclusions related to the aberrant development of the auditory tubercles.

9. What are the most common branchial cleft anomalies?
Second branchial cleft anomalies are the most common. First branchial cleft anomalies are the second most common; third and fourth branchial cleft anomalies are rare.

10. Describe the characteristic location and tract of second branchial cleft anomalies.
The ostium of the second branchial cleft sinus tract or fistula classically is identified along the anterior border of the middle-to-lower third of the sternocleidomastoid muscle. The tract penetrates the platysma and cervical fascia and ascends along the carotid sheath to the hyoid bone, where it courses medially, behind the posterior belly of the digastric and stylohyoid muscles and anterior to the hypoglossal nerve, to terminate in the tonsillar fossa.

11. Where are cartilaginous remnants of the second branchial cleft usually found?

They usually are found embedded in the anterior border of the sternocleidomastoid muscle.

12. What percentage of second branchial cleft anomalies are bilateral?

Approximately 10% are bilateral.

13. Describe the characteristic location and tract of third branchial cleft anomalies.

Third branchial cleft anomalies almost always occur on the left side of the neck. The ostium generally is located along the anterior border of the lower third of the sternocleidomastoid muscle, and the tract ascends lateral to the carotid artery rather than through its bifurcation, penetrates the thyrohyoid membrane, and terminates in the lower hypopharynx at the pyriformis sinus. Because of its intimate association with the upper left lobe of the thyroid gland, a left hemithyroidectomy may be required as part of en-bloc dissection.

14. Describe the clinical presentation of branchial cleft sinuses and cysts.

Branchial cleft sinuses, fistulas, and cartilaginous remnants typically occur in infancy, whereas branchial cleft cysts are encountered more commonly in childhood or early adulthood. Branchial cleft sinuses or fistulae are painless and may present with clear mucoid drainage. Branchial cleft cysts occur if the cutaneous opening of a sinus tract becomes occluded.

15. What is the most common complication associated with branchial cleft cysts and sinus tracts?

Branchial cleft cysts and sinus tracts commonly become secondarily infected. Indeed, it may be infection that brings the anomaly to the attention of the physician. Infection makes resection more difficult and increases the risk of recurrence.

16. How should infected branchial cleft cysts and sinus tracts be managed?

Management includes warm soaks, antibiotics, and, if fluctuant, needle aspiration or incision and drainage. Complete excision should follow resolution of the infection. Recurrent infections are common.

17. What are the key principles for excision of branchial cleft cysts and sinus tracts?

The neck should be hyperextended. A transverse incision generally is made. A lacrimal duct probe may be inserted into the sinus tract to aid in dissection. Stair-step counterincisions may be necessary to facilitate complete excision of the tract. Care must be taken to avoid injury to associated nerve structures (i.e., the facial nerve branches in first branchial cleft anomalies; the hypoglossal, glossopharyngeal, spinal accessory, and vagus nerves in second branchial cleft anomalies). The entire tract must be excised to prevent recurrence (i.e., to the external auditory canal in first branchial cleft anomalies; to the tonsillar fossa in second branchial cleft anomalies; and to the pyriform sinus in third branchial cleft anomalies).

18. What is the recurrence rate after excision of branchial cleft cysts/sinuses?

The recurrence rate is less than 7% in most series.

19. What factors predispose to recurrence?

Recurrence most commonly is due to infection and incomplete excision of the sinus tract.

20. Does malignant degeneration occur?

Malignant degeneration has been reported in branchial cleft remnants persisting to adulthood.

BIBLIOGRAPHY

1. Brown RL, Azizkhan RG: Pediatric head and neck lesions. Pediatr Clin North Am 45:889–905, 1998.
2. Fallat ME: Neck. In Oldham KT, Colombani PM, Foglia RP (eds): Surgery of Infants and Children: Scientific Principles and Practice. Philadelphia, Lippincott-Raven, 1997, pp 844–846.
3. Rowe MI: Neck lesions. In O'Neill JA, Grosfeld, Fonkalsrud EW, et al (eds): Essentials of Pediatric Surgery. St. Louis, Mosby, 1995.
4. Tapper D: Head and neck sinuses and masses. In Ashcraft KW, Holder TM (eds): Pediatric Surgery, 2nd ed. Philadelphia, W.B. Saunders, 1993, pp 923–926.
5. Telander RL, Deane SA: Thyroglossal and branchial cleft cysts and sinuses. Surg Clin North Am 57:779–791, 1977.
6. Telander RL, Filston HC: Review of head and neck lesions in infancy and childhood. Surg Clin North Am 72:1429–1447, 1992.

IX. Genitourinary

47. ACUTE AND CHRONIC RENAL FAILURE

Abubakr Imam, M.D., and Wayne R. Waz, M.D.

1. Define acute renal failure.

Acute renal failure (ARF) is defined as a sudden, sustained decline in glomerular filtration rate (GFR), usually associated with azotemia, elevated creatinine, and a fall in urine output (oliguria or, rarely, anuria). Normal urine output in children is 0.5–3 ml/kg/hr. A rapidly rising serum creatinine (i.e., > 0.5–0.7 mg/dl/day) indicates a GFR less than 10 ml/min/1.73m^2.

2. Can blood urea nitrogen or creatinine be elevated in the absence of renal failure?

Yes. Increase in blood urea nitrogen (BUN) without renal failure is noted in conditions such as gastrointestinal hemorrhage, severe catabolism (e.g., with infection or after surgery), intravascular volume depletion, and administration of certain drugs (e.g., corticosteroids or tetracycline). Similarly, the creatinine can be elevated in patients with large muscle mass (such as body builders), after acute muscle injury, or after administration of drugs that interfere with assays (cephalosporins).

3. What causes ARF?

Most cases of intrinsic ARF, as opposed to prerenal azotemia or postrenal obstruction, are caused by ischemic (50%) or nephrotoxic (35%) injury to the kidney. About 15% of cases are caused by acute tubular interstitial nephritis or acute glomerulonephritis. Some causes of ARF pertain to children of all ages (e.g., shock, nephrotoxins, and obstructive uropathy). During the first days and months of life, renal failure often develops in seriously ill infants with infection, shock, dehydration, or asphyxia. The pathogenesis may be vascular thrombosis, acute tubular necrosis, or urate nephropathy. In infants without systemic distress, obstructive uropathy or insufficient renal parenchyma (renal hypoplasia or dysplasia) is often the cause. From infancy to adolescence, hemolytic uremic syndrome and acute postinfectious glomerulonephritis are the most common causes of ARF. Other glomerular disorders that produce renal failure in this age group include Henoch-Schönlein purpura, IgA nephropathy, membranoproliferative glomerulonephritis, crescentic nephritis, and lupus nephritis.

4. How is hypoperfusion of the kidney differentiated from intrinsic renal damage?

Urinalysis and microscopy are helpful. Most children with intrinsic ARF have decreased concentration ability, which reflects the inability either to concentrate or to dilute the urine because of tubular cell damage. In cases of renal hypoperfusion, however, the urine is concentrated because of avid renal salt and water retention. The presence of red cell casts suggests that acute glomerulonephritis may be presenting as ARF. Renal tubular cells and pigmented, coarsely granular casts support the diagnosis of acute tubular necrosis. Other findings may point to other causes: oxalate crystals may be found in ethylene glycol ingestion, and eosinophiluria suggests acute interstitial nephritis. The fractional excretion of sodium (FENa), which represents the proportion of filtered sodium not absorbed, also may be helpful. If the FENa is less than 1% in the presence of concentrated urine and oliguria, the patient most likely has prerenal ARF. However, if the FENa is greater than 2–3%, intrinsic renal damage is the likely cause of ARF. (See table next page.)

Dehydration/Decreased Renal Perfusion Versus Acute Renal Failure

	DEHYDRATION/DECREASED PERFUSION		ACUTE RENAL FAILURE	
	CHILD	*NEWBORN*	*CHILD*	*NEWBORN*
U_{Na} (mEq/L)	< 10	≤ 20	> 50	> 50
FENa (%)*	≤ 1	≤ 2.5	> 2	> 3
U_{osm}	≥ 500	≥ 350	≤ 300	≤ 300
U/P_{osm}	≥ 1.5	≥ 1.2	0.8–1.2	0.8–1.2
BUN/creatinine	> 20	> 10	Both ↑	Both ↑
Fluid push	Urine ↑	Urine ↑	No change	No change

U_{Na} = urinary sodium, U_{osm} = urine osmolality.
* FENa = $[U_{Na}/P_{Na}]/[U_{Cr}/P_{Cr}] \times 100$, where P_{Na} = plasma sodium, U_{Cr} = urinary creatinine, and P_{Cr} = plasma creatinine.

5. What happens to the kidney in ARF?

Three main areas of dysfunction may be involved in the physiology of intrinsic ARF. At the hemodynamic level, decreased renal perfusion and resulting ischemia lead to decreased glomerular capillary permeability, back leak of glomerular filtrate, tubular obstruction, and hemodynamic imbalance. At the cellular level, once cells are damaged, they may undergo one of three fates: necrosis, apoptosis, or recovery. At the level of cell-to-cell interaction, the communication between cells of various types (endothelial, mesangial, epithelial) and their response to damage may determine the ultimate outcome in ARF. In patients with multiple-organ system failure, ARF may progress as part of a more generalized systemic inflammatory response syndrome (SIRS).

6. What are the keys to management of patients with ARF?

Despite the emerging understanding of the pathophysiology of ARF, current management remains largely supportive. Careful attention to fluid status, electrolytes, acidosis, uremia, and nutrition/metabolic support are the keys to eventual recovery from ARF. Future therapies, hopefully, will address the specific hemodynamic and cellular insults that lead to ARF and may include growth factors, atrial or other natriuretic peptides, treatment or prevention of SIRS to prevent multiple-organ system failure, blood purification, immunotherapy, nitric oxide synthase inhibition, and antioxidants.

7. How do you manage fluids in a patient with ARF?

The first step is to assess extracellular volume status by measuring pulse and blood pressure, body weight, skin turgor, and capillary refill, and, if necessary, through more invasive monitoring (central venous pressure). The physical examination should reveal the presence or absence of heart failure, peripheral or pulmonary edema, and third-spacing. Children who present with ARF and evidence of intravascular volume depletion require prompt and carefully monitored fluid resuscitation. However, ARF associated with fluid overload requires immediate fluid restriction, diuretic medications, or dialysis, depending on the underlying cause.

The use of low-dose dopamine (2-3 mg/kg/min) is controversial. Although a number of animal studies suggest that the use of low-dose dopamine before the initiation of ARF can ameliorate disease, little clinical evidence suggests that its use significantly alters the course of patients with ARF.

Once the normal intravascular volume has been established, its maintenance depends on balancing fluid losses with intake by replacing urine output and insensible water loss (400 ml/m²/day).

8. What are the electrolyte changes in ARF?

- Hyponatremia, which may be dilutional or secondary to hyponatremic dehydration.
- Hyperkalemia, which is the leading cause of death in ARF. It may be due to (1) marked reduction in GFR, (2) impairment of renal tubular potassium secretion, or (3) the presence of associated tissue catabolism and metabolic acidosis.

• Hypocalcemia, which may be due to (1) hyperphosphatemia, (2) skeletal resistance to parathyroid hormone, or (3) decreased production of 1,25 $(OH)_2$ vitamin D3.

9. Describe the emergency treatment of hyperkalemia.

Emergency Treatment of Hyperkalemia

DRUG	DOSE	COMPLICATIONS
Calcium gluconate 10%	0.5–1.0 ml/kg IV over 2–4 min (watch EKG while infusing)	Bradycardia, hypercalcemia
$NaHCO_3$	1–2 mEq/kg IV over 30–60 min	Hypernatremia, fluid overload, hypertension, alkalosis
Insulin + glucose	Bolus: glucose 0.5–1.0 gm/kg (D25W: 2–4 ml/kg) IV over 30 min + insulin 0.1 U/kg (IV or SQ) Infusion: D25W at 1–2 ml/kg/hr + insulin 0.1 U/kg/hr	Hyper- or hypoglycemia
Albuterol	5–10 mg via nebulizer	Tachycardia
Kayexalate	1 gm/kg PO/PR (with 2–4 ml 70% sorbitol or 10% dextrose if PR)	Constipation, hypernatremia

IV = intravenously, EKG = electrocardiogram, D25W = 25% aqueous dextrose solution, SQ = subcutaneously, PO = orally, PR = rectally.

10. What are the indications for dialysis in ARF ?

The most common indications for acute dialysis include uremic syndrome, hyperkalemia, acidosis, or fluid overload. In addition, dialysis is customarily initiated prophylactically in patients with ARF when the plasma urea level reaches 100 mg/dl or when creatinine clearance decreases to less than 7–10 ml/min/1.73m². However, in the absence of symptomatic uremia, with acceptable plasma levels of potassium and bicarbonate and without fluid overload, acute dialysis is not always necessary even when plasma urea or creatinine clearance crosses these boundaries.

On the other hand, in patients with decreased urea generation due to poor nutrition or liver disease, manifestations of uremic syndrome may appear when the plasma urea level is well below 100 mg/dl. Similarly, dialysis may be needed for fluid removal or hyperkalemia in many patients with relatively low plasma urea levels or relatively well-preserved creatinine clearance values.

In general, other less common indications for dialysis include drug intoxication, hyperuricemia, hypercalcemia, hyperammonemia (particularly in patients with urea cycle defects), hypothermia, and metabolic alkalosis.

11. What are the choices of therapeutic modalities for acute dialysis in ARF ?

Hemodialysis offers a more rapid change in plasma solute composition and the possibility of more rapid removal of excessive body water than other modalities. This feature may be an advantage or disadvantage, depending on the clinical setting. Rapid correction of electrolyte imbalance may predispose to cardiac arrhythmia, and removal of fluid often is tolerated poorly by patients in an intensive care setting. On the other hand, in hypercatabolic patients and patients needing rapid correction of an electrolyte imbalance, hemodialysis may be the therapy of choice.

Peritoneal dialysis is approximately one-eighth as efficient as hemodialysis in altering blood solute composition and about one-fourth as efficient in fluid removal. However, it can be applied continuously, 24 hours per day, whereas hemodialysis usually is given for a maximum of 4 hours per day. Thus, on a daily basis the efficacy of hemodialysis and peritoneal dialysis in effecting changes in solute and fluid removal is not markedly different. The continuous nature of peritoneal dialysis allows changes in blood solute and total body water to be made gradually; thus, it is the therapy of choice for hemodynamically unstable patients. However, in some patients it cannot be performed because of the state of the abdomen (e.g., recent abdominal surgery that involved a bowel anastomosis or the presence of extensive adhesions from previous abdominal surgery).

Slow continuous procedures, such as continuous arteriovenous hemofiltration (CAVH) and continuous venovenous hemofiltration (CVVH), allow gradual change in plasma solute composition and gradual removal of excessive fluid similar to the effects of peritoneal dialysis. The main disadvantage is the need for insertion and maintenance of catheters in a large artery and a large vein (for CAVH) and the need for extracorporeal blood pumps (for CVVH). Dialysis can be added to these techniques for increased solute clearances.

12. What does end-stage renal disease mean?

End-stage renal disease (ESRD) means that the GFR is less than 5 ml/min/1.73m² in patients with chronic renal failure, which in the pediatric age group usually is due to congenital defects (e.g., renal hypoplasia or posterior urethral valves) or acquired conditions, which include primary renal disease (e.g., focal segmental glomerulosclerosis, hemolytic uremic syndrome, IgA nephropathy, membranoproliferative glomerulonephritis), disease secondary to systemic illness (e.g., diabetes mellitus, lupus erythematosus), or complications of treatment (e.g., cancer chemotherapy). Regardless of the cause, when a patient is diagnosed with ESRD, the options for maintaining life are chronic dialysis (hemodialysis or peritoneal dialysis) or transplantation.

13. How do you estimate GFR in pediatric patients with chronic renal failure?

In pediatric patients, GFR can be estimated by the Schwartz formula, which is based on serum creatinine and patient height. The result can be factored by the average normal value for GFR, which is 125 ml/min/1.73m².

Schwartz formula: creatinine clearance (ml/min/1.73m²)= (K × L)/Cr, where K= constant of proportionality, which is age-specific; L = length in cm; and Cr = serum creatinine in mg/dl.

Age	K
Low birth weight: < 1 yr	0.33
Full term: > 1 yr	0.45
2–12 yr	0.55
Female: 13–21 yr	0.55
Male: 13–21 yr	0.7

14. How do you keep track of the multiple problems in patients with chronic renal insufficiency or ESRD on chronic dialysis?

Make up your own mnemonic based on the letters **A, A, B, B, F, K,** and **G**:

Anemia. The anemia of chronic renal failure responds only to blood transfusion or erythropoietin therapy. The main reason for transfusing patients is to relieve symptoms, not to raise the hematocrit to some arbitrary level. Although some patients develop symptoms when the hematocrit falls below 20%, others exhibit none when the hematocrit is 15%. In patients on hemodialysis, Epoetin alfa usually has been administered as an IV bolus 3 times/week. In patients on peritoneal dialysis, it may be given by intravenous or subcutaneous injection. Patients receiving erythropoietin therapy also require supplemental iron therapy.

General Therapeutic Guidelines for Epoetin Alfa

Starting dose	50–100 U/kg 3 times/week
Reduce the dose when	Target range is reached *or* Hematocrit increases > 4 points in any 2-week period
Increase the dose if	Hematocrit does not increase by 5–6 points after 8 weeks of therapy and hematocrit is below target range
Maintenance dose	Individualize; general dosage range is 25 U/kg 3 times/week
Target hematocrit	30–33% (maximum = 36%)

Acidosis. Hydrogen ions retained in the body because of decreased renal excretion should be neutralized by alkali therapy such as sodium bicarbonate or sodium citrate. Acidosis can be monitored by measuring serum total carbon dioxide concentration, which should be restored to and maintained within the range of age-related normal values: 22–24 mEq/L for infants, 24–26 mEq/L for young children, and 26–28 mEq/L for older children and adolescents.

Blood pressure. The failed kidney, more often caused by glomerular disease, exhibits an exaggerated, uninhibited release of renin in its final efforts to restore glomerular filtration. The blood pressure elevation in such patients is also related to fluid overload. It can be lowered initially by reduction of the blood volume through fluid restriction or dialysis; however, further volume reduction stimulates renin release. Sustained control of blood pressure can be accomplished with single or combination drug regimens, including calcium channel blockers, labetalol, clonidine, and other agents. Angiotensin-converting enzyme inhibitors generally are contraindicated because of the risk of hyperkalemia.

Bone disease. Measures should be taken to prevent secondary hyperparathyroidism and vitamin D deficiency, which cause renal osteodystrophy, hypocalcemic tetany, and soft tissue calcification. When the serum phosphorus level exceeds 5 mg/dl, a medication such as calcium carbonate or calcium acetate should be started as a source of calcium and for binding phosphorus in the gastrointestinal tract. Moreover, phosphorus intake must be restricted in the diet. As a rough estimate of relative risk from metastatic calcification of soft tissue , the product of calcium and phosphorus concentration in plasma (in mg/dl) should be less than 70. The higher the value, the more likely the complications. Vitamin D replacement with 1,25(OH) vitamin D (calcitriol) is also essential.

Fluid restriction. Patients on hemodialysis need fluid restriction between treatments to maintain good blood pressure control and to prevent fluid overload or pulmonary edema.

Growth. Growth should be observed closely. Referral to an endocrinologist for growth hormone therapy should be considered when necessary.

Potassium. When dietary potassium restriction alone or correction of metabolic acidosis fails to reduce plasma potassium concentration satisfactorily, a sodium-potassium cation exchange resin such as Kayexalate can be administered by mouth or enema. In a dose of 1–2 gm/kg, plasma potassium is expected to be lowered by approximately 1 mEq/L, whereas serum sodium is expected to be raised by 1 mEq/L. Chronic therapy in hypertensive or edematous patients can complicate blood pressure control.

BIBLIOGRAPHY

1. Breen D, Bihari D: Acute renal failure as a part of multiple organ failure: The slippery slope of critical illness. Kidney Int 53 (Suppl 66):S25–S33, 1998.
2. Nissenson AR: Acute renal failure: Definition and pathogenesis. Kidney Int 53 (Suppl 66):S7–S10, 1998.
3. Nolan CR, Anderson RJ: Hospital-acquired acute renal failure. J Am Soc Nephrol 9:710–718, 1998.
4. Pinsky MR: The critically ill patient. Kidney Int 53 (Suppl 66):S3–S6, 1998.
5. Schwartz GJ, Brion LP, Spitzer A: The use of plasma creatinine concentration for estimating glomerular filtration rate in infants, children, and adolescents. Pediatr Clin North Am 34:571–590, 1987.
6. Star RA: Treatment of acute renal failure. Kidney Int 54:1817–1831, 1998.
7. Zawada ET: Indications for dialysis. In Daugirdas JT, Ing TS (eds): Handbook of Dialysis, 2nd ed. Boston, Little, Brown, 1994, pp 3–9.

48. RENAL CYSTIC DISEASES

Julian Wan, M.D.

1. What are the major pediatric renal cystic diseases?
The major pediatric renal cystic diseases can be divided into two broad groups: heritable and nonheritable conditions:

Heritable conditions
- Autosomal recessive (infantile) polycystic kidney disease
- Autosomal dominant (adult) polycystic kidney disease
- Cysts associated with multiple malformations

Nonheritable conditions
- Multicystic dysplastic kidney
- Multilocular cysts
- Simple cysts
- Medullary sponge kidney
- Acquired cysts of renal failure
- Calyceal diverticuli

2. What is the most commonly reported cause of an abdominal mass in infants?
Multicystic dysplastic kidney (MCDK) usually is reported as the most common or second most common (after obstruction at the ureteropelvic junction [UPJ]) cause of a palpable abdominal mass in infants. It is a unilateral condition.

3. What is the natural history of MCDK? Is surgical excision ever recommended? What is the cause?
Most cases of MCDK regress spontaneously with time. By the age of 2 years many MCDKs are no longer detectable by ultrasound, although some take longer to resolve. Surgical removal is recommended in the rare cases associated with hypertension, hematuria, or uncertain diagnosis. MCDK is believed to be caused by ureteral atresia early in embryogenesis. Other theories postulate failure of the ureteric bud to meet the nephrogenic blastema appropriately.

4. How does an MCDK appear on ultrasound, intravenous pyelography, computed tomography (CT) scan, and nuclear medicine scan?
Ultrasound: The MCDK shows a unilateral affected kidney with several irregular cysts throughout the parenchyma.

Intravenous pyelography: The MCDK is nonfunctional and unable to concentrate the contrast material.

CT scan: numerous irregular-sized cysts are scattered throughout the kidney. In the rare adult patient whose MCDK did not regress, the scan reveals thin, shell-like calcification of the cysts.

Nuclear medicine scan: The MCDK is nonfunctional. The technetium dimercaptosuccinic acid (DMSA) scan shows no activity on the ipsilateral side.

5. MCDK can be confused with what noncystic entities?
UPJ obstruction and duplicated renal system. The dilated renal pelvis and calyces of a UPJ obstruction can mimic an MCDK. The duplicated system may have cysts in the upper pole segment with a dilated ectopic ureter.

6. How can MCDK be differentiated from UPJ obstruction and a duplicated system on ultrasound?
In MCDK ultrasound reveals:
- Interfaces between cysts
- Nonmedial location of the largest cysts
- Absence of an identifiable renal sinus
- No demarcation between the cysts and a region of normal renal parenchyma

In contrast, UPJ obstruction shows links between the dilated calyces and the centrally located pelvis. The pelvis is the largest single dilated space, and the renal pelvis is discernible. A duplicated system may have dilation and cysts in the upper-pole segment, but the lower-pole segment usually is normal. Demarcation between the upper and lower portions may be visible. There also may be a dilated upper ureter with an ectopic bladder insertion (possibly with a ureterocele).

7. What conditions can be found in the contralateral kidney of patients with MCDK?

Patients with MCDK have been noted to have an increased incidence of contralateral UPJ obstruction and vesicoureteral reflux. For this reason all patients with MCDK should have a voiding cystourethrogram and imaging of the contralateral kidney.

8. How does autosomal recessive (infantile) polycystic kidney disease (ARPKD) present? What are its salient features?

ARPKD usually presents within the first decade of life. Both kidneys are affected. ARPKD occurs in about 1 in 40,000 births. Small cysts develop within the collecting tubules. Large, palpable, poorly functioning kidneys may occupy most of the abdomen, displacing the peritoneal contents. In newborns it is often fatal. Oligohydramnios is commonly seen with concomitant respiratory distress. Cysts also are usually seen in the biliary tree as biliary ectasia and may lead to portal hypertension, varices, and hepatosplenomegaly. Liver cysts usually are not seen, nor are cerebral aneurysms.

9. How does ARPKD appear on imaging studies? What is its natural history?

In ARPKD ultrasound shows a multitude of small cysts. The interfaces of the cysts cause so many reflections that they increase echogenicity, leading to the appearance of large, "bright" kidneys. Because function is poor, both intravenous pyelography and nuclear scan may show few findings, although nephromegaly sometimes is seen. The natural history of ARPKD involves progressive renal failure in childhood. Dialysis and renal transplantation are the only treatments. Removal of the kidneys may be necessary because of infection and hypertension.

10. How does autosomal dominant (adult) polycystic kidney disease (ADPKD) present? What are its salient features?

ADPKD usually presents symptomatically later in life, although early detection is possible. Less than 10% of ADPKD cases are symptomatic in the first decade of life. This autosomal dominant condition with variable penetration affects about 600,000 people in the United States. Cysts of varying sizes occur at any point throughout the course of the nephrons. Most patients develop renal insufficiency and later failure, starting in their mid-forties and progressing into their sixties. Hypertension, hematuria, and increasing renal size leading to mechanical compression of the peritoneal contents are common symptoms. Because of variable expression, some patients have a mild form.

11. How does ADPKD differ from ARPKD?

Autosomal Dominant vs. Autosomal Recessive Polycystic Kidney Disease

CATEGORY	ARPKD	ADPKD
Age of onset	Usually < 10 yr	Usually > 20 yr
Inheritance mode	Autosomal recessive	Autosomal dominant; variable penetrance
Clinical course	Renal failure	Variable; renal failure is possible
Type of cyst	Multitude of small cysts in collecting system	Variable-sized cysts located anywhere on nephron
Associated cysts elsewhere	Cysts in biliary tree	33% with cysts in liver, pancreas, and lung; 20% with aneurysm in cerebral circulation

12. In addition to treating the patient, who else should be evaluated in ARPKD and ADPKD?

The parents of children with either condition should be counseled about the genetic risks. Patients with ADPKD and their immediate family should be considered for evaluation of aneurysms in the circle of Willis. Autopsy studies of patients with ADPKD found that 22% have cerebral aneurysms. About 9% of adult patients with ADPKD die of subarachnoid hemorrhage.

13. What major malformation syndromes are associated with renal cysts?

Tuberous sclerosis and Von Hippel-Lindau (VHL) syndrome are autosomal dominant conditions commonly seen with renal cysts. Down syndrome and Turner syndrome are chromosomal disorders linked with renal cysts.

14. What are tuberous sclerosis and Von Hippel-Lindau syndrome ?

Tuberous sclerosis is an autosomal dominant condition characterized by mental retardation, epilepsy, sebaceous acne, and renal masses. The masses may be renal hamartomas (usually angiomyolipomas), simple cysts, or both. VHL is an autosomal dominant condition characterized by cerebellar hemangioblastomas, retinal angiomata, cysts of the pancreas and kidney, epididymis, pheochromocytoma, and renal cell carcinoma (found in 30–40% of patients with VHL).

15. What is a multilocular cyst? What are its key features ?

A multilocular cyst, as the name suggests, is a complex cyst with multiple loculations. It may present at any age as a flank mass or be asymptomatic and found incidentally. It is benign but poses a diagnostic challenge because it may strongly resemble a cystic Wilms' tumor or cystic renal adenocarcinoma. It usually is treated with nephrectomy.

16. How does a multilocular cyst differ from MCDK?

Multilocular Cystic Kidney vs. Multicystic Dysplastic Kidney

FEATURE	MCDK	MULTILOCULAR KIDNEY
Age at presentation	Usually in infancy	Any age
Symptom	Abdominal mass	Abdominal mass
Contralateral anomalies	UPJ obstruction, vesicoureteral reflux	None; contralateral kidney usually is normal
Ipsilateral ureter	Atretic	Usually normal
Cyst description	Variable-sized cysts throughout kidney; little normal parenchyma, marked dysplasia	Variably sized, with cysts within cysts; usually a polar location and no dysplasia
Tumor risk	None	Rare, but included in differential diagnosis

17. What is medullary sponge kidney?

Medullary sponge kidney (MSK) is characterized by small (1–5-mm) cysts in the collecting tubules. On a cut surface the cysts give the kidney a sponge-like appearance. MSK is not believed to be a heritable disorder, although there is a familial predilection in about 5% of cases. MSK usually presents after 20 years of age but occasionally presents in children. It is usually a bilateral condition (75%) associated with notable radial stretching and puddling of contrast in the calyces on intravenous pyelography.

18. What conditions are associated with MSK?

Some patients with MSK exhibit hypercalciuria, which predisposes to stone formation.

19. What is a simple cyst?

Simple cysts are uncommon in children. They are usually solitary and are about 3–4 cm in size. They have a sharp outline on ultrasound with no loculations and a thin wall. Usually asymptomatic and found incidentally, simple cysts should not affect the patient's life.

20. What is included in the differential diagnosis of a simple cyst?

Cystic Wilms' tumor, multilocular cyst, duplication anomalies, calyceal diverticulum, and early presentation of genetic cyst disorders.

21. What are acquired renal cysts (ARCs) of renal failure?

Patients with renal failure on chronic hemodialysis have been noted to develop renal cysts, which may be multiple and remain small or become enlarged. Symptoms may resemble polycystic kidney disease: abdominal mass, pain, and hematuria.

22. Why is ARC a worrisome finding?

ARC is associated with a high incidence of kidney tumors. Up to 25% of patients with ARC develop a tumor. About 20% of the tumors are renal adenocarcinoma, whereas the other 80% are benign. It has been estimated that about 1 in every 23 patients on long-term hemodialysis will develop renal adenocarcinoma. This risk is about 7 times higher than in the general population.

23. What is a calyceal diverticulum?

A calyceal diverticulum is an outpouching from the fornix of the calyx, usually arising in the upper pole. It appears as a round cyst that extends from the calyx and fills with contrast on intravenous pyelography. A thin wall of parenchyma surrounds the cyst.

24. How does a calyceal diverticulum present? How is it treated?

Usually it is asymptomatic and appears when a stone or infection develops within it. The stones characteristically are composed of milk alkali. Operation is rarely needed and usually is done only in cases of recurrent infection or obstructing or infected stones. The cyst is unroofed, and its neck is ligated. The cyst cavity is collapsed and filled with fat from Gerota's fascia when possible.

BIBLIOGRAPHY

1. Glassberg KI, Filmer RB: Renal dysplasia, renal hypoplasia, and cystic disease of kidney. In Kelalis PP, King LR, Belman AB (eds): Clinical Pediatric Urology, 3rd ed. Philadelphia, W.B. Saunders, 1992, pp 1121–1184.
2. Lieberman E, Salinas-Madrigal L, Gwinn JL, et al: Infantile polycystic disease of the kidneys and liver: Clinical, pathological and radiological correlations and comparison with congenital hepatic fibrosis. Medicine 50:277, 1971.
3. Sayney S, Sandler MA, Weiss L, et al: Adult polycystic disease: Presymptomatic diagnosis for genetic counseling. Clin Nephrol 20:89, 1983.
4. Kleiner B, Filly R, Mack L, et al: Multicystic dysplastic kidney: Observations of contralateral disease in the fetal population. Radiology 161:27, 1986.

49. OBSTRUCTIVE UROPATHIES

Leslie D. Tackett, M.D., and Anthony A. Caldamone, M.D.

1. Name the most common sites of congenital urinary tract obstruction.
- Ureteropelvic junction (UPJ)
- Ureterovesical junction
- Posterior urethra

2. What is the most common presentation of urinary tract obstruction?
Since the advent of routine prenatal ultrasound screening, prenatal hydronephrosis is the most common presentation of urinary tract obstruction. Other common presentations include flank pain accompanied by vomiting, urinary tract infection, hematuria, or an abdominal mass due to hydronephrosis. Older children with posterior urethral valves or an ectopic hydronephrotic ureter may present with urinary incontinence.

3. How is prenatal hydronephrosis defined? How commonly is it identified during routine prenatal ultrasound screening?
Depending on how it is defined and at what stage of pregnancy screening is performed, dilation of the urinary tract is identified in approximately 1 in 50 to 1 in 100 pregnancies, although only 1 in 500 have a significant urologic abnormality. Prenatal hydronephrosis is defined by a renal pelvic anteroposterior diameter greater than 8 mm at or beyond 24 weeks gestation, or an anteroposterior pelvis-to-renal cortex ratio greater than 0.5.

4. Aside from the presence or absence of hydronephrosis, what other ultrasound findings are important in the genitourinary evaluation?
A systematic approach to prenatal ultrasound screening is of paramount importance. Assessment should include determination of the amount of amniotic fluid and overall fetal size and maturity as well as examination of the genitalia, evaluation of bladder fullness and wall thickness, and imaging to ascertain other structural anomalies. The echogenic characteristics of the renal parenchyma can be predictive of postnatal renal function. Prenatal ultrasound also provides serial monitoring of detected abnormalities for potential prognostic information as well as treatment planning.

5. What are the common causes of prenatal hydronephrosis?
- UPJ obstruction
- Posterior urethral valves
- Ureterocele
- Primary obstructive megaureter
- Vesicoureteral reflux (VUR)
- "Physiologic" dilatation

6. What postnatal studies are necessary to evaluate a patient with a history of prenatal hydronephrosis?
After physical examination of the newborn, which in most cases is normal, a postnatal ultrasound and voiding cystourethrogram are key in the postnatal evaluation of prenatal hydronephrosis. In children with severe bilateral hydronephrosis or a solitary kidney, a baseline blood urea nitrogen (BUN) and serum creatinine should be considered, keeping in mind that the baseline serum creatinine may not be achieved until 1 week of age or older.

7. When should one perform a postnatal ultrasound in a male infant with a history of unilateral hydronephrosis? Bilateral prenatal hydronephrosis?
Newborn infants are relatively oliguric for the first 48 hours, and a postnatal ultrasound may underestimate the presence of hydronephrosis (false negative). In the neonate with a history of

unilateral hydronephrosis, if the initial postnatal ultrasound before discharge from the hospital is normal, a follow-up ultrasound evaluation in 1–3 months should be performed. Alternatively, one may wait until 1 month of age for the initial postnatal ultrasound. In male infants with a history of bilateral prenatal hydronephrosis, an early postnatal ultrasound before discharge, followed by voiding cystourethrogram if hydronephrosis is present, is vital to evaluate possible posterior urethral valves.

8. How can one differentiate between hydronephrosis and multicystic dysplasia on renal ultrasound? What other studies may assist in the diagnosis?

Hydronephrosis is suggested on ultrasound by a large central "cyst" (renal pelvis) with interconnecting smaller peripheral "cysts" (calyces), a "catcher's mitt" appearance. Multicystic dysplastic kidneys demonstrate loss of the reniform shape with multiple cysts of varying sizes that do not appear to connect. Also in the multicystic dysplastic kidney, the septa between cysts are hyperechoic as a result of the dysplastic parenchyma, and no renal cortex is discernible. A Tc 99m dimercaptosuccinic acid (DMSA) renal scan can be used to demonstrate the presence (hydronephrotic kidney) or absence (multicystic dysplastic kidney) of renal function.

9. Describe Dietl's crisis.

More commonly seen in older children and adults, Dietl's crisis refers to an apparent intermittent obstruction at the UPJ, which during high rates of urine flow, as may occur with a large intake of fluids, leads to severe abdominal pain and vomiting. When the renal pelvis drains, the symptoms resolve.

10. Name three diagnostic studies used to demonstrate urinary tract obstruction.
- Diuretic nuclear renal scan
- Intravenous urogram (IVU)
- Whitaker test

11. How is a Whitaker test performed?

The Whitaker test, also known as the constant volume perfusion test, begins with placement of a nephrostomy tube or insertion of a spinal needle to access the hydronephrotic collecting system. A urethral catheter is also placed. A pump is used to provide flow at a constant rate into the kidney, and renal pelvic pressure and bladder pressure are measured. If the maximal difference between renal pelvis pressure and bladder pressure is greater than 22 cm H_2O, obstruction is suggested. For pressure differentials between 15 and 22 cm H_2O, the test is considered indeterminate. If the pressure remains below 15 cm H_2O, the system is considered nonobstructed.

12. How does one choose the radiopharmaceutical for a nuclear renal scan?

Technetium (Tc) 99m diethylenetriaminepentaacetic acid (DTPA) is cleared almost exclusively by glomerular filtration. This property allows estimation of glomerular filtration rate based on the activity during parenchymal transit between 1 and 3 minutes after injection of the radionuclide. DTPA is used in conjunction with furosemide to assess upper urinary tract obstruction.

Tc 99m dimercaptosuccinic acid (DMSA) is the most sensitive agent for imaging the renal parenchyma and provides functional information about the renal unit. Areas of decreased or absent function may be identified, including focal pyelonephritis, renal scarring, dysplasia, or a nonfunctioning unit of a duplex system.

Tc 99m mercaptoacetyltriglycerine (MAG-3) is secreted by the renal tubules more efficiently than DTPA, making it the agent of choice in neonates and patients with renal functional impairment. Like DTPA, MAG-3 is useful in demonstrating the presence of obstruction or confirming the lack of function in a presumed multicystic dysplastic kidney. MAG-3 is more expensive and has a shorter shelf life than DTPA.

13. What common pitfalls may confound the interpretation of the diuretic renal scan?

Several factors can affect the results and interpretation of the diuretic renogram, including the degree of renal function based on maturity or impairment, the state of hydration, the capacity of the collecting system, bladder fullness, patient positioning, choice of radiopharmaceutical, placement of the region of interest, and timing of diuretic administration. To standardize the technique of diuretic renography, the Society of Fetal Urology and the Pediatric Nuclear Medicine Council of the Society of Nuclear Medicine have reached a consensus methodology to define the "well-tempered" renogram.

14. Is the upper-pole moiety of a duplex collecting system more prone to reflux or obstruction? Why?

The ureteral orifice of the upper pole of a duplex collecting system is positioned in a more medial and caudal location compared with the more lateral and cephalad orifice of the lower-pole system. The result is that the lower-pole ureter has a shorter intramural tunnel and is more prone to reflux, whereas the upper-pole ureter is more prone to obstruction based on its ectopic location. This is the Weigert-Meyer law.

15. A neonate presents with unilateral prenatal hydronephrosis, and further evaluation with a DTPA-Lasix renogram confirms unilateral UPJ obstruction. Are any additional studies warranted?

Ipsilateral VUR occurs in approximately 10% of children presenting with UPJ obstruction, and contralateral reflux occurs in approximately 20%. A voiding cystourethrogram should be performed to exclude ipsilateral or contralateral VUR and to rule out urethral obstruction in male infants.

16. Name the major causes of UPJ obstruction.
  • Aperistaltic ureteral segment (muscular derangement)
  • Ureteral valve
  • Ureteral stricture
  • Secondary to high-grade reflux or distal obstruction
  • Fibroepithelial polyp
  Other causes of UPJ obstruction may include:
  • Fibrous bands or adhesions
  • High insertion of the UPJ
  • Crossing lower pole renal vessel

17. How does one classify megaureter?
  • Refluxing   • Nonrefluxing/nonobstructed
  • Obstructed   • Refluxing/obstructed

18. Describe posterior urethral valves of types I, II, and III. Which are the most common? The least common?

In 1919 three types of posterior urethral valves (PUV) were described by Hugh Young. Type I valves are leaflets, like sails, separated by a slit-like opening, that extend distally and laterally from the verumontanum and fuse anteriorly at the 12 o'clock position. Ninety-five percent of PUVs are type I. Type II valves extend proximally from the verumontanum. They are nonobstructing, thought to have little clinical significance, and therefore no longer included in the classification of PUV. Type III valves, 5% of PUVs, are described as a congenital urethral membrane that mimics a wind-sock.

19. What is VURD syndrome?

Valves, unilateral reflux, and renal dysplasia (VURD) syndrome affects approximately 15% of children with posterior urethral valves who have unilateral VUR associated with a nonfunctioning kidney. Because of the presumed "pop-off" mechanism of reflux into the dysplastic kidney, the prognosis for renal function is generally good.

20. What factors should be considered before prenatal intervention for hydronephrosis? What is the most common form of intervention?

The goals of prenatal intervention for hydronephrosis are to preserve or improve renal function and to prevent pulmonary hypoplasia. Although no solid evidence indicates that prenatal therapy can improve renal function, especially at the point in renal development when intervention is feasible, some clinical evidence suggests that in utero intervention to correct oligohydramnios does improve postnatal pulmonary function. Thus, normal amniotic fluid volume is a relative contraindication to in utero intervention. Prenatal intervention is unlikely to be indicated in a female fetus because lower urinary tract obstruction rarely occurs in females.

In a male fetus with high-grade hydronephrosis, a distended bladder, and low or decreasing amniotic fluid volume, urine electrolytes and beta$_2$-microglobulin should be evaluated via bladder tap. In patients diagnosed before 20 weeks gestation and patients with poor renal function based on fetal urine evaluation, the outcome of intervention is generally poor because of irreversible renal dysplasia. If fetal renal function is preserved by virtue of fetal urine evaluation, in utero intervention vs. early delivery (if greater than 32 weeks gestation) of the fetus may be contemplated. Placement of a vesicoamniotic shunt is the most common form of intervention with a complication rate of up to 45% and overall survival rate of 47%. Even with intervention, 40% of survivors have end-stage renal disease.

21. Once a diagnosis of UPJ obstruction is made, what are the important factors in deciding to proceed with operative correction?

Operative correction of UPJ obstruction should be considered to prevent renal functional impairment. Although kidneys with relative renal function as low as 25% of the total may recover function during periods of observation, experimental and clinical data support early pyeloplasty to relieve obstruction and potentially reverse its consequences in the newborn kidney. Patients with mild-to-moderate obstruction may be followed closely with radiographic evaluation. Approximately 30% of such children ultimately undergo pyeloplasty. Surgical treatment should be considered in any child with significantly impaired differential renal function (< 35%), thinned renal parenchyma, poor renal or somatic growth, a solitary functioning kidney, pyelonephritis, flank pain, stone disease, or suspected poor compliance with follow-up evaluation.

22. Describe the surgical options and the relative expected rate of success for treatment of UPJ obstruction.

Open pyeloplasty: 95–98%
Endopyelotomy: 82%
Laparoscopic pyeloplasty: 80% in adults; no data in children available

23. Outline the initial management of a child with posterior urethral valves.

Initial management of posterior urethral valves depends to some degree on the overall condition of the newborn. Adequate respiratory support and fluid resuscitation may be required. Prompt bladder drainage with a small (5- or 8-Fr) feeding tube should be performed in infants with significant hydronephrosis, acidosis, hyperkalemia, azotemia, or sepsis. Antibiotic therapy should be considered. A baseline serum creatinine level should be obtained after 24 hours. In infants with urosepsis and impaired renal function, early vesicostomy or supravesical diversion may be indicated. Children with good renal function and overall stable medical condition without infections may undergo primary valve ablation with postoperative voiding cystourethrogram and renal ultrasound to assure adequate relief of obstruction.

24. Is VUR common in children with posterior urethral valves? How does the presence of reflux change the management of PUV?

Vesicoureteral reflux occurs in approximately 50% of boys with PUV at presentation. The presence of reflux does not alter the initial management of these children. Furthermore, following relief of obstruction reflux may improve or resolve in 25% of the cases.

25. If a primary megaureter is diagnosed, what factors does one consider in determining whether operative intervention is indicated?

Preservation of renal function is the goal of surgical intervention. Loss of renal function may be due to persistent or progressive obstruction or infection. Surgical correction should be considered for children with impaired renal function, deterioration of renal function, or thinning of renal parenchyma as well as in children with pyelonephritis, stone disease, or flank pain.

COMPLICATIONS

26. What are the potential complications of untreated urinary tract obstruction?

The most serious complication of untreated urinary tract obstruction is progressive loss of renal function. Other complications include recurrent infection, stone disease, and failure to thrive.

27. Name prognostic factors relative to renal function in children with PUV.

Good Prognosis: • Serum creatinine of less than 1.0 mg/dl at 1 year of age
                           • Urinary ascites
                           • VURD syndrome

Poor Prognosis: • Presentation before 24 weeks gestation
                           • Nadir serum creatinine of 1 mg/dl or higher
                           • Echogenic kidneys, cystic renal parenchyma, or loss of corticomedullary differentiation by ultrasound
                           • Bilateral vesicoureteral reflux
                           • Significant proteinuria

28. What are the causes of a failed pyeloplasty for UPJ obstruction?

The key elements to a successful pyeloplasty are adequate dependent drainage of the collecting system and a water-tight, tension-free anastomosis, and maintenance of good vascularity to the ureter. Extravasation of urine through the anastomosis is thought to create a secondary inflammatory response which results in persistent obstruction in many patients. Additionally, devascularization of the ureter due to exuberant mobilization can result in postoperative stenosis.

29. What is the accepted approach to the failed pyeloplasty?

After failed pyeloplasty, the accepted approach is endopyelotomy. This endourologic technique has an overall success rate of 91% in pediatric patients with secondary UPJ obstruction. Alternatively, repeat open pyeloplasty or ureterocalycostomy can be considered.

30. What special considerations arise during the reimplantation of an obstructive megaureter?

Because of the increased ureteral diameter, a longer intramural tunnel must be created to achieve the recommended tunnel length to ureteral diameter ratio of 5:1 in order to prevent postoperative VUR. Tapering of the megaureter has led to reliably reproducible prevention of postoperative reflux. Postoperative ureteral obstruction is a potentially serious complication which is most commonly due to distal ureteral ischemia or angulation at the ureterovesical junction. Meticulous surgical technique can prevent these complications in most cases.

BIBLIOGRAPHY

1. Cendron M, Elder JS, Duckett JW: Perinatal urology. In Gillenwater JY, Grayhack JT, Howards SS, Duckett JW (eds): Adult and Pediatric Urology, 3rd ed. St. Louis, Mosby, 1996, pp 2075–2165.
2. Coplen DE: Prenatal intervention for hydronephrosis. J Urol 157:2270–2277, 1997.
3. DiSandro MJ, Kogan BA: Neonatal management: Role for early intervention. Urol Clin North Am 25:187–197, 1998.
4. Docimo SG, Silver RI: Renal ultrasonography in newborns with prenatally detected hydronephrosis: Why wait? J Urol 157:1387–1389, 1997.

5. Figenshau RS, Clayman RV: Endourologic options for management of ureteropelvic junction obstruction in the pediatric patient. Urol Clin North Am 25:199–209, 1998.
6. Gonzales ET Jr: Posterior urethral valves and other urethral anomalies. In Walsh PC, Retik AB, Vaughan ED Jr, Wein AJ (eds): Campbell's Urology, 7th ed. Philadelphia, W.B. Saunders, 1998, pp 2069–2092.
7. Koff SA: Neonatal management of unilateral hydronephrosis: Role for delayed intervention. Urol Clin North Am 25:181–186, 1998.
8. Society for Fetal Urology and Pediatric Nuclear Medicine Council: The "well tempered" diuretic renogram: A standard method to examine the asymptomatic neonate with hydronephrosis or hydroureteronephrosis. J Nucl Med 33:2047–2051, 1992.
9. Woodard JR: Megaloureter. In King LR (ed): Urologic Surgery in Infants and Children. Philadelphia, W.B. Saunders, 1998, pp 67–77.

50. VESICOURETERAL REFLUX

Saul P. Greenfield, M.D.

1. What is vesicoureteral reflux?

Vesicoureteral reflux (VUR) is the retrograde flow of urine from the bladder back up the ureters.

2. Is vesicoureteral reflux ever normal?

VUR is never normal in humans at any age, including premature newborns. In many species of animals, however, reflux occurs without apparent harm to the kidneys.

3. What is the incidence of VUR in the population?

Reflux occurs in under 1% of all people.

4. What is the incidence of VUR in children who present with a urinary infection?

The incidence of reflux in boys and girls with a history of urinary infection is 30–50%. This incidence is the same after only one infection. All children, therefore, who present with their *first* infection must be evaluated for reflux.

5. Does VUR present only as pyelonephritis?

Many children with acute pyelonephritis do not have reflux. More virulent forms of bacteria can ascend from the bladder to infect the kidney in the absence of reflux. VUR, however, has a significant incidence in populations who present with pyelonephritis as well as in children who present only with cystitis or asymptomatic bacteriuria.

6. Why do people with reflux have more urinary tract infections?

Reflux allows easy entrance of bacteria to the upper urinary tract. Furthermore, regurgitation of urine up the ureter during voiding means that bacteria in the bladder are not cleared with micturition. Not voiding to completion, therefore, promotes colonization of the urinary tract.

7. Can VUR cause symptoms in the absence of infection?

Reflux is asymptomatic, without abdominal or flank pain, and is not perceived by the patient.

8. Is reflux inherited?

VUR is inherited. The mechanism is believed to be autosomal dominant with variable penetrance.

9. What is the incidence of VUR in asymptomatic siblings?

Between 25–50% of asymptomatic male and female siblings also have VUR. Once a proband is identified, therefore, it is recommended that the siblings be screened, even if they have never had a documented urinary infection.

10. Should children with nocturnal enuresis be evaluated for VUR?

Children with monosymptomatic (nighttime only) bedwetting do not have a higher-than-normal incidence of congenital urinary tract abnormalities and need not be evaluated. Children with daytime wetting, especially with a history of urinary infection, should be screened for reflux.

11. How is VUR diagnosed?

Diagnosis requires a voiding cystourethrogram (VCUG). The child must be catheterized and awake so that he or she can void, because reflux may not be seen until bladder pressures are elevated during micturition. VCUGs can be performed with iodinated contrast and standard fluoroscopy or with a radionuclide agent.

12. Can a renal or bladder ultrasound diagnose reflux?

Ultrasound may show hydronephrosis or hydroureter in extreme cases of high-grade reflux. However, ultrasound also may be normal in high- and low-grade VUR. There is no reliable non-invasive means of diagnosing reflux; a VCUG must be performed.

13. How is VUR graded?

Most clinicians use the international scale, ranging from grades I to V. Grade I reflux goes up the ureter without filling the renal pelvis. Grade II reflux reaches the pelvis but does not cause ureteral dilatation or calyceal blunting. Grades III–V demonstrate progressive degrees of ureteral dilatation and tortuosity along with calyceal distortion. Grading can be done only with contrast VCUG; none of these features can be seen on a radionuclide VCUG.

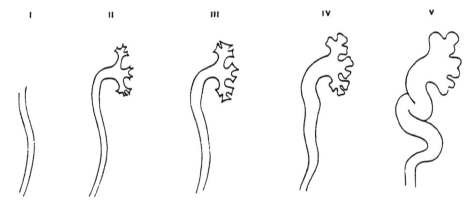

The international reflux classification from grades I to V. (From Walker RD: Vesicoureteral reflux. In Gillenwater JY, Grayhack JT, Howards SS, et al (eds): Adult and Pediatric Urology, Vol 2. Chicago, Year Book, 1987, pp 1676–1708; with permission.)

14. What prevents reflux in the normal person?

The ureters enter the bladder muscle and then travel for a distance between the bladder muscle and mucosa before opening on the trigone. This "tunnel" between the mucosa and muscle acts as a flap-valve mechanism. As the bladder fills, the roof of the tunnel is compressed, preventing the reflux of urine upward. People with VUR have abnormally short or absent tunnels and, therefore, deficient or absent valves. Higher grades of reflux are associated with shorter tunnels. Cystoscopy reveals that the more severe grades have more lateral and gaping orifices.

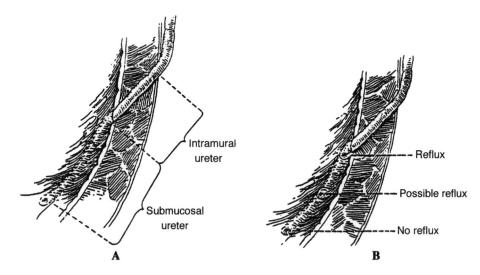

A, Normal ureterovesical junction with submucosal segment long enough to function as a "flap valve" to prevent reflux. **B**, Anatomic features of a shortened submucosal tunnel, allowing vesicoureteral reflux. (From Politano VA: Vesicoureteral reflux. In Glenn JF (eds): Urologic Surgery, 2nd ed. New York, Harper & Row, 1975, pp 272–293; with permission.)

15. How do children "outgrow" reflux?

As children grow toward adult height, the deficient tunnel elongates, and in many instances the flap-valve mechanism starts to function. In general, the lower grades of reflux have higher rates of resolution with growth. Approximate rates of resolution over time in the five grades are as follows:

Grade I: 90%	Grade IV: 25%
Grade II: 75%	Grade V: 0–5%
Grade III: 50%	

16. Is there a difference in the prognosis of high-grade reflux in newborns versus reflux diagnosed later in childhood?

Prenatal ultrasound detection of hydronephrosis has resulted in the identification of newborns with high-grade reflux before they have the chance to develop urinary infections. As opposed to older children, neonates with grade IV or V reflux have around a 35% chance of spontaneous resolution by the age of 2 years.

17. How long does it take for reflux to resolve?

It is impossible to predict when or whether reflux will resolve. The process is slow and takes years; resolution may not occur until adolescence.

18. How does reflux harm kidneys?

VUR does not harm kidneys except in the presence of infection with pyelonephritis. Sterile reflux can be tolerated for the life of the patient. Most renal "scars" occur after infection. Kidneys exposed to numerous infections may develop many scars and become atrophic. The morbidity of VUR—hypertension and renal insufficiency—results from these scars. Unrecognized and untreated reflux may lead to renal failure and the need for transplantation.

19. Are congenital renal "scars" associated with reflux?

Some infants with high-grade reflux who were identified with prenatal ultrasound appear to have scarred kidneys at birth before they have had any urinary tract infections. Such children are born with segmental renal dysplasia. Renal organogenesis, therefore, may be abnormal in association with high-grade reflux. Most scars seen in infants and children with reflux, however, are acquired postnatally and are due to infection.

20. How are renal scars diagnosed in children with VUR?

Scars are best seen with a radionuclide renal scan. Renal ultrasound misses many scars, as does an intravenous pyelogram. The imaging agents that should be used give the best representation of the outline of the renal parenchyma: technetium-99 dimercaptosuccinic acid and gluco-heptonate.

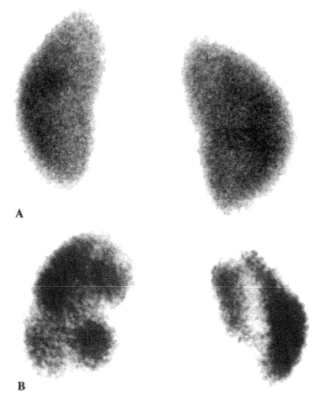

Radionuclide renal scan demonstrating normal kidneys without scarring (**A**) and severe bilateral scarring (**B**).

21. Describe the medical management of reflux.

Continuous low-dose antibiotic prophylaxis is the cornerstone of medical management for all grades of reflux. Maintaining sterile urine prevents the development of renal scarring. Merely observing patients without prophylaxis and treating infections as they occur has been shown to allow the development of scars and, therefore, is not optimal.

22. What are some of the indications for correcting VUR surgically?

This area is highly controversial. Most experts agree, however, that surgery should be discussed with families in the following situations:
- There are documented breakthrough infections with organisms resistant to prophylactic medication.
- Children and families are noncompliant and unwilling or unable to take prophylactic medication for many years.

• Grade IV or V reflux is present in an older child (the likelihood of spontaneous resolution is low).
• The child has reached adolescence, and the reflux has not resolved.

23. Are adult women with reflux at an increased risk for morbidity?

Pregnant women with uncorrected reflux have more urinary tract infections and pyelonephritis. Such episodes may lead to premature delivery and small-for-date newborns. It also has been shown that adult women with a history of successful surgery for reflux have similar rates of urinary infection during pregnancy. This finding suggests that such women are more susceptible to urinary infection, despite the fact that the reflux has been eradicated. Corrective surgery is recommended for adolescent girls with persistent VUR so that they can discontinue prophylaxis. They still should be advised of the increased risk of urinary infection during pregnancy.

24. How is reflux surgically corrected?

All open operations to correct reflux attempt to recreate the natural flap-valve mechanism and to restore the ureteral tunnel between the bladder mucosa and bladder muscle. Such procedures are termed "ureteral reimplantation." Success rates are close to 98% in low-grade reflux and exceed 90% in high-grade reflux.

25. What is the cystoscopic approach to correcting reflux?

Materials can be injected adjacent to the ureteral orifice through a cystoscope to stop reflux. These bulking agents narrow the ureteral orifice and cause the valve to function. Recently used materials include polytetrafluoroethylene paste (Teflon) and cross-linked bovine collagen. Unfortunately, neither agent is ideal. Teflon particles have been shown to migrate to other organ systems, including the lungs and central nervous system. The various collagen products are not durable; because they are resorbed, reflux may recur over time.

BIBLIOGRAPHY

1. Belman AB: Vesicoureteral reflux. In Rushton HG, Greenfield SP (eds): Pediatric Urology. Philadelphia, W.B. Saunders, 1997, pp 1171–1190.
2. Elder, JS, Peters CA, Arant BS, et al: Pediatric vesicoureteric reflux guidelines panel summary report on the management of primary vesicoureteral reflux in children. J Urol 157:1846–1851, 1997.
3. Greenfield SP, Ng M, Wan J: Experience with vesicoureteral reflux in children: Clinical characteristics. J Urol 158:574–577, 1997.
4. Greenfield SP, Ng M, Wan J: Resolution rates of low grade vesicoureteral reflux stratified by patient age at presentation. J Urol 157:1410–1413, 1997.
5. Greenfield SP, Wan J: Vesicoureteral reflux: Practical aspects of evaluation and management. Pediatr Nephrol 10:789–794, 1996.
6. Kramer SA: Vesicoureteral reflux. In Kelalis PP, King LR, Belman AB (eds): Clinical Pediatric Urology, 3rd ed. Philadelphia, W. B. Saunders, 1992, pp 441–499.

51. CIRCUMCISION AND DISORDERS OF THE PENIS

Jacob C. Langer, M.D., and Douglas E. Coplen, M.D.

1. How long has circumcision been performed?

Circumcision has been widely practiced since ancient times. In many cultures, including ancient Egypt and Sumeria, circumcision was done at puberty as a rite of passage into adulthood. Neonatal circumcision was first practiced by the ancient Hebrews. Many religious and cultural groups still practice circumcision. Jews perform the procedure in a ritual called *berit mila* on the eighth day of life, whereas in many other groups the procedure is done later during childhood.

2. What are the medical indications for circumcision?

Circumcision is an option for the management of phimosis, paraphimosis, and infections of the foreskin, such as balanitis and balanoposthitis.

3. What is the major contraindication to circumcision?

Circumcisions should not be done in children with hypospadias, because the foreskin is often used for reconstruction.

4. What are the risks of circumcision?

- Bleeding
- Infection
- Damage to the glans or urethra
- Removal of too little or too much foreskin

5. Should neonatal circumcision be performed routinely?

This issue is controversial for two reasons. Firstly, routine neonatal circumcision is widely practiced in North America (although not in Europe) because of cultural imperative. Secondly, the data supporting or opposing routine neonatal circumcision are difficult to interpret and often contradictory. In recent statements, both the Canadian Pediatric Society and the American Academy of Pediatrics recognize a balance between the potential health benefits and risks of circumcision. The decision should be made by the parents after they have been fully educated.

6. How is circumcision performed?

In neonates, circumcision usually is done with one of three kinds of clamps: the bell (Gomco), plastibell, or Mogen (see Fig. 1). General anesthesia generally is not used, although local anesthesia with a form of nerve block or an eutectic mixture of local anesthetics (EMLA cream) should be encouraged. In older children, circumcision should be done using a freehand approach under general anesthesia.

7. Define phimosis.

Phimosis often is defined as a nonretractable foreskin. However, this finding is normal and is not an indication for surgery unless it is associated with obstruction of the urinary stream. The incidence of retractability increases during childhood, the foreskin should be fully retractable by puberty.

8. What are the treatment options for phimosis?

Nonsurgical options include repeated forcible retraction and the use of topical steroid cream. Surgical options include dorsal slit, ventral slit, and circumcision.

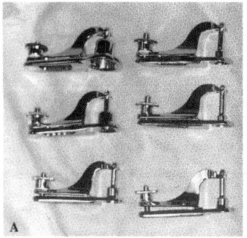

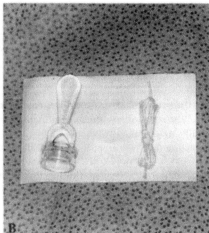

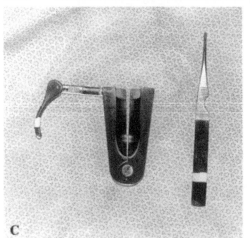

Figure 1.   The three most common clamps used for neonatal circumcision. *A*, Gomco, *B*, plastibell, *C*, Mogen.

9. Define paraphimosis.

In paraphimosis the foreskin is not replaced after retraction—for example, during a bath or shower or after catheterization. The preputial ring becomes tight, and the glans swells, leading to pain and ultimately to vascular compromise. A similar condition may occur as a complication of the plastibell clamp, if the plastic ring slips downward onto the penile shaft. Treatment involves placing the foreskin back into its normal position—a procedure that often requires general anesthesia.

10. Define balanitis.

Balanitis is defined as inflammation of the glans, which also may be associated with inflammation of the inner surface of the foreskin (balanoposthitis). Although relatively common in adults, both conditions are relatively rare in children. Most cases are infectious, although other causes, such as allergy, contact irritation, and trauma, also may be seen. Management involves treatment of the underlying problem; in recurrent cases, circumcision may be recommended.

11. What is meatal stenosis?

Meatal stenosis is an acquired narrowing of the glanular orifice that is found in circumcised males. It results from ammnoniacal dermatitis or ischemic injury at the time of circumcision.

The diagnosis is not made solely on the appearance of the meatus but also by observing the urinary stream.

12. Is meatal stenosis a cause of obstructive uropathy?

No. The urinary stream is misdirected, but the urethra is distensible and the kidneys and bladder are protected.

13. Does meatal stenosis require treatment?

When the urinary stream is sufficiently misdirected, a meatotomy should be performed. Best results are obtained when a V-shaped wedge of tissue is excised. This procedure can be performed safely under topical local anesthesia or with brief general anesthesia.

14. What are the typical findings in a patient with hypospadias?

- Meatus at a subcoronal location
- Flattened glans configuration
- Dorsally hooded foreskin
- Penile curvature
- Penile torsion

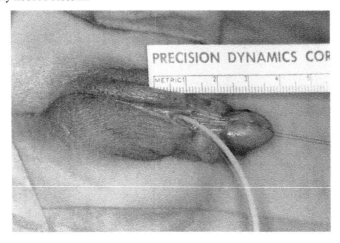

Figure 2.   Typical appearance of hypospadias (courtesy of A. Khoury, M.D.)

15. Do males with hypospadias require a complete genitourinary evaluation?

Hypospadias is usually an isolated abnormality. The incidence of undescended testes is higher (9%), but radiographic evaluation of the urinary tract is not indicated because the incidence of upper tract abnormalities with surgical significance is no greater than in the general population.

16. When should hypospadias be corrected?

Severe curvature or a proximal meatus that does not allow micturition while standing are significant functional abnormalities. More distal hypospadias is associated with meatal stenosis and deflection of the urinary stream; in such cases, surgery should be recommended.

17. How is hypospadias corrected?

Most cases of hypospadias are corrected on an outpatient basis using single-stage vascularized repairs. The goal is to normalize voiding and erectile function.

18. What are the complications of hypospadias repair?

- Subglanular meatus
- Meatal stenosis
- Urethrocutaneous fistula
- Poor cosmetic outcome

19. What is epispadias?

Isolated epispadias is extremely rare (1 in 200,000 births). In contrast to hypospadias, epispadias results from an abnormality in normal penile development. The meatus is located on the dorsal surface of the phallus at any point from the glans to the penopubic junction. This condition is usually a closed variant of bladder exstrophy and is associated with complete urinary incontinence.

BIBLIOGRAPHY

1. Cartwright PC, Snow BW, McNees DC: Urethral meatotomy in office using topical EMLA cream for anesthesia. J Urol 156:857–859, 1996.
2. Fetus and Newborn Committee, Canadian Pediatric Society: Neonatal circumcision revisited. Can Med Assoc J 154:769–780, 1996.
3. Harbinson M: The arguments for and against circumcision. Nurs Stand 11:42–47, 1997.
4. Khouri FJ, Hardy BE, Churchill BM: Urologic anomalies associated with hypospadias. Urol Clin North Am 8:565–571, 1981.
5. Lander J, Brady-Fryer B, Metcalfe JB: Comparison of ring block, dorsal penile nerve block, and topical anesthesia for neonatal circumcision. JAMA 278:2157–2162, 1997.
6. Langer JC, Coplen DE: Circumcision and pediatric disorders of the penis. Pediatr Clin North Am 45:801–812, 1998.
7. Noe HN, Dale GA: Evaluation of children with meatal stenosis. J Urol 114:455–456, 1975.
8. Rickwood AM, Walker J: Is phimosis overdiagnosed in boys and are too many circumcisions performed in consequence? Ann R Coll Surg Engl 71:275–277, 1989.

52. TESTICULAR PROBLEMS AND VARICOCELES

Gail E. Besner, M.D.

1. What is cryptorchidism?

Cryptorchidism ("hidden testis") is the most common congenital genitourinary anomaly in males and results when the testis does not descend into its normal intrascrotal position during development. It may be unilateral (90%) or bilateral (10%); 70% of unilateral cases occur on the right side. In full-term infants, the incidence is 2.7–5.9% at birth but decreases to 1.2–1.8% by 1 year of age. The incidence is 10-fold higher in premature infants.

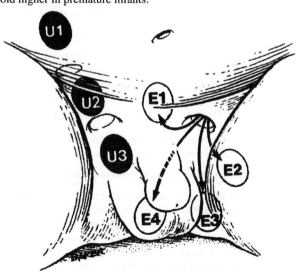

Locations of undescended (U) and ectopic (E) testes. U1, intraabdominal; U2, intracanalicular, U3, suprascrotal; E1, suprapubic; E2, femoral; E3, perineal; E4, contralateral. (From Pillai S, Besner G: Pediatric testicular problems. Pediatr Clin North Am 45:813–830, 1998; with permission).

2. Describe normal testicular descent.

Initially, in an androgen-independent transabdominal phase, the testes migrate from their site of development near the kidneys to the level of the internal inguinal ring. By 28 weeks of gestation, a rapid androgen-dependent inguinal-scrotal phase of descent occurs, with the left testis descending before the right (hence the higher incidence of right-sided undescended testes).

3. What is a retractile testis?

A testis that is normally descended but retracts into the upper scrotum or groin due to a hyperactive cremasteric response. Retractile testes are often bilateral and are most common in boys 5–6 years of age. As the child reaches early adolescence, the retractile testis should descend spontaneously into the normal scrotal position and usually has normal sperm production and size.

4. What is an ectopic testis?

Ectopic testes descend normally through the external inguinal ring but are then diverted to abnormal locations. At times groin exploration is needed to make the definitive distinction between ectopic and undescended testes.

5. Describe the physical examination of the pediatric scrotum.

Initially the child should be examined in the supine position. Visual inspection may reveal a hypoplastic or poorly rugated hemiscrotum, with or without inguinal fullness. The scrotum should be palpated. A finger placed across the top of the hemiscrotum will trap a normal but retractile testis before it has the chance to retract. The testis should be brought as far into the scrotum as possible with gentle traction. If the testicle is not palpable in the supine position, the patient should be examined in the seated cross-legged position (Taylor's position), which diminishes the cremasteric reflex.

6. Are radiologic examinations useful in the diagnosis of cryptorchidism?

Many modalities have been used, including ultrasonography, computed tomography, and magnetic resonance imaging. Most pediatric surgeons, however, probably operate without obtaining such tests. The options for radiologic work-up, therefore, should be left to the preference of the operating surgeon.

7. How can hormonal stimulation be useful in the diagnosis of cryptorchidism?

A short course of human chorionic gonadotropin (hCG) (2000 IU/day intramuscularly for 3–4 days) may be useful in distinguishing bilateral *anorchidism* from bilateral *cryptorchidism*. The test is based on the stimulatory effect of hCG on the testis to produce testosterone. With bilateral anorchidism, testosterone levels do not rise with hCG stimulation, whereas with bilateral cryptorchidism, testosterone levels increase. In addition, baseline levels of luteinizing hormone and follicle-stimulating hormone in males with anorchia are elevated. If a patient has both a negative testosterone response to hCG and elevated basal gonadotropin levels, the diagnosis of bilateral anorchia is assured and surgical exploration is unnecessary.

8. What are the major potential complications of cryptorchidism?

Infertility. The fertility potential of the testis correlates with the length of time that the testis remains outside the scrotum. Cryptorchid testes contain smaller seminiferous tubules, fewer spermatogonia, and increased peritubular tissue. These changes begin to appear during the first year of life.

Malignancy. Undescended testes have an increased incidence of malignant potential. The risk of developing testicular cancer is 20–40-fold greater in patients with cryptorchidism than in the general population. Abdominal testes are most likely to develop malignant transformation. Of interest, if testicular cancer develops in a patient with unilateral cryptorchidism, there is a 20% chance that the malignancy will occur in the contralateral, normally descended testis. Up to 60% of tumors that develop in cryptorchid testes are seminomas. Testicular cancer usually develops in the third-to-fourth decades of life. Orchidopexy does not decrease the chance of malignant transformation, but it does aid in earlier identification of the tumor.

Trauma. Undescended testes located in the inguinal canal are at higher risk of local trauma.

9. What is the treatment of cryptorchidism?

Surgery is indicated in cryptorchidism (1) to repair an associated hernia, (2) to improve future fertility, (3) to place the testis in an easily palpable position, and (4) to afford cosmetic and psychological benefit. Orchidopexy is best performed at 6–24 months of age.

10. How is monorchidism diagnosed?

Unilateral testicular absence occurs in 1 in 5000 males. Monorchidism may be due to total agenesis or to an intrauterine vascular accident such as torsion. Because monorchidism cannot be distinguished from cryptorchidism with a nonpalpable testis on examination, surgical exploration is needed for diagnosis.

11. Is laparoscopy useful in the differentiation of cryptorchidism and monorchidism?

Over the past several years, laparoscopy has been shown to be the most accurate method of localizing nonpalpable testes. Findings at laparoscopy may include the following:

- Intraabdominal testicle. If it is atretic, laparoscopic orchiectomy can be performed. If it is normal, either immediate orchidopexy can be performed via an inguinal approach or, for the very high abdominal testis, the testicular vessels can be ligated laparoscopically in preparation for orchidopexy as a second-stage procedure.
- Vas deferens and testicular vessels exiting through the internal inguinal ring. Inguinal exploration should be performed and may reveal a normal testicle (in which case orchidopexy is performed), an atretic testicle (in which case orchiectomy is performed), or no testicle (vanishing testis syndrome).
- Atretic spermatic vessels above the internal inguinal ring. It can be assumed that the testis has vanished, and inguinal exploration can be avoided.

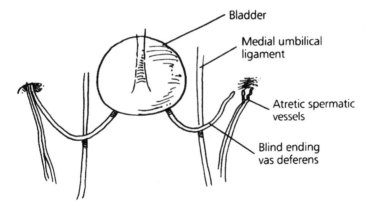

Pediatric pelvic anatomy of a patient with an absent right testis. (From Kavoussi L: Pediatric applications of laparoscopy. In Clayman RV, McDougall EM (eds): Laparoscopic Urology. St. Louis, Quality Medical Publishing, 1993, pp 209–224; with permission).

12. What is testicular torsion?

The testicle twists upon the spermatic cord, causing venous congestion, edema, and eventual arterial obstruction, which, if not treated, lead to gonadal necrosis. Testicular torsion affects approximately 1 in 4000 males under age 25; most cases occur in late childhood or early adolescence. It is one of the few pediatric urologic emergencies.

13. Describe the clinical findings of testicular torsion.

Testicular torsion presents clinically as acute unilateral scrotal swelling and pain. Palpation of the inguinal canal may reveal a thickened or twisted cord. The affected testis is elevated within the hemiscrotum from spermatic cord shortening due to the twist. It must be distinguished clinically from epididymitis, orchitis, and appendiceal (testis or epididymis) torsion.

14. How can the diagnosis of testicular torsion be confirmed?

Helpful diagnostic imaging studies include nuclear scintigraphy and Doppler sonography. However, urgent treatment of the patient believed to have testicular torsion should not be postponed if the availability of these tests is delayed. Do not hesitate to obtain radiologic imaging in patients in whom the diagnosis of epididymitis, orchitis, appendiceal torsion, or other acute scrotal conditions is equivocal.

15. What is the treatment of testicular torsion?

Surgery involves initial detorsion of the testis. If the testis is viable, it is fixated within the tunica vaginalis with multiple nonabsorbable sutures. If the testis is nonviable, it should be removed. In addition, contralateral testicular fixation should be performed to prevent future contralateral torsion. Maximal success rates are obtained when surgery is performed within 10 hours of torsion. After 24 hours, testicular salvage is almost nonexistent.

16. How is testicular appendiceal torsion diagnosed and treated?

Patients, usually prepubescent boys, present with scrotal pain that may be acute or gradual. Testicular tenderness may be localized to the superior pole of the testis. The torsed appendage may produce a bluish dot or discoloration in the wall of the scrotum, and a small tender nodule may be palpated on the testicular wall, but the testicle itself is normal. Treatment consists of analgesics for pain control with scrotal ice packs and elevation to reduce swelling. Most cases resolve spontaneously; surgery is reserved for patients with chronic pain.

17. How is epididymitis diagnosed and treated?

Epididymitis presents as acute scrotal swelling from inflammation of the epididymis. It is usually idiopathic and affects adolescent boys. Up to 50% of patients have fever and pyuria. A tender epididymis is palpated anterior to the testis, which itself is nontender. Laboratory tests should include urinalysis and white blood cell count, which may show pyuria and leukocytosis. Treatment consists of appropriate antibiotic coverage and scrotal elevation.

18. How is orchitis diagnosed and treated?

Many viral infections, especially mumps, may cause acute scrotal swelling. Mumps orchitis is unilateral in 80% of cases. Patients are usually adolescents who present with acute or gradual scrotal swelling and pain. Examination reveals a firm, tender testis. Associated symptoms may include fever, dysuria, or leukocytosis. Treatment includes scrotal elevation, ice packs, and analgesics. Approximately one-third of affected patients later develop testicular atrophy, with an increased risk of infertility and malignancy.

19. What is a varicocele?

A collection of venous varicosities within the scrotum. Venous stasis or retrograde flow within the spermatic veins causes dilatations within the pampiniform plexus. Varicoceles are usually asymptomatic and more pronounced upon standing. Obstruction of venous outflow leads to an increase in intrascrotal temperature that results in eventual decreased spermatogenesis.

20. How do varicoceles develop?

Ninety-five percent of varicoceles occur on the left side because of partial compression of the left renal vein as it passes between the aorta and superior mesenteric artery. In addition, the fact that the left spermatic vein joins the left renal vein at a 90° angle causes more turbulent flow. The right spermatic vein, on the other hand, tangentially drains directly into the inferior vena cava, allowing better flow dynamics.

21. What special consideration should be given to a young child with a varicocele?

In younger children, especially those less than 5 years of age, the presence of a varicocele may be the presenting finding of a neoplasm such as a Wilms' tumor, which often causes ipsilateral renal vein obstruction and secondary testicular vein varicosities. The young child with a varicocele, therefore, should undergo careful abdominal examination and abdominal ultrasonography to rule out the possibility of an intraabdominal tumor.

22. Describe the grading of varicoceles.

Grade I: very small and difficult to detect on exam. Color duplex ultrasonography assists in diagnosis.

Grade II: easily visualized on exam; 1–2 cm in diameter.

Grade III: diameter > 2 cm.

Grade II and III varicoceles feel like a "bag of worms" that decreases or disappears when the child is supine. Testicular volume should be measured and recorded.

23. How are varicoceles treated?

Grade I varicoceles with testes of equal volumes should be followed. Grade I varicoceles with testicular atrophy should be treated, as should grade II and III varicoceles. Treatment consists of spermatic vein ligation, either through an inguinal approach or laparoscopically. Results after surgery are extremely good, with return of testicular volume and improved semen quality in 90–95% of patients treated during early-to-mid adolescence.

BIBLIOGRAPHY

1. Cromie WJ: Cryptorchidism and malignant testicular disease. In Hadziselimovic F (ed): Cryptorchidism: Management and Implications. New York, Springer-Verlag, 1983, pp 83–92.
2. Hadziselimovic F, Herzug B, Segauchi H: Surgical correction of cryptorchidism at two years: Electron microscopic and morphometric investigation. J Pediatr Surg 10:19, 1975.
3. Hutson JM, Beasley SW: Embryologic controversies in testicular descent. Semin Urol 6:68, 1988.
4. Moore RG, Peters CA, Bauer SB, et al: Laparoscopic evaluation of the nonpalpable testis: A prospective assessment of accuracy. J Urol 151:728–731, 1994.
5. Pillai S, Besner G: Pediatric testicular problems. In Glick PL, Irish MS, Caty MG: (eds): Pediatr Clin North Am 45:813–830, 1998.
6. Sawczuk IS, Hensle TW, Burbige KA, et al: Varicoceles: Effect on testicular volume in prepubertal and pubertal males. Urology 41:467, 1993.
7. Sheldon CA: Undescended testis and testicular torsion. Surg Clin North Am 65:1303, 1985.

53. GYNECOLOGIC PROBLEMS

Kent Crickard, M.D.

OVARIAN TORSION

1. What are the typical findings in a young girl with ovarian torsion?

- Acute abdomen
- Complex adnexal mass on ultrasound
- Elevated white blood cell count with a left shift (frequently afebrile)

2. Is a total oophorectomy the treatment of choice for ovarian torsion?

Many cases can be treated conservatively by detorsing the ovary via the laparoscopic approach. Even if the ovary appears cyanotic, detorsing is still recommended. Early diagnosis is important.

3. Can ovarian torsion be predicted on the basis of the size of the fetal cyst?
Simple fetal ovarian cysts larger than 4 cm have a high probability of torsion. Cysts that enlarge rapidly or cysts that are noted to wander about the abdominal cavity on serial ultrasound are also at increased risk for torsion.

4. What ultrasound findings suggest ovarian torsion?
A cyst with fluid-debris level, a cyst with a retracting clot, or a septated ovarian cyst. Doppler studies may indicate little or no blood flow into the cyst.

5. How often does torsion of an ovarian cyst occur?
Torsion is the most common complication of an ovarian cyst. It may occur in up to 40% of fetal cases and 70% of neonatal cases.

6. What complications are associated with fetal ovarian torsion?
  • Urinary tract obstruction
  • Intestinal perforation
  • Ascites
  • Respiratory distress

OVARIAN CYSTS

7. Prenatal diagnosis of ovarian cysts is based on what criteria?
  • Presence of a cystic structure
  • Integrity of the GI and GU tracts
  • Female sex of the fetus

8. How common are fetal ovarian cysts?
With the advent of prenatal sonography, simple ovarian cysts smaller than 4 cm are frequently seen. In most cases, they regress as the estrogen stimulus associated with pregnancy decreases and generally resolve within 1–6 months after birth.

9. At what gestational age are fetal cysts diagnosed?
The average age at the time of diagnosis is 33 weeks gestation.

10. Describe the management of a simple fetal ovarian cyst larger than 4 cm.
Consideration should be given to antenatal percutaneous aspiration due to the significant risk of torsion unless the cyst resolves spontaneously or postdelivery aspiration or laparoscopic drainage is scheduled for persistent cysts.

11. What risks other than torsion are associated with fetal ovarian cysts?
Polyhydramnios is reported to occur in up to 18% of cases and is associated more commonly with cysts larger than 6 cm.

12. What is the optimal therapy for asymptomatic cysts in childhood?
Under 18 months of age, ovarian cysts are almost always nonpathologic functional cysts. In asymptomatic patients, ultrasound monitoring is the appropriate management. In symptomatic patients, ultrasound-guided aspiration or laparoscopic drainage of the cyst is warranted.

13. Can a simple ovarian cyst represent an epithelial ovarian cancer?
Epithelial ovarian cancers rarely present as simple cysts in children. Seventy percent of ovarian cancers within this age group are of germ cell origin and present as solid or complex ovarian masses.

14. How specific is ultrasound in diagnosing fetal and infant ovarian cysts?
The diagnosis is always presumptive. Mesenteric cysts, urachal cysts, and intestinal duplication, although less common, cannot be excluded.

ECTOPIC PREGNANCIES

15. Why is ectopic pregnancy called the great masquerader?
Because of its various presentations, ectopic pregnancy may be misdiagnosed. When in doubt, obtain a serum level of human chorionic gonadotropin (HCG).

16. What predisposing factors may place a patient at greater risk for ectopic pregnancy?
A prior history of pelvic inflammatory disease, tubal surgery, use of assisted reproductive technologies, exposure to diethylstilbestrol, and method of contraception.

17. What is the relationship of the intrauterine device (IUD) to ectopic pregnancy?
Modern IUDs (copper-bearing, progestin) and implantable hormone devices (Norplant) decrease the overall incidence of pregnancy, including ectopic pregnancy. However, in the few patients who become pregnant while using these devices, the pregnancy is more likely to be ectopic.

18. Where are ectopic pregnancies located most frequently?
• Within the fallopian tube

    Ampullary segment   80%

    Isthmic segment   12%

    Cornual, interstitial   2%

• Abdominal, ovarian, cervical locations 1.8%

19. How useful are quantitative HCG levels in diagnosing ectopic pregnancies?
• An appropriate rise in HCG level (50% per day) usually, but not always, is associated with intrauterine pregnancy.
• When HCG levels are around 2000 IU/L, the ultrasound should demonstrate an intrauterine pregnancy (except with multiple gestations).
• Abnormally rising HCG levels (< 50% per day) are consistent with nonviable or ectopic pregnancy.

20. What is the role of vaginal ultrasound?
• Intrauterine pregnancy can be identified.
• No intrauterine pregnancy with HCG levels around 2000 IU/L is consistent with ectopic pregnancy.
• Adnexal masses and cardiac activity outside the uterus can be identified.

21. What are the contraindications to using methotrexate for the medical treatment of ectopic pregnancy for which surgery is indicated?
• HCG titer greater than 10,000 IU/L (relative contraindication)
• Abdominal pain with evidence of intraabdominal bleeding
• Adnexal mass larger than 3 cm
• Evidence of cardiac activity in ectopic pregnancy
• Hemodynamic instability

22. What are the criteria for use of methotrexate?
The patient must have no contraindication for the use of methotrexate, and there must be no ultrasound evidence of an intrauterine pregnancy.

23. How is methotrexate administered?
• As a single injection: 50 mg/M_2 intramuscularly (repeat in 1 week if HCG titers do not drop appropriately).
• Multiple-dose regimen: 1 mg/kg intramuscularly every other day for 4 doses; citrovorum factor, 0.1 mg/kg, is given only the day after each methotrexate injection for 4 doses.

24. What is the failure rate with methotrexate?
It varies from 10% to 20%. If the patient becomes symptomatic, evidence of intraabdominal bleeding or tubal rupture is found, or HCG titers rise, surgery is indicated.

25. What is the role of laparoscopy?
Most surgical cases can be managed via laparoscopy. Occasionally a laparotomy is necessary.

26. Which procedures are indicated according to the location of the ectopic pregnancy?
- A linear salpingostomy along the antimesenteric border of the tube is the procedure of choice for ampullary ectopics.
- Segmental resection of the tube is preferred for isthmic ectopic pregnancies because of the poor results with linear salpingostomy.
- For unruptured interstitial ectopic pregnancies, methotrexate is the treatment of choice if the condition is diagnosed early enough. Surgery usually requires partial resection of the uterotubal junction and may even require hysterectomy if bleeding cannot be controlled. Risk of uterine rupture with subsequent pregnancy is a concern with the surgical approach.

27. What are the indications for total salpingectomy?
- Child-bearing complete
- Previous ectopic pregnancy in the same tube
- Fallopian tube damaged beyond repair
- Uncontrolled bleeding

28. Should removal of the ovary with the tube be avoided?
By all means. The patient may wish to undergo in vitro fertilization in the future.

29. Is it necessary to follow postoperative HCG levels after total salpingectomy?
HCG titers must be followed until they return to normal after all surgical procedures, including total salpingectomy. Persistent trophoblastic tissue has been reported, even for cases involving total salpingectomy. When HCG levels fail to return to normal after surgery, methotrexate is indicated.

HYDROMETROCOLPOS

30. What are the most common causes of hydrometrocolpos?
Imperforate hymen and transverse vaginal septum occasionally are diagnosed in the neonate. If significant mucous secretions develop, bulging of the membrane between the labia may occur.

31. Can secondary complications occur with hydrometrocolpos?
If significant mucus build-up develops, distortion of the bladder and urethra may lead to hydroureter and hydronephrosis.

32. What is the outcome of imperforate hymen?
In the neonate, the hymen often ruptures spontaneously because of mucous secretions. The diagnosis usually is made in adolescence when the onset of menses leads to hematometrocolpos and lower abdominal pain.

UTERINE ATRESIA

33. What is the most common syndrome associated with uterine atresia?
Müllerian agenesis (Mayer-Rokitansky-Kustner-Hauser syndrome) occurs in 1:5000 births. Patients have a 46 XX karyotype with normal ovarian function. Absence of the vagina, uterus, and fallopian tubes is the hallmark of this syndrome.

34. What other anomalies are associated with müllerian agenesis?
- 40% of cases have urinary tract anomalies
- 12% have musculoskeletal anomalies (lumbar sacral spine)

35. In addition to müllerian agenesis, what is the only other condition with an absent uterus in a normal-appearing female?
Androgen insensitivity syndrome. In the complete form, the karyotype is 46 XY with no virilization at puberty. The gonads are testes. Vaginal agenesis is also present.

36. Why must the gonads be removed?
Gonadal tumors develop (usually after age 25). Gonadectomy usually is performed around age 16 to 18 after puberty.

37. How do patients with androgen insensitivity syndrome present in childhood?
Occasionally the gonads are present in the inguinal canal. This scenario may present as inguinal hernia and/or inguinal masses in childhood.

UTERINE DUPLICATION

38. What are the most common uterine anomalies?
- Bicornuate uterus (37%)
- Incomplete or complete uterine septum (22%)
- Uterine didelphys (11%)
- Unicornuate uterus (5%)

39. How is the presence of various uterine anomalies associated with the presence or absence of various vaginal anomalies?
Fusion of the müllerian ducts begins near the uterine–cervix junction and extends both caudally and cephalad.

40. When is acute surgical intervention necessary for uterine anomalies associated with vaginal anomalies?
Occasionally, uterine didelphys, bicornuate uterus, or a uterus with a complete uterine septum is associated with an obstructed hemivagina. Excision of the vaginal septum is required because of hematocolpos and pelvic pain.

41. Is there an association between uterine anomalies and urogenital anomalies?
Ultrasound and intravenous pyelogram may be useful in detecting horseshoe kidneys or absent or hypoplastic kidneys which may be associated with uterine anomalies. In the case of noncommunicating hemivagina, ipsilateral renal agenesis is often present. The early diagnosis of renal anomalies often alerts the physician to the diagnosis of uterine and vaginal anomalies.

VAGINAL ATRESIA

42. How is vaginal atresia classified?
Vaginal atresia may be complete or incomplete. When associated with secondary urogenital and cloacal abnormalities, it may be proximal (high) or distal (low).

43. How do patients with complete vaginal atresia present?
The classic presentation is primary amenorrhea, at which time an absent vagina is noted on examination.

44. What two syndromes are associated most commonly with absent vagina?

Müllerian agenesis (absence of vagina, uterus, and fallopian tubes) and androgen insensitivity syndrome (46 XY phenotypic female with testes). In both syndromes, functional uterine tissue is absent.

45. What are the methods for creation of a neovagina in patients with vaginal agenesis without the presence of functional uterine tissue?

In selected cases with a motivated patient, vaginal dilators may be sufficient to create a neovagina. In the remainder of cases, a split-thickness skin graft (McIndoe technique) or colon graft has been used to create a neovagina.

46. Does it matter at what age the procedure to create a neovagina is performed?

Most surgeons delay the procedure until the patient is sexually active and old enough to be able to manage the postoperative use of vaginal dilators or other techniques.

47. Can vaginal agenesis be misdiagnosed on physical examination?

Transverse vaginal septum, vaginal atresia, and vaginal agenesis may be associated with a blind vaginal pouch. Magnetic resonance imaging, ultrasound, and other imaging studies are useful in making the correct diagnosis.

48. In evaluating vaginal atresia associated with urogenital sinus malformations, what diagnostic studies are needed before surgery?

• Ultrasonography
• Voiding cystourethrogram
• Careful cystoscopy

49. What is the incidence of stenosis of the vaginal introitus in patients with proximal or high vaginal atresia undergoing vaginal pull-throughout operations?

From 40% to 60% of patients may experience stenosis. Periodic dilatation may be needed to prevent vaginal stenosis and further vaginal surgery. This emphasizes the need for long term follow-up.

50. What is the treatment for distal (low) vaginal atresia?

Generally, the use of a perineal flap vaginoplasty is sufficient.

51. What is the approach for proximal (high) vaginal atresia with urogenital sinus?

There is no simple answer. Various techniques may be used, including abdominoperineal vaginal pull-through, use of various peritoneal flaps for reconstruction of the vagina, and use of a vascularized graft of sigmoid colon to create the distal portion of the vagina.

GENITAL WARTS

52. Describe the appearance of genital warts.

The appearance depends on the location. On mucosal surfaces, the warts take on the appearance of grape clusters. On keratinized skin surfaces, they have the classic wart appearance.

53. What are the treatments for genital warts?

Although podophyllin is somewhat effective, laser ablation under general anesthesia produces an excellent clinical response.

54. What postoperative measures minimize the child's discomfort?

• Local anesthesia (0.25% marcaine)
• Emla cream
• Frequent sitz baths

55. Are human papilloma virus subtypes helpful in identifying the mode of transmission?

Although certain subtypes are associated with sexual transmission, any papilloma viral subtype can be transmitted by sexual or nonsexual contact.

56. When do genital warts appear if they are due to vertical transmission in the birth canal from mother to infant?

The warts generally are present by 18 months but may appear as early as 6 months, presumably when maternal antibodies transmitted to the infant disappear.

PELVIC INFLAMMATORY DISEASE

57. Describe the standard evaluation for pelvic inflammatory disease (PID).
- Pelvic and abdominal examination
- Cervical cultures for gonorrhea and chlamydia
- Complete blood count
- Sedimentation rate
- Pregnancy test to rule out ectopic pregnancy

58. When, in relation to menses, do most patients present with symptoms?

Most patients present at the end of menses.

59. What percentage of cases of PID are iatrogenic?

Approximately 85% of cases are secondary to spontaneous infections. Another 15% follow procedures that allow vaginal flora to colonize in the upper genital tract. Examples include endometrial biopsy, hysterosalpingogram, curettage, hysteroscopy, placement of intrauterine devices, and intrauterine insemination.

60. Does a negative cervical culture for gonorrhea or chlamydia exclude the diagnosis of PID?

Negative cultures are relatively common in PID.

61. What findings are associated with PID?
- 90% of patients have abdominal pain, cervical motion tenderness, and/or adnexal tenderness.
- 75% of patients have an endocervical infection or coexistent purulent vaginal discharge.
- Less than 50% have white blood cell count greater than 10,000.
- 33% have a temperature greater than 38°C.

62. What are the indications for hospitalization?
- Adolescence
- Tubo-ovarian complex or abscess
- Uncertain diagnosis
- Peritonitis
- Inadequate response to outpatient antibiotic therapy
- Gastrointestinal symptoms

63. What is the chandelier sign?

Lateral movement of the cervix on pelvic examination causes intense pain due to the inflamed adnexa. The patient "reaches for the chandelier."

64. What is the role of laparoscopy?

The indications for laparoscopy are similar in adolescents and adults. If the diagnosis is not evident, laparoscopy may be indicated to diagnose PID vs. ectopic pregnancy, endometriosis, ovarian cysts, appendicitis, and other diagnoses. Correct diagnosis and early, aggressive antibiotic therapy offer the best opportunity to minimize the sequelae of PID.

65. Can laparoscopy be used in the diagnosis and therapy of pelvic abscess?

In selected cases, laparoscopy without laparotomy can be used to diagnose and drain pelvic abscesses. The skill, experience, and judgment of the surgeon determine whether laparoscopy alone can be used to manage a pelvic abscess safely.

66. What is Fitz-Hugh-Curtis syndrome?

Approximately 5–10% of women with PID develop perihepatic inflammation with resultant "banjo string" adhesions between the liver and anterior abdominal wall.

67. What is the incidence of false-positive clinical diagnosis of acute PID?

Approximately 20–25% of women with the clinical diagnosis of PID have no identifiable intraabdominal or pelvic disease at the time of laparoscopy. Another 10–15% have some other pathologic disorder (e.g., appendicitis, endometriosis, ovarian cyst, ectopic pregnancy).

BIBLIOGRAPHY

1. Armentano G, Dodero P, Natta A, et al: Fetal ovarian cysts: Prenatal diagnosis and management. Report of two cases and review of literature. Clin Exp Obstet Gynecol 25:88–91, 1998.
2. Brandt ML, Luks FI, Filiatrault D, et al: Surgical indications in antenatally diagnosed ovarian cysts. J Pediatr Surg 26:276–282, 1991.
3. Chambers S, Muir B, Haddad N: Ultrasound evaluation of ectopic pregnancy including correlation with human chorionic gonadotropin levels. Fr J Radiol 63:246–250, 1990.
4. Craighill MC: Pediatric and adolescent gynecology for the primary care pediatrician. Obstet Gynecol Clin North Am 45:1659–1688, 1998.
5. Crombleholme T, Craigo SD, Garmel S, D'Alton ME: Fetal ovarian cyst decompression to prevent torsion. J Pediatr Surg 32:1447–1449, 1997.
6. Donahoe P, Gustafson M: Early one-stage reconstruction of the extremely high vagina in patients with congenital adrenal hyperplasia. J Pediatr Surg 29:352–358, 1994.
7. Eggermont EE, Lecoutere D, Devlieger H, et al: Ovarian cysts in newborn infants. Am J Dis Child 142:702, 1988.
8. Frank R: The formation of an artificial vagina without operation. Am J Obstet Gynecol 35:1053–1055, 1938.
9. Girardini G, Segre A: Vaginal agenesis (Mayer-Rokitansky-Kuster-Hauser syndrome). Clin Exp Obstet Gynecol 19:98–102, 1982.
10. Hendren W: Construction of the female urethra from vaginal wall and perineal flap. J Pediatr Surg 123:657–664, 1980.
11. Hendren W, Donahoe P: Correction of congenital abnormalities of the vagina and perineum. J Pediatr Surg 15:751–763, 1980.
12. Karsdorf VHM, Van der Veen F, Schats R, et al: Successful treatment with methotrexate of five vital interstitial pregnancies. Hum Reprod 7:1164–1170, 1992.
13. Kim H, Laufer M: Developmental abnormalities of the female reproductive tract. Curr Opinion Obstet Gynecol 6:518–525, 1994.
14. Manuel M, Kayayama KP, Jones HW Jr: The age of occurrence of gonadal tumors in intersex patients with a Y chromosome. Am J Obstet Gynecol 124:293–298, 1976.
15. Meyers RL: Congenital anomalies of the vagina and their reconstruction. Clin Obstet Gynecol 40:168–180, 1997.
16. Rose PG, Cohen SM: Methotrexate therapy for persistent ectopic pregnancy after conservative laparoscopic management. Obstet Gynecol 76:947–952, 1990.
17. Sellers J, Mahony J, Goldsmith C, et al: The accuracy of clinical findings and laparoscopy in pelvic inflammatory disease. Am J Obstet Gynecol 164:113–118, 1991.
18. Serra J, Ballesteros A, Paloma V, et al: Surgical treatment for congenital absence of the vagina using tissue expansion. Surg Gynecol Obstet 177:158–162, 1993.
19. Simpson JL: Genetics of sexual differentiation. In Rock JA, Carpenter SE (eds): Pediatric and Adolescent Gynecology. New York, Raven Press, 1992, pp 1–37.
20. Skala EP, Leon ZA, Rouse GA: Management of antenatally diagnosed fetal ovarian cysts. Obstet Gynecol Surv 46:407–414, 1991.
21. Stassart J, Nagel T, Prem K, et al: Uterus didelphys, obstructed hemivagina, and ipsilateral renal agenesis: The University of Minnesota experience. Fertil Steril 57:756–760, 1992.
22. Strubbe E, Willemsen W, Lemmens J, et al: Mayer-Rokitansky-Kuster-Hauser syndrome: Distinction between two forms based on excretory urographic, sonographic, and laparoscopic findings. Am J Radiol 160:331–334, 1993.
23. Wee J, Joseph V: A new technique of vaginal reconstruction using neurovascular pudendal-thigh flaps: A preliminary report. Plast Reconstr Surg 83:701–709, 1989.
24. Yokoyama Y, Kagiya A, Ozaki T, et al: Two cases of twisted fetal ovarian cysts. J Obstet Gynaecol Res 22:85–89, 1996.

X. Trauma

54. TRAUMA—GENERAL APPROACH

Chatt A. Johnson, M.D., RVT, MAJ MC USA,
Kenneth S. Azarow, M.D., LTC MC USA, and
Richard H. Pearl, M.D., FACS, FAAP, FRCS(C)

1. What are the priorities of management in pediatric trauma? How do they differ from the management of adult trauma?
The priorities of management in pediatric trauma do *not* differ from the priorities in adults. Patent airway, breathing (ventilation and oxygenation), and circulation (perfusion) are the ABCs of evaluating and treating any patient in distress. Pediatric trauma has some unique characteristics, but priorities of initial management are not among them.

2. Name the major anatomic difference between the pediatriac and adult airways.
The narrowest portion of the airway in children less than 10 years old is at the level of the cricoid cartilage. The cricoid cartilage is nondistensible and gives the larynx a funnel shape. Teenagers and young adults have a cylinder-shaped larynx with the narrowest portion at the glottic inlet. Clinically, this shape magnifies the consequences of edema of the airway in small children and infants by significantly reducing the diameter and increasing airway resistance.

3. How does this difference affect what kind of endotracheal tube is placed?
In general, uncuffed tubes should be used in children younger than 8–10 years old. The normal anatomic narrowing at the cricoid cartilage provides a functional cuff. A cuff can be used as long as an audible air leak is present when ventilation to a presssure of 20–30 cmH$_2$O is provided. Too much pressure in this area (cuffed or uncuffed tube) can cause ischemia of the tissues with a resultant stricture. Subglottic stenosis secondary to prolonged endotracheal intubation from a tight-fitting tube can cause long-term chronic airway narrowing that requires surgical correction.

4. What sized endotracheal tube is ideal for newborns, infants, and children?
• Term newborns: 3.0, 3.5 mm (uncuffed) internal diameter
• 1 year old: 4.0, 4.5 mm (uncuffed) internal diameter
• 2 year old: 4.5, 5.0 mm (uncuffed) internal diameter
• > 2 years old: internal diameter = age (yr) ÷ 4 × 4
A rule of thumb is to check the pinky size and match it to a tube.

5. What is SCIWORA?
Spinal cord injury without radiologic abnormality. Children (especially those under 6 years old) have incomplete ossification centers, metabolically active growth centers, and a hypermobile cervical spine. These differences from the adult skeletal system provide a set-up for "normal" radiographs that may miss ligamentous injuries. Awareness of SCIWORA makes it absolutely critical to clear the cervical spine with normal radiographs and a reliable, unremarkable exam in a patient without complaints of cervical pain. For more details, see Chapter 55, "Neurosurgical Trauma."

6. What is the most common cause of cardiac arrest after trauma in children?
Respiratory arrest—i.e., hypoventilation causing cardiac arrest. After securing control of the airway, appropriate ventilation and oxygenation are the most important priorities.

7. What is the earliest measurable sign of shock?

Tachycardia. Understanding normal heart rates in pediatric patients is important.

	Standard (beats/min)	Range (beats/min)
Newborn to 3 mo	160	120–200
3 mo to 2 yr	140	100–190
2–10 yr	120	80–140
> 10 yr	90	60–100

Hypotension does not appear until 25–30% of the blood volume has been lost. When 45% of the volume has been lost, compensatory mechanisms fail and bradycardia with hypotension can ensue. At this point the patient is close to irreversible shock, and cardiac arrest may occur without prompt correction.

8. How do children maintain cardiac output?

Children do not have the ability to significantly increase stroke volume (end-diastolic volume). Because cardiac output = stroke volume + heart rate, and stroke volume remains relatively constant, the only way to increase cardiac output in response to volume loss is to increase the heart rate. Thus, pediatric cardiac output is almost exclusively rate-dependent. This is an important clinical difference in comparison with older patients, in whom it may be important to *lower* the heart rate to increase cardiac output. Atropine, a drug rarely indicated in the resuscitation of adult trauma patients, may be indicated in pediatric patients with heart rates less than 60 beats/min and poor perfusion. The vagolytic effect increases the heart rate (and thus cardiac output) while resuscitation continues.

9. Describe the initial intravenous fluid therapy in a child with blunt trauma.

An initial bolus of 20 ml/kg of lactated Ringer's or normal saline solution, which may be repeated three times. Blood products should be given with the third bolus (packed red blood cells at 10–20 ml/kg).

10. What is the goal of fluid resuscitation? How can you clinically assess the response to resuscitation?

The goal of fluid resuscitation is restoration of systemic perfusion at the organ and ultimately cellular level. This goal includes improvement in vital signs and clinical resolution of shock as demonstrated by improved capillary refill, adequate urine output, warm extremities, and improved mentation. In children with blunt trauma to the abdomen, operative exploration should be considered for failure to restore systemic perfusion after transfusion of 40 ml/kg of blood products during the initial resuscitation. One caveat to this rule is that other sources of blood loss must be ruled out (e.g., pelvic or femur fracture, hemothorax, and scalp or extremity hemorrhage).

11. Describe the method of choice in controlling hemorrhage.

Control of external hemorrhage is accomplished with direct pressure over the sight of bleeding and in some cases splinting or immobilization of long-bone fractures. Hemostatic clamps placed into the wound and tourniquets should not be used to control hemorrhage unless an operating room environment is available and lighting and exposure are optimal. Embolization of pelvic and deep muscle bleeding is also possible despite the patient's small size if skilled interventional radiologists are available.

12. Name an alternative site for intravenous access if the veins are difficult to cannulate.

An intraosseous line can be used for the administration of drugs, fluids, and blood products in children 6 years old or younger. This approach should be considered central access for any therapeutic intervention. The intraosseous line is a reliable site that can be accessed within 30–60 seconds in most cases. Intraosseous needles should be readily available in all trauma rooms.

13. What are the landmarks for placement of an intraosseous line?
The anteromedial surface of the tibia, 1–3 cm below the tibal tuberosity, provides a large narrow cavity for access and avoids the tibial growth plate. Specific training and mentoring are required to learn this technique.

14. Name two drugs used in the resuscitation of children in shock.
Epinephrine and atropine can be used for cardiac resuscitation in children who do not respond to fluid/blood administration. These drugs increase cardiac output and thus perfusion by increasing heart rate (see question 8). They also can be given via an endotracheal tube if vascular access has not been obtained. The use of resuscitative drugs in adult trauma victims rarely is indicated and emphasizes another important difference between pediatric and adult trauma treatment. However, these drugs do not replace resuscitation. Volume replacement is always the mainstay of treatment for traumatic shock. Drugs are a bridge to allow transient improvement in vital signs and perfusion until continued aggressive fluid therapy resolves the shock state.

15. How can the cause of severe blood loss be evaluated efficiently with radiographic studies?
Blood loss into the thorax and abdomen (cavitary hemorrhage) can be reliably evaluated initially with a chest radiograph and trauma ultrasound, respectively, while assessment and resuscitation are ongoing. A pelvic radiograph confirms or rules out pelvic fractures, which can account for significant blood loss. An abdominal computed tomography scan is the gold standard to evaluate solid organ injuries causing hemorrhage and shock.

16. Mortality is consistently lower in children than in adults for a given level of injury severity. How does a child's reaction to shock differ from an adult's?
Recent animal experiments suggest that young animals and weanlings produce fewer free radicals than mature animals with the same level of tissue ischemia. This finding explains the ability of infants and children to recover organ function more readily than adults with similar levels of traumatic injury. Prevention, early recognition, and treatment of shock, however, are essential because once a child is in hemorrhagic shock, the mortality rate is no different from that in adults.

17. What is one of the important consequences of adequate resuscitation after a period of hypoperfusion?
Reperfusion injury occurs after flow is restored to ischemic tissue. Free radicals are formed at the molecular level when oxygen is supplied to ischemic areas. They trigger a systemic inflammatory cascade as they gain access to the circulation, causing endothelial and parenchymal cell injury. Rebound from fluid loss at the cellular level results in capillary leak, which is manifested macroscopically as subcutaneous edema, pulmonary edema (with normal or decreased central venous pressure), and renal dysfunction (decreased urine output and concentrating ability).

18. How are free radicals formed?
Adenosine triphosphate is catabolized to adenosine and inosine during the ischemic period. This process leads to the accumulation of the purine bases hypoxanthine and xanthine. Xanthine dehydrogenase is converted to xanthine oxidase in ischemic tissue. Xanthine oxidase requires oxygen to metabolize the purine bases into uric acid. This process generates a superoxide free radical that initiates the microvascular and parenchymal cell injury associated with reperfusion injury. The two key steps in this process are the accumulation of purine bases and the conversion of xanthine dehydrogenase to xanthine oxidase. To date, attempts to block free radical formation have been unsuccessful.

19. How does basic science research on the inflammatory response affect trauma management?

We now understand the systemic response to trauma. The release of inflammatory mediators results in peripheral muscle catabolism and conversion of hepatic function to the acute-phase response. The metabolic response to injury is critical for recovery. Ongoing research is focused on stimulation of the hepatic response to allow increased production of acute-phase proteins and provide the building blocks for tissue repair. Although many inflammatory mediators have been identified (e.g., interleukins 1, 6, and 8; tumor necrosis factor), our ability to regulate and stimulate the systemic response to trauma is still in its infancy. Current trauma therapy is basically supportive, now matter how high-tech it becomes. Pharmacologic modulation of the immune response to trauma (particularly in patients manifesting a decreased ability to respond to this stimulus) will be the next quantum leap forward in our ability to stabilize and heal patients with severe multisystem traumatic injury.

BIBLIOGRAPHY

1. Airway and ventilation, vascular access, fluid therapy and medications, trauma resuscitation. In Chameides L, Hazinski MF (eds): Pediatric Advance Life Support. American Heart Association, 1997, pp 4.1–6.12, 8.1–8.7.
2. Clowes GHA Jr: Stresses, mediation and responses of survival. In Clowes GHA Jr (ed): Trauma, Sepsis and Shock. New York, Marcel Dekker, 1988, pp 1–54.
3. Montgomery RA, Venbrux AC, Bulkley GB: Mesenteric vascular insufficiency (reperfusion injury). Curr Probl Surg 34:968–969, 1997.
4. Pediatric trauma. In Advanced Trauma Life Support Program for Doctors, 6th ed. Chicago, American College of Surgeons, 1997, pp 353–377.
5. Ramenofsky ML: Infants and children as accident victims and their emergency management. In O'Neill JA, Row MI, Grosfeld JL, et al (eds): Pediatric Surgery, 5th ed. St. Louis, Mosby, 1998, pp 235–242.
6. Tepas JJ III: Resuscitation of the injured child. In Trunkey DD, Lewis FR (eds): Current Therapy of Trauma, 4th ed. St. Louis, Mosby, 1999, pp 81–84.
7. Tepas JJ III: Pediatric trauma. In Feliciano DV, Moore EE, Mattox KL (eds): Trauma, 3rd ed. Stamford, CN, Appleton & Lange, 1996, pp 879–899.
8. The threat of oxidant injury. In Marino PL (ed): The ICU Book, 2nd ed. Baltimore, Williams & Wilkins, 1998, pp 32–50.

55. NEUROSURGICAL TRAUMA AND CERVICAL SPINE INJURIES

William Olivero, M.D.

HEAD INJURY

1. What is the most common type of head injury requiring operative care?

Scalp lacerations, which in children (unlike in adults) may cause significant blood loss and hypovolemic shock.

2. What are the five distinct layers of the scalp?

S = Skin
C = Connective tissue subcutaneous
A = Aponeurotic layer or epicranium (strongest layer)
L = Loose connective tissue
P = Pericranium or periosteum

3. What is Battle's sign?
When a basilar skull fracture occurs through the temporal bone, blood may collect around the mastoid tip. The bruising is known as Battle's sign.

4. What is pediatric concussion syndrome?
A child with pediatric concussion syndrome cries immediately after a mild head injury (usually a short fall) and, minutes to hours later, becomes irritable, pale, cold, and clammy and begins to vomit. The fontanelle is soft. Such children do well.

5. What is the classic presentation for an epidural hematoma?
Brief loss of consciousness followed by a lucid period and then rapid deterioration.

6. Name the artery most commonly affected in epidural hematoma.
Middle meningeal artery.

7. Is a skull fracture necessary to cause an epidural hematoma?
No.

8. What is the classic presentation of an acute subdural hematoma?
A severe head injury followed immediately by depressed level or consciousness or coma.

9. Are cortical contusions more common with acute subdural hematoma?
Cortical contusions are more common with subdural hematoma. Although epidural hematomas may occur with relatively minor head injury, subdural hematomas require transmission of greater forces to the brain. These shear forces tear the bridging veins from the cortex to the dura and cause subdural hematomas. This force also may be transmitted directly to the brain itself, causing contusions.

10. How do chronic subdural hematomas present in children?
Usually a child less than 2 years old presents with a slowly enlarging head, full or bulging fontanelle, irritability, and vomiting.

11. Describe the clinical manifestations of uncal herniation.
When the uncus of the temporal lobe herniates through the tentorial notch, it compresses the third nerve and midbrain, resulting in an ipsilateral dilated pupil, decreased level of consciousness, and contralateral hemiparesis.

12. What type of epidural hematoma is more likely to cause uncal herniation?
A hematoma that develops in the low temporal fossa and causes herniation of the medial temporal lobe (uncus).

13. What is the definitive diagnostic radiologic examination for uncal herniation due to epidural hematoma?
Computed tomography (CT) scan.

14. Describe the whiplash-shaken baby syndrome.
A child with whiplash-shaken baby syndrome presents with altered consciousness, retinal hemorrhages, and evidence on CT or magnetic resonance imaging (MRI) of subdural hematomas. Caregivers typically relate no history of injury or an inappropriate history for the degree of injury observed.

15. Are retinal hemorrhages pathognomonic for shaken baby syndrome?
Not always. But they should arouse distinct suspicion.

SPINE INJURY

16. In children, what part of the cervical spine is more prone to fracture and dislocation?
The upper cervical spine (C1 and C2). Because children have a large head in relationship to the rest of their body, the head can act as a fulcrum, disrupting the ligaments in the upper cervical spine region.

17. Do normal spine films in children rule out the possibility of spinal cord injury?
No. Children have such lax and mobile ligaments that the spinal cord can be injured without radiologic abnormalities.

18. What is SCIWORA?
Spinal cord injury without radiologic abnormality.

19. Why does SCIWORA occur in children?
As mentioned above (see Question 17), the ligaments and joint capsules are lax, allowing mobility at the cost of stability. Excessive mobility can damage the spinal cord during trauma without sign of fracture or subluxation on plan cervical spine films or CT scan.

20. Is MRI abnormal in cases of SCIWORA?
Frequently MRI shows patterns of injury in the spinal cord at the anatomic level of suspicion. There may be abnormal signs in the ligamentous structures as well.

21. How do normal cervical spine films differ in children and adults?
The predental space (the space between the anterior arch of the atlas and the odontoid process) may be as high as 5 mm (3 mm in adults). Pseudosubluxation between the second and third cervical vertebrae is common in children (up to 45%).

22. Describe the neurologic exam in a patient with complete spinal cord injury.
Loss of motor, sensory, and autonomic function distal to the level of injury.

23. Describe the neurologic exam in a patient with anterior spinal artery syndrome.
Preservation of light touch and proprioception with loss of all other cord function distal to the level of injury.

24. Describe the neurologic exam in a patient with central cord syndrome.
A disproportional loss of motor power in the upper versus lower extremities is accompanied by varying degrees of sensory loss. Some degree of functional recovery is typically seen.

25. Describe Brown-Séquard syndrome.
Ipsilateral motor and proprioceptive loss with contralateral pain and temperature loss.

PERIPHERAL NERVE INJURY

26. What percentage of newborns with brachial plexus injuries due to birth trauma obtain full recovery?
75–95%.

27. A peripheral nerve is clearly transected with no or minimal bruising. The general condition of the patient does not contraindicate surgery. When should it be repaired?
The day of the injury.

CONTROVERSY

28. In a child with a brachial plexus injury who has shown no signs of recovery by 3 months, when should the plexus be explored?

Some authors recommend cord exploration at 3 months. Other authors, however, believe that because of the high percentage of patients with spontaneous recovery, which may occur after the first 3 months, a more expectant approach is warranted. They wait until around 12 months. Data supporting early vs. late repair are not definitive.

BIBLIOGRAPHY

1. Aldrich EF, Eisenberg HM, Saydjari C, et al: Diffuse brain swelling in severely head-injured children. A report from the NIH traumatic coma data bank. J Neurosurg 76:450–454, 1992.
2. Chan K-H, Mann KS, Yue CP, et al: The significance of skull fractures in acute traumatic intracranial hematomas in adolescents: A prospective study. J Neurosurg 72:189–194, 1990.
3. Duhaime AC, Alario AJ, Lewander WJ, et al: Head injury in very young children: Mechanisms, injury types, and ophthalmologic findings in 100 hospitalized patients younger than 2 years of age. Pediatrics 90:179–185, 1992.
4. Duhaime AC, Gennarelli TA, Thibault LE, et al: The shaken baby syndrome. A clinical, pathological, and biomechanical study. J Neurosurg 66:409–415, 1987.
5. Hahn YS, Raimondia AJ, McLone DG, et al: Traumatic mechanisms of head injury in child abuse. Child's Brain 10:229–241, 1983.
6. Pang D, Wilberger JE Jr: Spinal cord injury without radiographic abnormalities in children. J Neurosurg 57:114, 1982.
7. Söderström CE: Diagnostic significance of CSF spectrophotometry and computer tomography in cerebrovascular disease. A comparative study in 231 cases. Stroke 8:606–612, 1977.
8. Walden JN: Subarachnoid Hemorrhage. Edinburgh, Livingstone, 1956.

56. THORACIC TRAUMA

Nikola K. Puffinbarger, M.D., and Steven Stylianos, M.D.

1. In a child with documented chest injury, what should the trauma surgeon suspect?

Chest injury is often a marker for other injuries. More than two-thirds of children with chest injury have other organ system injuries, including closed-head injury, extremity fractures, and intraabdominal solid-organ damage.

2. Are rib fractures common in children?

No. Rib fractures are rare because of the compliance of the child's chest wall. When rib fractures do occur, they are an indication of severe impact.

3. What type of thoracic injury is common in children?

The compliance of the chest wall results in a higher frequency of pulmonary contusions and direct intrapulmonary hemorrhage, usually without overlying rib fractures. Injuries that disrupt the pleura, such as pneumothorax, hemothorax, or hemopneumothorax, have similar physiologic consequences in children and adults and usually require chest tube decompression.

4. What clinical signs raise the suspicion of a pulmonary contusion?

Evidence of a shunt with resultant hypoxia, indicative of a ventilation-perfusion mismatch.

5. What are the complications of pulmonary contusion?

• **Pneumonia** may develop in the injured lung segment. Frequent suctioning and physiotherapy may prevent the development of pneumonia.

• **Posttraumatic pseudocysts** within the lung. In children, posttraumatic pseudocysts may resolve over time; however, they may become infected and form lung abscesses.

6. What are the signs and symptoms of a tension pneumothorax?

Chest pain, respiratory distress, tachycardia, hypotension, tracheal deviation, unilateral breath sounds, and neck vein distention.

7. What hemodynamic changes occur with a tension pneumothorax?

The mediastinum shifts away from the collapsed lung, compresses the contralateral lung, and displaces the diaphragm downward. This shift of the mediastinum results in an angulation of the vena cava with decreased systemic venous return to the heart and cardiac output and increased central venous pressure, and may result in cardiovascular collapse.

8. Describe the treatment of a tension pneumothorax.

Immediate decompression by a large-bore needle inserted into the second intercostal space in the midclavicular line on the side of the chest with absent breath sounds. *Tension pneumothorax is a clinical diagnosis.* Valuable time may be lost in obtaining a chest film.

9. What is a "sucking" chest wound?

Penetrating trauma may cause an open pneumothorax. The opening of the chest wall allows air to enter and escape the thorax, resulting in paradoxical respirations.

10. How does an open pneumothorax compromise ventilation?

The chest wall can no longer generate a negative intrathoracic pressure, and ventilation is severely compromised. Treatment requires occlusion of the wound and chest tube insertion.

11. What is Beck's triad? Is it present in small children?

The typical adult patient with cardiac tamponade often has three physical findings: (1) markedly diminished heart sounds, (2) venous distension in the neck, and (3) decreased arterial pressure. These findings may be difficult to assess in an infant. Usually the child with cardiac tamponade presents with penetrating trauma to the mediastinum and shock.

12. What chest x-ray findings suggest pericardial effusion or hemorrhage?

Increase in size of cardiac silhouette and overall profile of the heart appearing more rounded than normal.

13. Describe the *immediate* treatment for suspected cardiac tamponade.

If tamponade is suspected, pericardiocentesis should be performed. An angiocatheter is passed upward and to the left of the xiphoid process. After a flash of blood the needle is removed, and a syringe is attached for aspiration. Aspiration of as little as 15-20 ml of blood results in immediate improvement. Valuable time may be lost in obtaining a chest film or echocardiogram before intervention.

14. What is indicated by the aspiration of blood that "clots" during pericardiocentesis?

The blood is from an intracardiac chamber rather than the pericardial space.

15. In what age group is cardiac contusion most common?

Adolescents, who typically are unrestrained drivers.

16. When should cardiac contusion be suspected?

Patients with blunt injuries to the anterior chest associated with diminished cardiac output despite adequate blood volume and fluid resuscitation should be suspected of having cardiac contusion. Important clinical signs and symptoms of cardiac contusion include hypotension, significant conduction abnormalities on EKG, or wall motion abnormalities on echocardiography.

17. How long should a patient with cardiac contusion be monitored?
Patients with cardiac contusion diagnosed by conduction abnormalities are at risk for sudden dysrhythmias and should be monitored for the first 24 hours after injury. After 24 hours the risk of sudden dysrhythmia decreases substantially.

18. What is the speculated mechanism of sudden death in a young athlete who sustains a blow to the chest from a projectile object (e.g., a baseball)?
Sudden death most likely is due to ventricular dysrhythmia induced by an abrupt, blunt precordial blow, presumably delivered at an electrically vulnerable phase of ventricular excitability.

19. Aortic injury in children is rare. Name two situations in which it may be suspected.
Deceleration injuries such as (1) motor vehicle crash with unrestrained adolescent driver and (2) fall from a great height.

20. Where does the aorta usually lacerate?
At the level of the ligamentum arteriosum where the aorta is fixed.

21. What is the gold standard for diagnosis of aortic injury?
Aortography.

22. What are alternatives to aortography to assess for an aortic injury?
Transesophageal echocardiogram or dynamic computed tomography.

23. What chest film findings indicate a possible thoracic aortic disruption?
- Widened mediastinum
- Obliteration of the space between the pulmonary artery and the aorta
- Depression of the mainstem bronchus
- Deviation of the esophagus (nasogastric tube) to the right
- Fractures of the first or second rib or scapula

24. When should a tracheobronchial injury be suspected in a child?
Tracheobronchial injuries are rare in children. Tracheal and bronchial tears occur after crushing injury from heavy objects falling or being pulled onto the chest. Clinical presentation may include subcutaneous air, hypoxia, and/or hemoptysis. Chest tube placement indicates a massive air leak that does not resolve.

25. Which tracheobronchial injuries require direct repair?
Tears of the intrathoracic trachea and major bronchi require direct repair.

26. What is the treatment of basilar bronchi tears?
Rents of basilar bronchi frequently respond to high-frequency, low-pressure ventilation. Distal bronchial leaks may be occluded with fibrin glue selectively placed via bronchoscope. If these measures fail, thoracotomy with segmental resection or lobectomy is required.

27. What is the most common cause of esophageal injury in infancy and childhood?
Almost all traumatic injuries to the esophagus in children are secondary to penetrating mechanisms and are usually iatrogenic (related to endoscopic or dilatation procedures).

28. What findings on a chest film may indicate esophageal injury?
Air in the mediastinum, subcutaneous emphysema, or pneumo/hemothorax.

29. Name the best study for esophageal injury.
Esophagram with a water-soluble contrast material.

30 What is the treatment of an acute esophageal injury?
Administration of broad-spectrum antibiotics and wide mediastinal drainage.

31. How is a diaphragmatic rupture diagnosed in children?
Diagnosis is usually suggested on plain chest films if a nasogastric tube is above the diaphragm.

32. In children, what incision is used to repair a blunt diaphragmatic injury?
The repair is done via laparotomy, which provides access to possible concomitant injury to abdominal viscera.

BIBLIOGRAPHY

1. Allen GS, Cox CS Jr, Moore FA,et al: Pulmonary contusion: Are children different? J Am Coll Surg 185:229–233, 1997.
2. American College of Surgeons Committee on Trauma: Advanced Trauma Life Support for Doctors Instructor Course Manual. American College of Surgeons, Chicago, 1997.
3. Black TL, Snyder CL, Miller JP, et al: Significance of chest trauma in children. South Med J 89:494–496, 1996.
4. Blostein PA, Hodgman CG: Computed tomography of the chest in blunt thoracic trauma: Results of a prospective study. J Trauma 43:13–18, 1997.
5. Cooper A, Barlow B, DiScala C, String D: Mortality and truncal injury: The pediatric perspective. J Pediatr Surg 29:33–38, 1994.
6. Mandal AK, Thadepalli H, Chettipalli U: Posttraumatic empyema thoracis: A 24-year experience in a major trauma center. J Trauma 43:764–771, 1997.
7. Maron BJ, Poliac LC, Kaplan JA, Mueller FO: Blunt impact to the chest leading to sudden death from cardiac arrest during sports activities. N Engl J Med 333:337–342, 1995.

57. ABDOMINAL TRAUMA

Richard H. Pearl, M.D.

1. Is abdominal trauma in children principally blunt or penetrating?
Blunt. In most pediatric series, blunt trauma is the mechanism of injury in over 90% of cases.

2. True or false: Of all major body systems (head, chest, abdomen, spine, extremities), abdominal injury has the highest mortality rate.
False. Spinal cord injury (43%) and chest trauma (25%) have the highest mortality rates in children sustaining significant multisystem injury. In this setting, the mortality rate for abdominal injury is 15%. These percentages represent the contribution of each body system to the overall death rate of children with multisystem injuries.

3. In sequence, what are the three most commonly injured organs in the abdominal cavity?
Spleen, liver, and kidneys. The solid organs are much more commonly injured when blunt forces are applied to the abdomen.

4. What is the test of choice for assessing a child with a significant abdominal injury?
Computed tomography (CT) scan is the gold standard for evaluating children with abdominal injuries. Although intravenous and oral contrast is recommended, recent studies have shown that a screening CT without oral contrast can be diagnostic in most circumstances, including injury to the small and large intestine.

5. True or false: Diagnostic peritoneal lavage (DPL) should be performed whenever intra-abdominal hemorrhage is suspected.

False. The presence of intra-abdominal blood is not an indicator for laparotomy in children. Spleen, liver, and kidney injuries frequently bleed and then stabilize without surgical intervention. Additionally, DPL produces free air in the abdomen, negating the value of CT in correctly quantifying abdominal free air.

6. True or false: The nonoperative management of splenic injury is well accepted.

True (sort of). Although observational management of splenic injury in children is universally accepted, as recently as 10 years ago senior surgeons in adult trauma centers were still debating its efficacy and rationale. Of note, these same surgeons now support the nonoperative treatment of splenic injuries in adults, proving that adults are really large children!

7. If the presence of blood on CT scan or lavage does not mandate surgery, how do you determine the requirement for laparotomy in patients with solid organ injury?

Transfusion requirements. In earlier articles, the 50/50 rule applied. If a child required replacement of 50% of blood volume by crystalloid, followed by 50% of blood volume in blood products, and did not become hemodynamically stable, a laparotomy was indicated (assuming blood loss from nonabdominal sources had been ruled out). Recently, the blood volume requirement has been reduced to 25–30% in some reports because of the concern of viral transmission from transfusions.

8. What is the circulating blood volume in a child?

A good rule of thumb is 80 ml/kg of body weight. For example, a 20-kg child is prepared for surgery if tachycardia and hypotension continue after administration of 800 ml of Ringer's lactate solution and 800 ml of packed red blood cells.

9. If peritoneal lavage is not routinely performed, how does one determine when it is required?

Response to resuscitation is the primary indicator for surgical intervention due to hemorrhage. CT scan is performed on all patients with significant abdominal trauma who are hemodynamically stable. The presence of solid organ injury (e.g., contusion, lacerations, fragmentation) defines what is observed but does not determine the requirement for surgery. The presence of free air on CT scan, however, frequently mandates surgery. Lavage is reserved for the following scenarios:
- Unexplained shock in the absence of significant blood loss
- Suspicion of intestinal injury without free air on plain film or CT
- Equivocal physical findings and a nondiagnostic abdominal CT in children about to have an anesthetic for neurologic or orthopedic injuries
- To rule out abdominal injury in the operating room in a child having emergent thoracic surgery without time for other diagnostic workup

10. True or false: Blunt hepatic trauma is managed the same as splenic injury in children.

True. Most blunt liver injuries (> 90%) stabilize without surgery. In injuries requiring surgery, minimal debridement with suture ligature of bleeders or simple packing frequently is all that is required. Major resections are rarely required and have a significant mortality rate. Transcaval shunting, although well described, is performed infrequently and should be avoided unless the surgeon is well versed in the technique. Packing, transfusion, and observation with planned reexploration frequently are curative and life-saving without the morbidity and mortality of more sophisticated interventions.

When aggressive surgical management is mandated by instability and ongoing hemorrhage, brief periods of vascular isolation of the liver can be tolerated, allowing a relatively bloodless field for rapid hepatic resection. Clamping of the suprahepatic vena cava, infrahepatic vena cava, and portahepatis (Pringle maneuver) is required. Central venous access with rapid infusion to maintain right-heart filling pressures is required during this procedure.

11. In what percentage of patients with blunt injury to the spleen is splenic conservation possible?

97%. Of patients with documented splenic injury, 85% recover without surgical intervention. Of the remaining 15%, most require simple packing, splenorrhaphy, or partial splenectomy. Rarely is splenectomy required (< 3% of cases)—usually in the setting of significant multisystem trauma when the time needed to repair the spleen would be excessive and rapid splenectomy is required for stability.

12. When splenectomy is performed, what is required during the postoperative period to prevent infectious complications?

Overwhelming postsplenectomy infection (OPSI) is well described; the incidence is low, but the case mortality rate is 50%. To prevent this sequela, postoperative immunization with polyvalent vaccines for encapsulated gram-positive organisms (e.g., pneumococci, meningococci, *Hemophilus influenzae*) is required. In addition, daily prophylaxis with penicillin is recommended.

13. True or false: Blunt trauma to the duodenum is common and always requires surgery.

False. Trauma to the duodenum represents < 5% of all injuries in the abdomen and does not always require surgery. Duodenal hematoma is the most common injury; observation usually suffices, with return to normal function in 2–3 weeks. Surgery is required in < 5% of cases for persistent obstruction or stenosis. Duodenal laceration or disruption requires immediate surgical repair; delay causes a significant increase in morbidity and mortality. CT scan with contrast can be diagnostic; an upper gastrointestinal (GI) series is performed in equivocal cases. Duodenal hematoma occurs 2–3 times more frequently than laceration or disruption of the duodenum.

14. What are the principles of repair of duodenal injury?

In simple lacerations with minimal disruption or soiling, primary repair with local drainage suffices. In more complicated injuries (loss of bowel wall continuity with disruption) or with significant soilage (delayed diagnosis), the keys to the repair are:
   a. Serosal patch or roux-en-Y duodenojejunostomy
   b. Pyloric exclusion
   c. Gastrostomy (tube)
   d. Jejunostomy (tube)
   e. Gastrojejunostomy to replace c and d above
   f. Decompressing duodenostomy tube (optimal)
   g. Wide drainage of the contaminated field
In the absence of injury to the biliary system, no manipulation or drainage of the common bile duct should be performed.

15. True or false: Significant blunt trauma to the pancreas with ductal disruption requires surgical intervention.

Controversial. Injury to the pancreas is caused by compression of the body of the pancreas across the spine. Contusion, laceration, fragmentation, or complete disruption of the pancreas can ensue. In a recent report, 35 children with significant documented pancreatic injury were treated nonoperatively. Ten developed pseudocysts treated with bowel rest and, in 6 cases, percutaneous drainage. Eight patients had complete duct disruption, which healed. The average length of stay for the entire group was 21 days. Many authors argue that with duct disruption a distal pancreatectomy decreases hospital stay and allows earlier return to oral feedings. This argument may be true, but complications such as pancreatic abscess, wound infection, and bowel obstruction do not occur with nonoperative management.

16. True or false: Pancreatic injuries frequently are diagnosed late because of the inadequacies of current diagnostic studies.

False. Contrast-enhanced CT scanning documented injury in all 35 cases of the previously mentioned report. Careful review of each study revealed abnormal fluid collections in multiple regions in and around the pancreas, which suggested injury. All of the parenchymal injuries (contusion through duct disruption) were imaged accurately by CT scan.

17. True or false: Small and large bowel injuries can occur by burst, shear, or crush.

True. Although jejunal, ileal, and colonic injuries occur less frequently than solid organ or duodenal injury, their contribution to operative interventions far exceeds their incidence. Rapid compression of a distended viscus (burst), deceleration (shear), or compression across the spine (crush) can cause bowel wall disruption with abdominal cavity soilage. Peritoneal findings (an acute abdomen), free air, or lavage fluids showing GI contents mandate surgery.

18. True or false: Lap belts save lives but cause injuries.

True. In all reports, restrained children have improved survival rates with decreased injuries. However, the triad of injuries caused by lap and shoulder belt compression is well described: abdominal wall contusions (lap belt marks), hollow viscous injury, and Chance fractures of the lumbar spine (flexion/compression). All children with lap belt contusions should have an abdominal CT scan and thoracic/lumbar spine imaging.

19. True or false: Penetrating trauma from gunshot wounds between the nipples and groin requires laparotomy.

True. Gunshot wounds can create cavitary and blast forces far beyond the direct path created by the bullet. Therefore, gunshots entering the abdominal cavity require surgical exploration. Entry and exit wounds should be assessed, with the trajectory and type of bullet considered in planning and performing surgery. In the past low-velocity pistol wounds were the norm. Sadly, this is no longer true; high-powered military weapons and shotguns are used with increasing frequency. Complete exploration and wide debridement with a systematic approach to performing each laparotomy are required.

20. True or false: Like gunshot wounds, stab wounds to the abdomen mandate surgical exploration.

False. A selective approach to stab wounds is reasonable and decreases the negative laparotomy rate. First, an exploration of the stab wound is performed under local anesthesia. If the peritoneum is intact, no further surgery is entertained. If the peritoneum has been entered, peritoneal lavage is performed. If the result is positive, a laparotomy follows; if it is negative, a triple-contrast CT scan completes the evaluation. Using this schema, only patients with documented peritoneal contamination are explored surgically. After admission and observation, a change in clinical status necessitates reevaluation and possible exploration.

21. True or false: Diaphragmatic rupture is difficult to diagnose and frequently missed.

False. Diaphragmatic rupture is rare, representing < 0.5% of all major abdominal traumas. However, with modern CT scanning virtually 100% of cases can be diagnosed quickly. In addition, careful review of the chest radiographs reveals specific (or subtle) signs of injury in most cases. Laparotomy with direct repair is required, and multiorgan injury usually is present.

22. After considering all factors, the decision to operate on a child who has sustained blunt abdominal trauma is based on which findings: clinical status, lab tests, or radiologic studies?

Clinical status. To review what has been stated several times, the clinical response to resuscitation (volume replacement) and physical exam findings are the most reliable and predictive indicators for surgery. Hemodynamic instability after one-half the blood is replaced, first by crystalloid and then by colloid solutions, or peritoneal findings on abdominal exam determine the urgent need for surgery in most cases. After stability is established, CT scanning follows after admission to determine the injury being observed and, occasionally, to diagnose injuries requiring surgical intervention. Likewise, the clinical exam in gunshot and stab wounds also determines the need for surgical intervention. The clinical judgment of the surgeon is paramount in evaluating abdominal injuries in children.

BIBLIOGRAPHY

1. Eichelburger MR, al Moront M: Abdominal trauma. In O'Neill JA, Rowe MJ, Grosfeld JL, et al (eds): Pediatric Surgery, vol. 1, 5th ed. St. Louis, Mosby, 1998.
2. Pearl RH, Wesson DE, Spence LJ, et al: Splenic injury: A 5 year update with improved results and changing criteria for conservative management. J Pediatr Surg 24:121–124, 1989.
3. Shilyansky J, Pearl R, Kreller M, et al: Diagnosis and management of duodenal injuries in children. J Pediatr Surg 32:880–886, 1997.
4. Shilyansky J, Kreller M, Sehna L, et al: Non-operative management of pancreatic injuries in children. J Pediatr Surg 33:1–9, 1998.
5. Snyder CL: Abdominal and genitourinary trauma. In Ashcraft KW, Murphy JP, Sharp RJ, et al (eds): Pediatric Surgery, 3rd ed. Philadelphia, W.B. Saunders, 2000.

58. GENITOURINARY TRAUMA

Churphena Reid, M.D.

Approximately 10% of all injuries due to external violence involve the genitourinary system, most commonly the kidney. Traumatic injuries to the genitourinary tract must be considered in children presenting with abdominal trauma because of the more intra-abdominal location of the kidney and bladder and the presence of undetected congenital anomalies, reportedly as high as 7% in some series.

1. What is the most common presentation of injury to the genitourinary tract?

Hematuria, microscopic or gross, is the most common presentation of injury to the urinary system. McAninch recommends that all children who sustain trauma and have greater than 5 red blood cells per high-power field on urinalysis should undergo radiographic imaging to assess potential renal injury. However, approximately 10–25% of urinary injuries present without hematuria, primarily those involving damage to the vascular system, particularly the renal pedicle.

2. What are the two main groups of renal injuries?

Penetrating abdominal injuries (20%) and blunt abdominal injuries (80%).

3. Describe the management of penetating renal injuries.

Penetrating renal injuries usually are associated with other intra-abdominal injuries and thus usually are explored surgically by the trauma team. Computerized tomography of the abdomen and pelvis should be done by the trauma team before taking the patient to the operating room to establish the status and function of the kidneys. If this is not possible, however, nephrotomograms must be obtained, even on the operating table, before opening any retroperitoneal hematomas because of the increased probability that renal exploration of penetrating trauma may result in partial or total nephrectomy. In the unstable patient, packing and further resuscitation can be performed, followed by on-table radiographic assessment of the kidneys.

4. What dose of intravenous contrast is appropriate for urgent renal imaging in children?

Intravenous injection of a 2-ml/kg bolus of noniodinated contrast, followed by a 10-minute "single-shot" abdominal film, should provide information about function, anatomy, and extravasation of contrast from the kidneys and drainage system.

5. What is the indication for surgical exploration in patients with renal trauma?

Penetrating injuries to the abdomen are generally explored. Any evidence of penetrating renal injury on radiographic imaging should be explored. An absolute indication for renal exploration is an expanding or pulsatile retroperitoneal hematoma. Relative indications include urinary extravasation, nonviable renal tissue, and arterial thrombosis. The decision to explore should be based on extent of injury, hemodynamic stability, and the need for operative repairs of associated injuries.

6. What is the surgical strategy for operative management of penetrating renal injuries?

Renal exploration should be accomplished through a midline abdominal or thoracoabdominal incision that allows exposure of the retroperitoneum and associated intra-abdominal injuries. Before the retroperitoneum is opened, control of the renal vessels should be obtained by identifying the renal vasculature at the aorta and inferior vena cava through an incision made in the posterior retroperitoneum at the level of the inferior mesenteric artery. The vessels should be secured with vessel loops. The retroperitoneum is then entered lateral to the colon and reflected medially. At this point the traumatized kidney is repaired. Early isolation and control of the renal vessels should minimize the possibility of nephrectomy.

7. Describe the initial management of blunt renal injuries.

Blunt renal injuries usually result from rapid deceleration, as in an automobile accident or fall. Children are especially vulnerable to blunt trauma to the kidneys, even from seemingly simple accidents, because of a higher incidence of undiagnosed congenital renal anomalies. Therefore, all children with blunt abdominal trauma, hematuria (microscopic or gross), and stable hemodynamic status should undergo renal imaging.

8. How are renal injuries classified?

Minor renal injuries (85%)
a. Renal contusion
b. Shallow cortical laceration
c. Subscapsular hematoma
d. Collecting system injury

Major renal injuries (15%)
a. Shattered kidney
b. Renal pedicle injury
c. Perirenal hematoma

9. How are blunt renal injuries staged?

CT has replaced intravenous urography because of better anatomic detail of the vascular, parenchymal, and drainage systems of the genitourinary tract. It also has the advantage of providing details about other organ systems that may be involved in the trauma. A spiral CT scan now can be done in a few minutes without orally administered contrast. Spiral CT imaging also provides excellent imaging of the renal vascular system to assess pedicle injury, thus replacing the need for angiography at most trauma centers.

Intravenous urography may be done with noniodinated contrast at a dosage of 2 ml/kg. Nonvisualization of the kidney should be followed by arteriography to rule out renovascular pedicle injury.

10. How are blunt renal injuries treated?

Minor renal injuries (subtypes a, b, and c) and **some perirenal hematomas** are best treated conservatively with bedrest until urine grossly clears and the patient is hemodynamically stable. Hematocrit should be followed closely until it remains stable.

Injuries to the collecting system, which usually involve extravasation, are best treated with stenting and bedrest.

Major renal injuries usually demand immediate surgery, either revascularization or nephrectomy.

All injuries involving a solitary kidney should be treated as conservatively as possible to maximize preservation of the kidney.

11. What are the complications of renal trauma?

• Hypertension
• Abscess formation
• Delayed hemorrhage, which may occur 1–4 weeks after injury

- Obstruction of the collecting system
- Arteriovenous fistula

12. How do ureteral injuries occur in children?

Ureteral injuries rarely occur in children and generally are associated with renal trauma proximally and/or bladder injuries distally.

13. Describe the management of ureteral injuries.

Most ureteral injuries are easily managed with stenting unless the ureter is transected completely. If a stent cannot be passed, the next step consists of urinary diversion with placement of a nephrostomy tube until the patient's clinical status stabilizes. Final repair of the ureter (if still indicated) depends on the location of the injury. Low ureteral injuries near the ureterovesical junction are easily managed with antirefluxing ureteral reimplantation using a psoas hitch or Boari flap, if indicated. Options for mid-ureteral injuries include primary ureteroureterostomy over a stent or transureteroureterostomy. Proximal urteral injuries are best treated with primary ureteroureterostomy. Other options include ileal segment interposition, autotransplantation, and, finally, nephrectomy.

All ureteral injuries should be stented and drained extraperitoneally. Patients should receive antibiotic coverage.

14. How do bladder injuries occur in children? How are they classified?

Until puberty, the bladder is an intra-abdominal organ and thus may be easily involved in penetrating or blunt abdominal trauma. Blunt bladder injuries are more common than penetrating bladder injuries. Blunt bladder injuries are divided into two groups: intraperitoneal rupture and extraperitoneal rupture.

Intraperitoneal rupture occurs with increased frequency in children because the bladder is largely an intra-abdominal organ before puberty. Intraperitoneal rupture occurs when a patient with a full bladder receives a sudden blow to the lower abdomen.

Extraperitoneal rupture, which accounts for only 10% of pediatric bladder trauma, results from laceration of the bladder with a bony spicule from associated pelvic fracture.

Combined intra- and extraperitoneal injuries do occur, but they account for less than 10% of all bladder trauma.

15. What diagnostic test is usually done to establish bladder injury?

Gross hematuria and abdominal pain are the most common findings on physical examination. A distention cystogram using dilute contrast to bladder capacity and postdrainage films detect the majority of disruptions to the bladder. The child is best catheterized with smooth non-latex catheters (i.e., 8-French feeding tubes) to avoid further trauma to the lower urinary tract. The appearance of a teardrop-shaped bladder on cystogram indicates a massive extraperitoneal hematoma.

The diagnosis of intraperitoneal rupture is established when contrast extravasates into the peritoneal cavity and outlines the configuration of the bowel.

16. How are bladder injuries managed?

Intraperitoneal ruptures are treated with surgical exploration and closure of the defect in two or three layers with absorbable suture. The bladder should be drained with non-latex Foley or suprapubic catheters, depending on the severity and type of associated injuries.

Extraperitoneal ruptures are associated most commonly with pelvic fractures; often they also are associated with urethral injuries. Extraperitoneal ruptures are managed conservatively with non-latex Foley catheter drainage. A follow-up cystogram in 7–10 days is indicated before catheter removal.

17. How do pediatric urethral injuries occur? How are they classified?

Urethral injuries are more common in males than females. They may result from pelvic injuries or fractures (posterior urethra) or straddle-type injuries to the perineum (anterior urethra).

The primary site of injury in prepubertal boys is more likely to be at the bladder neck and prostatic base because the prostate is not fully developed. In postpubertal boys urethral disruption most often occurs at the prostatomembranous junction.

Most patients with **posterior urethral injuries** present with blood at the meatus and inability to void. Rectal examination of the high-riding or floating prostate is not a specific finding in prepubertal compared with postpubertal boys.

Patients with **anterior urethral injuries** are usually able to void. They tend to have a bloody urethral discharge and a butterfly-shaped perineal hematoma.

18. How is the diagnosis of urethral injury established?

Posterior urethral injuries are associated with pelvic rami fractures. Retrograde urethrogram demonstrates extravasation of contrast above and/or below the urogenital diaphragm.

Anterior urethral injuries result from straddle-type injuries to the perineum. Retrograde urethrogram demonstrates an intact but usually stretched urethra with minimal or no extravasation.

19. How are urethral injuries managed?

Posterior urethral injuries are best managed initially by placement of a suprapubic catheter. Attempted placement of a urethral catheter often worsens the urethral rupture and thus complicates a later final repair. After 2 weeks, when associated trauma is stable, a cystogram through the suprapubic catheter is done. It not surprising to see continuation of the urethra reestablished. Otherwise, primary alignment may be attempted with the so-called duelling cystoscopes procedure or with open urethral reconstruction.

Anterior urethral injuries are managed with either non-latex Foley or suprapubic catheter drainage (if extravasation is present) until the perineal hematoma resolves. A voiding cystourethrogram is obtained before the catheter is removed.

20. What are the long-term complications of urethral injuries?

Complications of **posterior urethral injuries** include stricture, incontinence, and impotence. Delayed primary repair is reported to decrease the incidence of incontinence from 30% to less than 5% and the incidence of impotence from 50% to less than 15%. However, timing of the repair, because of various advantages and disadvantages, remains controversial.

The major complication of **anterior urethral injuries** is stricture formation, which may occur several years after injury.

21. What is the main cause of external genital injuries in children?

Trauma from physical or sexual abuse accounts for the majority of injuries to the external genitalia of both boys and girls. Burns to the genitalia result when the child is placed in scalding water. Forceful vaginal penetration in young girls may result in extensive lacerations of the external genitalia.

Burn injuries require extensive monitoring because the full extent of the injury is usually greater than what is initially apparent. Non-latex Foley catheter or suprapubic bladder drainage is necessary in children with extensive burns. Debridement of devitalized tissue along with topical application of sulfasilverdene ointment is recommended. Occasionally skin grafting may be required.

Extensive lacerations of the external genitalia in girls usually require suturing. Superficial lacerations usually respond to nonoperative management with application of topical antibacterial creams. Urinary diversion with non-latex Foley or suprapubic catheter drainage may ease patient discomfort.

All injuries involving the external genitalia should be reported to law enforcement agencies.

BIBLIOGRAPHY

1. Connor JP, Hensle TW: Systematic case of the traumatized kidney in children. Contemp Urol 3(6):60–70, 1991.
2. Lee JY, Cass AS: Renal injuries in children. In McAninch JW (ed): Traumatic and Reconstructive Urology. Philadelphia, W.B. Saunders, 1996, pp 127–133.

3. Morse TS: Renal injuries. Pediatr Clin North Am 22:379–391, 1975.
4. Peters PC, Sagalowsky AI: Genitournary trauma. In Walsh PC, et al (eds): Campbell's Urology, 6th ed. Philadelphia, W.B. Saunders, 1992, pp2571–2593.
5. Wessells H, CC, McAninch JW: Upper urinary tract trauma. American Urologic Association Update XV(14):110–115, 1996.

59. SOFT TISSUE INJURIES

Holly L. Hedrick, M.D., and Perry W. Stafford, M.D.

CRUSH INJURIES

1. What is the crush syndrome?
The crush syndrome occurs when the products of devitalized tissues enter the circulation. Signs and symptoms include severe hyperkalemia with possible arrhythmia and acute oliguric renal failure from myoglobinuria. Supportive treatment includes aggressive hydration, maintenance of high urine output, and alkalinization of the urine with intravenous sodium bicarbonate.

2. True or false: The most important part of the physical exam in assessing a patient for the presence of a compartment syndrome is the presence or absence of distal pulses.
False. Distal pulses are frequently palpable in an acute compartment syndrome. Capillary refill also is within normal limits. The classic symptom of a patient with an impending compartment syndrome is pain out of proportion to the injury. The first clinical sign is a tense, swollen compartment that produces pain with palpation or passive extension of the distal extremity. Sensation and motor nerve ischemia are the next symptoms to appear. Disturbance of capillary refill and diminished arterial pulses are late symptoms and usually signify irreversible tissue death.

3. What is the pressure threshold at which a fasciotomy is indicated?
Decompressive fasciotomies are recommended at pressures exceeding 40 mmHg or within 30 mmHg of the patient's diastolic pressure. Pressures in the range of 30–40 mmHg are most likely also an indication to proceed with fasciotomies because of the morbidity of an incorrect decision. Delay of diagnosis for 6–8 hours can lead to irreversible death of muscle and nerve.

4. Describe where to measure the four compartments of the lower leg.
All compartments should be measured in the middle to upper third of the leg. The anterior compartment is entered 1 cm lateral to the tibia. The lateral compartment is entered directly lateral to the fibula. The superifical posterior compartment is measured in the posterior calf. The deep posterior compartment is entered by introducing the needle 1 cm from the posteromedial tibia and advancing parallel to the posterior cortex of the tibia until it is felt to pop through the deep fascia.

5. What are the late sequelae of lower extremity compartment syndrome?
- Equinus contracture secondary to gastrocsoleus infarct
- Varus foot secondary to posterior tibial infarct
- Claw toes with ankle dorsiflexion secondary to infarct of the flexor digitorum longus
- Footdrop secondary to anterior compartment infarct
- Renal failure secondary to myoglobinuria

6. Describe the double-incision fasciotomy technique for the lower extremity.
The first incision extends from knee to ankle and is centered over the anterior and lateral compartments between the tibia and fibula. The subcutaneous tissues are dissected away from the

fascia to identify the intermuscular septum. A fasciotomy of the anterior compartment is performed 1 cm anterior to the septum, whereas the lateral compartment is fasciotomized 1 cm posterior to the septum. The superifical peroneal nerve must be carefully identified in the lateral compartment. The posteromedial incision is centered 1–2 cm posterior to the posteromedial border of the tibia. The saphenous vein and nerve should be avoided. The fascia overlying the gastrocnemius and soleus muscle is released. The deep posterior compartment is decompressed by detaching part of the soleus muscle from the posterior tibia. The wounds are left open and covered with sterile dressings.

7. What is the most common cause of Volkmann's contracture in children?

Supracondylar fracture of the humerus. Ischemia with supracondylar fractures may be due to (1) vascular injury, which requires surgical repair; (2) vascular entrapment, which usually resolves with reduction; or (3) compression from marked elbow flexion, tissue edema, hemorrhage, tight casts, or tight bandages. If left to progress, ischemia causes Volkmann's contracture, with loss of motor and sensory function and necrosis of some of the forearm flexor muscles. The muscles contract and are replaced by scar so that the wrist develops a flexion contracture and the fingers become clawed. Irreversible muscle necrosis results after 4–6 hours of ischemia.

LACERATIONS

8. Are radiologic studies useful in the evaluation of a laceration?

Yes. Radiologic evaluation may be useful to determine the presence of a foreign body in the wound. Ninety percent of all glass fragments are radiopaque. Gravel, wood, and 10% of glass fragments are not visible on radiographs. If a foreign body is suspected but not visible on plain films, careful local exploration of the wound is mandatory.

9. True or false: Tissue loss is more common in children.

False. Because of the elastic quality of the dermis in children and young adults, even superficial wounds can result in significant spreading of the wound edges, giving the impression of significant tissue loss.

10. What is the role of a tourniquet in the prehospital setting or emergency department?

A tourniquet should be used only as a last resort to prevent exsanguination. Hemostasis is best achieved by direct external pressure. Tourniquets or blindly used clamps or suture ligatures can significantly damage the vessels or surrounding nerves.

11. Where is the use of local anesthetic with epinephrine contraindicated?

Epinephrine should not be used with local anesthetics when it may interfere with end-arterial perfusion (e.g., digits, penis).

12. What are the potential complications of a digital block?

Excessive local infiltration can cause distortion of anatomic landmarks, local ischemia by arterial compression and impairment of venous return. Direct intravenous injection can cause rapid systemic toxicity.

13. Which is more important in determining the timing of wound closure and incidence of infection: the age of the wound or the number of bacteria in the wound?

The bacterial count determines the safety of closure. In general, younger wounds tend to have fewer bacteria. Wounds with greater than 10^5 organisms per gram of tissue are on average at least 5 hours old. The vascularity of the tissue and the mechanism of injury also affect bacterial proliferation. Animal and human bites contain high bacterial counts and therefore should not be closed primarily. Crush injuries also increase the amount of devitalized tissue and bacterial count and therefore have a higher likelihood of becoming infected. Finally, the presence of a hematoma increases the incidence of wound infection.

14. What are the current recommendations for tetanus prophylaxis?

For nontetanous-prone wounds, tentanus immune globulin (TIG) is never indicated. If a patient has not completed the three-dose immunization schedule or has not received a tetanus booster dose within the past 10 years, a booster dose of tetanus and diphtheria toxoids adsorbed (Td) is advised. For a tetanous-prone wound, no further treatment is required if the patient has been completely immunized and has received a tetanus booster within the past 5 years. If a patient with a tetanus-prone wound was not immunized or was incompletely immunized, TIG is given along with a dose of Td.

15. What are the characteristics of a tetanus-prone wound?

- Age of wound > 6 hours
- Stellate wound, avulsion, abrasion
- Depth > 1 cm
- Mechanism: missile, crush, burn, frostbites
- Signs of infection
- Devitalized tissue
- Contaminants such as dirt, feces, soil, or saliva

16. True or false: Betadine and hydrogen peroxide are good wound irrigants.

False. In general, wounds should not be irrigated with any solution not deemed suitable for one's own eyes. Tissue irritation, damage to cells, and interference with the healing process can result from the use of Betadine, alcohol, and hydrogen peroxide. The bacterial count in wounds is best reduced by vigorous use of large volumes of saline under pressure.

17. When should prophylactic antibiotics be used in the treatment of skin lacerations?

- Surrounding cellulitis
- Contaminated or dirty wounds in immunocompromised patients
- Extensive injuries to the center of the face (to prevent spread to meninges)
- Patients with cardiac valve disease
- Patients with prostheses
- Lymphedematous extremities
- Stool-contaminated wounds
- Human and animal bites

18. When should sutures be removed?

- Face: 3–4 days
- Abdomen or chest: 7 days
- Hands, feet, legs: 10–14 days
- Areas of movement or immunocompromise: 3 weeks

19. What is appropriate therapy for abrasions?

Superficial abrasions require only local cleaning and wound protection with a light, nonadhering dressing. The wound should be kept clean with gentle soaking and cleaning with soap twice daily. Antibacterial ointment may minimize eschar formation and prevent dressing adherence, but wound care is paramount.

Deep abrasions with embedded foreign matter are far more problematic and may result in permanent tattooing and significant scarring. Wound care requires removal of the embedded material with scrubbing or saline pressure jet lavage, often under general anesthesia. The resultant wound is equivalent to a burn wound and needs aggressive daily dressing changes with topical antibiotic coverage.

20. Should a wound caused by an animal bite be closed?

Most minor animal bite wounds can be closed after adequate irrigation and debridement. Exceptions include bites in areas of poor blood supply, such as the pretibial area, cat bites of the hand in proximity to tendon sheaths, and human bites. These potentially complicated wounds require consideration for inpatient care and/or referral for consultant options.

21. When should rabies vaccine be administered?

In many areas of the U.S., rabies has been virtually eradicated by vaccination and animal control. In such areas, only bat bites require treatments. In other areas, any unprovoked bite of a wild animal should be treated if the animal belongs to a species known to be a rabies host, such as skunk, fox, raccoon, bat, or coyote. Rodents are unusual carriers of the rabies virus in the U.S. If the bite is from a domesticated dog or cat, the decision rests on the condition of the animal, if apprehended, and its vaccination status. Difficulty arises when an animal makes an unprovoked attack and escapes.

22. How should animal bites suspected of rabies be treated?

ANIMAL	ANIMAL EVALUATION	TREATMENT OF EXPOSED HUMAN
Wild (skunk, fox, raccoon, coyote, bat)	Regard as rabid	HRIG + vaccine
Domestic (dogs and cats)	Healthy (vaccinated)	None
	Escaped (unknown)	HRIG + vaccine (may not be indicated in rabies-free area)
	Rabid: euthanasia with exam of brain for rabies antigen	HRIG + vaccine

All animal bite wounds should be treated locally with prompt mechanical wound cleaning with soap and water. Passive immunization with human rabies immune globulin (HRIG) (20 IU/kg) is given at the time of initial evaluation with half the dose infiltrated subcutaneously at the site of the bite and half given intramuscularly in the arm or buttocks. Active immunization with human diploid cell vaccine should be given in 5 doses at 0, 3, 7, 14, and 28 days.

BIBLIOGRAPHY

1. Gulli B, Templeton D: Compartment syndrome of the lower extremity. Orthop Clin North Am 25:677–684, 1994.
2. Lawrence WT, Bevin AG, Sheldon GF: Acute wound care. In Wilmore DW, Cheung LY, Harken AH, et al (eds): Scientific American Surgery, 3rd ed. New York, Scientific American, 1993, pp 1–17.
3. McBride AF, Hays JT: Compartment syndrome. In Cameron JL (eds): Current Surgical Therapy, 2nd ed. St. Louis, Mosby, 1998, pp 974–978.
4. Milford L: Volkmann's contracture and compartment syndromes. In Crenshaw A (ed): Campbell's Operative Orthopedics, 7th ed. St. Louis, Mosby, 1987, pp 409–418.
5. Wilson RF, Balakrishnan C: General principles of wound care. In Wilson RF, Walt AJ (eds): Management of Trauma: Pitfalls and Practice, 2nd ed. Baltimore, Williams & Wilkins, 1996, pp 70–84.

60. ORTHOPEDIC TRAUMA AND SPORTS INJURY

Carl R. St. Remy, M.D., William R. Puffinbarger, M.D., and David P. Roye, Jr., M.D.

1. What is the physis? Why is it important in trauma in children?
Otherwise known as the growth plate, the physis is the site of longitudinal growth of bone. Trauma to the physis may cause growth disturbance or arrest, resulting in angular deformity and/or limb length discrepancy.

2. Describe the Salter-Harris classification of physeal fractures.

Type I	Fracture line passes along the physis (extra-articular)
Type II	Fracture line passes along the physis and through the metaphyseal cortex (extra-articular)
Type III	Fracture line passes along the physis and through the epiphysis (intra-articular)
Type IV	Fracture that extends through the metaphysis, physis, and epiphysis (intra-articular)
Type V	Crush injury of the physis

3. A 6-year-old girl falls on her outstretched right hand and complains of right wrist pain with tenderness over the distal radius. Initial radiographs are "negative." What is your diagnosis?
Because wrist sprains are rare in children, a Salter-Harris type I fracture is the likely diagnosis. Comparison plain radiographs of the contralateral wrist are helpful in diagnosing injuries of the physis. The patient should be treated with casting of her wrist.

4. What is an open fracture?
An open fracture is associated with a wound communicating directly with the fracture site or hematoma. Because of the risk of complications (infection, malunion, and nonunion), open fractures require emergent surgical debridement and stabilization. All fractures with an associated soft tissue wound should be considered open until proved otherwise.

5. What is the most common long bone fractured in the upper extremity of children?
The clavicle. In utero it is the first long bone to ossify. Clavicle fractures usually are treated with a figure-of-eight wrap or a sling.

6. What is the most common elbow injury in children? How is it classified?
The most common elbow injury in children is supracondylar humerous fracture. There are two major types of mechanism of injury: (1) extension injury (> 95%), which results from falls on an outstretched hand, and (2) flexion injury, which results from direct trauma to the elbow.

7. What nerve is injured most commonly in association with supracondylar humerus fractures? What are the other immediate complications?
Some authors believe that the radial nerve is most commonly injured, followed by the median nerve. Others report that median nerve injury is more common. The ulnar nerve also may be affected. Other complications include vascular compromise and Volkmann's ischemic contracture (the chronic sequelae of compartment syndrome in the forearm). Hence, a complete neurovascular exam is essential at initial evaluation, and the patient must be followed closely after treatment.

8. What is a "gunstock" deformity of the elbow?

It is the cubitus varus deformity, a long-term complication, secondary to malunion, of supracondylar fractures.

9. What is a Monteggia fracture?

Fracture of the ulnar shaft in the proximal third with radial head dislocation. It is important to obtain plain radiographs of the elbow and to assess the radiocapitellar articulation in patients with a fracture of the ulna alone.

10. What percentage of pediatric forearm fractures involves the distal radius?

About 75–85%. Most distal radius fractures are metaphyseal and in children usually can be managed with closed reduction and casting.

11. Describe the difference between plastic deformation, torus fracture, and greenstick fracture.

These fracture patterns are common in children because of the unique biomechanical properties of pediatric bone in comparison with adult bone. Plastic deformation occurs when a bending force results in microfailure (fracture) over a broad area of the bone. The bone appears bent. A torus fracture occurs when the cortex of a long bone fails in compression and "buckles." A greenstick fracture occurs when one cortex fractures in tension while the other remains intact but plastically deformed.

12. What is a toddler's fracture?

A toddler's fracture is a fracture of the tibia due to low-energy forces in children 9 months to 3 years of age. It is usually a minimally or nondisplaced spiral fracture of the distal metadiaphysis. Often no episode of trauma is observed. The child suddenly refuses to stand or bear weight and may resume crawling.

13. What differences in healing between adult and pediatric fractures permit less accuracy in pediatric fracture reduction?

Generally, children demonstrate rapid and predictable healing. In addition, with growth and remodeling normal anatomy can be restored despite initial healing with some angulation and displacement. These characteristics diminish with the increasing age of the child.

14. Name the commonly fractured bones in abused children.

- Femur
- Humerus
- Tibia

The most common fracture pattern is transverse.

15. What is the most significant cause of femoral shaft fractures in children less than 3 years of age?

Child abuse (70%).

16. Why is significant pelvic ring disruption less common in children than adults in similar traumatic settings?

The flexibility of the pediatric pelvis allows single breaks in the pelvic ring.

17. What is Waddell's triad of injury?

Ipsilateral femur fracture, thoracic injury, and contralateral head injury. Waddell's triad describes the association of injuries in children (6–10 years old) struck by automobiles.

18. List the treatment options for pediatric femoral shaft fractures.

Spica casting (with or without traction), external fixation, compression plating, and intramedullary rodding.

19. What is FOOSH?

Fall on outstretched hand—the usual mechanism of injury for pediatric wrist fractures.

20. Why is it important not to transport infants and small children with suspected cervical spine injuries on a flat spine board?

Because the head of infants and small children is disproportionately large in relation to the torso, positioning on a flat board results in flexion of the neck. The most common level of injury in the small child involves the occiput–C1 and C1–C2 complexes. If the atlantoaxial ligaments have been disrupted but the odontoid process is intact, the flexed position results in spinal cord compression. Thus, elevation of the torso relative to the head keeps the neck in neutral position on a flat spine board.

21. What is the "lap-belt" sign in motor vehicle accidents?

The lap-belt sign is a linear ecchymosis on the abdomen. Lap-belt injuries are a common cause of thoracic and lumbar fractures and/or dislocations in children under the age of 13. Injury is due to improper positioning of the lap belt. The lap belt, which properly crosses the thighs of an adult, may improperly cross the abdomen of a child. Whenever the lap belt sign is seen, suspicion for neurologic, spinal, and/or visceral injuries should be high.

22. What is SCIWORA?

Spinal cord injury without radiographic abnormality. The osseous and ligamentous components of the pediatric cervical spine tolerate as much as four times the stretch allowed by the spinal cord. Thus, normal radiographs may be seen in children with severe cervical spinal cord injuries.

23. How common are hip fractures in children? What are the complications?

Hip fractures account for less than 1% of pediatric fractures and usually are secondary to high-energy trauma. The most common complication is avascular necrosis of the femoral head, which has an incidence as high as 40%. Other complications include malunion, nonunion, growth disturbance, and leg length discrepancy.

24. An obese 13-year-old boy presents with a 2-week history of right knee pain and limping. His parents report that he has had the pain since he fell while playing football and that radiographs of his knee were negative at the time of injury. How should you approach this patient?

The initial step is careful physical examination. A focused orthopedic exam should include at least the joint above and below the area of reported pain. If physical findings support injury in the knee, repeat plain radiographs of his knee are appropriate to rule out physeal injury. Because hip pain is commonly referred to the knee, however, radiographs of the hips should be done if abnormalities are noted on hip exam. Overweight adolescents are at risk for developing a slipped capital femoral epiphysis (SCFE), a displacement through the physis of the femoral neck relative to the epiphysis. SCFE is commonly associated with knee pain only.

25. What type of acute knee injury should you expect in a 14-year-old boy injured during strenuous jumping while playing basketball?

Tibial tubercle avulsion fracture. It is important to distinguish this fracture from the more chronic condition, Osgood-Schlatter disease, an aleration in the development of tibial tuberosity secondary to repeated application of tensile forces.

26. What is little leaguer's elbow?

Little leaguer's elbow is a valgus stress reaction of the medial epicondylar physis. It tends to occur in children 10 years of age or younger who participate in throwing sports. Medial epicondylar fractures tend to occur in adolescents as the medial epicondyle begins to fuse.

27. At what age do meniscal injuries begin to occur? How do they present?

Under age 14, a torn meniscus is rare. Meniscal tears in adolescents (> 14 years) usually result from significant trauma. Patients may present with pain, effusion, limping and inability to bear weight, or a locked knee. In this setting, meniscal injury commonly is associated with ligament injuries (cruciate and/or collateral ligament).

28. An 8-year-old boy complains of recurrent dramatic "popping" of his right knee with intermittent episodes of locking. He reports no history of injury. The knee exam reveals no ligamentous injury, and plain radiographs are negative. What is the diagnosis?

Such symptoms, termed snapping knee syndrome, are associated with a discoid meniscus, which is a congenital abnormality. Magnetic resonance imaging is the diagnostic modality of choice. Some discoid menisci are asymptomatic and require no treatment. Symptomatic discoid menisci are treated surgically; the type of discoid meniscus defines the specifics of surgical intervention.

29. Where does the anterior cruciate ligament insert on the tibia?

The anteror cruciate ligament (ACL) inserts on the tibial eminence. Intrasubstance tears of the ACL are uncommon in children under the age of 14. An avulsion fracture of the tibial eminence is an ACL-equivalent injury in a child. Generally, the mechanism of injury is hyperextension, sudden deceleration, or a valgus rotational force.

30. What is swimmer's shoulder?

Impingement syndrome of the shoulder. Adolescent swimmers may develop anterior shoulder pain after long swimming sessions. The tendons of the rotator cuff muscles are impinged between the humeral head and the anatomic ceiling created by the acromion, acromioclavicular joint, and coracoacromial ligament. Athletes in sports that require repetitive overhead shoulder activity, such as baseball and tennis, are also at risk. Impingement syndrome of the shoulder is treated with rest and rehabilitation, including modification of shoulder mechanics in activity.

31. What may be revealed in the pelvic radiograph of an adolescent track athlete presenting for evaluation of a pulled muscle?

Avulsion fracture of an apophysis. The rapid and forceful contraction of the muscles about the hip during sport activities can avulse an apophysis from its parent bone. Examples include avulsion of the lesser trochanteric apophysis by the iliopsoas muscle, of the ischial apophysis by the hamstring muscle, and of the apophysis of the anterior inferior iliac spine by the rectus femoris muscle. Rest, symptomatic measures, and crutch ambulation, followed by rehabilitation and gradual return to activies, are recommended.

32. How do distal femoral physeal fractures vary with the age of the child?

The juvenile-type injuries (age 2–10 years) are due to high-energy trauma (e.g., motor vehicle accidents) and may be associated with other skeletal, vascular, abdominal, and thoracic injuries. In contrast, adolescent-type injuries (> 11 years) usually result from low-energy trauma, as in sports participation.

BIBLIOGRAPHY

1. Andrish JT: Mensical injuries in children and adolescents: Diagnosis and management. J Am Acad Orthop Surg 4(5):231–237, 1996.
2. Beaty JH: Femoral shaft fractures in children and adolescents. J Am Acad Orthop Surg 3(4):207–217, 1995.
3. DaSilva MF, Williams JS, et al: Pediatric throwing injuries about the elbow. Am J Orthop 27(2):90–96, 1997.
4. Edwards PH, Grana WA: Physeal fractures about the knee. J Am Acad Orthop Surg 3(2):63–68, 1995.
5. Green NE, Swiontkowski MF (eds): Skeletal Trauma in Children, Vol. 3, 2nd ed. Philadelphia, W.B. Saunders, 1998.
6. Richards BS (ed): Orthopaedic Knowledge Update: Pediatrics. Rosemont, IL, American Academy of Orthopaedic Surgeons, 1996.
7. Skaggs DL: Eblow fractures in children: Diagnosis and management. J Am Acad Orthop Surg 5(6):303–312, 1997.
8. Stanitski CL: Acute slipped capital femoral epiphysis: Treatment alternatives. J Am Acad Orthop Surg 2(2):96–106, 1994.
9. Stanitski CL: Anterior cruciate ligament injury in the skeletally immature patient: Diagnosis and treatment. J Am Acad Orthop Surg 3(3):146–158, 1995.

61. BURNS

Gail E. Besner, M.D.

1. How common are pediatric burns?
Each year approximately 440,000 children receive medical treatment for burns in the United States. Over 20,000 of these children require hospitalization, 10,000 suffer severe permanent disability, and 2500 die from thermal injury.

2. What are the most common causes of pediatric burns?
Two-thirds of pediatric burns are from scalds due to household accidents or child abuse. Scald burns are the most common types of burns in children under the age of 3 years. In older children, flame burns become more common. Because 20% of child abuse cases present as burns, child abuse must be ruled out in caring for burn patients.

3. What factors determine the severity of burns in children?
The severity of the burn is related directly to the depth of the burn and the percentage of body surface area that is injured.

4. How is the depth of burn classified?

PARTIAL VS. FULL THICKNESS	DEGREE	APPEARANCE	RESULT
Partial thickness: very superficial with injury to epidermis only	First	Wounds are dry but extremely erythematous and painful	Heals spontaneously within 1 wk without scarring
Partial thickness: superficial with injury to epidermis and superficial dermis	Second	Ruptured, weeping blisters, erythematous, painful	Heals spontaneously within 2–3 wk, usually without scarring
Partial thickness: deep with injury to epidermis and deeper dermis, but some viable dermis remains	Second	Wound appears whiter and less erythematous as depth into dermis increases. May be hard to distinguish from full-thickness burns initially	Heals spontaneously, but often after 3–4 wk. Degree of hypertonic scarring related to length of time needed for re-epithelialization
Full thickness: injury to epidermis and entire dermis	Third	White, brown, or black, leathery, insensate eschar	Will not heal (except for very small wounds that heal by contraction)

Children under 2 years of age have disproportionately thin skin. As a result, burns that initially appear to be of partial thickness may turn out to be full thickness in depth. Thus, the child's thin skin makes initial determination of the severity of the burn difficult.

5. How is the percentage of involved body surface area calculated in children with burns?
Pediatric rule of nines. This method is the most useful initially, because it gives a quick estimate of the percentage of body surface area (% BSA) involved. An adaptation of the adult rule of nines, the pediatric rule of nines takes into consideration that in children the relative size of the head is larger and the relative size of the lower extremities is smaller.

Lund and Browder charts. The most accurate method of determining % BSA is to map the injured areas on a Lund and Browder chart. These charts detail more precisely the % BSA represented by each area of the body, according to the age of the patient.

246

Estimate based on the patient's palm. This method is useful for small, scattered burns and is based on the estimate that the patient's palm represents approximately 1% BSA.

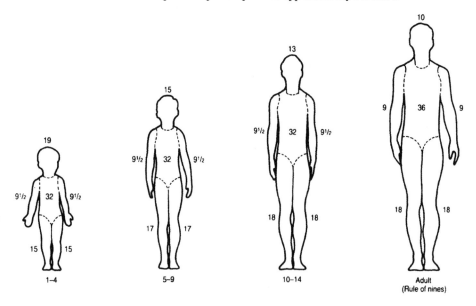

The pediatric rule of nines. Numbers = % BSA. (From Herndon DN (ed): Total Burn Care. Philadelphia, W.B. Saunders, 1996, p 351; with permission.)

6. What are the priorities in the treatment of pediatric burns?

The first priority, as with all trauma victims, is rapid assessment and treatment of immediate life-threatening conditions. The ABCs of trauma must be followed: an airway is established, breathing is maintained, and circulation is assessed. Endotracheal intubation is indicated in children with significant respiratory distress or airway compromise due to glottic or upper airway edema. Because the smaller diameter of the pediatric airway predisposes it to obstruction, a low threshold for intubation should be maintained to avoid potential disaster. Children with burns greater than 10% BSA should receive intravenous fluid resuscitation. Attention must be paid to keeping the pediatric burn patient warm, because thermoregulation is limited by greater body surface area, lesser body muscle mass, and inability of infants under 6 months of age to shiver. Once the ABCs are covered, a secondary survey is done, including a complete history and physical exam. The burn wounds themselves initially need to be covered only with dry sterile sheets in the emergency department. Tetanus immunization should be administered as needed.

7. How does the pediatric airway differ from the adult airway?

The infant's larynx is located more cephalad than the adult's, resulting in more acute angulation of the glottis. Repeated unsuccessful attempts at intubation may create additional edema, leading to complete airway obstruction. Thus, someone experienced in intubation of the pediatric airway is needed to intubate such patients.

A quick estimate of the size of the endotracheal tube that is needed is given by the diameter of the child's small finger or external nares. Cuffed endotracheal tubes are rarely needed in children, because the narrowest part of the airway is in the subglottic region. Open cricothyroidotomy is discouraged in children under 12 years of age. A large-bore needle placed through the cricothyroid membrane also may be used to obtain an emergent airway, if needed.

8. How does fluid resuscitation differ in pediatric and adult burn patients?

Because of the large ratios of body surface area to body mass in children, fluid losses are proportionately greater in children than in adults. Consequently, children have relatively greater needs for resuscitation fluids and greater evaporative water loss relative to weight than adults.

Ringer's lactate solution should be used initially in pediatric patients of all ages at 3–4 ml/kg/% BSA burned for the first 24 hours. One-half of the calculated fluid needs are administered in the first 8 hours, and the remaining half is administered over the next 16 hours. Maintenance fluids also should be administered. Maintenance requirements are 100 ml/kg/day for the first 10 kg of body weight plus 50 ml/kg/day for each kg of body weight from 11 to 20 kg plus 20 ml/kg/day for each kg body weight above 20 kg. Most importantly, rates of fluid administration are altered according to the patient's response. Very young patients are at risk of developing hypoglycemia due to limited glycogen reserves; therefore, blood glucose levels should be monitored and Ringer's lactate solution with 5% dextrose used as needed.

9. How is the response to fluid administration best assessed in pediatric burn patients?

By measurement of urine output via an indwelling urinary catheter. In children weighing less than 30 kg, urine output should be 1 ml/kg/hour. In children weighing greater than 30 kg, a urine output of 30–50 ml/hour should be maintained. Adequacy of resuscitation also is assessed by monitoring sensorium, blood pH, and peripheral circulation.

10. Identify useful routes of fluid administration in pediatric burn patients.

Intravenous access may be obtained percutaneously or by cutdown, either peripherally or centrally. Peripheral access in an unburned area is preferred. Intraosseous infusion may be lifesaving in severely burned patients if intravenous access is problematic.

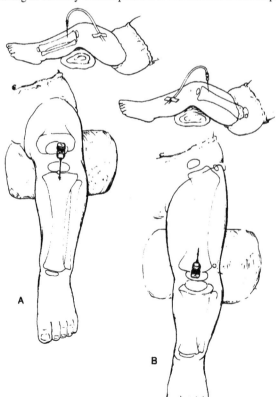

Intraosseous line placement in the proximal tibia *(A)* and distal femur *(B)*. (From Fleisher G, Ludwig S (eds): Textbook of Pediatric Emergency Medicine. Baltimore, Williams & Wilkins, 1998, p 1268; with permission.)

11. What are the complications of inhalation injury in pediatric patients?

Upper airway injury. Clues to inhalation injury above the glottis include facial burns, singed nasal hairs, soot in the mouth, carbonaceous sputum, hoarseness, coughing, labored breathing, wheezing, stridor, and confusion. Upper airway obstruction is treated with endotracheal intubation until airway edema resolves.

Lower airway injury. Smoke inhalation also may cause a chemically induced inflammatory reaction in the airways, leading to microbial colonization and pneumonia. Affected patients may need ventilatory support. In severe cases, the oscillating ventilator and even extracorporeal membrane oxygenation have been used successfully.

Carbon monoxide toxicity. All patients with actual or suspected inhalation injury should be treated for carbon monoxide toxicity with 100% inspired oxygen until carbon monoxide toxicity is ruled out or carboxyhemoglobin levels return to normal (< 5%).

12. What are the indications for admission of pediatric burn patients?
- Partial-thickness burns greater than 10% total BSA
- Full-thickness burns greater than 2% total BSA
- Inhalation injury
- Significant burns of face, hands, perineum, and feet
- Circumferential burns
- Burns over major joints
- Electrical burns (except for minor low-voltage injuries)
- Chemical burns
- All burns caused by child abuse

13. When is an escharotomy needed?

Escharotomy may be needed to relieve vascular compromise (extremity escharotomy) or ventilatory impairment (chest wall escharotomy). Vascular compromise to an extremity results from circumferential, full-thickness, inelastic eschar. Underlying tissue edema results in impaired venous outflow, followed by impaired arterial inflow if not treated. All extremity burns at risk should be monitored with at least hourly vascular checks of palpable or audible Doppler pulses. One should treat the condition immediately and not wait for loss of pulses, for by that time neurovascular damage is already occurring. Decreased Doppler signals or direct measurement of compartment pressures with pressures > 40 mmHg necessitates extremity escharotomy.

The chest wall and lungs are more compliant in children than in adults. Children, therefore, may become rapidly exhausted by the edema and restriction of a circumferential chest wall burn. Impaired ventilation, with progressive increase in ventilatory requirements, may signal the need for chest wall escharotomy.

14. How is escharotomy performed?

Escharotomy is typically performed in areas of full-thickness injury; therefore, analgesics are not needed. Incisions can be made with a scalpel, but the electrocautery device is preferable. Extremity escharotomy is begun with a longitudinal incision medially or laterally in the extremity, beginning above the burned area and extending below the inferior aspect of the burn. The incision is carried down to the subcutaneous fat, which bulges into the wound once an adequate incision is made. If pulses do not return with one incision, a second incision on the opposite side of the extremity is made. Adequate escharotomy should produce return of arterial pulses. Chest wall escharotomy is performed with incisions along the anterior axillary lines bilaterally, extending onto the abdomen, with transverse bridging incisions across the chest. Adequate chest wall escharotomy improves thoracic compliance and ventilation.

15. When and how should nutritional support be administered?

Nutritional support should be started as soon as possible after injury. Enteral feeds are preferred. Calorie counts should be recorded by a dietitian and daily weights obtained. A high-calorie, high-protein diet should be ordered. Many pediatric burn patients, however, cannot ingest enough calories by mouth to meet nutritional goals. In such cases, a postpyloric feeding tube should be placed and tube feeds administered.

16. How should the cutaneous injury be treated?

Devitalized skin and ruptured blisters should be debrided. Topical antibiotic therapy should be used to delay bacterial colonization. Silver sulfadiazine cream (Silvidine) is the most commonly used first-line agent because of its broad spectrum of activity, relatively painless application, and few side effects. It is applied as a thin layer with gauze dressings twice daily. Facial burns usually are treated with Neosporin ointment because Silvidine cream on the face may enter the eyes and cause severe irritation. Ear burns should be treated with the more potent Sulfamylon cream, because the thin subcutaneous tissue in the ears predisposes to the development of chondritis. To avoid the need for painful dressing changes, a number of artificial skin substitutes, including Biobrane, may be used for the treatment of partial-thickness burns in either the inpatient or outpatient setting. Once adherent to the burn surface, the dressing stays in place until re-epithelialization is complete.

17. When should a burn undergo skin grafting?

Full-thickness burns (with the exception of very small injuries that are allowed to heal by contraction) should be grafted. Early excision and grafting are used to decrease the incidence of invasive burn wound sepsis. The goal is to excise the wound within the first week of injury. In addition, deep partial-thickness burns that take longer than 3 weeks to heal usually benefit from grafting, with less hypertrophic scarring and better cosmetic result. Burn excision involves tangential removal of serial thin layers of devitalized tissue until a healthy well-vascularized wound bed is obtained. Skin grafting involves harvesting partial-thickness pieces of skin (autografts) from donor sites on unburned areas using a dermatome. The harvested grafts then are applied to the excised wound bed and secured in place.

18. What other options are available for wound closure?

Autograft skin is always preferred for skin grafting. Unfortunately, in large burns, the availability of enough donor site skin may be a limiting factor. In such cases, burns can be excised and temporarily covered with a number of biologic dressings (cadaver skin, pigskin) or skin substitutes. As autograft donor sites become available, the temporary wound coverings are removed and the wounds regrafted.

19. What is the difference between meshed and nonmeshed autografts?

Meshed autografts are harvested from the donor sites and then passed through a meshing machine that cuts a series of parallel offset slits in the grafts at various expansion ratios (e.g., 1:1, 2:1, 3:1, 4:1). This techniques allows the grafts to be expanded so that a greater surface area can be covered with each autograft. In addition, the interstices in the meshed grafts allow any fluid or blood that accumulates under the graft to extrude through the interstices into the overlying dressings so that the grafts do not lift off their beds. Unfortunately, the meshed patterns of the grafts persist after the grafts heal, often leading to a suboptimal cosmetic result.

Nonmeshed or sheet grafts are harvested from the donor sites in the same way but are not passed through a meshing machine. The use of sheet grafts leads to a better cosmetic result. Because the grafts cannot be expanded, however, it is difficult to cover major areas of injury with sheet grafts alone. Nonetheless, sheet grafts should be used whenever possible, especially in highly visible and functional areas such as the face, hands, neck, and joints. Meticulous attention to hemostasis is necessary, and the grafts should be inspected after approximately 48 hours so that any underlying fluid collections can be aspirated.

20. How are chemical burns treated?

Chemical burns are treated in children as in adults. Saturated clothing should be removed, powdered chemicals should be brushed off the skin, and the contaminated area shold be irrigated with copious amounts of water for at least 20 minutes until the patient experiences a decrease in pain in the wound. Chemical injuries to the eyes are treated by forcing the eyelid open and flushing the eye with water or saline. Petroleum products may cause severe full-thickness cutaneous tissue damage, and absorption of the hydrocarbon may cause pulmonary, hepatic, or renal failure.

21. How are pediatric electrical burns classified?

Low-voltage injuries, which result from sources of < 1000 volts, include oral injuries from biting an electrical cord, outlet injuries from placing an object into a wall socket, or injuries from contacting a live wire or appliance indoors.

High-voltage injuries, which are caused by sources of > 1000 volts, result from contact with a live wire outdoors or being struck by lightning.

22. How are pediatric electrical burns managed?

Children who have sustained **high-voltage electrical injury** require admission to the hospital (often initially to the intensive care unit), with cardiac monitoring, serial electrocardiograms, urinalysis, and determination of creatine phosphokinase and urine myoglobin levels. Myoglobinuria and hemoglobinuria should be treated aggressively with hydration, osmotic diuretics, and alkalinization of the urine to avoid renal failure. Extremities should be monitored carefully for the development of compartment syndromes, and escharotomy or fasciotomy should be carried out as needed.

Many pediatric patients who have sustained **low-voltage electrical injuries** can be treated on an outpatient basis. Hospital admission can be avoided when (1) the patient has no cardiac dysfunction, loss of consciousness, or history of tetany or wet skin during the accident; (2) the patient remains asymptomatic after 4 hours of observation in the emergency department; (3) the cutaneous wounds can be managed appropriately in the outpatient setting; and (4) the patient can return for a wound check on the following day. Parents of patients with oral commissure burns need to be instructed in the application of pressure to the lip in the event that the burn erodes into the labial artery, a complication that usually does not develop until several days after the injury.

23. How is frostbite recognized and treated?

Frostbite usually involves the ears, nose, hands, and feet and results from prolonged exposure to severe cold. Ice crystal formation in the tissues results in cellular dehydration, venous dilation and vasoconstriction result in peripheral blood pooling, and the end result is tissue necrosis. Signs and symptoms include red, blue, or pale skin, a prickling sensation with superficial frostbite, painless rigid skin with deep frostbite, and functional impairment. Treatment involves placing the patient in a warm environment, removing articles of clothing from the affected region, and rewarming the affected area by immersion in water at 100–105°F for up to 30–45 minutes. Do not rewarm the frozen part with massage or dry heat.

24. How can accidental scald burns in the home be avoided in children?

Water temperature of 130°F is tolerated for up to 30 seconds before an adult is burned. However, because of the thinner skin in children, only 10 seconds of exposure at the same temperature is required for injury. At 140°F, the common setting of home water heaters, burning occurs in less than 5 seconds in children and instantaneously in infants. Therefore, home water heaters should be set at less than 120°F to avoid such injuries. If the home water heater is inaccessible, various safety devices are available to indicate safe water temperatures for home use.

25. When are systemic antibiotics used?

Prophylactic systemic antibiotics are not used in the treatment of burn patients because they increase the risk of infection with resistant organisms. Systemic antibiotics are reserved for the treatment of specific infections and are administered at the first sign of clinical infection. Antibiotic regimens are modified as culture and antimicrobial sensitivity results become available.

26. How are hypertrophic scarring and contractures treated in burn patients?

The best treatment is to avoid the development of such problems. Burns that take more than 2 weeks to heal and all grafted burns should be treated with compression garments that apply about 30 mmHg pressure to the wounds, which has been found to decrease hypertrophic scar formation. In addition, silicone gel pads may be placed in specific areas under the garments to apply extra pressure to difficult areas.

Burns over joints should be treated with stretching and range-of-motion exercises during the healing process. A splinting regimen is often useful as well. Aggressive attention to physical and occupational therapy is necessary to ensure optimal results.

27. What is the prognosis in pediatric burns?

With the exception of infants, the prognosis for survival in children and adolescents is quite good. In the past decade the size of a survivable injury has increased from 70% BSA to > 95% BSA in children under 15 years of age.

Intraosseous line placement in the proximal tibia *(A)* and distal femur *(B)*. (From Fleisher G, Ludwig S (eds): Textbook of Pediatric Emergency Medicine. Baltimore, Williams & Wilkins, 1998, p 1268, with permission.)

BIBLIOGRAPHY

1. Demling RH, LaLonde C (eds): Burn Trauma. New York, Thieme, 1989.
2. Herndon DN, Rutan RL, Alison WE, Cox CS: Management of burn injuries. In Eichelberger MR (ed): Pediatric Trauma: Prevention, Acute Care and Rehabilitation. St. Louis, Mosby, 1993, pp 568–590.
3. McDonald WS, Sharp CW, Deitch EA: Intermediate enteral feeding in burn patients is safe and effective. Ann Surg 213:177–183, 1991.
4. Rutan R, Benjamin D: Special considerations of age: The pediatric burned patient. In Herndon DN (ed): Burn Care. Philadelphia, W.B. Saunders, 1993, pp 350–356.
5. Zubair M, Besner G: Pediatric electrical burns: Management strategies. Burns 23:413–420, 1997.

62. CHILD ABUSE

Paula Mazur, M.D.

1. What does child abuse have to do with pediatric surgery?

Head injury, abdominal trauma, broken bones, and burns in children are usually managed by pediatric surgical subspecialists. These injuries may be accidental or inflicted by the child's caretaker.

2. How can I tell the difference between accidental and inflicted injury?

First, ask yourself if the injury that you see on physical or radiologic exam could have resulted from the mechanism described by the child's caretaker.

3. What if the caretaker does not know how the injury occurred?

It is hard to know whether the caretaker is telling or avoiding the truth. These aspects of the history should raise the suspicion of child abuse:
- The history of injury is vague and/or changes over time.
- There was a delay in seeking treatment for the injury.
- The child's developmental stage does not match the caretaker's account of the injury.

4. Do I tell the family that I am concerned about child abuse?

Yes. Tell them that this is one of your concerns. The child will need to undergo additional medical and social evaluation because of your suspicions of abuse. Families are more cooperative if approached honestly and nonjudgmentally early in the medical investigation of suspected abuse. They also should understand that you are a mandated reporter, bound by law to report suspected cases of abuse to child protective services.

5. Can I be penalized if I report a case, but the injury is ultimately believed to be accidental?

No. A mandated reporter is any person dealing with children in a professional capacity. A mandated reporter can be punished by law for *failure to report* suspected abuse or neglect but is immune from litigation for making an unfounded report. Clearly, state law encourages you to make the report.

6. Where do I call to make a report?

The state's child protection hot line. Any facility that cares for children should have this phone number readily available.

7. What further medical evaluation needs to be done when I suspect child abuse?

Your investigation becomes forensic. Regardless of the child's presenting injury, you must identify and document all new and old injuries suffered by the child. This requires a careful physical exam with inspection of the skin for scars, bruising, or burns; inspection of the genitalia for evidence of sexual abuse; and radiologic and laboratory studies to identify occult injuries. Photographs of all visible injury should be taken. If a formal rape exam is conducted, a chain of custody must be established for the evidence.

Family court, in particular, bases its judgment on the "preponderance of the evidence." The more evidence collected, the stronger is the argument for child abuse.

8. Is the color of a bruise helpful in determining time of injury?

Recently this question has become controversial. Although bruises undergo a predictable sequence of color change during resolution (red-blue-green-yellow-brown), the rate of resolution varies with the depth of the bruise, the part of the body bruised, and the age of the child. A resolving bruise may demonstrate several colors at the same time. Child abuse specialists have moved away from using bruise color to date an injury. Instead, they emphasize bruise pattern and distribution on the body.

9. How do inflicted bruises differ from accidental bruises?

Accidental bruises usually are found on bony prominences (shins, knees, elbows, forehead) and tend to be unilateral in distribution. Inflicted bruises are often bilateral in distribution, occur in soft fleshy parts of the body that are unlikely to be struck during a fall (facial or buttock cheeks, thighs, calves), and may assume the pattern or shape of the inflicting object (e.g., hand print, bite mark, belt buckle, electrical cord loop, hairbrush bristles). Inflicted bruises are frequently found on the posterior side of the child's body, because the victim usually tries to run away from the perpetrator during the beating.

	ACCIDENTAL BRUISES	INFLICTED BRUISES
Location	Bony prominences	Soft, fleshy body areas
Distribution	Unilateral	Bilateral
	Front and back of body	Concentrated on posterior side of body (victim runs away from perpetrator)
Appearance	Nonspecific shape	Assumes pattern of inflicting object (hand print, belt, cord, brush)

10. How can you tell that a bite mark is from an adult perpetrator and not another child?

You cannot tell by visual inspection. There may be as little as a 7-mm size difference between the dental arch of an adult and a child. A dentist with forensic training can determine if the bite is from an adult or child by studying the depth of the bite mark at various points along the arch. Primary and secondary teeth bite at different depths along the dental arch. Bite marks may be associated with sexual abuse.

11. What are the physical findings in a child who has been sexually abused?
You may see evidence of trauma in the perineal area. The hymen may be thickened and scarred. The posterior fourchette may be torn or scarred. However, most victims of sexual abuse have no gross physical findings. They should be referred to a child abuse specialist trained in colposcopic examination and forensic interview techniques.

12. When are burns suspicious for abuse?
The distribution of the burn on the child's body and a history incompatible with this distribution or with the child's developmental abilities are clues to abuse. Common sense plays a great role. For an infant to pull a cup of hot liquid over, he or she has to have some ability to grasp objects willfully. For a child to reach up and pull a cup of hot liquid off the tabletop, he or she would have to be able to stand, creep, or walk. And no self-respecting toddler voluntarily holds the hands under hot water long enough to sustain a full-thickness burn.

	ACCIDENTAL BURNS	INFLICTED BURNS
Pattern	Random with splash marks	Immersion pattern: the burn margin is at a uniform level on the body and is circumferential on the trunk or limbs
	Body creases are burned`	Body creases are spared as the child tries to withdraw limbs from hot water (withdrawal sign)
Depth	Varies because liquid cools as it runs down the body	Uniform throughout

13. Which radiologic studies are used in the medical investigation of abuse?
The skeletal survey is the most widely used screening test in child abuse evaluations. This study should include two views of each bone in the body, and each section of the skeleton must be x-rayed separately. A "babygram," in which the infant's entire skeleton is viewed on one x-ray plate, does not provide an adequate survey for fractures that are highly specific for abuse. Roughly 30% of all skeletal surveys show additional stigmata of abuse.

14. Should all children with suspicious injuries receive a skeletal survey?
Skeletal survey has the highest yield in the youngest children. Roughly speaking, the easier it is to pick up, shake, or throw a child, the more you expect to find on survey. It is recommended in children 5 years of age or less and highly recommended in children less than 2 years of age.

15. Which fractures are highly specific or suspicious for abuse?
Posterior rib fractures, metaphyseal fractures, healing fractures that were not brought to medical attention, large bone fractures for which no significant mechanism of injury is offered by the caretaker (femur, sternum, scapula), and long-bone fractures in nonambulatory infants. It is particularly concerning if you find fractures of different ages in the same skeletal survey. This finding suggests that abuse has occurred on more than one occasion.

16. Can posterior rib fractures occur accidentally?
It is widely postulated that a posterior rib fracture occurs when the rib cage is rocked or shaken around the vertebral column. The transverse vertebral process acts as a fulcrum for the posterior rib at its articulation, and the rib fractures on its pleural surface, not its ventral surface. Posterior rib fractures are not commonly seen when a blunt external force is applied to

the rib cage. They do not occur as a result of chest compression during cardiopulmonary resuscitation (CPR).

17. Why is a metaphyseal fracture highly suspicious for abuse?

The metaphysis is the region of newly formed bone adjacent to the growth plate. This area contains the most delicate bone trabeculae. Ironically, in a pediatric long bone the periosteum is most tightly attached at the metaphysis. When a long bone is forcefully pulled or twisted, periosteal tension is transmitted to the delicate metaphyseal region, where a fine linear fracture occurs through the metaphysis. A metaphyseal fracture implies a forceful twisting or pulling of the long bone. This fracture appears as a corner fracture or a bucket-handle fracture next to the growth plate on radiographs.

18. What is the difference between a bucket-handle fracture and a corner fracture?

They are the same fracture caught in different planes by the x-ray beam. They are alternate terms for the metaphyseal fracture.

19. Are spiral long bone fractures also suspicious for abuse?

A spiral configuration to a fracture implies that a twisting force has broken the bone, but spiral fractures do occur accidentally in ambulatory children. If a long-bone shaft fracture of any configuration (spiral, transverse, oblique) occurs in a nonambulatory infant or child, abuse should be considered.

20. Do some children have brittle bones?

The existence of temporary brittle bone disease, a proposed collagen enzyme-processing deficiency, is highly controversial. Keep in mind that child abuse is far more common than any condition resulting in fragile bones. In rickets you see osteopenia, cupping at the ends of the long bones symmetrically, and widened ribs at the costochondral junction (rachitic rosary). Osteogenesis imperfecta types I and IV are most often misdiagnosed as child abuse, but their overall incidence is less than 1 per 30,000 live births. They are usually autosomal dominant and may be associated with osteopenia, blue sclera, deafness, short stature, and abnormal dentition.

21. How accurately can fractures be dated?

Radiographs usually distinguish between fresh and healing fractures, but fractures cannot be dated exactly. The timing of bone changes in a healing fracture varies with the nature of the fracture and the age of the child. On radiographs a fresh fracture has sharp margins and is surrounded by soft tissue swelling. Loss of the sharp fracture line begins 10–14 days after injury. Bone callous forms at 14–42 days.

22. Do bone scans help in the dating of fractures?

No. A bone scan highlights an area of the skeleton within hours of the injury but cannot differentiate multiple-aged fractures. Bone scan is most useful for identifying areas of the skeleton that require more detailed radiography to rule out occult fracture. Because fresh posterior rib fractures are difficult to see on plain radiograph, bone scan is helpful. A positive bone scan must be verified by subsequent radiographs.

23. What is shaken baby syndrome?

Shaken baby syndrome (SBS) is a constellation of clinical and radiologic findings that are believed to have resulted from a violent shaking episode with or without impact of the infant's head against a surface. SBS is the subcategory of child abuse with the highest mortality rate and neurologic morbidity. Approximately 25% of shaken infants die early in their hospitalization, and most survivors have permanent neurologic disability, ranging from a complete vegetative state to mental retardation with motor disabilities.

24. How does a shaken infant present to the hospital?

It is believed that upon violent shaking, usually in an attempt to stop crying, infants immediately lose consciousness. The perpetrator then places or throws the now quiet infant into its crib and waits for the infant to return to a normal state. Intracranial injury from the shaking episode progresses, and eventually the caretaker calls for help or brings the infant to the hospital because the infant remains lethargic, stops breathing, or seizes secondary to intracranial injury. The infant often displays no obvious signs of physical abuse on presentation.

25. If there are no signs of abuse on exam, how can we begin to identify a shaken infant?

It is easy to miss the diagnosis of SBS. Pediatric subspecialists always must keep trauma in the differential diagnosis of infants with altered mental status. A computed tomography (CT) scan of the head must be obtained early in the hospital course to look for intracranial hemorrhage. **Subdural hematomas** are markers of SBS in infants with altered mental status.

26. Is the subdural hematoma primarily responsible for neurologic injury in SBS?

No. Subdural hematoma is a marker of SBS. Diffuse axonal injury (DAI) is believed to be the major pathology. Shaking an infant's head produces acceleration and deceleration forces that combine to exert shearing or tearing forces on intracranial structures. The cerebral bridging vessels tear and bleed into the subdural space. More significantly, neurons are torn along their axons. The torn neurons die, resulting in permanent loss of brain tissue. DAI has been identified microscopically at autopsy of shaken infants.

27. Is subdural hematoma the only easily identified finding of SBS?

SBS is a constellation of clinical and radiologic findings. There may be evidence of cerebral contusion or skull fracture on CT or at autopsy if the infant's head was impacted during the assault, but these findings are not essential to the diagnosis of SBS. **Retinal hemorrhages** are usually seen on ophthalmologic examination of the shaken infant. Retinal hemorrhages are considered diagnostic of SBS.

28. Can other conditions cause retinal hemorrhages?

The retinal hemorrhages of SBS are simultaneously of several different configurations and in several layers of the retina. They are seen in the vitreous, intraretinally, and subretinally. They appear as boat-shaped, flame, and dot-and-blot hemorrhages. No other medical condition has been associated with these retinal findings. CPR does not cause retinal hemorrhage. It is estimated that 30% of newborn infants have retinal hemorrhages at birth regardless of the method of delivery. Birth hemorrhages resolve within the first 3–4 weeks of life.

29. Are the retinal hemorrhages of SBS easily seen with a direct ophthalmoscope?

They may be. However, indirect ophthalmoscopy should be performed by an ophthalmologist to document definitively the presence of retinal hemorrhage. Indirect ophthalmoscopy allows visualization of the peripheral retina for hemorrhage that may be missed with a direct ophthalmoscope, and indirect ophthalmoscopy enables photography of the retina for legal documentation.

30. What else should be considered when SBS is suspected?

The shaken infant is a victim of child abuse; therefore, all of the previously mentioned stigmata of abuse should be looked for as well. Many shaken infants have suffered previous episodes of abuse and are found to have resolving bruises and healing fractures. In addition, many shaken infants also have been battered and may have serious intrapulmonary and/or intraabdominal injury that must be identified.

31. Should the victim of child abuse be considered a multiple trauma victim?

Absolutely. The same trauma protocol applied to the victim of a motor vehicle accident applies to the child who has been severely physically abused.

BIBLIOGRAPHY

1. Bergen R, Margolis S: Retinal hemorrhages in the newborn. Ann Ophthalmol 8:53–56, 1976.
2. Dalton HJ, Slovis T, et al: Undiagnosed abuse in children younger than 3 years with femoral fracture. Am J Dis Child 144:875–878, 1990.
3. Langlois NEI, Gresham GA: The ageing of bruises: A review and study of the colour changes with time. Foren Sci Int 50:227–238, 1991.
4. Kleinman PK: Diagnostic Imaging of Child Abuse, 2nd ed. St. Louis, Mosby, 1998.
5. Reece RM: Child Abuse: Medical Diagnosis and Management. Philadelphia, Lea & Febiger, 1994.
6. Stephenson T: Ageing of bruising in children. J R Soc Med 90:312–314, 1997.
7. Thomas SA, Rosenfield NS, et al: Long-bone fractures in young children: Distinguishing accidental injuries from child abuse. Pediatrics 88:471–476, 1991.
8. Tosi L: Osteogenesis imperfecta. Curr Opin Pediatr 9:94–99, 1997.

63. INJURY PREVENTION

David E. Wesson, M.D.

1. Who was William Haddon, Jr.? What is Haddon's matrix?

Haddon was an orthopedic surgeon who pioneered the scientific approach to injury prevention. He combined the classic epidemiologic model of the causes of disease—host, agent, and environment—and the idea that injuries can be prevented before, during, and after the event into a matrix that greatly clarifies the approach to injury prevention. Interventions directed at the host, agent, and environment before, during, and after the event can produce beneficial results.

	HOST	AGENT	ENVIRONMENT
Before the event	Age Experience Alcohol Drugs Speed	Defects Brakes Tires Avoidance systems	Visibility Pavement Signals Constructions
During the event	Belt use Helmet use Tolerance	Air bag Automatic belts Crash-worthiness	Guardrails Medians Breakaway posts
After the event	Age Physical condition	Fire Fuel leaks	Emergency medical service (EMS) First responder Bystander care

2. Name the three main categories of injury prevention strategies that correspond to Haddon's before-, during-, and after-the-event phases.

- Primary: eliminate crashes through better highway design.
- Secondary: reduce injuries in crashes by better car design.
- Tertiary: improve outcome for crash victims by improving the EMS system.

3. What is the underlying mechanism in pediatric trauma?

The basic mechanism is energy transfer from the environment to the host (i.e., the child).

4. Describe the public health approach to injury prevention.

There are five essential steps:
- Surveillance: what is the problem?
- Risk identification: what are the causes from the perspective of host, agent, and environment?

- Intervention: what is the best prevention strategy?
- Implementation: how can you apply the best strategy to the population at risk?
- Outcome: did it work?

5. What are the four Es of injury prevention?
- Education
- Enactment/enforcement
- Engineering
- Economic

These measures complement each other. For example, voters will not accept legislation until they have been educated. This principal was true for seat belt laws and probably will be true for gun control.

6. What is meant by active and passive injury prevention?

Active prevention requires an action on the part of the host, whereas passive prevention works automatically. Seat belts are active; air bags are passive.

7. Which works better—active or passive injury prevention?
Passive.

8. Name five factors that affect injury risk.
- Age
- Gender
- Family income
- Parental education
- Race

9. Are there any exceptions to the preponderance of boys in pediatric trauma?
Yes. In young children girls and boys are equally at risk for motor vehicle occupant injuries.

10. Name six proven injury prevention strategies.
- National highway speed limits
- Cycle helmet use
- Child passenger restraint laws
- Apartment window guards
- Smoke detectors
- Violence prevention programs

11. Do the causes of fatal unintentional injury vary with age throughout childhood?

Yes. The leading causes of death from unintentional injuries for the standard statistical age groups are:
- < 1 year: suffocation
- 1–4 years: drowning
- 5–9 years: motor vehicle occupant
- 10–14 years: motor vehicle occupant

12. What is the most common environment for childhood injury?
The home.

13. What is the most lethal agent in the child's environment?
The motor vehicle.

14. Who is Robert Saunders? Why is he famous?

Saunders is a pediatrician from Tennessee who started the ball rolling for child motor vehicle occupant protection laws. Such laws are now in force in all 50 states, the District of Columbia, and all U.S. territories.

15. What is the safest seat position for children up to 12 years of age riding in cars?
The back seat. Front-seat air bags can be dangerous for children younger than 12 years.

16. What type of restraint is appropriate for a newborn, a 2-year-old who weighs 12 kg, and a 7-year-old who weighs 22 kg?
- Newborn: rear-facing child safety seat
- 2-year-old: forward-facing child safety seat
- 7-year-old: booster seat with seat belt

17. What is the difference between a hockey helmet and a bike helmet?
A hockey helmet is designed to absorb multiple low-energy blows. A bike helmet is designed to absorb a single high-energy impact and is damaged or destroyed in a crash. Hockey helmets are used repeatedly; bike helmets should be discarded after a significant impact.

18. What is the most lethal sport in America?
Fishing. More people die while engaged in this sport than in any other, usually by drowning and often under the influence of alcohol or other drugs.

19. How do you install a child safety seat?
With great care and only after reading several times the instructions that come with the seat and the vehicle owner's manual.

20. Are death rates for homicide of children in the U.S. increasing or decreasing?
Decreasing. In 1998 the rate was 37% below the peak reached in 1991.

21. What is the leading cause of death among children 0–14 years of age in the U.S.?
Motor vehicle crashes account for 18% of all deaths and 37% of all injury-related deaths.

22. Are injury death rates higher in urban or rural communities?
Rural.

23. What can an individual physician do to prevent injuries?
- Be a role model; walk the talk.
- Look for injury patterns and prevention opportunities in your own practice.
- Participate in well-planned community-based prevention programs.
- Lobby for legislation to prevent injuries.
- Lobby for support of injury prevention research.
- Conduct research on the effectiveness of injury prevention strategies and programs.

BIBLIOGRAPHY

1. American College of Surgeons Web Site: <http://www.facs. org/about college/acsdept/trauma dept/in-jread.html >
2. Guyer B, Hoyer DL, Martin JA, et al: Annual Summary of Vital Statistics–1998. Pediatrics 104:1229, 1999.
3. National Center for Injury Prevention and Control Web Site: <http://www.cdc.gov/ncipc/factssheets/childh.htm>
4. Rivara FP, Grossman DC, Cummings P: Injury prevention. N Engl J Med 337:543, 1997.
5. Rivara FP, Grossman DC, Cummings P: Injury prevention. N Engl J Med 337:613, 1997.
6. Stevenson JE, Spurlock C, Nypaver M: Factors associated with the higher traumatic death rate among rural children. Ann Emerg Med 27:625, 1996.

XI. Tumors and Oncology

64. NEUROBLASTOMA

Michael P. La Quaglia, M.D.

1. What is neuroblastoma?
Neuroblastomas are tumors derived from primordial neural crest cells. These cells normally populate the adrenal medulla, sympathetic ganglia, and a number of other sites. Neuroblastomas demonstrate a broad spectrum of biologic behavior from highly malignant to benign. Ganglioneuromas, neoplasms related to neuroblastomas, are benign tumors consisting of ganglion cells that are the endpoint of differentiation of primitive neural crest cells. Neuroblastoma is categorized as a small, round, blue cell tumor of childhood.

2. What is the incidence of neuroblastoma in childhood?
The overall rate is 9.1 per million children, according to Surveillance Epidemiology and End-Results (SEER) data. The incidence for males is 9.4 per million; for females, is 8.9 per million. These figures translate into about 650 new cases in the United States per year.

3. At what age is neuroblastoma most likely to occur?
Neuroblastoma has a much higher incidence in infancy, as can be appreciated in the figure below.[4]

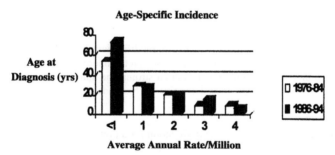

Age-Specific Incidence

Age at Diagnosis (yrs)

□ 1976-84
■ 1986-94

Average Annual Rate/Million

4. How do patients present clinically?
The clinical presentation may be related to the effects of the primary tumor or metastatic deposits. An abdominal primary tumor may cause pain or a mass effect. A large thoracic primary can cause respiratory distress. Transforaminal epidural extension may cause paralysis or bladder and bowel dysfunction. A cervical primary tumor can result in Horner's syndrome due to stellate ganglion involvement. Metastatic deposits also can be symptomatic, depending on the site. Bilateral orbital metastases can cause "raccoon's eyes," which result from periorbital ecchymoses due to intraorbital hemorrhage. Extensive hepatic metastases can result in severe abdominal distention and respiratory embarrassment in stage 4S patients. Long-bone metastases result in pain on ambulation or limping.

5. Where can neuroblastoma present anatomically? To which sites does it metastasize?
The most common primary anatomic site is the adrenal gland (35%) followed by the retroperitoneum (30%), mediastinum (19%), pelvis (2%), neck (1%), and miscellaneous primary

sites (12%). The most common metastatic site is the bone marrow. Other common sites of dissemination include cortical bone, lymph nodes, liver, and skin. Hepatic and skin metastases usually are observed in infants with stage 4S disease.

6. What staging system is used for neuroblastoma?

At present the universally accepted staging system is the International Neuroblastoma Staging System (INSS).

7. Define stage 1 neuroblastoma. At what age are patients with stage 1 neuroblastoma most likely to present?

INSS stage 1 is defined as a localized tumor confined to the area of origin and completely excised with or without a positive microscopic margin. Ipsilateral and contralateral lymph nodes are microscopically negative. Stage 1 disease usually occurs in newborns or infants.

8. Define stages 2a and 2b neuroblastoma.

Stage 2a neuroblastoma is a unilateral tumor with incomplete gross excision but without lymph node involvement. Stage 2b is a unilateral tumor that is either completely or incompletely excised and with positive ipsilateral but negative contralateral lymph nodes.

9. Define stage 4 and stage 4S neuroblastoma.

Stage 4 involves tumor dissemination to distant sites such as bone, bone marrow, distant lymph nodes (4N), and liver. Stage 4S is defined as a localized primary tumor with dissemination limited to the bone marrow, skin, and/or liver. The amount of marrow infiltration is less than 10%. Stage 4S usually occurs in infants, whereas most stage 4 tumors occur in patients older than 12 months.

10. What is the Shimada classification?

The Shimada histopathologic classification with modifications by Joshi is similar to a grading system that seeks to define prognostic groups based on the microscopic characteristics of the untreated primary tumor. The amount of extracellular stroma, the number of mitoses and karyorrhexis per 5000 cells, and age at diagnosis determine the Shimada classification.

11. What is *MYCN*?

MYCN (pronounced "miccans") is the designation for a proto-oncogene of important prognostic significance in neuroblastoma. Normally we have two copies of the *MYCN* gene. Human neuroblastoma tumors can have more than 100 (about 25% of stage 4 and fewer lower-stage tumors). *MYCN* amplification, defined as more than 10 copies, is associated with poor prognosis; patients require intense therapy.

12. What are *Trk* genes? How do they relate to human neuroblastoma?

Trk genes (pronounced "track") are related to the nerve growth factor receptor. Increased expression of *Trk-A* mRNA or protein in neuroblastoma tumor cells is associated with a good prognosis.

13. What prognostic factors are clinically used to assess risk in human neuroblastoma?

Age at diagnosis, INSS stage, and *MYCN* amplification are the most significant factors in multivariate analysis. Other factors include loss of heterozygosity on the short end of the first chromosome (LOH 1p), gain of DNA on chromosome 17q, tumor ploidy, *Trk-A* expression, and serum ferritin and lactic dehydrogenase (LDH) levels at diagnosis. Older age (> 12 months), higher stage, increased *MYCN* copy number (> 10 copies), the presence of DNA loss on chromosome 1p or gain on 17q, a diploid tumor, lack of *Trk-A* expression, serum LDH > 1500, and a high serum ferritin (usually > 147–150 ng/ml) are associated with worse prognosis.

14. How are high-, low-, and intermediate-risk neuroblastomas defined?

VARIABLE	LOW RISK	INTERMEDIATE RISK	HIGH RISK
Karyotype or ploidy	Hyperdiploid/ triploid	Near-diploid or near-tetraploid	Near-diploid, near-tetraploid
MYCN	Normal (< 3 copies)	Normal	> 10 copies
Chromosome 1p	Normal	± 1p LOH	± LOH
Age at diagnosis	Usually < 12 mo	Usually > 12 mo	Usually > 12 mo
INSS stage	Usually 1, 2, 4S	Usually 3, 4	Usually 3, 4
Survival	95%	25–50%	~5%

From Brodeur GM, Castleberry RP: Neuroblastoma. In Pizzo PA, Poplack DG (eds): Principles and Practice of Pediatric Oncology, vol. 1. Philadelphia, Lippincott-Raven, 1997, pp 761–792, with permission.

15. What is the current treatment for stage 1 and stage 2 neuroblastoma?

The answer must be qualified by assuming that these patients have biologically favorable stage 1 and 2 tumors. This assumption usually is valid, but occasionally an adverse biologic factor can place a stage 2 patient into an unfavorable category. If the biology is favorable, however, the treatment of stage 1 and 2 tumors is excision alone. The importance of assessing adverse biologic factors cannot be overemphasized.

16. What is the present treatment for stage 3 neuroblastoma?

If the stage 3 tumor is of low biologic risk, surgery alone may be adequate treatment. If the biology is not favorable, preoperative chemotherapy is administered first, followed by complete excision. Considerable evidence in the literature indicates that gross total resection of stage 3 tumors correlates with better survival.

17. How are patients with stage 4 neuroblastoma treated?

Almost all stage 4 patients are high risk biologically. Treatment consists of neoadjuvant chemotherapy followed by second-look resection of the primary tumor. High-dose chemotherapy with combinations of active agents such as doxorubicin, cyclophosphamide, cisplatin, and etoposide is administered. Second-look surgery is usually done after four cycles of multiagent chemotherapy.

18. How does treatment differ for patients with stage 4S neuroblastoma?

Stage 4S patients can be distinguished from stage 4 patients by a younger age at diagnosis (often under 6 months) and pattern of metastases. Stage 4S tumors usually resolve without treatment. The exceptions are cases with massive hepatic enlargement and subsequent respiratory embarrassment. Such infants usually require chemotherapy and sometimes external-beam radiotherapy to control hepatic enlargement. They also may require placement of an abdominal wall silo to relieve an abdominal compartment syndrome.

19. Are biologic therapies used to treat neuroblastoma?

Yes. Retinoic acid and monoclonal antibody therapy are two examples of biologic agents presently used in the treatment of neuroblastoma.

20. Is autologous bone marrow transplant of use in the treatment of neuroblastoma?

Yes. Autologous bone marrow or stem-cell transplant is now accepted as an important component in the treatment of high-risk stage 3 or 4 neuroblastoma.

21. When is radiotherapy used to treat patients with neuroblastoma?

Neuroblastoma is fairly radiosensitive. Low-dose radiotherapy (2100 cGy) is often used after surgical excision for local control of the primary tumor or involved lymph node chains in patients with high-risk neuroblastoma. Newborns and small infants with rapidly enlarging hepatic metas-tases in stage 4S often receive whole-liver external-beam radiation as well.

22. What is the overall survival rate for stage 4 (high-risk) neuroblastoma?
With modern therapy stage 4 patients have an overall survival rate of approximately 40–50% at 5 years from diagnosis.

23. What is the objective of diagnostic biopsy in neuroblastoma?
Assessment of biologic factors is of great importance in determining the appropriate treat-ment of a child with neuroblastoma. Many of these factors can be assessed only with gross tissue samples from the tumor (Shimada, *MYCN*, ploidy, 1p LOH, *Trk-A*)—not on fine-needle aspira-tion cytology. The surgeon should obtain at least a cubic centimeter of tissue (preferably more) at the primary biopsy.

24. When is definitive resection performed in high-risk neuroblastoma?
Usually after the fourth cycle of chemotherapy. Resection at diagnosis usually is associated with more complications, such as nephrectomy, and a lower likelihood of gross total excision.

25. Does resecting the primary tumor require negative microscopic margins?
No. The objective of neuroblastoma surgery is gross total resection. Obtaining a negative mi-croscopic margin is rarely feasible. Most tumors are wrapped around or adjacent to major unre-sectable vascular structures, including the aorta and vena cava. No layer of normal tissue that might constitute a margin is interposed.

26. What are the results of mass screening for neuroblastoma?
Mass screening by analysis of urinary catecholamines has been performed in Japan and Quebec for a number of years. The data from these studies suggest that neuroblastomas of low biologic risk are detected by screening but not aggressive tumors. Mass screening does not seem to have an effect on neuroblastoma-associated mortality.

BIBLIOGRAPHY

1. Brodeur GM, Castleberry RP: Neuroblastoma. In Pizzo PA, Poplack DG (eds): Principles and Practice of Pediatric Oncology, vol. 1. Philadelphia, Lippincott-Raven, 1997, pp 761–792.
2. Cheung NKV, Kushner BH, Cheung IY, et al: Anti-GD2 antibody treatment of minimal residual stage 4 neuroblastoma diagnosed at more than 1 year of age. J Clin Oncol 16:3053–3060, 1998.
3. Combaret V, Gross N, et al: Clinical relevance of TRKA expression on neuroblastoma: Comparison with N-MYC amplification and CD44 expression. Br J Cancer 75:1151–1155, 1997.
4. Goodman MT, Gurney JG, Smith MA, Olshan AF: Sympathetic nervous system tumors. In Ries L, Smith MA, Gurney JG, et al (eds): Cancer Incidence and Survival among Children and Adolescents: United States SEER Program 1975–1995. Bethesda, MD, National Cancer Institute SEER Program, 1999.
5. Haase GM, Atkinson JB, et al: Surgical management and outcome of locoregional neuroblastoma: Comparison of the Childrens Cancer Group and the International Staging Systems. J Pediatr Surg 30:289–294; discussion, 295, 1995.
6. Joshi VV, Rao PV, et al: Modified histologic grading of neuroblastomas by replacement of mitotic rate with mitosis karyorrhexis index. A clinicopathologic study of 223 cases from the Pediatric Oncology Group. Cancer 77:1582–1588, 1996.
7. Kushner BH, Cheung NK, et al: Survival from locally invasive or widespread neuroblastoma without cy-totoxic therapy. J Clin Oncol 14(2):373–381, 1996.
8. La Quaglia MP, Kushner BH, et al: Stage 4 neuroblastoma diagnosed at more than 1 year of age: Gross total resection and clinical outcome. J Pediatr Surg 29:1162–1165, 1994.
9. Powis MR, Imeson JD, et al: The effect of complete excision on stage III neuroblastoma: A report of the European Neuroblastoma Study Group. J Pediatr Surg 31:516–519, 1996.
10. Seeger RC, Brodeur GM, et al: Association of multiple copies of the N-myc oncogene with rapid pro-gression of neuroblastomas. N Engl J Med 313:1111–1116, 1985.
11. Shamberger RC, Allarde-Segundo A, et al: Surgical management of stage III and IV neuroblastoma: Resection before or after chemotherapy. J Pediatr Surg 26:1113–1117; discussion, 1117–1118, 1991.

65. WILMS' TUMOR

Daniel M. Green, M.D.

1. What is the incidence of Wilms' tumor?
The incidence of Wilms' tumor is 11.1 cases per million in white males less than 15 years of age and 9 cases per million in white females less than 15 years of age. The incidence is approximately 3 times higher for blacks in the United States and Africa than for East Asians.

2. What is WAGR syndrome?
WAGR syndrome is the association of Wilms' tumor, aniridia, genitourinary malformation, and mental retardation.

3. What is Denys-Drash syndrome?
Denys-Drash syndrome is the association of male pseudohermaphroditism and/or renal disease (glomerulonephritis or nephrotic syndrome) with Wilms' tumor.

4. What tumors may occur in Beckwith-Wiedemann syndrome?
Beckwith-Wiedemann syndrome, which includes macroglossia, omphalocele, and visceromegaly, is associated with Wilms' tumor, hepatoblastoma, rhabdomyosarcoma, and adrenal cortical carcinoma.

5. What is WT1?
WT1 is the Wilms' tumor suppressor gene located at 11p13. The gene is deleted in WAGR syndrome and has point mutations in Denys-Drash syndrome. Point mutations in this gene occur in approximately 5% of sporadic Wilms' tumors.

6. From which parent are new germ-line deletions of the WT1 gene transmitted in WAGR syndrome?
With one exception, all new deletions of the WT1 gene in the WAGR syndrome have been transmitted from the father.

7. What other chromosomal loci contain Wilms' tumor-associated genes?
Additional Wilms' tumor-associated genes are located at 16q (disease progression gene), 11p15.5 (Wilms' tumor-associated tumor suppressor gene), 17q12-q21 (familial Wilms' tumor gene), and 7p13 (Wilms tumor-associated tumor suppressor gene.

8. Where is the earliest known Wilms' tumor specimen located?
The earliest known specimen of Wilms' tumor is on display in the Hunterian Museum of the Royal College of Surgeons in London. This specimen of bilateral renal tumors from a young infant was prepared by John Hunter, who died in 1793.

9. From what tissue is Wilms' tumor derived?
Wilms' tumor is thought to be composed of or derived from primitive metanephric blastema. In addition to expressing a variety of cell types and aggregation patterns in the normally developing kidney, these neoplasms often contain tissues not found in the normal metanephros, such as skeletal muscle, cartilage, and squamous epithelium.

10. What are the most frequent histologic patterns in childhood renal tumors?
The most frequent histologic patterns in childhood renal tumors are Wilms' tumor, Wilms' tumor with focal or diffuse anaplasia, clear cell sarcoma of the kidney, and rhabdoid tumor of the kidney.

11. What childhood renal tumor frequently metastasizes to bones?
Clear cell sarcoma of the kidney.

12. What childhood renal tumors frequently metastasize to the brain?
Rhabdoid tumor of the kidney and clear cell sarcoma of the kidney.

13. What are the most frequent signs and symptoms at initial presentation in children with Wilms' tumor?
The most frequent signs and symptoms at initial presentation in children with Wilms' tumor are abdominal mass (75%), abdominal pain (28%), hypertension (26%), gross hematuria (18%), microscopic hematuria (24%), fever (22%), and urinary frequency (4%).

14. What are the signs of obstruction of the spermatic vein or inferior vena cava?
A varicocele secondary to obstruction of the spermatic vein may be associated with the presence of a tumor thrombus in the renal vein or inferior vena cava. Persistence of the varicocele when the child is supine is highly suggestive of venous obstruction.

15. What initial radiographic examination should be performed for the evaluation of an abdominal mass?
The initial radiographic study should be an abdominal ultrasound examination, which demonstrates whether the abdominal mass is solid or cystic and may allow identification of the organ of origin as well as measurement of the maximal diameter of the mass. It also allows assessment of the patency of the inferior vena cava.

16. What radiographic study should be performed to determine whether pulmonary metastases are present?
A plain chest radiograph should be obtained to determine whether pulmonary metastases are present. Computed tomography of the chest is not reliable because of substantial interobserver variation in interpretation. In addition, the finding of pulmonary nodules on chest computed tomography does not mandate modification of treatment for Wilms' tumor.

17. Are a bone scan and skeletal survey required for the pretreatment evaluation of a child with a renal tumor?
A bone scan and skeletal survey are required only for children who have clear cell sarcoma of the kidney.

18. Is a magnetic resonance imaging scan of the brain required for the pretreatment evaluation of a child with a renal tumor?
A magnetic resonance imaging scan of the brain is required only for children who have a clear cell sarcoma of the kidney or rhabdoid tumor of the kidney.

19. What surgical approach is used for nephrectomy and abdominal staging of a child with Wilms' tumor?
The transperitoneal approach to the tumor is the standard procedure because it allows inspection and biopsy of the regional lymph nodes, even if they appear normal, and permits mobilization of the opposite kidney, which should be inspected on all its surfaces for evidence of a synchronous bilateral tumor or evidence of nephrogenic rests, which may not be identified on preoperative imaging studies.

20. What is the rate of intestinal obstruction if the contralateral kidney is or is not explored during the laparotomy at which the nephrectomy for Wilms' tumor is performed?
In the National Wilms' Tumor Study 3, the frequency of intestinal obstruction was 5.6% in patients who had not undergone contralateral renal fossa exploration after Gerota's fascia was

opened compared with 6.9% among all patients evaluated for surgical complications. No patient suffered renal injury as the result of contralateral renal exploration.

21. Which patients with Wilms' tumor should receive prenephrectomy chemotherapy?
Prenephrectomy chemotherapy should be administered to patients who have intravascular extension of tumor thrombus to the intrahepatic vena cava or more proximally, including to the right atrium, and children with bilateral Wilms' tumor.

22. How often does Wilms' tumor present with involvement of both kidneys?
Synchronous bilateral Wilms' tumor occurs in 4.4–7.0% of patients.

23. What is the treatment for children with stage I or II Wilms' tumor and favorable histology?
The treatment for children with stage I or II Wilms' tumor and favorable histology is nephrectomy followed by 18 weeks of combination chemotherapy with vincristine and dactinomycin.

24. What is the treatment for children with stage III Wilms' tumor and favorable histology?
The treatment for children with stage III Wilms' tumor and favorable histology is nephrectomy followed by tumor-bed or whole-abdomen irradiation and 21 weeks of combination chemotherapy with vincristine, dactinomycin, and doxorubicin.

25. What is the treatment for children with stage IV Wilms' tumor and favorable histology?
The treatment for children with stage IV Wilms' tumor and favorable histology is nephrectomy followed by whole-lung irradiation and 21 weeks of combination chemotherapy with vincristine, dactinomycin, and doxorubicin. Tumor-bed or whole-abdomen irradiation is given if the intraabdominal tumor is stage III.

ACKNOWLEDGMENT

The author thanks the investigators of the Pediatric Oncology Group and the Children's Cancer Group and the many pathologists, surgeons, pediatricians, radiation oncologists, and other health professionals who managed the children entered in the National Wilms' Tumor Studies.The author also thanks Diane Piacente for preparation of the manuscript. Supported in part by USPHS Grant CA-42326.

BIBLIOGRAPHY

1. Diller L, Ghahremani M, Morgan J, et al: Frequency of constitutional mutations in the WT1 gene in patients with Wilms tumors. J Clin Oncol 16:3634–3640, 1998.
2. Green DM: Wilms tumor. Eur J Cancer 33:409–418, 1997.
3. Green D, Breslow N, Beckwith J, et al: A comparison between single dose and divided dose administration of dactinomycin and doxorubicin. A report from the National Wilms Tumor Study Group. J Clin Oncol 16:237–245, 1998.
4. Green DM, Breslow NE, Beckwith JB, et al: The effect of duration of treatment on outcome and cost of the treatment for Wilms tumor. A report from the National Wilms Tumor Study Group. J Clin Oncol 16:3744–3751, 1998.
5. Green DM, Coppes MJ, Breslow NE, et al: Wilms' tumor. In Pizzo PA, Poplack DG (eds): Principles and Practice of Pediatric Oncology, 3rd ed. Philadelphia, Lippincott-Raven, 1997, pp 733–759.
6. Meisel JA, Guthrie KA, Breslow NE, et al: Significance and management of computed tomography detected pulmonary nodules. A report from the National Wilms Tumor Study Group. Int J Rad Oncol Biol Phys 44:579–585, 1999.
7. Wilimas JA, Kaste SC, Kauffman WM, et al: Use of chest computed tomography in the staging of pediatric Wilms' tumor: Interobserver variability and prognostic significance. J Clin Oncol 15:2631–2635, 1997.

66. HEPATIC TUMORS

Scott C. Boulanger, M.D., Ph.D., and Michael G. Caty, M.D.

1. What percentage of primary liver tumors in children are malignant? What are the most common types?

Approximately 70% of primary pediatric liver tumors are malignant. They account for 2% of all childhood malignancies. Most are hepatoblastomas (HB) and hepatocellular carcinomas (HCC); mesenchymal sarcoma (mesenchymoma) is quite rare.

2. At what age do HB and HCC commonly occur?

Most HBs develop in children between the ages of 1 and 3 years; two-thirds occur by 24 months of age. The incidence appears fairly constant throughout the world. There is a slight male preponderance (1.5:1). HCC generally presents in the adolescent years, with a mean age of onset of 12 years. The male-to-female ratio is approximately 2:1.

3. HB and HCC occur with increased frequency in which diseases?

Although HB generally occurs sporadically, it has been found in association with Beckwith-Weidemann syndrome and hemihypertrophy. HB also has been found in children with kidney or renal agenesis and children whose parents are afflicted with familial adenomatous polyposis (FAP). These observations may be explained by certain genetic abnormalities that are commonly seen in HB. Examples include trisomy of chromosomes 2 and 20 and loss of heterozygosity of the short arm of chromosome 11 (11p). Beckwith-Weidemann syndrome also has been localized to the short arm of 11. Of interest, Wilms' tumor and rhabdomyosarcoma also map to chromosome 11p. Genetic mapping and the increased incidence of HB in families with FAP suggest that chromosome 11p probably is home to a tumor suppressor gene.

HB also is associated with fetal alcohol syndrome, maternal ingestion of oral contraceptives and gonadotropins, and parental exposure to some paints, metals, and petroleum products. Other associated factors include Fanconi's syndrome, cirrhosis, type I glycogen storage disease, tyrosinemia, and cholestasis induced by total parenteral nutrition. HB also has been seen many years after successful treatment of right-sided Wilms' tumor with chemotherapy and radiation.

HCC commonly is associated with cirrhosis due to hepatitis B infection, familial cholestasis, and alpha$_1$-antitrypsin deficiency, all of which lead to a nonspecific reaction called giant cell hepatitis.

4. What radiologic tests should be obtained?

Several radiographic tests are obtained routinely in the evaluation of a liver mass. All patients should get abdominal and chest radiographs. The chest radiograph is obtained to rule out pulmonary metastases. Abdominal radiographs may demonstrate a mass effect in the right upper quadrant, as well as calcifications. Ultrasound examination of the abdomen reliably determines the tumor's organ of origin and differentiates solid from cystic lesions. In addition, the kidneys, hepatic veins, portal vein, and vena cava can be evaluated for tumor involvement.

Abdominal imaging using contrast-enhanced computed tomography (CT) or magnetic resonance imaging (MRI) provides valuable information about tumor relationship to the regional vasculature. Some studies suggest that MRI is superior to CT in determining resectability and detecting recurrent disease. CT of the chest should be obtained to evaluate for metastases.

5. Should arteriography be routinely performed?

In the past, arteriography was obtained routinely to evaluate the hepatic vasculature. However, better understanding of liver anatomy and better imaging with spiral CT and MRI make this test generally unnecessary.

6. What is the most valuable lab test in the evaluation of HCC? Why?

Serum alpha-fetoprotein (AFP) level probably provides the most information, both diagnostically and therapeutically. Ninety-three percent of patients with hepatic epithelial malignancy have an elevated AFP. However, elevated AFP also can be seen in malignant teratomas and germ-cell tumors of the ovaries and testes. In addition, both HB and HCC occur in association with low AFP. Therefore, it is not currently recommended to initiate chemotherapy on the basis of elevated AFP and imaging studies alone.

Ferritin levels also have been shown to increase in HCC as well as in cirrhosis. Perhaps the most valuable role for AFP and ferritin levels is to detect recurrence. Additionally, the absolute level of AFP may have prognostic significance in HCC, although this does not appear to be the case for HB.

7. What are the staging systems for HB and HCC?

Staging of HB and HCC according to the Children's Cancer Group and Pediatric Oncology group is based on findings at surgery, results of the initial operation, and pathology. Of interest, tumor size is not part of the staging criteria.

Stage I   Complete resection of primary tumor
Stage II   Complete resection of gross tumor with residual microscopic disease
Stage III   Gross residual disease after surgery of unresectable tumor
Stage IV   Metastatic disease

8. What are the histologic subtypes of HB? Which is associated with a more favorable outcome?

HB is classified as pure epithelial or mixed epithelial/mesenchymal. Pure epithelial HB can be subdivided into fetal, embryonal, macrotrabecular, and small cell. Mixed tumors are subdivided into teratoid or nonteratoid. Nonteratoid is the most common (34%), followed by fetal (31%) and embryonal (19%). In several series, the fetal subtype has been associated with improved outcomes in patients with completely resectable tumors. A review of 105 cases at the Armed Forces Institute of Pathology failed, however, to confirm this finding.

9. Which histologic variant of HCC may have a more favorable outcome?

A variant of HCC, known as fibrolamellar carcinoma, occurs primarily in noncirrhotic livers. Patients generally range in age from 5 to 23 years. This tumor is characterized by polygonal cells associated with dense fibrous stroma, which sometimes give the tumor an appearance similar to that of focal nodular hyperplasia. Several studies suggest prolonged survival in patients with fibrolamellar carcinoma. Five-year survival rates up to 62% have been reported in small series of patients. The CCG/POG series failed to confirm significant survival advantage, however. Complete resection also appears to be more common in this histological subtype.

10. What is the treatment of choice for malignant liver tumors?

Complete resection is the treatment of choice. This approach involves formal lobectomy or trisegmentectomy. Advances in pre- and postoperative care and improvements in technique have lowered the mortality rate for liver resection to less than 5%.

Laparotomy can be performed through an abdominal approach or through a liver transplant incision. Large tumors may require a thoracoabdominal incision. The tumor then is evaluated for resectability. If the tumor is unresectable, a biopsy should be performed. Because survival is clearly improved in patients with complete resection, it should be performed if at all possible. Even in the case of bilobar disease, complete lobectomy with wedge resection of up to three nodules is reasonable.

11. Does liver transplantation have a role in the treatment of malignant tumors?

Experience with hepatic transplantation for patients with unresectable disease confined to the liver is limited. Of interest, recent reports of transplantation from the Children's Hospital of Pittsburgh, among others, seem to be encouraging. Survival rates of 83% for HB and 44% for

HCC after a mean of 21 months follow-up have been reported. Currently, transplantation is considered for children with unresectable disease limited to the liver after chemotherapy.

12. What is the role of laparoscopy in the management of malignant liver tumors?

For tumors deemed unresectable by CT or MRI, a biopsy specimen is required before initiation of chemotherapy. The specimen can be obtained by CT- or ultrasound-guided biopsy or by laparoscopy. It may be reasonable in the future to explore all patients with laparoscopy to ascertain resectability, much as for adult pancreatic cancer.

13. Adjuvant therapy is advisable for which stage of HB and HCC?

Currently adjuvant therapy is used for all stages of HCC and HB. The best survival rate is obtained with stage I disease treated with chemotherapy (85–95%). Complete resection alone achieves a survival rate of approximately 66%. Unfortunately, stage II disease carries a much worse prognosis even with chemotherapy. Unresectable disease is incurable.

Chemotherapy regimens for stage I disease include doxyrubicin and cisplatin or cyclophasphamide, vincristine, and 5-fluorouracil. Results of early trials by the Children's Cancer Study Group revealed that the combination of cisplatin and doxorubicin was effective in shrinking initially unresectable tumors to allow complete resection. Twenty five of 26 patients with HB had either partial or complete response. Twenty two underwent second-look laparotomy, and complete resection was done in 16 cases. Only one of the 16 developed recurrent disease. Unfortunately, patients with HCC fared much worse; only 14% of patients undergo complete resection of tumor at second look. Based on this study, aggressive chemotherapy is advised even for stage IV.

14. Are paraneoplastic syndromes associated with malignant hepatic tumors?

Yes. For example, male and female precocity as a result of gonadotropins and polycythemia as a result of erythropoietin have been described.

15. What is the most common presenting symptom of benign liver tumors?

Most benign lesions present as a painless mass in the right upper quadrant. Other common symptoms include pain (usually dull and aching), vomiting, anorexia and constipation.

16. What is the most common benign liver tumor in infants and children?

Hemangiomas are probably the most common benign tumor. They certainly are the most common benign lesion in adults. In children, they are found incidentally; because the treatment is nonoperative, usually no specimen is obtained to confirm pathology.

17. The triad of hepatomegaly, cutaneous hemangiomas, and congestive heart failure is seen in which tumor?

This triad of symptoms can be seen in hemangiomas of the liver. Cardiac failure results from arteriovenous shunting in the tumor. In addition, coagulopathy also may develop as a result of platelet trapping within the tumor (Kasabach-Merritt syndrome). Hemangiomas of the liver generally present before 6 months of age. CT scan often confirms the diagnosis. Tumors presenting with heart failure or coagulopathy may be treated medically with diuretics, steroids, and digoxin. Refractory tumors involving a single lobe can be resected. However, diffuse involvement of the liver requires alternative therapies, such as hepatic artery ligation or embolization and even transplantation. With these modalities, the mortality rate has been reduced to approximately 30% in severely symptomatic patients.

18. An abdominal ultrasound of a 6-month-old infant reveals a liver mass of both solid and cystic components that is well-demarcated from the surrounding tissue. Hepatic scintigraphy reveals reduced uptake. AFP is normal. What is the most likely diagnosis?

These findings are characteristic of a mesenchymal hamartoma, which most often presents within the first 2 years of life. These tumors more commonly are found in the right lobe and are solitary. They may be primarily cystic or solid and can present in a fashion similar to vascular tumors (i.e., with congestive heart failure). Treatment is resection, if possible. Large cystic lesions can be treated with unroofing and marsupialization.

19. What is the treatment of hepatic adenoma? Why?
Resection is the treatment of choice for patients in whom it can be performed safely. Resection is chosen because adenomas often are not distinguishable from HCC. Enucleation is a reasonable option during exploration if the lesion is clearly an adenoma. Although in adults adenomas have a propensity to rupture and bleed intraperitoneally, this problem is less common in children. However, it can be a reason for emergent operation.

Adenomas are unusual in children and appear to be related to anabolic steroid use, multiple transfusions for chronic anemia, and type I glycogen storage disease. Estrogen use is common in adults with this lesion and may be a consideration in teenage girls.

20. What is the classic finding on CT scan of focal nodular hyperplasia?
Focal nodular hyperplasia may be diagnosed on CT scan by the presence of a characteristic central stellate scar. These lesions are usually found incidentally and are much more common in females (4:1). Expectant management is the rule if the diagnosis can be made by CT and fine-needle biopsy.

BIBLIOGRAPHY

1. Bellanti FA, Massimino M: Liver tumors in childhood: Epidemiology and clinics. J Surg Oncol 3(Suppl):119–121, 1993.
2. Berman MM, Libbey NP, Foster JH: Hepatocellular carcinoma: Polygonal cell type with fibrous stromas—an atypical variant with a favorable prognosis. Cancer 46:702, 1980.
3. Conrad RM, et al: Hepatoblastoma: The prognostic significance of histological type. Pediatr Pathol Lab Med 12:167, 1992.
4. Guzzetta PC Jr, Raleigh Thompson W: Nonmalignant tumors of the liver. In O'Neill JA Jr, Rowe MI, Grosfeld JL, et al (eds): Pediatric Surgery. St. Louis, Mosby, 1998.
5. Haas JE, et al: Histopathology and prognosis in childhood hepatoblastoma and hepatocarcinoma. Cancer 64:1082, 1989.
6. King DR: Liver tumors. In O'Neill JA Jr, Rowe MI, Grosfeld JL, et al (eds): Pediatric Surgery. St. Louis, Mosby, 1998.
7. Pazdur R, Bready B, Cangir A: Pediatric hepatic tumors: Clinical trials conducted in the United States. J Surg Oncol 3(Suppl):127–130, 1993.
8. Weinberg AG, Finegold MJ: Primary hepatic tumors in childhood. Hum Pathol 14:512–537, 1983.

67. ENDOCRINE TUMORS

James D. Geiger, M.D.

THYROID DISORDERS

1. When should ectopic thyroid tissue be considered?
In every child with a midline neck mass such as thyroglossal duct remnants. Consider a preoperative ultrasound or thyroid scan for further evaluation, especially in the setting of hypothyroidism.

2. What cells form the lateral lobes of the thyroid?
C cells from the fourth ultimobranchial pharyngeal pouches, which contain and secrete calcitonin. They give rise to medullary thyroid cancer.

3. What are the most common causes of congenital hypothyroidism?
• Sporadic thyroid dysgenesis (75%)
• Thyroid enzyme deficits (10%)

• Transient hypothyroidism (10%)
• Hypothalamic pituitary dysfunction (5%)

4. What is the most common cause of hyperthyroidism in children?
Graves' disease, manifested by goiter, thyrotoxicosis, exophthalmos, and, rarely, pretibial myxedema.

5. What are the possible therapies for Graves' disease?
• Antithyroid drugs: thionamides (propylthiouracil); usually not definitive therapy.
• Radioactive iodine (^{131}I): used commonly in adolescents and adults.
• Surgical treatment: total or occasionally subtotal thyroidectomy may be the best therapy for young children.

6. Are solitary thyroid nodules common in children?
No. Thyroid nodules are rare compared with adults. A palpable thyroid nodule is of great concern because of an estimated 25–55% incidence of malignancy.

7. What is the number-one risk factor for thyroid cancer?
Radiation exposure associated with the treatment of head and neck malignancies (e.g., Hodgkin's disease) or fallout, as in the Chernobyl disaster in Belarus, has led to increased rates of thyroid cancer.

8. Describe the clinical presentation of childhood thyroid cancer.
• More common in teenage girls than teenage boys
• One or more firm nodules in the neck (often metastasis to a lymph node)
• 10–25% present with lung metastasis at diagnosis

9. List the three most common types of thyroid cancer in children in order of frequency.
• Papillary
• Follicular
• Medullary

10. How is differentiated thyroid cancer treated?
• Thyroidectomy (extent controversial)
• Radioactive iodine therapy (used to treat metastatic and recurrent disease)
• Thyroid hormone replacement (lifelong)

11. Do children die of thyroid cancer?
Yes, but rarely and usually not until they are adults. Survival rates exceed 90–95%.

12. Name two pediatric diseases associated with mutations in the *RET* proto-oncogene.
• Hirschsprung's disease
• Multiple endocrine neoplasia (MEN) 2A and 2B: medullary thyroid cancer (MTC)

13. How has identification of the *RET* proto-oncogene affected treatment of MEN2A/2B?
Prophylactic thyroidectomies now are performed at a young age in all patients with MEN 2A/2B found to have a mutation of the RET proto-oncogene.

14. How is medullary thyroid cancer treated?
Total thyroidectomy with central compartment lymph node dissection.

15. Describe the differences between MEN 2A and 2B.
• MEN 2A: parathyroid disease is common, occurring in about one-third of patients.
• MEN 2B: parathyroid disease is rare; characteristic facies, multiple mucosa neuromas, aggressive MTC.

16. What features do MEN 2A and 2B have in common?
Autosomal dominant, MTC, and pheochromocytomas.

PARATHYROID DISORDERS

17. Does primary hyperparathyroidism occur in children?
Yes, but it is rare. The incidence of hyperparathyroidism (HPT) is greater in adolescents and adults.

18. Does primary HPT occur in neonates?
Yes. Primary HPT can be fatal and usually is of the familial type.

19. Name the familial syndromes associated with HPT.

MEN 1	Familial hypocalciuric hypercalcemia
MEN 2A	Familial HPT

20. What is the treatment for primary hyperthyroidism.
Surgery. A simple adenoma is cured with excision; familial cases require more complex management, including subtotal parathyroidectomy ($3\frac{1}{2}$ glands) or four-gland thyroidectomy with immediate autograft.

PANCREATIC DISORDERS

21. Name the pancreatic disorder associated with high insulin levels and hypoglycemia.
Persistent hyperinsulinemic hypoglycemia of infancy or neonatal hyperinsulinemia, formerly and incorrectly known as nesidioblastosis.

22. What are the treatment options for neonatal hyperinsulinemia?
- Diazoxide
- Somatostatin analog
- Pancreatectomy (95%) in most cases; in some patients, partial pancreatectomy may be adequate if focal disease is localized by venous sampling.

23. Name the tumor that causes hyperinsulinism.
Islet cell adenoma (insulinoma). A functioning beta-cell adenoma is the most common tumor arising from the islet cells. Ninety percent are benign.

24. How is an insulinoma treated?
- Surgery
- Enucleation if the tumor is localized or in combination with distal pancreatectomy for non-localized lesions

25. A teenage girl without history of trauma has a cystic mass in the tail of the pancreas. What is the most likely diagnosis?
Mucinous cystadenoma. Mucinous cystic neoplasms of the pancreas usually are large and multilocular and should be excised completely because of a small chance of malignancy.

ADRENAL DISORDERS

26. Does the "rule of tens" apply to pediatric pheochromocytoma?
No. The rule of tens applies only to adults.

LESIONS	CHILDREN	ADULTS
Bilateral	25–50%	~10%
Extra-adrenal	~30%	~10%
Malignant	< 5%	~10%

27. Pheochromocytoma is one of the causes of nonessential hypertension that can be cured with surgery. Name the others.
- Cushing's syndrome
- Conn's syndrome (aldosteronoma/hyperplasia)
- Hyperthyroidism
- Renal artery stenosis/compression
- Coarctation of the aorta

28. What is the best test for a child suspected of having pheochromocytoma?
Urinary catecholamines. Order a 12–24 hour urine collection for vanillylmandelic acid and metanephrine.

29. Describe the management of a child with positive catecholamines.
- Preoperative alpha-adrenergic blocking with or without beta-adrenergic blocking agents
- Tumor localization with imaging studies (computed tomography, magnetic resonance imaging, metaiodobenzylguanidine study)
- Surgical excision of true pheochromocytoma with exploration of the opposite adrenal gland

30. What are the noniatrogenic causes of Cushing's syndrome in children?
- Cushing's disease (pituitary-dependent hypercortisolism): 85%
- Adrenocortical tumors: 10%
- Nonendocrine tumors producing corticotropin: 5%

31. How do children with Conn's syndrome (primary aldosteronism) present?
- Hypertension
- Weakness
- Polyria and polydipsia
- Hypokalemia

32. What is the treatment of Conn's syndrome?
Unilateral adrenalectomy for adenomas and spironolactone for idiopathic hyperplasia.

BIBLIOGRAPHY

1. Decker RA, Geiger JD, Cox CE, et al: Prophylactic surgery for MEN 2a following genetic diagnosis: Is parathyroid transplantation indicated? World J Surg 20:814–820, 1995.
2. DeLonlay-Debeney P, Poggi-Travert F, Fournet JC, et al: Clinical features of 52 neonates with hyperinsulinism. N Engl J Med 340:1169–1175, 1999.
3. Farahati J, Parlowsky T, Mader U, et al: Differentiated thyroid cancer in children and adolescents. Langenbecks Arch Surg 383:235–239, 1998.
4. Gillis D, Brnjac L, Perlman K, et al: Frequency and characteristics of lingual thyroid not detected by screening. J Pediatr Endocrinol Metabol 11:229–233, 1998.
5. Hundahl SA, Fleming ID, Fremgen AM, Menck HR: A National Cancer Database report on 53,856 cases of thyroid carcinoma treated in the U.S., 1985–1995. Cancer 83:2638–2648, 1998.
6. Nikiforov Y, Gnepp DR, Fagin JA: Thyroid lesions in children and adolescents after the Chernobyl disaster: Implications for the study of radiation tumorigenesis. J Clin Endocrinol Metabol 81:9–15, 1996.
7. O'Neill JA Jr, Rowe MI, Grosfeld JL, et al (eds): Pediatric Surgery, 5th ed. St. Louis, Mosby, 1998.
8. Shilyanski J, Fisher S, Cutz E, et al: Is 95% pancreatectomy the procedure of choice for treatment of persistent hyperinsulinemic hypoglycemia of the neonate? J Pediatr Surg 37:342–346, 1997.
9. Stringel G, et al: Pheochromocytoma in children: An update. J Pediatr Surg 15:496, 1980.
10. Turner MC, Lieberman E, DeQuattro V: The perioperative management of pheochromocytoma in children. Clin Pediatr 31:583, 1992.
11. Vassilopoulou-Sellin R, Goepfert H, Raney B, Schultz PN: Differentiated thyroid cancer in children and adolescents: Clinical outcome and mortality after long-term follow-up. Head Neck 20:549–555, 1998.
12. Wells SA Jr, Skinner MA: Prophylactic thyroidectomy based on direct genetic testing in patients at risk for the multiple endocrine neoplasia type 2 syndromes. Exp Clin Endocrinol Diabetes 106:29–34, 1998.

68. GERM CELL TUMORS

David A. Rodeberg and Charles Paidas, M.D.

1. What is the origin of a germ cell tumor?
Germ cell tumors originate from primordial germ cells, which originate from the zygote. The primitive germ cells migrate through the dorsal mesentery of the hind gut and reside in the gonadal ridges. For unknown reasons, abnormal migration results in a nest of cells in a midline ectopic position. Germ cell tumors commonly are located in the sacrococcygeal, retroperitoneal, and cervical regions as well as in the mediastinum and pineal gland.

2. What are the histologic types of germ cell tumors?
Germ cell tumors originate from the zygote, which differentiates into three types of tissue (yolk sac, fetus, and placenta). All germ cell tumors are derived from some combination of these three tissues. Germ cell tumors are classified as follows:
- Germinoma, gonadoblastoma, seminoma
- Embryonal carcinoma
- Yolk sac tumor (endodermal sinus tumor)
- Choriocarcinoma
- Teratoma (mature, immature)

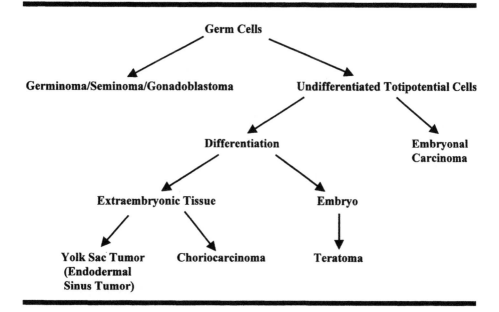

3. What are the most common types of malignant and benign germ cell tumors?
The yolk sac derivative (endodermal sinus tumor) is the most common malignant tumor, and teratoma is the most common benign tumor.

4. At what age are germ cell tumors diagnosed?
The answer depends on the type of tumor. As a general rule, extragonadal tumors occur in infants and young children, whereas gonadal tumors usually occur in adolescents. Sacrococcygeal

tumors are frequently found in infants < 2 years old, whereas mediastinal and retroperitoneal tumors are present in children > 2 years old. Ovarian tumors occur in girls 10–15 years old. The exception to this general rule is testicular tumors, which usually present in 2-year-old boys.

5. Are germ cell tumors more common in males or females?
They are much more common in females; 80% of cases occur in young girls.

6. What percentage of germ cell tumors are malignant?
20–30%.

7. List germ cell tumors from most to least aggressive.
The term *aggressive* denotes the capacity for tumor invasion and the development of metastatic lesions. Using these criteria, the most aggressive tumor is choriocarcinoma, followed by embryonal cell, yolk sac, germinoma, and teratomas (least aggressive).

8. Which tumors secrete markers? What are their half-lives?
- Alpha fetoprotein (αFP) is produced by yolk sac tumors and has a half-life of 4 days; it is normally high in neonates. Thus, check the measured value against a nomogram for the infant's age.
- Beta human choriogonadotropin (βHCG) is secreted from choriocarcinoma and testicular tumors. Any positive value is abnormal.
- Alkaline phosphotase and lactate dehydrogenase (LDH) may be elevated in children with germinoma-type tumors.

9. What is the definition of malignancy for germ cell tumors?
Malignant germ cell tumors contain any combination of the histologic subtypes of yolk sac carcinoma, embryonal carcinoma, germinoma, or choriocarcinoma. Most such tumors contain a component of yolk sac carcinoma and therefore have an elevated αFP. Malignancy should not be confused with tissue immaturity and the presence of neuroepithelial tissue. The histologic type of malignant tissue does not significantly affect outcome. All extragonadal malignant tumors receive the same therapy regimen, which depends only on staging.

10. What is the best predictor of outcome?
Extent of tumor as defined by stage is the best predictor of outcome. Patients' age, location of primary tumor, and tumor grade also should be considered. Grading of tumors is based on degree of immaturity and presence of neuroepithelium. The tumor is given a numerical value from 0 for mature with no neuroepithelium to 3 for immature with significant neuroepithelium.

11. Define the staging of germ cell tumors.
Stage I: localized disease completely resected.
Stage II: microscopic residual disease, capsular invasion, or microscopic involvement of the lymph nodes.
Stage III: gross residual disease, gross disease in the lymph nodes (> 2 cm or positive cytology in washings).
Stage IV: metastatic disease.

12. Who should receive adjuvant therapy?
A chemotherapy regimen consisting of cisplatin, etoposide, and bleomycin (PEB) is used for the treatment of stage I or II malignant nongerminomatous germ cell tumors. A regimen with a higher dose of cisplatin is used for patients with stage III or IV disease, although the higher dose is associated with a higher incidence of ototoxicity (74% compared with 10% for standard PEB). These regimens have increased overall 5-year survival from 20% to 60–80%. It is controversial to treat immature tumors with chemotherapy because 90% of children do well with operative resection alone. X-ray therapy may be beneficial in local control.

13. Who should undergo a second-look operation for germ cell tumors?

Children whose imaging studies demonstrate residual mass after chemotherapy or a subsequent new mass need a second look. In addition, a tumor marker that does not return to normal after resection or subsequently rises, even if radiographic studies are negative, mandates operation.

14. Describe adequate follow-up for all germ cell tumors.

Radiographic studies (ultrasound or computed tomography [CT]) and tumor markers every 6 months for 2 years and then annually for 3 years.

15. What is a Currarino triad?

It is not the next Three Tenors concert. This triad includes a presacral tumor, anal stenosis, and a scimitar type sacral anomaly. It is inherited in an autosomal dominant pattern with incomplete penetrance. The presacral tumor may be benign or malignant. Not all patients present with all three components of the triad.

16. When is emergency operation indicated for sacrococcygeal teratoma (SCT)?

When there is significant hemorrhage into the tumor in neonates, in the presence of congestive heart failure secondary to shunting, and at the onset of diffuse intravascular coagulation.

17. What is the preoperative work-up for SCT?

These children should have spine films and an MRI of the abdomen and pelvis. The germ cell tumors are frequently calcified. A chest radiograph should be obtained to rule out pulmonary metastases. And, of course, blood should be analyzed for tumor markers.

18. How is age related to the incidence of malignancy for SCT?

Usually the tumors in neonates (< 1 month) are benign (95%). In contrast, children older than 1 year have a much higher incidence of malignancy (80%).

19. What is the surgical treatment for SCT?

Operative excision. The incision is either a chevron over the tumor or a posterior sagittal approach. The middle sacral artery is ligated. The surgeon must remember to remove the coccyx, which frequently contains pleuripotential cells. Failure to remove the coccyx results in a 40% recurrence rate. The levator muscle complex is reconstructed after tumor removal. When a significant abdominal component is present, patients require separate incisions for the abdominal and sacral potions. The abdominal portion of the operation should be performed first.

20. What percentage of SCTs have an intraabdominal component?

The amount of tumor in the abdomen is described by the type of the tumor. Type I is predominately external, type II has some intraabdominal component, type III is predominantly intraabdominal, and type IV is exclusively intraabdominal. A total of approximately 55% have some intraabdominal component (45% are type II or III, and 10% are type IV). The tumors with an intraabdominal component are more likely to be malignant because of the late stage at diagnosis.

21. What is the most common location for nongonadal germ cell tumors?

Tumors originating from the sacrococcygeum account for approximately 50% of all germ cell tumors. These lesions are also the most common tumors in newborns.

22. What is the differential diagnosis for sacral masses?

The differential diagnosis includes SCT, meningocele, lipomeningocele, lipoma, chordoma, rectal duplication, and epidermoid cyst.

23. What percentage of patients with SCT have associated anomalies?

Approximately 20% of children have associated anomalies. Musculoskeletal anomalies are the most common. However, central nervous system, genitourinary, gastrointestinal, or cardiac systems also may be involved.

24. What are the presenting symptoms of SCT?

Most children are asymptomatic, but tumors may cause gastrointestinal or genitourinary obstruction due to compression. A neurologic deficit may indicate spinal involvement and/or malignancy.

25. Can SCT tumors recur?

Yes. About 25% recur locally. Risk factors for recurrence are age > 1 year, tumor immaturity, and elevated αFP. Sometimes a benign SCT can mutate and recur as a malignancy. All recurrences should be resected, followed by chemotherapy with ifosfamide, carboplatin, and etoposide.

26. What are the most common postoperative complications of SCT?

Approximately 20% of children experience fecal and urinary incontinence, probably secondary to either sacral plexus or pudendal nerve injury.

27. What determines malignancy in SCT?

About 25% of tumors are malignant. Malignancy is determined by the presence of malignant tissue such as yolk sac carcinoma, embryonal carcinoma, germinoma, or choriocarcinoma. Most commonly the SCT contains malignant tissue derived from the yolk sac. Such children frequently have an elevated αFP.

28. What is the blood supply to an SCT?

The middle sacral artery, which arises from the aorta at the iliac bifurcation.

29. What is the second most common site for nongonadal germ cell tumors?

The mediastinum. Mediastinal tumors usually are located in the anterior compartment and have a 20% malignancy rate because of a yolk sac component. They present most commonly with airway symptoms. Germ cell tumors account for 20% of all mediastinal tumors.

30. What test should be done in a boy with a mediastinal mass that is βHCG-positive?

Such patients require karotyping, because they frequently have Klinefelter's syndrome (XXY). A CT scan is the best test for assessing the mass and its effect on the airway.

31. What is the differential diagnosis for mediastinal masses in young children?

This list is long and includes anterior tumors (thymoma, thymic cyst, teratoma, cystic hygroma, lipoma), middle tumors (lymphoma, bronchogenic cyst), and posterior tumors (esophageal duplication, neurogenic tumors).

32. How do cervical germ cell tumors present? Where are they found?

Patients usually have antenatal polyhydramnios and some degree of respiratory distress due to pulmonary hypoplasia and airway compression. Cervical germ cell tumors are located beneath the strap muscles and extend posteriorly to the pretracheal fascia. They are usually benign (80%). Not infrequently, affected neonates require an EXIT procedure, which is performed by cesarean section with delivery of the infant onto the operative field and control of the airway. Only then is the umbilical cord clamped and divided. This procedure allows the newborn to be oxygenated through the placenta for approximately 50–60 minutes, while the airway is managed.

33. What percentage of germ cell tumors occur in the gonads?

Gonadal tumors occur most commonly in older children and adults; they account for about 50% of all germ cell tumors.

34. How do ovarian germ cell tumors present?

Ovarian germ cell tumors are usually asymptomatic. More commonly they present as vague abdominal or pelvic pain with increasing abdominal girth in girls between 5 and 15 years of age. Rare patients present with acute abdominal pain secondary to ovarian torsion.

35. How are ovarian germ cell tumors diagnosed and treated?

An abdominal ultrasound is usually diagnostic for ovarian masses. Like any other ovarian tumor, these lesions are treated by salpingo-oophorectomy, omentectomy, peritoneal washings, and peritoneal biopsies. Bivalving the other ovary is no longer necessary. Surgical resection is adequate for benign disease. All children with malignant germ cell tumors should receive PEB chemotherapy.

36. At what ages do testicular germ cell tumors occur? How do they present?

The age distribution is bimodal and includes children less than 2 years old as well as adolescents. Tumors present as asymptomatic nontender masses that progressively increase in size. On examination they are easily confused with hydrocele, appendix testis, varicocele, and hernia.

37. What is the preoperative work-up for a testicular mass?

Patients should be evaluated by obtaining serum markers (αFP, βHCG, LDH, and alkaline phosphatase), chest radiograph, and an abdominal CT with oral and intravenous contrast.

38. What operative approach is indicated for testicular masses?

The procedure should begin with an inguinal incision, followed by a radical orchiectomy with excision of the spermatic cord at the internal ring. A transscrotal approach should not be used.

39. Which boys with testicular tumors should receive a unilateral retroperitoneal lymph node resection and adjuvant therapy?

If retroperitoneal lymph nodes are enlarged on CT or markers remain elevated postoperatively, patients should undergo a unilateral retroperitoneal lymph node resection. All patients with germinoma tumors should receive 3–5 cycles of PEB. Patients with seminomas do not require this aggressive treatment and do well with single-agent therapy. All other malignant histologies receive PEB if they are stage II or greater or if they are recurrent tumors. The use of x-ray therapy is no longer recommended becauseof the undesirable long-term side effects.

40. Can you make a table giving the current treatment strategies for all germ cell tumors?

HISTOLOGY	PRIMARY SITE	STAGE	TREATMENT
Teratoma (mature and immature)	All sites	Localized	Surgical resection
Germinomas, dysgerminomas, seminomas	Testicular	Stage I	Surgery
	Testicular	Stage II	Surgery + PEB*
	Testicular	Stage III-IV	Surgery + PEB
	All other sites	All stages	Surgery + PEB
Nongerminatous tumors	Testicular	Stage I	Surgery
	Testicular	Stage II-IV	Surgery + PEB
	Ovarian	Stage I-IV	Surgery + PEB
	Extragonadal	Stage I–II	Surgery + PEB
	Extragonadal	Stage III-IV	Surgery + HD-PEB

PEB = cisplatin, etoposide, and bleomycin; HD-PEB = high-dose PEB.

* Seminomas in children are rare. They probably are more common in adolescents, in whom adult guidelines with less aggressive therapy should be used. Use of PEB for stage II testicular seminoma may be overtreatment.

BIBLIOGRAPHY

1. Ablin AR, et al: Results of treatment of malignant germ cell tumors in 93 children: A report from the Children's Cancer Study Group. J Clin Oncol 9:1782, 1991.
2. Altman RP, Randolph JG, Lilly JR: Sacrococcygeal teratomas: American Academy of Pediatrics Surgical Section Surgery. J Pediatr Surg 9:389, 1974.
3. Davidoff AM, et al: Endodermal sinus tumor in children. J Pediatr Surg 31:1075, 1996.

4. Grosfeld JL, Billmire DR: Teratomas in infancy and childhood. Curr Probl Cancer 11:3, 1985.
5. Hawkins E, Isaacs H, Cushing B, et al: Occult malignancy in neonatal sacrococcygeal teratomas: A report from a combined pediatric oncology group and children's cancer group study. Am J Pediatr Hematol Oncol 15:406, 1993.
6. Marina N, et al: Treatment of childhood germ cell tumors. Cancer 70:2568, 1992.
7. Marina NM, et al: The role of second-look surgery in the management of advanced germ cell malignancies. Cancer 68:309, 1991.
8. Pinkerton CR et al. "JEB": A carboplatin based regimen for malignant germ cell tumours in children. Br J Cancer 62:257, 1990.
9. Shih GH, Boyd GL, Vincent RD, et al: The EXIT procedure facilitates delivery of an infant with a pretracheal teratoma. Anesthesiology 89:1573–1575, 1998.
10. Skinner MA: Germ cell tumors. In Oldham KT, Foglia RP, Colombani PM (eds): Surgery of Infants and Children: Scientific Principles and Practice. Philadelphia, Lippincott-Raven, 1997, pp 653–662.
11. Wu JT, Book L, Sudan K: Serum alpha fetoprotein (AFP) levels in normal infants. Pediatr Rev 15:50, 1981.

69. MISCELLANEOUS TUMORS

Amanda J. McCabe, FRCS, and Philip L. Glick, M.D.

1. Small round blue cells are commonly seen in which six pediatric tumors?
• Neuroblastoma
• Rhabdomyosarcoma
• Ewing's tumor
• Lymphoma
• Peripheral primitive neuroectodermal tumor (PNET)
• Wilms' tumor

These cells are seen by light microscopy arranged in clusters or diffuse sheets. Differentiation of the tumor cell type is made possible by considering the age of the patient and the site of the tumor and by immunohistochemical and electronmicroscopy techniques.

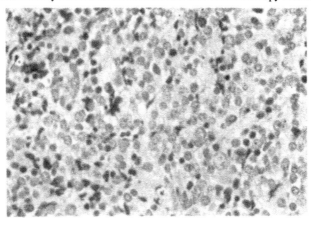

Small round blue cells.

2. Which tumors have been reported in association with Meckel's diverticulum?
Carcinoid tumors are the most common tumors in Meckel's diverticula. They have a greater metastatic potential than appendiceal carcinoids, and tumors > 5 mm are associated with a

markedly increased risk of spread. Sarcoma, lymphoma, adenocarcinoma, and leiomyoma also have been reported in Meckel's diverticulum.

3. What is thought to be the origin of the carcinoid tumor?

An amine precursor uptake and decarboxylation (APUD) neoplasm, presumably of neuroectodermal origin. Most appendiceal carcinoid tumors lack the serotonin-containing cells that are typical of midgut carcinoid tumors; thus they are rarely symptomatic and typically present incidentally at appendectomy.

4. How is an appendiceal carcinoid treated?

Tumors larger than 2 cm in diameter, those that have obviously metastasized, and those at the appendix base require right hemicolectomy. Tumors smaller than 1 cm in diameter that have not obviously metastasized are treated by appendectomy alone. The treatment of tumors in the 1–2-cm domain remains controversial.

5. Colonic obstruction may be the presenting feature of which neoplastic processes?

- Intraluminal: polyps, neurofibromas, or adenocarcinoma
- Extrinsic compression: non-Hodgkin's lymphoma, retroperitoneal sarcomas, or teratomas
- Intraluminal infiltration: neurofibromatosis

6. How do colorectal tumors differ in children and adults?

Location. Childhood colorectal cancer lesions are evenly distributed throughout the colon, whereas two-thirds of adult lesions are in the rectosigmoid region.

Stage at diagnosis. In children, more than 80% of the tumors are Dukes' C or 'D,' in contrast to 40% in adults.

Histologic type. The mucinous type of adenocarcinoma is found in over one-half of children with colorectal tumors. This subtype has an aggressive course and is known to metastasize early. Only about 5% of adult cases present with this tumor subtype.

7. What predisposes children to colorectal cancer?

- Familial polyposis syndromes
- Inflammatory bowel disease (especially ulcerative colitis)
- Hereditary nonpolyposis syndromes
- Previous ureterosigmoidostomy
- Chronic parasitic infection
- Previous radiation therapy
- Diet high in fat and low in fiber
- Exposure to environmental chemicals

The overall incidence of colorectal cancer in children is 1.3–2 cases per million lives; however, 25% of childhood cases are associated with a predisposing condition.

8. What is the risk of colonic carcinoma in patients with ulcerative colitis?

The risk is approximately 20 times that of the general population and is related to the duration of disease. After the first 10 years the likelihood of developing colonic carcinoma increases from 1% to 2% per year. Groups at particular risk include younger patients and patients with pancolitis.

9. What is the relative frequency of pulmonary neoplasms in childhood?

The approximate ratio of primary pulmonary tumors to metastatic neoplasms to nonneoplastic lesions of the lung is 1:5:60. Although primary pulmonary tumors (e.g., bronchial adenoma, bronchogenic carcinoma, and, pulmonary blastoma) are rare in children, most are malignant.

10. What is the most common benign tumor of the lung in childhood?

Plasma cell granuloma (inflammatory pseudotumor) accounts for 50% of all benign lesions and 20% of all primary lung tumors. The natural history is that of a slow-growing mass with a tendency to local invasion.

11. Which childhood tumors commonly metastasize to lung?

Wilms' tumor, rhabdomyosarcoma, osteogenic sarcoma, Ewing's sarcoma, and primary hepatic tumors.

12. Should lung metastases be surgically excised?

In general, operative removal of metastatic disease should be undertaken in the context of a significant tumor response at the primary site. Ideally, it also should be demonstrated that the metastases have responded to systemic chemotherapy before resection to ensure that undetectable micrometastases do not result in early relapse. Aggressive pulmonary metastasectomy is indicated in osteogenic sarcoma, but not in most embryonal soft tissue sarcomas.

13. Are bronchial adenomas benign?

No. Bronchial adenomas are the most frequently encountered malignant primary pulmonary tumor in childhood. There are three histologic types: carcinoid (80%), mucoepidermoid carcinoma, and adenoid cystic carcinoma. They present with incomplete bronchial obstruction with cough, recurrent pneumonitis, and hemoptysis. Rarely, the classic carcinoid syndrome is a feature, usually in the presence of metastases. This tumor is associated with an excellent prognosis in children, even in the presence of local invasion.

14. Patients with congenital cystic adenomatoid malformation (CCAM) are at risk of developing which tumor?

The literature reports a few cases of rhabdomyosarcoma in association with CCAM. There are also cases of rhabdomyosarcoma within congenital bronchogenic cysts and congenital pulmonary cysts. A single pediatric case of bronchioalveolar carcinoma is reported in the lung parenchyma adjacent to a CCAM. These few cases suggest that pulmonary cystic malformations may be intrinsically susceptible to neoplastic transformation; therefore, early removal of all cystic lesions may be advisable.

15. How common is rhabdomyosarcoma?

Rhabdomyosarcoma accounts for approximately one-half of all pediatric soft-tissue sarcomas and 15% of all pediatric solid tumors. There are approximately 250 new pediatric cases of rhabdomyosarcoma each year in the United States (annual incidence of 4.35 cases per million children aged 0–14).

16. In what head and neck sites do rhabdomyosarcomas arise? What clinical features are associated with each?

Orbital: proptosis, chemosis, eye-lid or conjunctival mass, blindness, and ophthalmoplegia.

Parameningeal: nasopharynx, paranasal sinus, middle ear mastoid, and pterygoid-infratemporal sites. Lesions in these areas can cause cranial bone erosion, resulting in cranial nerve palsies and meningeal symptoms. Nasopharyngeal tumors may cause voice changes, airway obstruction, dysphasia, nasal discharge, and epistaxis.

Nonparameningeal: scalp, external ear, parotid sites, face, buccal mucosa, pharynx, tonsil, larynx, and neck. Symptoms of hoarseness, bleeding, discharge, or a mass lesion result. Cervical node metastasis can be anticipated in 5–20% of cases.

17. What tumor features help to predict survival in cases of rhabdomyosarcoma?

Site (superior outcome in orbital tumors), size, tumor invasiveness, regional node involvement, and distant metastasis have the most significant impact on survival. Site and distant metastasis are the most powerful predictors. Although histologic type (superior outcome with botryoid types) is another important factor, it does not influence prognosis more than the other variables.

18. What is a desmoid tumor?

Also termed aggressive fibromatosis, this rare tumor of childhood involves musculoaponeurotic tissue. It presents as a solid, painless, enlarging mass around the age of 13 years. It may present in postsurgical locations, and when present on the abdomen, it is often associated with

Gardner's syndrome (an autosomal-dominant disease manifested by desmoid tumors, familial adenomatous polyposis, and osteomas). Wide local excision is the chosen therapy, but recurrences are common. Adjuvant therapies such as high-dose irradiation, chemotherapy, antiestrogens, and inflammatory agents have been used with some success for unresectable or recurrent tumors.

19. What distinguishes infantile fibrosarcoma (IF) from adult-type fibrosarcoma (AF)?

Histologically, IF has abundant atypical mitoses with associated hypercellularity and spindle cells but lacks the anaplasia of AF. Genetic analysis reveals that the infant form has numerical chromosomal abnormalities, whereas the adult form displays random structural chromosomal abnormalities.

20. What is a teratoma?

Embryonal neoplasms derived from totipotential cells that contain tissue from at least two and more often three germ layers (ectoderm, endoderm, and mesoderm).

21. How are sacrococcygeal teratomas (SCT) classified?

The American Academy of Pediatrics Surgical Section has classified SCT as follows:

Type I	Tumors are predominantly external, attached to the coccyx, and may have a small presacral component (46% of cases).
Type II	Tumors have both an external mass and a significant presacral pelvic extension (34% of cases)
Type III	Tumors are visible externally, but the predominant mass is pelvic and intraabdominal (9% of cases).
Type IV	Tumors are not visible externally but are entirely presacral (10% of cases).

22. Which mechanisms place the fetus diagnosed with SCT at risk?

Currently, 52% of infants diagnosed with SCT die in utero or at birth. This high mortality rate relates to tumor mass and physiology. The mass effect may cause an abnormal lie, or dystocia may result in traumatic tumor rupture and hemorrhage during vaginal or cesarean delivery. The mass, with or without polyhydramnios, may cause uterine distension and result in the delivery of a neonate with lung immaturity. SCT has the potential to steal blood from the middle sacral artery (fetus) or the placenta, resulting in fetal anemia, high-output heart failure, and possibly hydrops. Demand for blood by the tumor can be increased by minor trauma in utero or necrotic/cystic degeneration of the tumor. The anemic, hydropic fetus with SCT thus may benefit from in utero transfusion, whereas a fetus with vascular steal requires tumor resection or in utero ligation of the middle sacral artery.

23. What anomalies are associated with type IV SCT?

Congenital anomalies are seen in 12–15% of cases. Examples include anorectal malformations, such as anorectal stenosis or imperforate anus with an occasional rectovaginal fistula.

Spinal abnormalities include a central sacral defect, sacral hemivertebrae, absence of the sacrum, and coccyx (Currarino triad).

24. What are the operative principles for removing a SCT?

Treatment of a SCT is complete excision as soon as possible. Baseline alpha fetoprotein level is determined for postoperative comparison. Blood is crossmatched, and intraoperative blood loss is kept to a minimum with a low threshold for early transfusion. Fifty percent of the neonate's blood volume is composed of fetal hemoglobin with reduced oxygen-carrying capacity, and a significant proportion of the total blood volume is lost in the tumor. Large-bore intravenous lines are placed in the upper extremities as opposed to the groin or lower extremities. The use of intraoperative laser or harmonic scalpels also may help to decrease intraoperative blood loss. An inverted-V incision is made in the skin over the lower sacrum. The dissection is continued in the midline directly down to the fourth or fifth sacral vertebra. The sacrum is divided, and the tumor is displaced inferiorly to expose, ligate, and divide middle sacral vessels. Failure to remove the coccyx is associated with a 35% recurrence rate. Anatomy is distorted as the presacral mass pushes the perineal structures forward. The rectum must be delineated during dissection with a rectal pack or Hegar dilator. The tumor is dissected outside the capsule from thinned levator and gluteus muscles and then out of the pelvis. The pelvic floor is reconstructed with muscle and fascia. Abdominal exploration is necessary if an abdominal component is involved.

25. What moles should be removed?

Any mole that increases in size, changes color (either darker or lighter), itches, or ulcerates should be removed for histologic examination. In children < 12 years a brief general anesthetic often is required.

26. What is a Spitz nevus?

A dome-shaped firm papule or nodule with a smooth surface, often pink rather than melanotic in color and most commonly located on the head and neck. Spitz nevi range from 1 mm to 3 cm in diameter and are more common in children than in adults. The natural history is benign, but local recurrence after excision is seen in 5% of cases. Histologically Spitz nevi are composed of spindle cells, epithelioid cells, or a mixture of both. Nuclear atypia is seen in both Spitz nevi and melanomas, making their distinction difficult.

27. Name five groups at high risk of developing malignant melanoma.

- Xeroderma pigmentosa
- Familial atypical mole and melanoma syndrome
- Neurocutaneous melanosis
- Immunosuppression
- Transplacental spread and giant congenital nevus (risk higher in nevi covering > 5% of the body surface area)

28. What are Clark's levels? What is their importance?

Clark described five levels of melanoma thickness in the skin:

Level I: an intradermal melanoma that does not metastasize.
Level II: a melanoma that penetrates the basement membrane into the papillary dermis.
Level III: a melanoma that fills the papillary dermis and encroaches on the reticular dermis in a pushing fashion.
Level IV: a melanoma that invades the reticular dermis.
Level V: a melanoma that invades subcutaneous fat.

Excised melanoma are assessed by both Clark's level and the Breslow method, which measures the actual depth of melanoma skin invasion and is accepted as a more exact measure of tumor invasion. Lesions less than 1 mm have a cure rate of over 99% with excision. Intermediate lesions (1–4 mm) have a risk of metastasis and death. Lesions over 4 mm are high-risk and have a relatively poor cure rate. Thin lesions may show a low Breslow measurement with a deeper Clark level, indicating a greater risk of recurrence and spread.

29. Knee pain may be the presenting feature of which tumors?

Benign: osteocartilaginous exostosis, nonosseous fibromas, chrondroblastoma, desmoid tumor. Osgood Schlatter's disease, although not a true tumor, is a common cause of knee pain in adolescents and may be associated with swelling.

Malignant: osteosarcoma, rhabdomyosarcoma, synovial sarcoma, fibrosarcoma.

30. Which sites are commonly affected in osteogenic and Ewing's sarcomas?

Osteogenic sarcoma: a tumor of the metaphyseal part of the bone, especially the distal femur, proximal tibia, and proximal humerus.

Ewing's sarcoma: a tumor of the diaphysis or midshaft of the bone. Any bone can be affected, but the femur, humerus, ribs, and flat bones such as the scapula are more commonly involved.

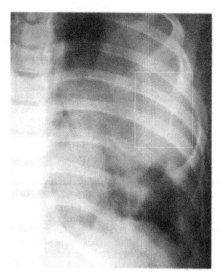

Ewing's sarcoma of the anterior end of the fourth rib.

31. How are osteogenic and Ewing's sarcomas differentiated on radiographs?

Osteogenic sarcoma: varied osteolysis and elevated periostium with a sunburst pattern of soft-tissue calcification

Ewing's sarcoma: extensive cortical involvement with layers of new periosteal bone formation giving an onionskin appearance.

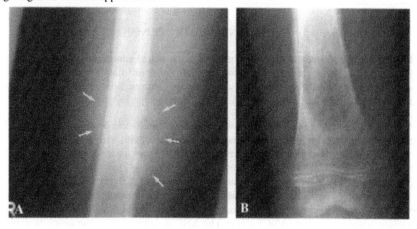

A, Osteogenic sarcoma causing osteolysis of the distal femur. *B,* Typical sunburst appearance of an osteogenic sarcoma of the distal femur.

32. What are the prognostic indicators for Ewing's sarcoma?

Five-year survival rates currently approach 60%. Stage is the most important predictor of outcome. Patients presenting with metastatic disease to bone or bone marrow fare poorly. Other adverse prognostic factors include older age, increased lactate dehydrogenase, tumor volume > 100 cm^3, tumor length of 5–10 cm, and increased neuroectodermal features. The latter include (1) expression of catachol acetyl transferase (an enzyme involved in neurotransmitter biosynthesis), (2) expression of neuron-specific enolase, and (3) formation of primitive dendrites and expression of neural-associated proteins in response to differentiating agents.

BIBLIOGRAPHY

1. Ceballos PI, Ruiz-Maldonado R, Mihm MC: Melanoma in children. N Engl J Med 332:656–662, 1995.
2. d'Agostino S, Bonoldi E, Dante S, et al: Embryonal rhabdomyosarcoma of the lung arising in cystic adenomatoid malformation: Case report and review of the literature. J Pediatr Surg 32:1381–1383, 1997.
3. Denny CT: Ewing's sarcoma: A clinical enigma coming into focus. J Pediatr Hematol Oncol 20:421–425, 1998.
4. Flake AW: Fetal sacrococcygeal teratoma. Semin Pediatr Surg 2:113–120, 1993.
5. Granata C, Gambini C, Balducci T, et al: Bronchioloalveolar carcinoma arising in congenital cystic adenoid malformation in a child. Pediatr Pulmonol 25:62–66, 1998.
6. La Quaglia MP: The surgical management of metastases in pediatric cancer. Semin Pediatr Surg 2:75–82, 1993.
7. Murphy JJ, Blair GK, Fraser GC, et al: Rhabdomyosarcoma arising within congenital pulmonary cysts: Report of three cases. J Pediatr Surg 27:1364–1367, 1992.
8. Nesbit ME, Gehan EA, Burgert EO, et al: Multimodality therapy for the management of primary nonmetastatic Ewing's sarcoma of bone: A long term follow-up of the first intergroup study. J Clin Oncol 8:1664–1674, 1990.
9. O'Neill JA, Rowe MI, Grosfeld JL, et al (eds): Pediatric Surgery, 5th ed. St. Louis, Mosby, 1998.
10. Puri P (ed): Neonatal Tumors. London, Springer, 1996.
11. Swerdlow AJ, English JSC, Qiao Z: The risk of melanoma in patients with congenital nevi: A cohort study. J Am Acad Dermatol 32:595–599, 1995.
12. Wiener ES: Rhabdomyosarcoma: New dimensions in management. Semin Pediatr Surg 2:47–58, 1993.

70. PEDIATRIC MEDICAL ONCOLOGY

Ashraf Abdel-Monem, M.D., and Sharon H. Smith, M.D.

FEVER AND NEUTROPENIA

1. True or false: A febrile neutropenic patient is a medical emergency.

True. A febrile neutropenic patient should be evaluated immediately with a good history and thorough physical examination, followed by appropriate cultures. Broad-spectrum IV antibiotics should be started immediately after the collection of cultures, pending results.

2. A 5-year-old boy diagnosed with acute lymphocytic leukemia develops a fever of 38.7°C during induction therapy. His white blood cell count is 10,000, with 55% blasts, 42% lymphocytes, 1% segmented neutrophils, and 2% bands. Does he meet the criteria for fever and neutropenia?

Patients with cancer are considered immunocompromised secondary to the disease itself as well as the effects of chemotherapy. The patient in this scenario meets the criteria of febrile neutropenia, which is a temperature $\geq$ 38.5°C once or 38–38.4°C three times in a 24-hour period and an absolute neutrophil count (ANC) < 500. The ANC is calculated by the absolute number of segmented and band neutrophils, which in this case is $1\% \times 10,000 + 2\% \times 10,000 = 300$.

3. What should the empiric antibiotic coverage include in febrile neutropenic patients?

Broad-spectrum IV antibiotics with good coverage against gram-positive and gram-negative organisms should be used; anaerobic coverage may be added initially, depending on the clinical situation (e.g., suspected abdominal or perirectal sepsis). Third-generation cephalosporins and carbepenem are used extensively as monotherapy.

4. When do you consider antifungal coverage in febrile neutropenic patients?

The risk of developing fungal infection in patients with cancer is directly proportionate to the length and degree of neutropenia. Patients are considered at very high risk if they have neutropenia for more than 7 days and the ANC nadir is under 200. Patients in relapse or after bone marrow transplant are also at high risk. Empiric broad-spectrum antifungal therapy (e.g., amphotericin B) usually is started in patients who are persistently febrile and neutropenic after 5–7 days on broad-spectrum antibiotics with negative cultures. Patients at high risk for fungal infection may be treated with prophylactic fluconazole.

5. True or false: Antibiotics can be discontinued when neutropenic patients with negative cultures become afebrile.

False. Antibiotics in febrile neutropenic patients with negative cultures should continue even when the patient becomes afebrile until the ANC recovers (i.e., > 500). Discontinuing antibiotics before that time has been associated with recurrence of fever and positive cultures in about one-third of patients.

6. How do you treat fever in patients with a central line?

The incidence of catheter-related infections with the need for subsequent line removal has been estimated at 20% in patients with central lines. *Staphylococcus epidermidis* is the primary infecting organism. Treatment should include good coverage against both gram-negative and gram-positive organisms, especially *S. epidermidis* (for which the drug of choice is vancomycin). Blood cultures should be obtained from all lumens of the central line, and antibiotics should be rotated through the lumens to ensure avoidance of colonization. Central lines must be removed in cases of tunnel infection, persistent infection, repeated infection with the same organisms, or fungal infection.

7. What are the recommendations for vaccinating a patient with cancer?

Live attenuated vaccines, such as the measles, mumps, and rubella vaccine and polio vaccine, are contraindicated during active disease and/or immune suppression secondary to chemotherapy. Close household contacts (such as siblings) should not receive the oral polio vaccine but should be given the injectable vaccine to avoid feco-oral transmission of the polio virus to the patient. Killed vaccines or capsular polysaccharides, such as diphtheria-pertussis-tetanus vaccine or *Haemophilus influenzae* type B vaccine, can be given without additional risk.

LONG-TERM COMPLICATIONS AND OUTCOMES

8. What are the two most important organ-specific side effects of cisplatinum?
- Nephrotoxicity with azotemia and electrolyte wasting can be minimized by vigorous hydration during the drug infusion. It may be reversible.
- Irreversible hearing loss, mainly in the high-frequency range.

9. Does cancer therapy result in infertility?

Gonadal dysfunction is a well-known side effect of cancer therapy. The risk of infertility depends on more than one variable for a given drug dose. The age and sex of the patient, the disease itself, and, finally, the specific therapy are important factors in assessing risk. Children sustain less gonadal damage than adults. Males have a greater incidence of infertility than their female counterparts. Hodgkin's disease and its systemic therapy, especially nitrogen mustard and procarbazine-containing regimens, lead the list for infertility. Low doses of irradiation are known to produce azospermia in males (as in total body irradiation preparative regimen for bone marrow transplant), whereas females may escape infertility with oophropexy.

10. In counseling a teenage girl about the long-term side effects of cancer treatment, she asks about teratogenicity in her offspring. How should you respond?

Some reports show an increased risk of prematurity and still-births in the offspring of cancer survivors. But no evidence of mutagenesis in human fetuses among survivors of cancer is available. Similarly, no increase in the incidence of congenital malformation has been found. Cancer survivors are encouraged to have children after completion of therapy, with close monitoring and evaluation antenatally and postnatally.

11. Will the children of cancer survivors get cancer?
The risk of cancer in the offspring of cancer survivors was not found to be increased in two large studies, unless the parent's cancer was genetically determined, as in retinoblastoma.

12. What is the estimated risk of secondary malignancy in survivors of childhood cancer?
Survivors of childhood cancer have a 10- to 20-fold increase in life-time risk of developing a secondary malignancy. This figure varies with the primary cancer (Hodgkin's disease leads the list, followed by genetic Wilms' tumor and retinoblastoma) as well as the treatment modality. The highest incidence of secondary cancer occurs in radiation and alkylating agent-based therapy. Acute myeloblastic leukemia is the leading type of secondary malignancy related to chemotherapy, whereas radiation-field sarcomas are the most common solid tumor.

13. A teenage survivor of stage IV Wilms' tumor presents to the emergency department with shortness of breath. Besides pneumonia, what could the diagnosis be?
The patient may have a recurrence of the Wilms' tumor with pulmonary metastases. The more likely causes, however, are treatment-related. Therapy for stage IV Wilms' tumor usually includes doxorubicin hydrochloride as well as lung irradiation. Doxorubicin has cumulative, dose-related cardiotoxicity; significant toxicity occurs in approximately 11% of patients when the total dose exceeds 500 mg/m^2. Cardiotoxicity may present as congestive heart failure with shortness of breath. Another treatment-related cause of shortness of breath may be the chronic effects of lung radiation, which result in restrictive or obstructive lung disease.

14. What factors should be considered when deciding between surgery and radiation for local control of solid tumors?
Surgery, radiation therapy, and chemotherapy are complementary in the management of many patients with cancer. Occasionally, you may have the option to choose between surgery or radiation therapy in the local control of malignant disease. The following points should be considered:
   • Is the tumor radiosensitive? For example, Ewing's sarcoma is radiosensitive, but osteosarcoma is not.
   • Is it possible to achieve negative margins using surgery alone without compromising organ functions? If negative microscopic margins are not achieved, radiation is still necessary.
   • What are the acute and long-term morbidities of each modality? Examples include ileus and postoperative intestinal obstruction in case of abdominal surgery or secondary malignancy within the field in case of radiation. The decision needs to be made in a team-based setting with input from the pediatric surgeon, radiation oncologist, pathologist, radiologist, and pediatric oncologist.

15. Summarize the mechanisms of action and side effects of common pediatric chemotherapeutic agents.

DRUG	MECHANISM OF ACTION	TOXICITY
Antimetabolites (e.g., methotrexate, 6-mercaptopurine)	Inhibition of nucleotide synthesis	Bone marrow suppression
Alkylating agents (e.g., cyclophosphamide)	Alkylation of DNA/RNA	Bone marrow suppression, hemorrhagic cystitis, sterility
Bleomycin	DNA strand scission	Pulmonary fibrosis, fever, chills

Table continued on following page

DRUG	MECHANISM OF ACTION	TOXICITY
Anthracyclines	Formation of complex with DNA	Bone marrow suppression, cardiac damage
Plant alkaloid	Mitotic spindle disruption	Peripheral neuritis, constipation
Asparaginase	Inhibition of protein synthesis	Anaphylaxis, pancreatitis, hypercoagulability
Epipodyphyllotoxin (e.g., VP-16)	Topoisomerase inhibitor Failure of cell cycle progression	Bone marrow suppression, secondary malignancy

BIBLIOGRAPHY

1. Ariceta G, Rodriguez-Soriano J, Vallo A, et al: Acute and chronic effects of cisplatin therapy on renal magnesium homeostasis. Med Pediatr Oncol 28:35, 1997.
2. Bossi G, Cerveri I, Volpini E, et al: Long-term pulmonary sequelae after treatment of childhood Hodgkin's disease. Ann Oncol 8(Suppl):19, 1997.
3. Freifeld A, Walsh T, Pizzo P: Infectious complications in the pediatric cancer patient. In Pizzo P (ed): Principles and Practice of Pediatric Oncology, 3rd ed. Philadelphia, J.B. Lippincott, 1997, pp 1069–1114.
4. Freifeld A, Walsh T, Marshall D, et al: Monotherapy for fever and neutropenia in cancer patients: A randomized comparison of ceftazidime versus imipenem. J Clin Oncol 13:165–176, 1995.
5. Green DM, Fiorello A, Zevon MA, et al: Birth defects and childhood cancer in offspring of survivors of childhood cancer. Arch Pediatr Adolesc Med 151:379, 1997.
6. Grossi M: Management and long-term complications of pediatric cancer. Pediatr Clin North Am 45:1637, 1998.
7. Heikens J: Irreversible gonadal damage in male survivors of pediatric Hodgkin's disease. Cancer 78:2020, 1996.
8. Robinson LL, Mertens A: Second tumors after treatment of childhood malignancies. Hematol Oncol Clin North Am 7:401, 1993.
9. Seligmann H, Podoshin L, Ben-David J, et al: Drug-induced tinnitus and other hearing disorders. Drug Safety 14:198, 1996.
10. Shan K, Lincoff AM, Young JB: Anthracycline induced cardiotoxicity. Ann Intern Med 125:47, 1996.
11. Walsh TJ, Lee J, Lecciones J, et al: Empiric therapy with amphotericin B in febrile granulocytopenic patients. Rev Infect Dis 13:496–503, 1991.

XII. Special Topics

71. PEDIATRIC RADIOLOGY

David Martin, M.D., and James Backstrom, M.D.

1. What diagnosis may be demonstrated by ultrasound examination of the right lower quadrant in an 8-year-old boy with nausea, vomiting, and abdominal pain?

Appendicitis (Fig. 1).

Sonography using a graded compression technique is useful in the diagnosis of appendicitis. A noncompressable tubular mass with a diameter of 6 mm or greater is suspicious. Fluid, mesenteric thickening, or frank abscess also may indicate appendicitis. In addition, sonography is useful in diagnosing clinically equivocal cases as well as excluding or diagnosing diseases in other organs in the right side of the abdomen and pelvis. Computed tomography (CT) is a useful adjunct in cases that have negative ultrasonography but remain suspicious clinically and also in some cases with complications, such as perforation and smaller fluid collections including interloop abscess.

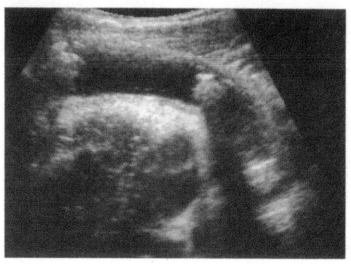

Figure 1. Right-lower-quadrant ultrasound. A fluid-filled appendix containing a fecolith is seen inferiorly, projecting from the cecum.

2. What diagnosis may be found on ultrasound in a 1-year-old boy with colicky abdominal pain and blood per rectum?

Intussusception (Fig. 2). An intussusception occurs when the intussusceptum (proximal bowel) invaginates into the more distal bowel segments (intussuscepiens).

The first line of treatment in a child who is not frankly septic and does not have peritonitis or free air on abdominal plain films is an an enema examination. Over the past several years, the air enema examination (Fig. 2C) has replaced the standard barium examination as the first line of treatment. Both barium and air enema examinations can be diagnostic and therapeutic. The radiologic literature would be reduced considerably in recent years without the various imaging controversies around the diagnosis and treatment of intussusception. Fortunately, the controversies have little effect on the care of the patient. Clearly, ultrasound, barium enema and air enema examinations serve quite well as diagnostic modalities for intussusception. Consideration of the individual child's circumstances often works better than dogmatic statements. We have converted to air enema reduction treatment techniques with excellent results. We revert to barium enema if atypical findings are present or if reduction is unsuccessful with air reduction techniques. The child must be closely monitored during the procedure. In addition, the surgical team must be involved with the child and be available with every reduction attempt. Communication and teamwork between the radiologist and surgeon result in optimal care.

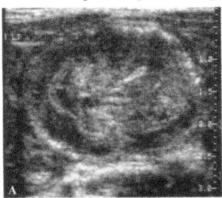

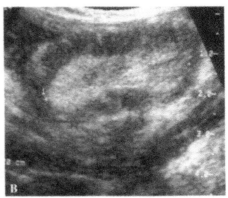

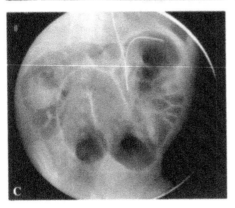

Figure 2.   Abdominal ultrasound showing a mass in the left lower quadrant which represents an intussusception. The longitudinal appearance (*A*) of the intussusception is often described as a "kidney-like" mass and the tangential view (*B*) as "target-like." *C*, Air contrast enema on the same patient shows a rounded mass in the descending colon representing the intussusception. The intussusception eventually was reduced completely with the air enema technique.

3. What may be demonstrated by upper abdominal sonogram in a 4-week-old boy with projectile vomiting?

Hypertrophic pyloric stenosis (Fig. 3). The pylorus is well defined by liquid in the gastric antrum and duodenal cap. The objective sonographic criteria for pyloric stenosis are:

Canal length	> 16 mm
Muscle thickness	> 3 mm
Pyloric diameter	> 11 mm
Pyloric volume	> 1.4 mm

Sonography for pyloric stenosis is a dynamic examination. Ingestion of water during the examination may help to demonstrate the inability of the antral peristaltic wave to travel effectively through the pyloric canal. Retrograde gastric peristalsis also may be seen under real-time observation. Measurements are an adjunct to the physiological study and may be used to confirm the condition (Fig. 3B).

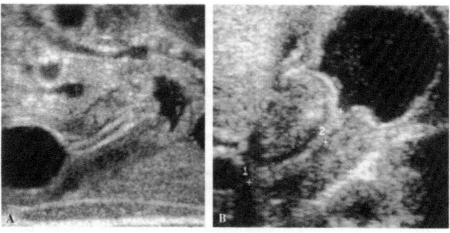

Figure 3. *A*, Ultrasound of pyloric stenosis. Note the elongated and curved pyloric channel with parallel walls and the thickened muscle with "shoulder" projecting into the antrum. *B*, Longitudinal sonogram of the pylorus in a patient with pyloric stenosis. 1 = canal length, 1.7 cm; 2 = muscle wall thickness, 0.6 cm.

4. **What may be the diagnosis in a 4-week-old child with abdominal pain and bilious emesis?**
   Malrotation (Fig. 4).

   Malrotation refers to any variation of intestinal rotation that deviates from normal. It is a serious cause of obstruction in newborns. Many attempts have been made to subclassify malrotation, but the subclasses carry little importance. Anatomic variations of the duodenum help with the interpretation of the upper gastrointestinal (GI) series. In a child with symptoms, any malrotation requires prompt surgical evaluation and treatment. The cecum is in a normal location (Fig. 4) in 16–20% of patients, and normal barium enema exam does not exclude malrotation. Rarely, malrotation can be present with a normal upper GI series. A small bowel series with a colonic exam should be performed if the clinical suspicion remains high after a normal upper GI exam. Ultrasound examination for malrotation is not recommended because it is neither sensitive nor specific for the diagnosis.

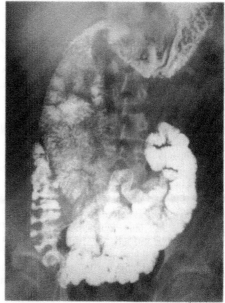

Figure 4. Upper GI series. The jejunum and ligament of Treitz are clearly to the right of the spine, and the cecum is situated in the right lower quadrant.

5. What may be the diagnosis in a 6-year-old boy with painless hematochezia?

Meckel's diverticulum, as diagnosed by a Meckel's scan utilizing ^{99m}Tc pertechnetate (Fig. 5).

There are many cases of asymptomatic Meckel's diverticula in the general population. It is estimated that only 25–30% of these diverticula cause symptoms. Fortunately, those that cause symptoms typically contain ectopic gastric mucosa. Pertechnetate, used in the Meckel's scan, is concentrated by mucous cells in the stomach as well as the ectopic gastric mucosa Meckel's diverticula. The Meckel's diverticulum will usually be faintly seen when the gastric mucosa is seen early in the scan. The activity in the diverticulum will typically become more intense as time progresses. If the patient is actively bleeding during the scan, one can see activity "flow" downstream inside the lumen of the small bowel and colon. Watching the images in the cine mode with your favorite radiologist will help clarify this confusing event.

6. A right-upper-quadrant ultrasound was obtained in a 4-month-old child with progressive jaundice. What is the diagnosis? What additional studies may be obtained to support the diagnosis?

Choledochal cyst, type 1A (Fig. 6).

The child was referred from an outside hospital with the diagnosis of "gallstones." Do you agree? Echogenic material is seen on ultrasound (Figs. 6A–D) both within the gallbladder and an adjacent cystic structure that can be followed to the level of the ampulla of Vater. This cystic dilatation is the common bile duct. The material within the gallbladder and common duct is sludge. Note the lack of acoustic shadowing that indicates the presence of stones.

Choledochal cysts are a heterogeneous collection of anatomic dilatations of the biliary ductal system. Various classification systems have been proposed to categorize choledochal cysts. The most common classification system divided choledochal cysts into five categories:

Type 1A   Isolated dilatation of the common bile duct below the cystic duct.

Type 1B   Dilatation of the common duct and hepatic ducts.

Type 2   Diverticulum off the common duct.

Type 3   Dilatation of the distal portion of the common duct as it enters the duodenum (choledochocele).

Type 4   Cystic dilatations involving intrahepatic and extrahepatic bile ducts (Caroli's disease).

Hepato-iminodiacetic acid (HIDA) nuclear medicine scans often are used to demonstrate communication of the cystic periportal area with the biliary tree (Fig. 6E). Magnetic resonance imaging (MRI) is becoming increasingly important in all phases of hepatobiliary imaging, including the imaging of choledochal cysts.

7. What is the differential diagnosis in a 2-day-old neonate with emesis and failure to pass meconium? What further radiographic studies are appropriate? Is the abnormal loop of bowel in the right side of the abdomen on plain film colon or ileum? How can they be differentiated?

Failure to pass meconium, abdominal distention, and emesis suggest obstruction in the neonate. The differential diagnosis includes meconium ileus/plug, colonic or small bowel atresia, Hirschsprung's disease, and malrotation.

In the absence of peritonitis the study of choice after plain radiography (Fig. 7A) is a barium enema. In this patient, a microcolon suggests either meconium ileus or small bowel atresia. A family history of cystic fibrosis would aid in the differential diagnosis. Ultrasonography is useful in demonstrating thick echogenic material in multiple loops of bowel in meconium ileus; only air or fluid in dilated loops is seen in ileal atresia. Provided no perforation is present, Gastrograffin enema (Fig. 7B) should be performed as the next diagnostic test. Both ileal atresia and meconium ileus show a microcolon. However, if one can reflux contrast into the terminal ileum, patients with meconium ileus demonstrate viscid meconium filling the terminal ileum. This finding is not seen with ileal atresia. A Gastrograffin enema is often therapeutic in cases of meconium ileus. The enema exam also serves to exclude colonic atresia. Intramural calcifications may be associated with ileal atresia. Peritoneal calcifications (meconium peritonitis, cyst) may be seen with either condition and are associated with antenatal perforation. This infant had ileal atresia.

It is not possible to distinguish small from large bowel with any certainty at this age.

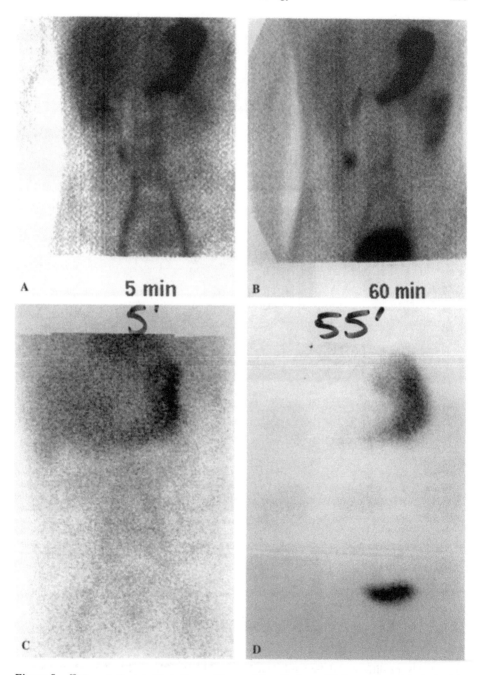

A 5 min

B 60 min

C

D

Figure 5. ^{99m}Tc pertechnetate Meckel's scan. The panel from 5 minutes (*A*) shows faint activity in the right lower quadrant just as gastric mucosa is beginning to become apparent. At 60 minutes (*B*) this activity is quite intense and diagnostic for Meckel's diverticulum. As is often the case, knowing what a normal Meckel's scan (*C* and *D*) shows can help with the interpretation of an abnormal scan. The exam typically lasts an hour. The 5-minute scan (*C*) shows the gastric mucosa beginning to blush. Over the next 50 minutes, the gastric blush intensifies, and the kidneys can be faintly seen as pertechnetate is excreted through the renal system (*D*). the bladder shows concentrated activity, and occasionally one needs to empty the bladder to avoid confusion.

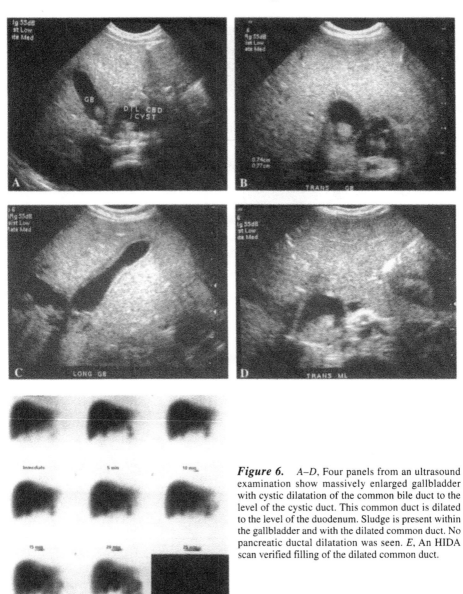

Figure 6. *A–D,* Four panels from an ultrasound examination show massively enlarged gallbladder with cystic dilatation of the common bile duct to the level of the cystic duct. This common duct is dilated to the level of the duodenum. Sludge is present within the gallbladder and with the dilated common duct. No pancreatic ductal dilatation was seen. *E,* An HIDA scan verified filling of the dilated common duct.

8. What is the differential diagnosis in a 7-year-old boy with persistent cough and a mass in the posterior mediastinum? What further studies are warranted?

The differential diagnosis includes: ganglioneuroma, neuroblastoma (especially if calcified), neurofibroma, paraspinal abscess, chest wall tumor, neurenteric cyst, and lateral meningocele.

Often the important clinical question in dealing with posterior mediastinal masses (Fig. 8A) is the extent of neuroforaminal/extradural involvement. MRI is the study of choice. A myelogram (Fig. 8B) was obtained in the work-up of this child, who has a neuroblastoma.

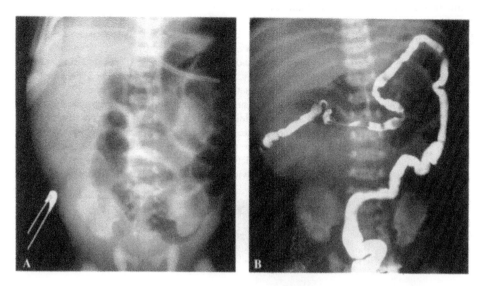

Figure 7.   *A*, Anteroposterior view of the abdomen shows a dilated loop of bowel with small bowel content interspersed with air in the right flank. Mildly dilated air-filled loops of small bowel are seen in the remainder of the abdomen. Absence of gas in the rectum is consistent with obstruction. *B*, A contrast enema confirms a small (micro) but patent colon.

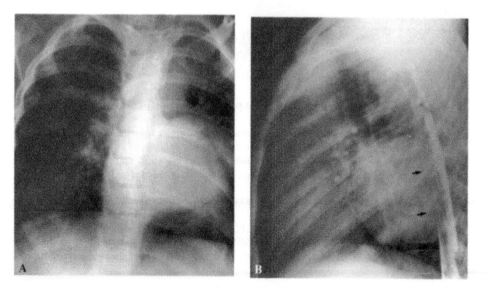

Figure 8.   *A*, Anteroposterior view of the chest shows a left paravertebral mass that is widening the left paravertebral soft tissues. Erosions of the left seventh rib is seen posteriorly. An associated finding is minimal mid-thoracic scoliosis convex to the right. *B*, The lateral view and myelogram confirm the tumor position and indicate the tumor's extension into the extradural space. Arrows indicate the region of effacement of the contrast column. Myelography is rarely performed today because of the widespread availability of MRI.

9. What may be the diagnosis in a child with diffuse abdominal pain, guarding, increased white blood cell count, fever, and anorexia?

Basilar pneumonia with diaphragmatic irritation (Fig. 9).

Clearly, there is a difference in the way that clinicians and radiologists approach radiography. The different approaches often are complimentary, but only with appropriate communication. The patient was seen in the emergency department and evaluated surgically. Ultrasound examinations were ordered to rule out appendicitis. Fortunately, no further imaging was ordered when the diagnosis of pneumonia was made after careful evaluation of the acute abdominal series.

The important teaching points of this case are to ensure that a chest radiograph is included with all pediatric acute abdominal series. In addition, surgical and radiologic consultation and communications are vital to cost-effective care. This communication must go beyond simply writing "pain" on the radiology requisition. The chest radiograph is still the most complex and subtle radiologic exam. It is often the most difficult to interpret well. Some causes of nonbasilar pneumonias present as abdominal pain. Simple views of the lung bases on an abdominal film are not adequate in a child.

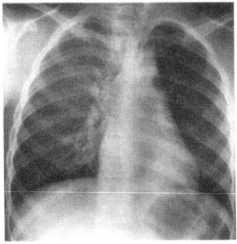

Figure 9.   Anteroposterior chest radiograph shows subtle left basilar, retrocardiac pneumonia. The patient presented with a "surgical" abdomen.

10. What bladder lesion may be present in a patient with flank pain and fever?

Ectopic ureterocele (Fig. 10).

An ectopic ureterocele represents the termination of the ureter from the upper pole collecting system of a duplex kidney. This abnormality most commonly presents as a urinary tract infection; however, one may encounter difficulty with voiding, urinary retention, and flank pain. The associated ureter may be dilated and tortuous. Reflux into the lower pole ureter is frequent.

11. A 1-year-old boy presents with acute scrotal pain. What radiologic study should you order?

Ultrasonography with color Doppler (Fig. 11).

Ultrasound with color Doppler allows the differentiation of testicular torsion from the more common pediatric condition of torsion of the testicular appendages (frequently the appendix epididymis). This particular case demonstrates testicular torsion.

12. What is the differential diagnosis of the right-sided abdominal mass in a female neonate?

Ovarian cyst, maternal hormonal stimulation (Fig. 12).

Sonography provides a ready vehicle to follow ovarian pathology. In the case of follicular stimulation by maternal hormones, one expects to see the ovary diminish to normal size in a few months. Duplication cysts of the duodenum or ileum and developmental cysts of the mesentery or omentum also should be considered in the differential diagnosis but do not diminish in size.

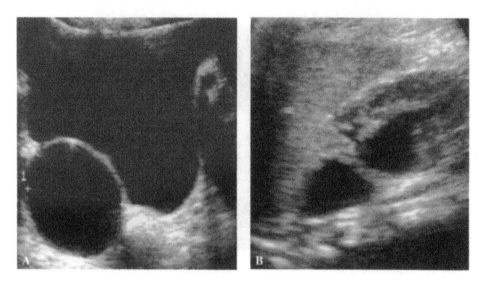

Figure 10. *A,* Transverse sonogram of the bladder shows a large right ectopic ureterocele measuring 3 cm in diameter. *B,* Coronal sonogram of the right kidney shows duplication of the renal collecting system with dilatation of the upper pole moiety due to the presence of the ureterocele. In addition, there is dilatation of the lower moiety related to severe reflux disease.

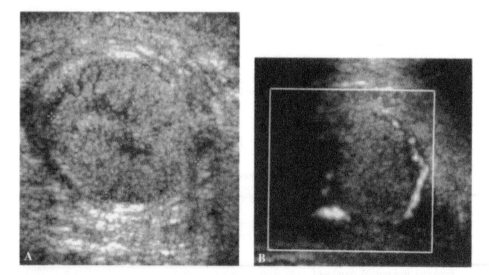

Fugure 11. *A,* Longitudinal sonogram of the left scrotal sac. The scan shows a massively enlarged testis with distinct swelling of the scrotal wall. The central hypoechoic area is consistent with necrosis. *B,* Transverse sonogram using power Doppler shows hyperemia in the swollen peripheral tissues. The lack of evidence of blood flow within the testis is distinctly abnormal.

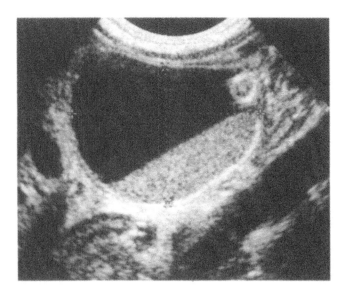

Figure 12.   Ultrasound of the right ovary. It is enlarged and contains one large cyst with a fluid-debris level probably representing an episode of previous hemorrhage. In addition, a small peripheral cyst can be identified. Note the thin rim of normal ovarian tissue that is seen medially. This constellation of findings proved to be benign, resulting from follicular stimulation by maternal hormones.

BIBLIOGRAPHY

APPENDICITIS

1. Galin DO, Gallego M, Fadrique B, et al: Evaluation of ultrasonography and clinical diagnostic scanning in suspected appendicitis. Br J Surg 85:37–40, 1998.
2. Jabra AA, Shalaby-Rana EI, Fishman EK: CT of appendicitis in children. J Comput Assist Tomogr 21:661–666, 1997.
3. Sivit CJ: Imaging children with acute right lower quadrant pain. Pediatr Clin North Am 44:575–589, 1997.

INTUSSUSCEPTION

4. Alan DM, Alton MD: Intussusception: Issues and controversies related to diagnosis and reduction. Radiol Clin North Am 34:743–756, 1996.
5. Carlos J, Savit M: Gastrointestinal emergencies in older infants and children. Radiol Clin North Am 35:865–877, 1997.
6. William H, McAlister M: Intussusception: Even Hippocrates did not standardize his technique of enema reduction. Radiology 206:595–598, 1998.

PYLORIC STENOSIS

7. Rohnschneider WK, Mittnachl H, et al: Pyloric muscle in asymptomatic infants: Sonographic evaluation and discrimination from idiopathic hypertrophic pyloric stenosis. Pediatr Radiol 28:429–434, 1988.
8. Stunden RJ, Le Quesne GW, et al: The improved ultrasound diagnosis of hypertrophic pyloric stenosis. Pediatr Radiol 16:200–205, 1986.
9. Westra SJ, de Groot CJ, et al: Hypertrophic pyloric stenosis: Use of pyloric volume measurements in early US diagnosis. Radiology 172:615–619, 1989.

MALROTATION

10. Carlo Buonomo M: Neonatal gastrointestinal emergencies. Radiol Clin North Am 35:845–853, 1997.
11. Frederick R, Long M, Sandra M, et al: Radiographic patterns of intestinal malrotation in children. Radiographics 16:547–556, 1986.

MECKE'S DIVERTICULUM

12. Mettler FA, Guiberteau MJ: Essentials of Nuclear Medicine Imaging. Philadelphia, W.B. Saunders, 1991.
13. Rossi P, Gourtsoyiannis N, et al: Meckel's diverticulum: Imaging diagnosis. AJR 166:567–573, 1996.
14. Sara M, O'Hara M: Pediatric gastrointestinal nuclear imaging. Radiol Clin North Am 34:849–851, 1996.
15. Sara M, O'Hara M: Acute gastrointestinal bleeding. Radiol Clin North Am 35:884–888, 1997.

CHOLEDOCHAL CYST
16. Chan YL, Yeung CK, et al: Magnetic resonance cholangiography: Feasibility and application in the paediatric population. Pediatr Radiol 28:307–311, 1998.
17. Kirks DR, Caron KH: Gastrointestinal tract. In Kirks DR (ed): Practical Pediatric Imaging: Diagnostic Radiology of Infants and Children. Boston, Little, Brown, 1991, pp 783–786.
18. Lane F, Donnelly M, Bisset MGS III: Pediatric hepatic imaging. Radiol Clin North Am 36:422–424, 1998.
ILEAL ATRESIA AND MECONIUM ILEUS
19. Irish MS, et al: Meconium ileus: Antenatal diagnosis and perinatal care. Fetal Matern Med Rev 8:79–83, 1996.
20. Irish MS, et al: Prenatal diagnosis of the fetus with cystic fibrosis and meconium ileus. Pediatr Surg Int 12:434–436, 1997.
21. Neal MR, Siebert JJ, Vandergalin T, Wagner CW. J Ultrasound Med 16:263–266, 1997.
22. Steinfeld JR, Harrison RB: Extensive intramural intestinal calcification in a newborn with intestinal atresia. Radiology 107:405–406, 1973.
NEUROBLASTOMA
23. Dietrich RB, Kanganloo H, Lenarsky C, Feig SA: Neuroblastoma: The role of MR imaging. AJR 148:937–942, 1987.
PNEUMONIA AND ABDOMINAL PAIN
24. Kanegaye J, Harley J: Pneumonia in unexpected locations: An occult cause of pediatric abdominal pain. J Emerg Med 13:773–779, 1995.
25. Ravichandran D, Burge DM: Pneumonia presenting with acute abdominal pain in children. Br J Surg 83:1707–1708, 1996.
ECTOPIC URETEROCELE
26. Bisset GS, Strife JL: The duplex collecting system in girls with urinary tract infection: Prevalence and significance. AJR 148:497, 1987.
27. Nussbaum AR, et al: Ectopic ureter and ureterocele: Their varied radiographic manifestations. Radiology 159:227, 1986.
TESTICULAR TORSION
28. Kadish HA, Bolte RG: A retrospective review of pediatric patients with epididymitis, testicular torsion and torsion of testicular appendages. Pediatrics 102:73–76, 1998.
OVARIAN CYST, MATERNAL HORMONAL STIMULATION
29. Ros PR, Olmstead WW, Moser RP: Mesenteric and omental cysts: Histological classification with imaging correlation. Radiology 164:327–332, 1987.
30. Schmahmann S, Haller JO: Neonatal ovarian cysts: Pathogenesis, diagnosis, and management. Pediatr Radiol 27:101–105, 1997.
31. Zeele RL, Henschke CI, Zapper D: The radiographic and ultrasonographic evaluation of enteric duplication cysts. Pediatr Radiol 10:9–14, 1980.

72. HEMANGIOMAS AND VASCULAR MALFORMATIONS

Steven J. Fishman, M.D.

1. Are all lesions resembling strawberries hemangiomas?

No. Many fruit-like lesions are vascular malformations rather than hemangiomas.

2. Do all hemangiomas look like strawberries?

No. Hemangiomas have a variety of appearances. They may be raised or flat, smooth or bosselated, superficial or deep. Subcutaneous (deep) lesions have a bluish appearance under normal skin.

3. What difference does it make whether a lesion is called a hemangioma or a vascular malformation?

Imprecise nomenclature is responsible for a widespread lack of understanding of these lesions. Improper diagnosis commonly leads to improper treatment (or lack thereof). Keep reading.

4. How many hemangiomas spontaneously involute?
Essentially all.

5. How many vascular malformations spontaneously involute?
Essentially none.

6. How many hemangiomas respond to angiogenesis inhibitors?
Corticosteroids (systemic or intralesional) lead to accelerated regression in approximately one-third of cases, stabilization in one-third, and no response in one-third. Alpha interferon induces accelerated involution in almost all hemangiomas, but because of its serious potential toxicity in infants, this drug should be reserved for patients with lesions that pose significant threat to life, vital functions, or tissue.

7. How many vascular malformations respond to angiogenesis inhibitors?
Essentially none. Responses, at best, are limited to rare case reports.

8. Summarize the difference between hemangiomas and vascular malformations.
Hemangiomas are the most common tumor of infancy. They are benign neoplasms of proliferative endothelium. Vascular malformations are the result of errors of vascular morphogenesis. They can derive from capillary, venous, arterial, or lymphatic channels or combinations thereof. In fact, hemangiomas and vascular malformations have nothing in common except sometimes a somewhat similar appearance.

9. What is the typical natural history of vascular anomalies?

Hemangiomas	Vascular Malformations
Usually not visible at birth; appear at 1–2 weeks of age	Usually visible (and always present) at birth
Proliferate rapidly over first year	Grow at rate approximately proportional to body
Involute over 5–7 years	Never involute

10. If hemangiomas involute during childhood, why do so many adult women have liver hemangiomas?
They don't. Liver "hemangiomas" in adults are really venous malformations.

11. Explain the difference between cystic hygroma and lymphangioma.
There is none. Both terms should be abandoned. The suffix -*oma* suggests a neoplastic tumor, either benign or malignant. The preferred term is lymphatic malformation (LM). Macrocystic LMs used to be called cystic hygromas, whereas microcystic LMs were called lymphangioma. LMs frequently have mixed macrocystic and microcystic components.

12. Should biopsy always be performed to distinguish a hemangioma from a malformation or to determine the type of malformation?
No. With experience, most lesions can be diagnosed by history and physical examination. Imaging studies, primarily ultrasound and magnetic resonance imaging, if properly interpreted, usually differentiate the others. Biopsy should be necessary infrequently. However, you should not hesitate to biopsy a lesion if malignancy cannot be excluded. Indeed, infantile fibrosarcoma has been confused with both hemangiomas and lymphatic malformation.

13. What is the Kasabach-Merritt phenomenon?
Severe thrombocytopenia (usually 2,000–10,000 platelets/mm^3), which usually occurs in association with kaposiform hemangioendothelioma. This lesion, only recently recognized as distinct from classic hemangioma, has a diffuse edematous, ecchymotic appearance. It usually is located on the torso and/or proximal extremity. Kasabach-Merritt thrombocytopenia does not occur with typical hemangioma.

14. Does the Kasabach-Merritt phenomenon ever occur with vascular malformations?
No. However, large venous malformations can cause a consumptive coagulopathy with diminished fibrinogen and prolonged prothrombin time.

15. What are the primary therapeutic options for venous malformations?
Intralesional sclerotherapy, performed under fluoroscopy with outflow occlusion, often obliterates the dilated anomalous channels. Repeated sessions may be necessary. Some lesions are amenable to surgical excision, contouring, or debulking. Preoperative sclerotherapy can be useful to diminish intraoperative bleeding.

16. How useful is ligation or embolization of the arterial feeding vessels of arteriovenous malformations?
Proximal inflow occlusion should be avoided. An arteriovenous malformation recruits flow from surrounding smaller vessels. Embolization must be performed deep in the nidus of the lesion to have any chance of success. Proximal vessel embolization is useful only as a preoperative measure to diminish bleeding during attempted surgical excision.

17. What is the blue-rubber-bleb nevus syndrome?
Multifocal venous malformations, most prominent on the skin and throughout the gastrointestinal tract. The visceral lesions can cause chronic gastrointestinal bleeding and/or intussusception.

BIBLIOGRAPHY

1. Enjolras O, Mulliken JB: The current management of vascular birthmarks. Pediatr Dermatol 10:311–333, 1993.
2. Fishman SJ, Mulliken J: Vascular anomalies: A primer for pediatricians. Pediatr Clin North Am 45:1455–1477, 1998.
3. Meyers JS, Hoffer FA, Barnes PD, Mulliken JB: MRI-correlation of the biological classification of soft tissue vascular anomalies. AJR 157:559–564, 1991.
4. Mulliken JB, Glowacki J: Hemangiomas and vascular malformations in infants and children: A classification based on endothelial characteristics. Plast Reconstr Surg 69:412–420, 1982.
5. Mulliken JB, Young AE: Vascular Birthmarks: Hemangiomas and Malformations. Philadelphia, W.B. Saunders, 1988.
6. Sarkar M, Mulliken JB, Kozakewich HPW, et al: Thrombocytopenic coaguloapathy (Kasabach-Merritt phenomenon) is associated with kaposiform hemangioendothelioma and not with common hemangioma. Plast Reconstr Surg (in press).

73. TRANSPLANTATION

Jorge Reyes, M.D.

1. List the clinical milestones of successful transplantation of the various solid organs.
Clinical transplantation of whole organs has spanned 40 years and includes the successful (and mostly contemporaneous) engraftment of the following organs:
- Kidney (from identical twins by Murray in 1954 and from nonidentical twins by Merrill in 1960)
- Liver (by Starzl in 1968)
- Heart (by Barnard in 1968)
- Lung (by Derom in 1971)
- Pancreas (by Kelly in 1967)
- Multiple abdominal viscera (by Starzl in 1989)
- Intestine (by Goulet in 1992)

2. What are the cornerstones for successful clinical transplantation?

Successful short- and long-term survival after whole-organ transplantation depends on the following factors:

- Preservation technology
- Surgical technique
- Histocompatibility
- Immunosuppression
- Development of varying degrees of tolerance (less or no immunosuppression)

3. What are the present standards of organ preservation?

Static preservation of all cadaveric organ allografts is accomplished with rapid in situ core cooling with special solutions instilled into the vascular system (aorta) after preliminary separation and cannulation. The Collins solution was used for 20 years before it was replaced with the University of Wisconsin solution developed by Belzer. The safe and longer preservation times for the kidney (48 hours) and liver (24 hours) allowed the development of national organ sharing.

4. Define rejection.

Rejection has not been defined precisely. However, its immunologic nature was first demonstrated in 1944 by Medawar, who showed that inhibition of allo-activated T-cells resulted in prolongation of allograft survival. The central role of this host lymphocyte, which bears the specific capability to differentiate self from nonself, is based on disparities in predetermined genetic barriers between donor and recipient. The major histocompatibility complex (MHC) became serologically measurable after identification of the HLA antigens.

5. What are the mechanistic events in host cell activation to donor antigen?

Histocompatibility antigens on the cells of the transplanted organ are presented to resting host lymphocytes by the host's antigen-presenting cells (bone marrow-derived dendritic cells, macrophages, monocytes, and B-cells, all of which express class 2 MHC antigens). These cells operate in a milieu of cytokines, transforming the resting CD4-positive T-lymphocyte into two potential subsets:

- T-helper-1 cells (secretion of interleukin [IL]-2, interferon-gamma, IL-3, and granulocyte-macrophage colony-stimulating factor [GM-CSF])
- T-helper-2 cells (secretion of IL-4, IL-5, IL-10, IL-3, and GM-CSF)

CD8-positive T-cells interact with MHC class 1 antigen-bearing cells and function as cytotoxic cells.

6. What is graft-versus-host disease?

Originally described in 1957 in the mouse and alternatively known as "runt disease," graft-versus-host disease (GVHD) occurs when the immunologically active allograft rejects the recipient, using a similar genetically predetermined repertoire of immunocytes.

7. Describe the basis for successful bone marrow transplantation.

- Recipient immunosuppressison and cytoablation with total body irradiation or cytotoxic drugs
- Transplantation of donor hematopoietic cells with adequate HLA matching
- Achievement of stable chimerism (endowing the recipient with a donor immune system). This provides graft versus malignancy effect. A mixed chimera state protects the host against lethal GVHD and, with successful engraftment, allows discontinuation of maintenance immunosuppression.

8. What are the strategies for clinical immunosuppression?

Effective clinical immunosuppression focuses on inhibition of antigen-induced T-lymphocyte activation and cytokine production and interruption of the allo-MHC recognition or effector responses.

9. What is the clinical toll of chronic immunosuppression?

To varying degrees, survival rates after liver, heart, kidney, and pancreas transplantation are quite good, whereas survival rates after lung and intestinal transplantation are lower. Survival includes relatively good quality of life and modest morbidity. However, the long-term impact of morbidity due to chronic immunosuppression is still unknown and includes infections (principally Epstein-Barr virus–induced), degenerative diseases, drug toxicities, and chronic rejection.

10. Is it necessary to remove the native kidney and place the donor kidney in the same location?

No, although on rare occasions it may be an option. Kidney allografts are placed heterotopically, usually in the iliac fossa. The vascular anastomoses are to the iliac artery and vein; in small children, they may be to the aorta and inferior vena cava. The ureteral connection usually is directly to the bladder and occasionally to the recipient ureter.

11. Does the presence of two kidneys per cadaveric donor and the ability to perform living related kidney transplants allow transplantation in all potential candidates?

No. Presently 40,000 patients are awaiting kidney transplantation, with a yearly accrual of approximately 2,500 candidates. About 13,000 kidney transplants are performed per year in the United States, of which 25% are from living related donors. Because of the large numbers of patients awaiting kidney transplantation, the total number of deaths on the waiting list is larger than for any other organ type.

12. Is laparoscopic donor nephrectomy replacing the traditional open approach?

Yes—but slowly. The development of laparoscopic donor nephrectomy is applied in many transplant centers, with similar outcomes but substantial improvement in length of hospital stay.

13. What are the most common indications for liver transplantation in children?

Biliary atresia is by far the most common indication, followed by inborn errors of metabolism, fulminant hepatic failure, and familial cholestatic disorders. The number of patients transplanted for primary hepatic malignancy is small; in selected patients, however, it has provided long-term survival and cure.

14. What clinical syndromes are indications for liver transplantation?

The term *end-stage liver disease* encompasses various clinical scenarios, including variceal hemorrhage, intractable ascites, hepatorenal syndrome, recurrent infection, and encephalopathy.

15. What specific laboratory parameters support the diagnosis of end-stage liver disease?
- Evidence of hepatic synthetic dysfunction (elevated prothrombin time, hypoalbuminemia, elevated serum ammonia)
- Portal hypertension (hypersplenism with thrombocytopenia and leukopenia)

16. Is liver transplantation the only recourse for patients with end-stage liver disease and variceal hemorrhage?

No. All variceal hemorrhages are managed initially with resuscitation, followed by measures to control bleeding with nasogastric decompression and lavage, endoscopic sclerotherapy or banding, splanchnic vasoconstrictors (somatostatin analog), Blakemore tube insertion, and, finally, portosystemic shunting procedures. Selected patients with well-compensated Child's A cirrhosis and variceal hemorrhage may show long-term benefit from surgical portosystemic shunting only.

17. Is transplantation indicated in a child who is not suffering life-threatening complications of end-stage liver disease?

Yes. Life-disabling complications of liver disease that are severely incapacitating or compromise growth and development are accepted indications for liver transplantation.

18. What is an auxiliary liver transplant?

The standard liver transplant involves removal of the diseased liver and replacement of the liver allograft in the orthotopic position. Auxiliary liver transplantation preserves the native diseased liver and provides a small liver allograft placed in a heterotopic position (usually the right sub-hepatic space) or orthotopic position (after partial removal of the native liver, usually the left lateral segment). This type of procedure is used only in selected cases of fulminant hepatic failure and inborn metabolic errors.

19. What are the basic principles of total hepatectomy?

Total hepatectomy and liver transplantation demand control of the hepatic hilum and the supra- and infrahepatic inferior vena cava. This portion of the vena cava may be preserved (routine approach in children).

20. What are the most common variations in arterial supply to the liver? How do they affect vascular reconstruction?

Donor or recipient anomalies of the hepatic artery (one-third of cases) include anomalous branches directly from the aorta, from the left gastric artery, or from the superior mesenteric artery. These anomalies can be reconstructed as a bench procedure, providing a single arterial anastomosis to a recipient vessel or using a vascular homograft implanted into the recipient infrarenal aorta.

21. Does total hepatectomy require replacement of a whole liver?

No. The success of liver transplantation after the early 1980s has produced a crisis in organ availability. Strategies to increase supply led to the ability to transplant hepatic segments. In children this approach has involved living related donations of left lateral liver segments, reduction of whole cadaveric liver allografts, and, most recently, splitting of a cadaveric liver allograft to allow transplantation of two patients with one liver (usually one adult and one child). This approach presently allows the development of split liver transplantation for two adults as well as adult living related donor liver transplantation.

22. What are the most common indications for intestinal transplantation?

Intestinal transplantation generally is indicated for patients who have intestinal failure and depend on total parenteral nutrition (TPN). Most of these patients have surgical short gut as a consequence of volvulus, gastroschisis, necrotizing enterocolitis, or intestinal atresias. Functional disorders of the intestine with or without normal intestinal length include Hirschsprung's disease and psuedoobstruction.

23. What clinical syndromes mandate listing for intestinal transplantation?

Of interest, intestinal failure produces clinical syndromes related not to the bowel structures, but to the use of TPN. Examples include progressive vascular thrombosis and lack of venous access, life-threatening catheter infections, and TPN-related cholestatic liver disease.

24. What are the technical challenges of intestinal transplantation?

Transplantation of the intestine may involve replacement of other organs such as the liver, stomach, and duodenopancreatic complex. Selection of the organ complex follows the functional assessment of other organs. Three principal procedures have been established: isolated intestine, liver/intestine, and multivisceral organ allografts.

25. Is it rational to transplant a heart into a 1-year-old infant?

The textbook answer is yes. The 3- and 5-year survival rates are 95% and 80%, respectively. However, follow-up reports after 5 years have shown an increase in patient and graft loss due to chronic rejection, the impact of which is still unknown in children.

26. What are the general indications for any cardiopulmonary transplant procedure?
- Severe symptoms (New York Heart Association class III–IV)
- Expected survival < 2 years

27. List the specific indications for heart transplantation.
- Cardiomyopathy
- Coronary artery disease
- Valvular disease
- Congenital heart disease

28. List the specific indications for lung transplantation.
- Cystic fibrosis
- Emphysema
- Alpha-1-antitrypsin deficiency
- Pulmonary hypertension
- Pulmonary fibrosis

29. When is combined heart/lung transplantation indicated?
- Congenital heart/lung disease
- Pulmonary hypertension
- Cystic fibrosis
- Emphysema
- Pulmonary fibrosis
- Alpha-1-antitrypsin deficiency

30. List the most common complications after heart transplantation.
- Primary nonfunction of the heart allograft
- Technical problems (bleeding, vascular thrombosis)
- Rejection
- Atherosclerosis
- Sepsis (bacterial, viral, fungal, protozoal)
- Stroke

31. What are the most common complications after liver transplantation?

Short-term complications include vascular strictures and thrombosis (hepatic artery, portal vein. and vena cava), biliary strictures, biliary leaks, and bleeding. **Longer follow-up complications** include rejection (acute and chronic) and infection (bacterial, viral, fungal, and protozoal).

BIBLIOGRAPHY

1. Barnard CN: What we have learned about heart transplants. J Thorac Cardiovasc Surg 56:457, 1968.
2. Belzer FO, Southard JH: Principles of solid-organ preservation by cold storage. Transplantation 45:673, 1988.
3 Billingham R, Brent L: A simple method for inducing tolerance of skin homografts in mice. Trans Bull 4:67, 1957.
4. Billingham RE, Brent L, Medawar PB: Actively acquired tolerance of foreign cells. Nature 172:603, 1953.
5. Broelsch CE, Emond JC, Whitington TF, et al: Application of reduced-size liver transplant as split grafts, auxiliary orthotopic grafts, and living related segmental transplants. Ann Surg 212:368–377, 1990.
6. Collins GM, Bravo-Shugarman M, Terasaki PI: Kidney preservation for transportation: Initial perfusion and 30 hours ice storage. Lancet 2:1219–1224, 1969.
7. Dausset J: The HLA Adventure In Teraskai PI (ed): History of HLA: Ten Recollections, Los Angeles, UCLA Tissue Typing Laboratory, 1990.
8. Derom F, et al: Ten-month survival after lung homotransplantation in man. J Thorac Cardiovasc Surg 61:835, 1971.
9. Goulet O, et al: Successful small bowel transplantation in an infant. Transplantation 53:940, 1992.
10. Johnson RB: Immunology: Monocytes and macrophages. N Engl J Med 318:747, 1988.
11. Kelly WD, et al: Allotransplantation of the pancreas and duodenum along with the kidney in diabetic nephropathy. Surgery 61:827, 1967.
12. Medawar PB: The behavior and fate of skin allografts and skin homografts in rabbits. J Anat 78:176–199, 1944.
13. Merrill JP, et al: Successful homotransplantation of the human kidney between identical twins. JAMA 160:277, 1956.
14. Merrill JP, et al: Successful homotransplantation of the kidney between non-identical twins. N Engl J Med 262:1251, 1960.

15. Mosmannn TR, Coffman RL: Heterogeneity of cytokine secretion patterns and functions of helper T cells. Adv Immunol 46:111, 1989.
16. Reyes J, Starzl TE: Principles of transplantation. In O'Neill JA, Rowe MI, Grosfeld JL, et al (eds): Pediatric Surgery, 5th ed. St. Louis, Mosby, 1998 pp 547–561.
17. Rogiers X, et al: In situ splitting of cadaveric livers: The ultimate expansion of a limited donor pool. Ann Surg 224:331–341, 1996.
18. Starzl TE, et al: Transplantation of multiple abdominal viscera. JAMA 261:1449, 1989.
19. Starzl TE, et al: Orthotopic homotransplantation of the human liver. Ann Surg 168:392, 1968.
20. Terasaki PI (ed): History of HLA: Ten Recollections, Los Angeles, UCLA Tissue Typing Laboratory, 1990.

74. NEONATOLOGY

Robert C. Dukarm, M.D.

HYPERBILIRUBINEMIA

1. What is physiologic jaundice?

Physiologic jaundice is the normal elevation of unconjugated bilirubin in healthy neonates. The timing of physiologic jaundice and the level of bilirubin differ slightly by race. In white and black infants the peak level of bilirubin is ~ 6 mg/dl at 72 hours of age. In Asian infants the bilirubin level peaks later (3–5 days) at a higher level (~ 12 mg/dl). In preterm neonates, the level is ~ 12 mg/dl on the fifth day of life.

2. What are the major causes of unconjugated hyperbilrubinemia?

GENERAL DISORDER	CAUSE	DIAGNOSIS
Production	Hemolysis	Rh incompatibility; major/minor blood group incompatibility
	Enzyme defects	G6PD deficiency; pyruvate kinase deficiency; hexokinase deficiency; congenital porphyria
	Structural defects	Hereditary spherocytosis; hereditary elliptocytosis
	Increased RBC mass	Polycythemia
	RBC sequestration	Hematoma, extensive bruising; hemangiomas
Hepatic uptake	Decreased	Gilbert syndrome
Conjugation	Decreased	Crigler-Najjar syndrome I/II; Lucey-Driscoll syndrome; hypothyroidism; pyloric stenosis
Enterohepatic circulation	Increased	Breast feeding, breast milk

RBC = red blood cell.

3. What is the basic laboratory work-up of a healthy newborn with increased unconjugated bilirubin?

The basic laboratory work-up for unconjugated hyperbilirubinemia includes a blood type/Rh and Coombs' test, a complete blood count with examination of the blood smear and reticulocyte count, and a total and direct bilirubin level. If direct hyperbilirubinemia is present, liver function tests and prothrombin and partial thromboplastin times should be obtained. The remainder of the work-up should be individualized based on the above tests, history, and physical examination.

4. In a healthy full-term newborn, when should phototherapy be started? When should an exchange transfusion be performed?

The American Academy of Pediatricians (AAP) published the following guidelines for phototherapy and exchange transfusion in 1994. Total bilirubin levels are expressed in mg/dl.

AGE (HR)	PHOTOTHERAPY	EXCHANGE TRANSFUSION + INTENSIVE PHOTOTHERAPY
25–48	≥ 15	≥ 25
49–72	≥ 18	≥ 30
>72	≥ 20	≥ 30

Jaundice in a newborn ≤ 24 hours of age is considered pathologic and requires at least a total serum bilirubin level and possibly other laboratory tests for detection of hemolysis or other disease processes.

5. What is the difference between breast-feeding jaundice and breast-milk jaundice?

In breast-feeding jaundice (early-onset breast-milk jaundice), the hyperbilirubinemia is multifactorial but basically results from starvation and dehydration. In late-onset breast-milk jaundice, the hyperbilirubinemia probably results from chemical changes in the milk that increase enterohepatic circulation. Both syndromes are caused by an increase in the enterohepatic circulation. Up to 4% of all breastfed infants have a serum bilirubin concentration > 10 mg/dl at 3 weeks of age. Recently bilirubin has been shown to be an antioxidant and may be potentially beneficial in protection against free radical damage.

6. How does phototherapy decrease bilirubin?

Phototherapy decreases bilirubin by photo-oxidation (small fraction) and configurational and structural isomerization. These processes make bilirubin more water-soluble and increase excretion in bile and urine.

7. What are the side effects of phototherapy?

Phototherapy causes diarrhea, skin rashes, and overheating. It increases insensible water loss and in the presence of direct hyperbilirubinemia may cause the bronze-baby syndrome. It may adversely affect the mother-infant relationship and the process of breast-feeding.

8. Is the majority of circulating bilirubin in the free form or protein-bound form?

Over 99% of circulating bilirubin is bound to albumin; the other 1% circulates in the free form.

9. If a healthy full-term neonate appears yellow from the face to the ankles, what is the approximate bilirubin level?

The cephalocaudal progression of jaundice is a useful clinical tool.

BODY PART	BILIRUBIN LEVEL (MG/DL)
Face	6
Neck to umbilicus	9
Umbilicus to knees	12
Knees to ankles	15
Hands and feet	> 15

10. What maternal blood type is a potential set-up for ABO incompatibility?

A mother with blood type O does not possess an A or B antigen and is therefore at risk for developing anti-A or anti-B antibody after exposure to that particular antigen. Sensitization may occur after a transfusion, first-trimester abortion, ectopic pregnancy, amniocentesis, chorionic blood sampling, normal pregnancy, manual extraction of the placenta, or any type of procedure.

11. What antigen causes classic erythroblastosis fetalis?

Classic erythroblastosis fetalis is due to maternofetal incompatibility of the D antigen (Rh-negative mother and Rh-positive infant). The degree of hydrops fetalis (severe erythroblastosis fetalis) becomes more severe with subsequent pregnancies. The discovery and widespread use of the anti-D immunoglobulin (Rhogam) to prevent maternal sensitization has made the condition uncommon. Before the advent of Rhogam, the most common cause of hydrops fetalis was hemolytic anemia caused by D antigen incompatibility; now the most common cause of hydrops fetalis is nonimmune.

12. What is kernicterus?

Kernicterus is a histologic diagnosis that refers to bilirubin staining of the basal ganglia, thalamus, cerebellum, hippocampus, and cranial nerve nuclei. It often is used to describe the long-term sequelae in children with evidence of bilirubin encephalopathy in the newborn period.

13. Do most pediatric surgeons have vigintiphobia or fear of the number 20?

No. By definition a surgeon fears nothing (especially a pediatric surgeon). Most pediatricians have vigintiphobia because much of the older literature (before Rhogam, when classic erythroblastosis fetalis was still common) advocated performing an exchange transfusion at a bilirubin level of 20.

METABOLIC PROBLEMS

14. What is the most common metabolic problem in the newborn?

Hypoglycemia is the most common metabolic problem in the newborn.

15. Define hypoglycemia.

In the early 1960s the definition of hypoglycemia depended on gestational age. Full-term newborns were considered hypoglycemic with a glucose level of < 30 mg/dl, whereas newborns with low birth weight were considered hypoglycemic with glucose levels < 20 mg/dl. Our understanding of antenatal/neonatal glucose metabolism has increased over the past 30 years, and most neonatologists define hypoglycemia as a glucose level < 35 or 40 mg/dl, regardless of gestational age. In a normal newborn glucose decreases to a physiologic nadir at approximately 1 hour of age.

16. What is the clinical presentation of a newborn with hypoglycemia?

The presentation is often nonspecific and may be confused with several other neonatal problems. The infant usually has some or all of the following symptoms: respiratory distress, tachypnea, tachycardia, apnea, desaturations/dusky spells, irritability, tremors, jitteriness, seizures, hypotonia, lethargy, and hypothermia. If the child is not hypoglycemic, other potential diagnoses need to be pursued.

17. What maternal condition predisposes to neonatal hypoglycemia?

Diabetes mellitus. Although the human fetus depends on the mother for glucose and other nutrients for energy, the fetus is hormonally independent of the mother. When the mother has inadequately controlled diabetes (or even with adequate control) during pregnancy, the fetus uses the available glucose for growth and stores the excess as fat and glycogen. The high glucose results in fetal islet cell hyperplasia.

18. What neonatal conditions are associated with hypoglycemia?

- Diabetic mother
- Small size for gestational age
- Beckwith-Wiedemann syndrome
- Hydrops fetalis

- Prematurity
- Birth asphyxia
- Hypothermia
- Polycythemia
- Sepsis
- Large size for gestational age
- Inborn errors of metabolism

- Maternal medications (beta sympathomimetics and beta blockers)
- Nesidioblastosis
- Endocrine problems (pituitary insufficiency, deficiency of glucagon, epinephrine, or cortisol)
- Exchange transfusion

19. What is the normal physiologic range of glucose production in a newborn? How do you calculate the amount of exogenous dextrose delivery in mg/kg/min?

The normal range of glucose production in a newborn is about 5–8 mg/kg/min. In initiating intravenous fluid therapy, the goal is to deliver this amount. The delivery of dextrose (mg/kg/min) = % dextrose concentration × fluid input × 10 ÷ 1440. In other words, a 10% aqueous dextrose solution (D10W) at 100 ml/kg/day delivers about 6.9 mg/kg/min of dextrose or $10 \times 100 \times 10 \div 1440$.

20. Describe the immediate management of a newborn with hypoglycemia.

In a newborn with a glucose < 35–40 mg/dl, many neonatologists repeat the measurement in 15 minutes, especially if the infant is less than 2 hours of age. If the repeat measurement is the same, the appropriate intervention is to give glucose. One approach is to establish intravenous access and give a 2-ml/kg bolus of D10W followed by an infusion of dextrose that delivers 5–8 mg/kg/min. If the infant remains hypoglycemic, the delivery of dextrose should be increased by 1–2 mg/kg/min with every subsequent low value until the dextrose equals 40–45 mg/dl. Another approach initially is to give nasogastric or oral formula or D10W and to repeat the serum glucose. Finally, if intravenous access is a problem, an intramuscular or subcutaneous injection of 0.1 mg/kg of glucagon in a newborn who is not preterm or growth-retarded can normalize glucose levels until intravenous access can be obtained.

21. Define hypocalcemia.

In a full-term neonate a total calcium < 8.0 mg/dl or an ionized calcium < 4.4 mg/dl is considered hypocalcemic. In a preterm neonate the definition is less well established; however, a total calcium < 6.5–7.0 mg/dl or an ionized calcium < 4.0–4.28 is a reasonable definition of hypocalcemia.

22. What are the clinical manifestations of hypocalcemia?

Hypocalcemia produces jitteriness secondary to increased neuromuscular irritability and seizures. Newborns with hypocalcemia also may be asymptomatic.

23. When is the majority of calcium transferred from the mother to the fetus?

Approximately 30 grams of calcium have been accrued in a full-term neonate. The majority (~70%) is transferred in the third trimester of pregnancy.

24. True or false: The majority of calcium is found circulating in a newborn.

False. Ninety-nine percent of calcium in the body is found in the skeletal system. The other 1% is found in the intracellular fluid and other body tissues. In the circulating pool of calcium, ~ 55% circulates as free ionized calcium. The remainder circulates bound to protein/albumin (majority) or as a complex with bicarbonate, citrate, lactate, and phosphate (minority).

25. A 10-day-old infant presents to the emergency department with seizures. The mother says that she cannot afford formula and has been feeding her baby whole milk. What is the diagnosis? Why?

The infant probably has hypocalcemic seizures related to the ingestion of cow's milk. Cow's milk is high in phosphate, and the phosphate load results in hypocalcemia and seizures.

26. A 7-week-old (former 25-week) infant with bronchopulmonary dysplasia requiring steroids and diuretics and necrotizing enterocolitis requiring long periods of total parenteral nutrition has a routine chest radiograph that reveals multiple-aged rib fractures and long-bone fractures. Should the surgical house staff notify child protective services?

No. The infant has multiple fractures related to osteopenia secondary to rickets of prematurity. The majority of calcium accretion occurs in the third trimester, and a 25-week infant accretes about 15% of the calcium accreted by a full-term infant. This infant probably was getting inadequate amounts of dietary calcium and phosphorus and was given medications, such as dexamethasone and diuretics, that cause calcium-wasting in the urine. The serum calcium is usually normal, the serum phosphate is decreased, and the serum alkaline phosphatase is elevated.

27. Define hypo- and hypermagnesemia.

Hypomagnesemia is a serum magnesium (Mg) < 1.6 mg/dl; hypermagnesemia is a serum Mg > 2.8 mg/dl.

28. What causes hypo- or hypermagnesemia?

Hypomagnesemia is seen in infants of diabetic mothers and newborns with intrauterine growth retardation, hypoparathyroidism, severe malabsorption, or renal tubular defects. Hypermagnesemia is usually iatrogenic and related to administration of magnesium sulfate to the mother (i.e., for preeclampsia or tocolysis) or excessive amounts of magnesium to the infant (i.e., hyperalimentation and experimental treatment for persistent pulmonary hypertension).

INTRAVENTRICULAR HEMORRHAGE

29. How many infants are born each year in the United States with a birth weight < 1500 grams?

According to the vital statistics published by the AAP for 1997, the total number of live births in the United States was 3.9 million. Of these infants, 1.41% weighed < 1500 gm or had a very low birth weight. In other words, more than 54,000 infants weighed < 1500 gm in the U.S in 1997.

30. What percentage of neonates weighing < 1500 grams survive?

According to the 1997 vital statistics, about 75% of neonates weighing < 1500 gm survive the first year of life. However, there is a large discrepancy for individual 250-gm birth weight categories. About 9 of 10 neonates weighing < 500 gm die within the first year of life, whereas about 95% of neonates weighing 1250–1499 gm survive the first year of life.

31. What percentage of newborns weighing < 1500 gm have intraventricular hemorrhage?

Approximately 20% of newborns weighing < 1500 gm have intraventricular hemorrhage (IVH).

32. At what gestational age are infants at risk for IVH?

Infants of ≤ 34 weeks gestation are at risk for IVH. The risk is inversely proportional to birth weight and gestational age. An infant born at < 28 weeks gestation has a threefold higher risk of IVH than an infant born at 28–31 weeks gestation.

33. How do neonatologists grade IVH?

Most neonatologists use the grading system published by Papile and colleagues:

GRADE	DESCRIPTION
I	Subependymal hemorrhage
II	Intraventricular hemorrhage without ventricular dilatation
III	Intraventricular hemorrhage with ventricular dilatation
IV	Intraventricular hemorrhage with parenchymal hemorrhage

Other grading systems include *small* hemorrhage (grades I and II in the Papile system), *moderate* hemorrhage (grade III), and *severe* hemorrhage (grade IV).

34. Which neuroimaging modality is used most frequently for diagnosing IVH?

The bedside cranial ultrasound. Other modalities include computed tomography (CT) scan or magnetic resonance image (MRI) of the head. These modalities are not practical because the premature infant must be taken to the imaging suite. Before neuroimaging techniques were available, lumbar puncture was used to diagnose IVH.

35. On which postnatal day should the first cranial ultrasound be done in a premature infant?

A cranial ultrasound on the first postnatal day detects about 50% of all IVHs. A cranial ultrasound on the second day detects another 25%, and a cranial ultrasound on the third day detects another 10–15%. Therefore, a cranial ultrasound on day three of life detects about 90% of all IVHs. A cranial ultrasound between day 10 and 14 detects nearly 100% of all IVHs and about 80–90% of infants with posthemorrhagic hydrocephalus.

36. Describe the clinical presentation of a catastrophic IVH.

Clinical features include coma, generalized seizures, decerebrate posturing, fixed pupils, respiratory disturbances (including apnea), bradycardia, temperature instability, metabolic acidosis, falling hemoglobin and hematocrit, a bulging anterior fontanel, and syndrome of inappropriate secretion of antidiuretic hormone.

37. What causes IVH?

The cause of IVH is multifactorial. The two most important factors are prematurity and acute respiratory failure requiring assisted ventilation. Other factors include alterations in cerebral blood flow caused by asphyxia, hypoxemia, and hypercapnia. Other critical neonatal events include pneumothorax, hypotension, hypertension, acidosis, coagulopathy, outborn status, volume expansion, and bicarbonate infusion.

38. What is the prognosis of a grade I, II, III, or IV IVH?

The risk of long-term neurodevelopmental sequelae exists with any grade of IVH. The table below shows the percentage of children at 2-year follow-up with long-term neurodevelopmental sequelae in two studies. In the study by Vohr, et al., grade I and II IVHs were analyzed together, as were grades III and IV.

GRADE IVH	PAPILE, ET AL. (1978)	VOHR, ET AL. (1989)
I	9%	7%
II	11%	7%
III	36%	25%
IV	76%	25%

39. What are the major ways to prevent IVH prenatally? Postnatally?

The most effective way to prevent IVH prenatally is to prevent preterm labor. Finding a way to prevent preterm labor would be worthy of a Nobel Prize—and might force neonatologists to seek residency in surgery. Antenatal corticosteroid therapy significantly decreases the risk of IVH independently of its effects on respiratory distress syndrome. Other more controversial antenatal therapies include phenobarbital and parenteral vitamin K administration to the mother.

Postnatal pharmacologic interventions for decreasing IVH include agents such as phenobarbital, indomethacin, ethamsylate, vitamin E, and pancuronium. Several studies with phenobarbital have reported inconsistent results, and the largest trial actually found an increase in IVH in the phenobarbital-treated group of infants. Indomethacin has been used in several clinical trials with varying results, including a decrease in the risk of IVH in several studies and no change in IVH in a few. Ethamsylate is currently unavailable in the U.S. but has had promising results in other countries. Vitamin E has been used in several studies, with most demonstrating a beneficial effect in decreasing IVH. However, one study showed an increase in the frequency of IVH. Pancuronium has been used in one trial and showed no significant decrease in IVH. In extremely premature infants, pancuronium has serious side effects, including edema and renal failure.

RESPIRATORY DISTRESS SYNDROME

40. Define respiratory distress syndrome.
Respiratory distress syndrome (RSD) refers to surfactant deficiency, which may be primary or secondary. Primary surfactant deficiency usually occurs in a preterm infant or an infant of a diabetic mother. Secondary or acquired surfactant deficiency occurs in an infant with adequate surfactant production, but for various reasons (i.e., pulmonary hemorrhage, meconium aspiration, and pneumonia) the surfactant has been inactivated.

41. What percentage of premature newborns ≤ 28 weeks gestation develop RDS?
Approximately 55% of infants ≤ 28 weeks develop RDS. Like IVH, the risk is inversely proportional to gestational age and birth weight. In an infant weighing 500–750 gm at birth, the incidence of RDS is about 85%; in an infant weighing 1250–1500 gm at birth, the incidence is about 25%.

42. Do full-term infants develop RDS?
Yes, but it is rare. The two groups of full-term infants that develop RDS are infants of diabetic mothers and infants with perinatal asphyxia. In fact, infants of diabetic mothers have RDS six times more frequently than infants born to mothers without diabetes.

43. Which cell produces pulmonary surfactant? What is the biochemical make-up of surfactant?
The type II pneumocyte in the lung is responsible for the synthesis and secretion of surfactant. The composition of surfactant is about 80% phospholipids, 10% neutrolipids, and 10% proteins. Sixty-five percent of the phospholipids are phosphatidylcholine, the majority of neutrolipids are cholesterol, and the proteins are made up of surfactant proteins A, B, C, D, and others.

44. What prenatal tests are used to assess lung maturity?
The standard against which all other tests are compared is the **lecithin/sphingomyelin (L/S) ratio.** The lecithin component is derived from phosphatidylcholine, which increases with lung maturity, and the sphingomyelin component is a general membrane lipid, which is a nonspecific component of amniotic fluid unrelated to lung maturation. With an L/S ratio > 2, RDS is unlikely. With an L/S ratio ≤ 1, RDS is very likely. Values between 1 and 2 are equivocal.

Another method to assess lung maturity is to look for the presence of **phosphatidylglycerol** (PG) in the amniotic fluid. In the premature lung, less than 1% of the phospholipids are PG, whereas in the mature lung approximately 10% of the phospholipids are PG. A positive PG correlates with lung maturity.

The **lung profile** is a test that combines the L/S ratio and PG to define lung maturity more accurately.

Another test is the **lung maturity index**, which is calculated by dividing surfactant (mg) by albumin (gm) in the amniotic fluid. A lung maturity index > 50 in normal pregnancies and > 75 in pregnancies complicated by diabetes is considered mature.

45. Do antenatal corticosteroids change the incidence of RDS?
Yes. Several studies have shown that antenatal corticosteroids given at < 32–34 weeks gestation, > 24 hours before delivery, and < 7 days before delivery significantly decrease the incidence

of RDS. Other studies have shown a benefit to antenatal corticosteroids even if delivery takes place before 24 hours after the initiation of steroids. Antenatal administration of thyroid-releasing hormone (TRH) also decreases the incidence of RDS but probably acts synergistically with corticosteroids.

46. Which law is important in understanding the pathophysiology of RDS?

Laplace's law, which states that pressure (dynes/cm^2) = 2 × tension (dynes/cm) ÷ radius (cm). In the absence of pulmonary surfactant, smaller alveoli are expected to collapse into larger alveoli. This collapse does not occur in the presence of pulmonary surfactant because of its surface tension–lowering properties. Alveolar interdependence also has some role in preventing collapse.

47. What is the clinical presentation of a newborn with RDS?

Usually in the first 6 hours the infant develops tachypnea, grunting, intercostal retractions, nasal flaring, cyanosis, hypoxia, increasing requirements for the fractional concentration of oxygen in inspired gases (FiO$_2$), and a characteristic appearance on chest radiograph.

48. What is the differential diagnosis of tachypnea in the newborn?

T	=	**T**ransient tachypnea of the newborn
A	=	**A**spiration (meconium, amniotic fluid, blood)
C	=	**C**ardiac failure, **c**ongenital malformations (e.g, congenital diaphragmatic hernia, congenital cystic adenomatoid malformations of the lung))
HY	=	**Hy**aline membrane disease
P	=	**P**neumonia
N	=	**N**erve damage (phrenic nerve)
E	=	**E**ffusions (pleural/chylous)
A	=	**A**ir leak syndromes, **a**cidosis

49. What are the chest radiographic findings in a newborn with RDS?

The characteristic chest radiograph in an infant with RDS has a diffuse reticulogranular pattern (areas of atelectasis alternating with superimposed areas of hyperinflation) with air bronchograms. In addition, the radiograph usually has low intrathoracic volume.

50. Are there biochemical differences in exogenous surfactant preparations?

The two basic types of surfactant preparations are mammalian (Surfacten, Survanta, Curosurf, and Infasurf) and synthetic (ALEC and Exosurf). Surfacten and Survanta are organic extracts of homogenized whole lung with further extraction of the neutral lipids. Dipalmitylphospatidylcholine, palmitic acid, and triglyceride are added to improve surface activation. Curosurf is an organic extract of homogenized whole lung "purified" by column chromatography. Infasurf is an organic extract of a bronchoalveolar lavage obtained from newborn lambs. The phospholipid profile of each differs. All four contain detectable SP-B and SP-C apoproteins, but Infasurf is the only one with physiologic levels of SP-B. ALEC and Exosurf contain dipalmitylphospatidylcholine and other components to facilitate surface adsorption. The dose is 3–5 ml/kg, depending on the preparation; dosage is based on the amount of phospholipid/kg.

51. Has surfactant replacement changed the management and mortality of RDS?

Yes. Surfactant replacement has significantly decreased the mortality and the incidence of air leak (i.e., pneumothorax and pulmonary interstitial emphysema) in patients with RDS. The incidence of other complications of prematurity and RDS, such as pulmonary hemorrhage, IVH, necrotizing enterocolitis, patent ductus arteriosus, and sepsis, has not changed with surfactant replacement.

52. Has surfactant decreased the incidence of bronchopulmonary dysplasia?

The severity, but not the incidence, of bronchopulmonary dysplasia (BPD) is probably decreased with exogenous surfactant. A few studies have shown a decreased incidence of BPD with exogenous surfactant, but this finding has not been consistent.

BRONCHOPULMONARY DYSPLASIA

53. Who provided the first definition or description of BPD?

In 1967, Northway used the term bronchopulmonary dysplasia to describe a chronic pulmonary syndrome associated with the use of mechanical ventilation in premature infants with RDS. His initial report described the orderly progression of clinical, pathologic, and radiographic changes from the early findings of severe RDS, which he termed stage I disease, to severe chronic bronchopulmonary insufficiency, which he termed stage IV disease. The infants in his study were more mature and larger at birth than most survivors of RDS today.

54. Do other descriptions or definitions of BPD exist?

Yes. Two more recent definitions have been used for BPD or chronic lung disease. The first combines clinical signs of chronic respiratory distress, an oxygen requirement, and an abnormal chest radiograph at 28 days postnatal age. The second definition is an infant with initial respiratory distress requiring mechanical ventilation and an oxygen requirement at 36 weeks postconceptional age.

55. What are the major pathologic findings in the lung of a patient with BPD?

Pathologic findings in BPD include medial muscular hypertrophy, elastic degeneration, marked decrease in the number of alveoli, mucosal hyperplasia and metaplasia, airway injury with a loss of epithelium and cilia, interstitial fibrosis and edema, and emphysema alternating with areas of atelectasis.

56. What causes BPD?

The cause of BPD is multifactorial. It begins as acute lung injury in a susceptible host (usually a premature infant). The many contributing factors include oxygen toxicity, oxygen free radical toxicity, barotrauma/volutrauma, infection and chronic inflammation, and pulmonary edema related or unrelated to a patent ductus arteriosus.

57. What is the incidence of BPD?

The incidence of BPD is inversely related to gestational age and birth weight. In infants born after 32–34 weeks, BPD is uncommon, with an incidence less than 2%. In a multicenter trial studying the prevention of RDS with surfactant prophylaxis, the incidence of BPD was between 12% and 18% (mean birth weight, 900 gm; mean gestational age, 26.5 weeks).

58. What are the risk factors for developing BPD?

The risk of developing BPD decreases with increasing gestational age and birth weight. Risk factors include prematurity, RDS, white race, male sex, infant of a diabetic mother, and family history of reactive airway disease.

59. What is the expected pulmonary function in a patient with BPD?

Infants with BPD characteristically have a marked increase in airway resistance and airway reactivity along with a decrease in dynamic compliance. Minute ventilation is usually increased, but because of lower dynamic compliance tidal volume is smaller and respiratory rate higher than normal. This results in an increase in dead-space ventilation and explains the alveolar hypoventilation and carbon dioxide retention in patients with chronic lung disease or BPD.

60. What is the treatment of BPD?

The first step in treatment, when indicated, is to provide mechanical ventilation in a way that minimizes barotrauma.

MEDICATION	BENEFICIAL EFFECTS	SIDE EFFECTS
Albuterol	Bronchodilator	Hypertension, tachycardia, possible arrhythmias
Theophylline	Bronchodilator, mild diuretic, respiratory stimulant, improves diaphragm contractility	Same as for albuterol
Furosemide, spironolactone	Diuresis, improve pulmonary compliance	Metabolic alkalosis, hypocalcemia, hypercalciuria, nephrocalcinosis, electrolyte disturbances
Chlorothiazide	Beneficial effects of diuretics	Side effects of diuretics
Antibiotics	Treat pulmonary and tracheal infections	Resistant bacteria, increased risk of fungal infections
Corticosteroids	Enhanced surfactant production, decreasd bronchospasm, decreased pulmonary and bronchial edema, decreased response of inflammatory cells and mediators in injured lung	Mask signs of infection, hyperglycemia, hypertension, adrenal cortical suppression, hypertrophic cardiomyopathy, gastroduodenal perforation, somatic growth suppression, increased proteolysis

Last and not least, treatment includes adequate nutrition. Patients with BPD often have an increased metabolic rate that requires more calories for growth.

61. How can BPD be prevented?

Because the incidence of BPD is inversely related to gestational age, the obvious answer is to prolong gestation. Other potential ways to decrease BPD are antenatal steroids and/or antenatal steroids combined with thyroid-releasing hormone. In the neonatal period it is important to minimize barotrauma and volutrauma. Early identification and treatment of a patent ductus arteriosus and nosocomial pulmonary and tracheal infections are important, along with adequate nutrition. Other methods currently under investigation are antioxidants and high-frequency ventilation. Vitamin A supplementation in the early neonatal period may be beneficial in preventing BPD because vitamin A deficiency has been known to cause BPD.

62. An infant born at 30 weeks gestation is in what stage of fetal lung development?

Fetal lung development is divided into pseudoglandular, canalicular, and terminal sac or saccular stages based on the descriptive characteristics of airway development. The canalicular stage of lung development starts at about 16 weeks gestation and lasts through 25 weeks gestation. The terminal sac or saccular stage of lung development takes place from about 25 weeks to term.

63. An infant born at 30 weeks gestation has how many alveoli?

At 30 weeks gestation the infant should have about 50 million alveoli. A normal full-term infant has about 100–150 million alveoli, and the normal adult has about 300 million alveoli. An infant born at 30 weeks who develops BPD will continue to repair and grow "new lung" until about 8 or 9 years of age.

64. Are there any biochemical markers for BPD?

Several markers have been shown to be increased in the bronchoalveolar and tracheal lavage fluid in patients with BPD, including neutrophils, elastase, fibrinonectin, certain leukotrienes, and platelet-activating factor. Their clinical relevance needs to be defined.

NEONATAL SEPSIS

65. Define sepsis neonatorum.
Strictly speaking, sepsis neonatorum describes any bacterial infection in the first month of life as documented by a positive blood culture. The incidence varies from report to report but is estimated at 0.1–0.5%.

66. What are the risk factors for neonatal sepsis?
Race is important in neonatal sepsis. Blacks have a higher incidence of sepsis than whites. Other factors include prematurity, fetal tachycardia, low birth weight, low socioeconomic status, maternal colonization with group B streptococci, maternal fever, prolonged rupture of membranes (> 12–24 hours), clinical evidence of chorioamnionitis, untreated or partially treated maternal infection, and any type of instrumentation in a newborn (e.g., umbilical artery line, umbilical vein line, endotracheal tube).

67. Is there a difference in the characteristics of early-onset vs. late-onset sepsis?
Yes. Early-onset sepsis usually occurs within the first several days of life, is usually transmitted vertically, and has a fulminant multiorgan system course with a mortality rate approaching 50%. Late-onset sepsis occurs after day 5, is usually transmitted vertically (but may be postnatal via fomites or other environmental sources), is usually less fulminant, and has a much lower mortality rate.

68. What are the most common bacteria in early-onset sepsis?
Pathogens associated with sepsis vary by geographic location. In the United States, the most common cause of early-onset sepsis is group B streptococci. Other common bacteria include gram-negative bacilli with the most common being *Escherichia coli*. Less common bacteria include *Listeria monocytogenes*, coagulase-negative staphylococci, *Staphylococcus aureus*, and *Enterococcus* species.

69. What are the most common bacteria in late-onset or nosocomial neonatal sepsis?
The most common pathogen in late-onset sepsis is coagulase-negative staphylococci. Other common bacteria include group B streptococci, gram-negative bacilli, and *S. aureus*. In extremely low-birth-weight infants, fungal sepsis is a possibility.

70. What is the best choice for empiric antibiotic coverage for early-onset neonatal sepsis? Late-onset neonatal sepsis? Nosocomial late-onset neonatal sepsis?
For **early-onset neonatal sepsis** a good choice for empiric antibiotic coverage is a combination of ampicillin and an aminoglycoside. Ampicillin has good coverage against group B streptococci and *Listeria* species, whereas the aminoglycoside (e.g., gentamicin) has good coverage against most gram-negative bacilli, in particular *E. coli*. Gentamicin also has been found to act synergistically with ampicillin against group B streptococci and *Listeria* species. Although meningitis is uncommon in early-onset disease, in patients with evidence of meningial involvement many physicians replace the aminoglycoside with a third-generation cephalosporin (e.g., cefotaxime) for better penetration of the central nervous system.

Empiric therapy for **late-onset neonatal sepsis** should provide adequate coverage for community-acquired pathogens such as *Haemophilus influenzae* type B, *Neisseria* species, and streptococcal pneumonia. Ampicilllin provides adequate coverage for *S. pneumoniae*, group B streptococci, and *Listeria* species, whereas a third-generation cephalosporin, such as cefotaxime or ceftriaxone, provides adequate coverage for the other usual pathogens. The third-generation cephalosporin has appropriate central nervous system penetration, which is important in late-onset sepsis because meningitis is common.

In **nosocomial late-onset sepsis,** the coverage of coagulase-negative staphylococci and other gram-positive bacteria is important. A therapy combining vancomycin with an aminoglycoside or a third-generation cephalosporin is usually adequate. If *Pseudomonas* species are a concern, coverage with ceftazidime and/or an aminoglycoside is appropriate. If fungus is a concern, coverage with amphotericin B is appropriate. Most hospitals publish microbial susceptibility patterns for the most common nosocomial pathogens. All physicians should be familiar with the susceptibility profiles for the most common neonatal pathogens isolated in their community and their neonatal unit.

71. What is "gray baby syndrome"?

Gray baby syndrome is a cardiovascular collapse reaction that occurs in infants receiving chloramphenicol. It is characterized by vomiting, refusal to suck, respiratory distress, metabolic acidosis, abdominal distention, and passage of loose, green stools. This syndrome has been documented with extremely high chloramphenicol levels (> 70 μg/ml). At many institutions chloramphenicol is no longer routinely used for coverage of neonatal sepsis. However, it still provides excellent coverage for many pathogens, including *H. influenzae*, *S. pneumoniae*, and *Neisseria meningitidis*. Chloramphenicol levels should be monitored closely and kept within the desired therapeutic range of 15–25 μg/ml.

72. What are the major clinical manifestations of neonatal sepsis?

Clinical manifestations of neonatal sepsis include changes in affect, feeding pattern or tolerance, level of activity or alertness, respiratory status or effort, muscle tone, and peripheral perfusion. Temperature instability (hypothermia, hyperthermia), dextrose stick instability, blood pressure instability, abdominal distention, vomiting, diarrhea, and seizures are also manifestations of sepsis.

73. Is fever or temperature elevation a good marker for neonatal sepsis?

Unfortunately, temperature elevation in full-term infants with sepsis is less common than hypothermia, especially in infants < 5 days of age. Noninfectious causes of hyperthermia include dehydration, extensive hematomas, and acute neonatal drug withdrawal.

74. What is the differential diagnosis for neonatal sepsis?

The differential diagnosis for neonatal sepsis depends on the age at presentation. Initially sepsis may present with or without pneumonia and may appear as respiratory distress, transient tachypnea of the newborn, or meconium aspiration syndrome. Other differential diagnoses should include intracranial hemorrhage, subarachnoid hemorrhage, intracranial catastrophe, child abuse, drug withdrawal, and inborn errors of metabolism. Any type of intestinal perforation or obstruction and necrotizing enterocolitis may present like sepsis. Overwhelming viral sepsis (i.e., herpes) also must be considered.

75. What laboratory tests should be done in the work-up for neonatal sepsis?

The most important specimen is a blood culture. Other body fluids should be cultured, including urine (not necessary in the work-up of early-onset sepsis) and cerebral spinal fluid (CSF). If CSF is obtained, a CSF Gram stain with cell count and differential and CSF glucose and protein levels should be measured. A complete blood count with manual differential to determine the total leukocyte count is important because absolute leukopenia has a higher correlation with sepsis than leukocytosis. The absolute neutrophil count (ANC) and number of immature neutrophils are also important. An ANC < 1000 at any age is considered abnormal. The I/T ratio is expressed as the number of immature neutrophils ÷ the total number of neutrophils. An I/T ratio > 0.2–0.25 is considered abnormal and is a risk factor for sepsis.

76. An 18-day-old infant is hospitalized with a second episode of *E. coli* sepsis. What test should be done?

First of all, the house officer should check the newborn screen for galactosemia. This task, however, may be difficult. A quicker test, which can help to establish the diagnosis, is checking the urine for reducing substances. The patient probably has the classic form of galactosemia—deficiency of galactose-1-phosphate uridyl transferase. Such infants are prone to gram-negative bacilli sepsis, probably as a consequence of impaired neutrophil function. Galactose should be removed immediately from the patient's diet.

77. Which surgical problem has been described as a result of group B streptococcal pneumonia?

Right-sided congenital diaphragmatic hernia is a late complication of group B streptococcal pneumonia.

78. What are the current recommendations about intrapartum penicillin for prevention of early-onset group B streptococcal disease?

Intrapartum penicillin is recommended by the Centers for Disease Control and Prevention and the American College of Obstetricians and Gynecologists for a woman with one or more of the following:

- Previous infant with invasive group B streptococcal disease
- Group B streptococcal bacteriuria during the current pregnancy
- Delivery at < 37 weeks gestation
- Rupture of membranes ≥ 18 hours
- Intrapartum temperature ≥ 38° C

If membranes rupture at < 37 weeks and the mother is not in labor, collect a group B streptococcal culture and either administer antibiotics until the culture results are negative or begin antibiotics when the culture is positive. If no risk factors are present, antibiotic prophylaxis is not necessary.

79. What is Waterhouse-Friderichsen syndrome?

Waterhouse-Friderichsen syndrome is a catastrophic cause of acute adrenal cortical insufficiency classically seen with meningicoccal infection. This syndrome can be seen with other bacterial infections due to *Pneumococcus*, *Staphylococcus*, and *Haemophilus* species. The patient usually has circulatory collapse, overwhelming bacteremia/toxemia, cardiac failure, and acute adrenal cortical insufficiency. Histologically the adrenal glands appear hemorrhagic and necrotic. If this condition is recognized promptly, appropriate treatment with large doses of antibiotics and steroids may save the patient's life.

THERMAL REGULATION

80. Who is Martin Couney? Who is Baby Qbata?

Martin Couney was a German-born pediatrician who trained under Pierre C. Budin. Couney conducted many exhibits in the late 1890s–1920s to show the Budin technique of keeping premature infants warm. He was known informally as the "incubator doctor" and had many exhibits in which he displayed premature infants. Incubator care for premature infants started about 20 years before the first Couney show.

Baby Qbata was the smallest infant ever born who lived. He weighed 2 pounds 9 ounces and was cared for in the infant incubator building at the Pan American Exposition in Buffalo, New York in 1901.

81. Does providing an environment that protects against heat loss change the survival rate of premature infants?

Yes. Many studies published in the late 1950s and early 1960s showed that keeping premature infants warm and decreasing the amount of heat loss improve survival. According to the Neonatal Resuscitation Program guidelines, the first step in resuscitation of a newborn is to dry the infant. However, even with drying in the delivery room, the heat produced by the infant is still 2–3 times less than the rate of heat loss. Therefore, it is important to dry and swaddle the infant and to provide radiant heat or skin-to-skin contact with the mother. These techniques decrease the infant's need to produce his or her own heat and markedly decrease the problems associated with rewarming.

82. Do newborn infants shiver?

No. Most of the heat in newborn infants is produced by nonshivering thermogenesis and metabolism of brown fat.

83. What is the best way to rewarm an infant with hypothermia?

This topic involves much debate, and almost all of the published literature is based on uncontrolled studies. Rewarming infants too quickly may cause apnea; therefore, it should be done carefully in a controlled environment. The first step in rewarming is to eliminate further heat loss. The patient should be placed in an incubator, and the temperature of the air in the incubator should be approximately 36°C. Evaporative loss may be decreased by raising the incubator humidity. If the infant's temperature continues to decrease or does not begin to increase, the incubator temperature should be raised about 1° every 15–30 minutes. If the infant still does not warm, swaddling and a radiant warmer over the incubator may help.

84. Where is brown fat located? How does it produce heat?

Brown fat is located primarily in the intrascapular, axillary, perirenal, mediastinal, perispinal, and nuchal regions. In response to cold stress, norepinephrine and thyroid hormone stimulate brown fat and generate heat. This heat is generated when triglycerides and brown fat are broken down and enter the mitochondria.

85. Explain servo and nonservo heating.

Servo-controlled heating refers to heat provided for a premature infant by placing a probe on the skin and programming the desired skin temperature into the probe. The probe senses the skin temperature and appropriately increases or decreases the amount of heat required to maintain the desired temperature. In nonservo heating, no probe is placed on the patient. A temperature is set on the radiant warmer or in the incubator (i.e., 37.0°C or 33.5°C), and the amount of heat is constant with no adjustment based on skin temperature.

86. What is a neutral thermal environment?

A neutral thermal environment is the range of ambient temperatures within which body temperature is normal, metabolic rate is minimal, and temperature regulation can be achieved by nonevaporative physical processes alone. For each gestational age, weight, and postnatal age, the range of temperature is different. A chart is usually available in the nursery with the appropriate range of temperatures.

87. Explain conductive, convective, evaporative, and radiation heat loss.

Conductive heat loss refers to transfer of heat between solid objects of different temperatures. **Convective heat loss** refers to the transfer of heat from a solid object to the surrounding gaseous environment. **Radiation heat loss** occurs at the speed of light between a warmer object and a cooler object with which it is not in contact (e.g., nurse, doctor, wall, window). **Evaporative heat loss** refers to the heat lost when water evaporates. A radiant warmer decreases radiant and conductive heat loss. A heat shield decreases convective and evaporative heat loss. Warm humidified air decreases evaporative heat loss. Humidifying a convective incubator decreases all types of heat loss except radiation heat loss.

MICROPREEMIES

88. What is a micropreemie?

By definition, low birth weight refers to a neonate weighing < 2500 gm, very low birth weight refers to a neonate weighing 1000–1500 gm, and extremely low birth weight refers to a neonate weighing < 1000 gm.

89. How many infants are born each year in these three birth-weight categories?

According to the 1997 vital statistics published by the AAP, about 290,000 infants were born in the United States with a birth weight < 2500 gm, and about 55,000 infants were born with a birth weight < 1500 gm. For infants with extremely low birth weight, data are not subdivided into a class of infants weighing < 1 kg at birth.

90. What is the overall mortality rate for infants with a birth weight < 750 gm?

The mortality rate for neonates weighing < 750 gm (which correlates with ≤ 24 weeks gestation) is about 50%. The rate varies among centers and within centers from year to year, but in general it is 40–60 %.

91. What is the morbidity rate for infants with a birth weight < 750 gm?

About 80–85% of surviving infants with a birth weight < 750 gm have some degree of long-term neurodevelopmental sequelae (e.g., deafness, blindness, mental retardation, cerebral palsy).

92. What is retrolental fibroplasia?

Retrolental fibroplasia (RLF) is an old term, initiated in the 1940s, for severe late sequelae of retinopathy of prematurity (ROP). Approximately 65% of all infants born with a birth weight < 1250 gm have some degree of ROP. The incidence is inversely proportional to gestational age (i.e., about 90% with a birth weight < 750 gm and about 50% with a birth weight of 1000–1250 gm).

In the mid 1980s the International Classification of Retinopathy of Prematurity (ICROP) was published. The classification is threefold. The first part refers to the **location** of the disease. The retina is divided into three distinct zones (posterior to anterior), each covering successive 360° concentric cones. The second refers to the **extent** of disease as defined by the number of clock hours. The third refers to the level of **aggression** with the designation of "plus disease." The staging of ROP, according to the ICROP, is similar to previous classifications. Stage 1 shows a demarcation line, stage 2 has three dimensions and represents an elevated ridge, stage 3 represents extraretinal neovascularization, and stage 4 represents retinal detachment (partial or total). In earlier systems, stage 5 (not included in the ICROP classification) represents complete retinal detachment.

Oxygen toxicity is important in the etiology of ROP, although other factors play a role. Exposure to ambient light has been studied and does not appear to be a risk factor for ROP. Laser surgery and cryotherapy to ablate the avascular retina have been used to treat stage 3 or greater disease with "plus disease."

Currently the AAP and American Academy of Ophthalmology recommend screening all infants with a birth weight < 1500 gm or a gestational age < 28 weeks and all infants > 1500 gm with an unstable course who are believed to be at high risk by the attending physician. The exam should be performed at 4–6 weeks of age and usually is repeated every 2 weeks unless aggressive disease is present, in which case it is repeated more frequently.

93. What are the maintenance fluid requirements for an infant with extremely low birth weight? What is insensible water loss? How is it calculated?

Maintenance fluid requirements for an infant < 1 kg are variable but generally tend to be 100–120 ml/kg/day. For infants < 750 gm, the maintenance fluid requirement tends to be 120–140 ml/kg/day. However, fluid requirements are extremely variable from patient to patient because of insensible water loss (IWL). IWL (ml/kg) = (total fluid intake – urine output) + (previous weight – current weight) ÷ birth weight (kg).

94. What are the differences between preterm and full-term formula?

Comparing 24 calories/oz of preterm formula with 24 calories/oz of full-term formula, the amounts of calcium, phosphorus, protein, and vitamins are greater in the preterm formula. The amounts of carbohydrate and sodium are slightly higher, and the osmolality is lower in preterm formula. Medium-chain triglyceride oil and glucose polymers are added to preterm formula.

95. In the stabilization of a 1-kg, 27-week infant, what size of endotracheal tube should be placed? Where should it be secured at the lip?

As a rule of thumb, the gestational age divided by 10 provides an estimate for the appropriate size of the endotracheal tube (ETT). In this particular infant, a 2.5 ETT is appropriate. As a rule of thumb, one should take 6 cm + birth weight (in kg) as an estimate of where the ETT should be secured at the lip; in this particular infant, about 7 cm.

96. How far should an umbilical arterial and an umbilical venous catheter be advanced for appropriate position in a 1-kg infant?

Placement depends on the desired position of the umbilical arterial line. For a high umbilical arterial line (which is in good position between thoracic vertebrae 6 and 9), the sum of [body weight (kg) × 3] + 9 indicates a good position; in this particular patient, about 12 cm. For adequate placement of a low umbilical arterial line (between lumbar vertebrae 3 and 4) or placement of a high umbilical venous line (in the right atrium), the rule of thumb is to measure from the umbilicus to the shoulder and multiply by 0.6.

97. What is the total circulating blood volume of a 750-gm premature infant?

The total circulating blood volume of a premature infant equals 90 ml/kg. Therefore, the total circulating blood volume of a 750-gm premature infant is 65–70 ml.

98. When should an infant under 1 week of age be transfused?

As a rule of thumb, an infant should be transfused whenever about 10% of blood volume is withdrawn or the hematocrit is < 35–40%. The transfusion should be 10–15 ml/kg of leukocyte-poor packed red blood cells. The red cells are filtered through a leukocyte filter to remove the white cells and therefore decrease greatly the risk of transmission of cytomegalovirus (CMV). Some physicians prefer to transfuse premature infants with CMV-negative cells, but this approach may be difficult because the majority of the donating pool is CMV-positive. Some experts advocate irradiating blood products given to premature infants to decrease the risk of graft-versus-host disease. However, this approach is probably of theoretical benefit only in a premature infant.

99. What therapies decrease the number of transfusions in an infant with anemia of prematurity?

Recombinant human erythropoietin given at various times in a neonate's life decreases the need for subsequent red blood cell transfusions. Which population of patients has the greatest response and the exact timing, dosage, and frequency of erythropoietin remain controversial. A patient taking erythropoietin must have adequate amounts of vitamin E and enteral iron or be supplemented with intravenous iron (iron dextran) to achieve normal erythropoiesis. Whether such infants require supplementation with vitamin B_{12} and folate is controversial.

BIBLIOGRAPHY

1. American Academy of Pediatrics: Practice parameter: Management of hyperbilirubinemia in the healthy term newborn. Pediatrics 94:558–565, 1994.
2. Creasy RK, Resnik R: Maternal-Fetal Medicine, 4th ed. Philadelphia, W. B. Saunders, 1999.
3. Fanaroff AA, Martin RJ: Neonatal-Perinatal Medicine: Diseases of the Fetus and Infant, vols. I and II, 6th ed. St. Louis, Mosby, 1997.
4. Guyer B, MacDorman MF, Martin JA, et al: Annual summary of vital statistics—1997. Pediatrics 102:1333–1349, 1998.
5. Hudak ML, Martin DJ, Egan EA, et al: A multicenter randomized masked comparison trial of synthetic surfactant versus calf lung surfactant extract in the prevention of neonatal respiratory distress syndrome. Pediatrics 100:39–50, 1997.
6. Jobe AH: Pulmonary surfactant therapy. N Engl J Med 328:861–868, 1993.
7. Northway WH Jr, Rosan RC, Porter DY: Pulmonary disease following respirator therapy of hyaline-membrane disease: Bronchopulmonary dysplasia. N Engl J Med 276:357–368, 1967.
8. Papile L, Burstein J, Burstein R, Koffler H: Incidence and evolution of subependymal and intraventricular hemorrhage: A study of infants with birthweights less than 1500 gm. J Pediatr 92:529–534, 1978.

9. Polin RA, Fox WW: Fetal and Neonatal Physiology, 2nd ed. Philadelphia, W. B. Saunders, 1998.
10. Remington JS, Klein JO: Infectious Disease of the Fetus and Newborn Infant, 4th ed. Philadelphia, W. B. Saunders, 1995.
11. Silverman WA: Incubator-baby side shows. Pediatrics 64:127–141, 1979.
12. Vohr BR, Garcia-Coll C, Mayfield S, et al: Neurologic and developmental status related to the evolution of visual-motor abnormalities from birth to 2 years of age in preterm infants with intraventricular hemorrhage. J Pediatr 115:296–302, 1989.
13. Volpe JJ: Neurology of the Newborn, 3rd ed. Philadelphia, W. B. Saunders, 1995.

75. ORTHOPEDIC SURGICAL DISEASE

Douglas G. Armstrong, M.D.

SCOLIOSIS

1. A pediatrician refers an 11-year-old girl with no complaints but asymmetry of the back in the bending forward position. What should be your primary concern?

Scoliosis. Lateral curvature of the spine results in deformity of the back—a rib hump, flank hump, or both—that is most apparent when the patient bends forward (Adams forward-bend test). Scoliosis often can be detected at an early stage by routine physical examination. Because it is seen most often in prepubertal girls, screening often is done by school nurses or primary care physicians. Once a deformity is detected, referral to a pediatric orthopedic specialist is reasonable; the diagnosis then may be confirmed by radiogram.

2. What is scoliosis?

Scoliosis is a three-dimensional deformity of the spine that results from abnormal development or abnormal vertebral formation. The deformity is produced by tilting, rotation, and lateral translation of the spinal column. It may involve any region but is most common in the thoracic spine.

3. What causes scoliosis?

There are several types of scoliosis but most patients fall into one of three basic categories: congenital, neuromuscular, or idiopathic.

Adolescent idiopathic scoliosis (AIS) is the most common type. Its cause remains a mystery, although research is progressing. Small curves are seen in about 2% of teenagers, but only 10% require treatment. AIS begins during the prepubertal years and by definition is detected at age 10 or older. AIS is 5–8 times more common in girls than boys, and about one-half of patients have a positive family history. **Juvenile idiopathic scoliosis** occurs between ages 3 and 10 years and **infantile idiopathic scoliosis** from 0 through 3 years. Both types are uncommon, occur equally in both sexes, and are likely to require treatment.

Neuromuscular scoliosis is associated with neurologic or muscular conditions, particularly those that render the patient nonambulatory. Examples include cerebral palsy, spina bifida, and Duchenne muscular dystrophy.

Congenital scoliosis is associated with vertebral malformations. About 10% of patients may have an underlying cord anomaly such as syringomyelia, Chiari malformation, or tethered or split cord.

4. How is scoliosis diagnosed?

History and physical exam, including neurologic exam, are followed by radiographs from which the angle subtended by the curve is measured. Magnitude of the curvature and skeletal maturity are used to guide treatment.

5. What is the treatment of AIS? Explain the rationale.

In general, curves that are 30° or less at maturity do not tend to cause problems, whereas curves that are 50° or more progress relentlessly and lead to increased deformity and ultimately pain. In children and adolescents with 2 or more years of growth remaining, curves of 30° or more almost always worsen, whereas curves of 20° or less progress in about only 1 of 3 patients. Furthermore, smaller (25–30°) curves can be kept from worsening by using a special brace, whereas curves of 45° or more are likely to worsen despite bracing. At present, the following treatment is recommended for most cases:

• Observation: curves of 20° or less, with 2 or more years of growth remaining
• Bracing: 25–40° curves, with 2 years or more of growth remaining
• Surgery: 50° or greater curve

6. What is involved in surgery for scoliosis?

Techniques continue to evolve. Surgery is considered a major procedure. The general goals are (1) to halt progression, (2) to restore the natural balance of the spinal column, (3) to correct the curvatures as much as safely possible, and (4) to leave the lower lumbar spine mobile. To achieve these goals, spinal fusion with instrumentation is performed. The vertebrae are exposed either through a posterior midline incision or via an anterior thoracic and/or lumbar approach. Soft tissues and cartilage are removed from the bone and intervertebral joints. Corrective forces are applied to the deformed part by attaching metal rods to the vertebrae with hooks and/or screws. The vertebrae are decorticated, and bone graft is applied. Over the ensuing 6 months the bone graft incorporates, thus healing the vertebrae together (fusion). Thus, progression is halted and correction maintained.

DEVELOPMENTAL DYSPLASIA OF THE HIP

7. A newborn girl has a "clunk" at the left hip when it is abducted by the examining physician. What may be the problem?

Developmental dysplasia of the hip (DDH). Children may be born with or develop instability of the hip. The condition is fairly common. Breech babies, females, and first-borns are at increased risk. The greatest risk factor is a positive family history. The incidence among blacks and Chinese is low, whereas the incidence among North American aboriginals is high.

8. How is DDH detected?

Most, but not all, cases can be found by screening newborns with simple physical examination. The **Ortolani test** detects dislocated hips. With the child relaxed and supine, the hip is flexed to 90° while holding the thigh gently with the thumb on the medial side and the long finger over the greater trochanter. The hip then is abducted gently and lifted anteriorly. A "clunk" indicates that the hip was dislocated initially and has relocated with the maneuver (positive Ortolani test). The hips should be examined one at a time.

The **Barlow test** detects hips that are dislocatable or subluxable. The patient must be relaxed and in the supine position. The examiner stabilizes the pelvis with one hand and performs the test with the other. The examining hand is kept in the same position as for the Ortolani test. The hip is flexed to 90°, then adducted a little. Gentle posteriorly directed pressure is applied. Instability may be detected as the hip subluxates or dislocates.

Ultrasound of the hips may be used to confirm the physical finding. Radiographs are not routinely used and are inaccurate in newborns.

9. What is the initial treatment for an infant with DDH?

In infants 6 months of age or less, the Pavlik harness is the most widely used device. The harness allows motion of the lower limbs while stabilizing the hips. It has an excellent success rate. The harness maintains the hips flexed to 90–100° by straps along the legs, which are attached to a chest strap (rather like a brassiere with leg straps). The harness is worn full-time for 3 months, then part-time for several weeks. Close monitoring is required to ensure that the harness is fitted properly and that the hip is stabilizing. If the hip is not located after 2–3 weeks, another treatment must be used. If treatment is successful, the child must be followed to skeletal maturity.

10. What is the treatment for late-presenting DDH or failed initial treatment?

The hip must be reduced by either closed or open reduction. The goals are (1) to achieve a fully located hip (concentric reduction); (2) to avoid complications (chiefly avascular necrosis of the femoral head; and (3) to reduce the hip as early as reasonably possible. The acetabulum will not develop normally as long as the femoral head is not fully located, and if the hip is not reduced before age 3½ years, it cannot fully remodel. Further surgery is required. Closed reduction under anesthesia may be preceded by a period of traction.

During surgery an arthrogram is performed to ensure that the hip is reduced concentrically. The reduction must be gentle, and the hip must be stable when held in a position of flexion of 100–110°, abduction (no more than 50°), and neutral rotation (the "human" position). Extreme positions cause loss of blood flow to the femoral head. If these criteria are not met, the hip must be reduced under direct vision, removing the anatomic obstacles and stabilizing it (i.e., open reduction must be performed). The child then is placed into a hip spica cast. Generally, casting is necessary for at least 3 months; the cast is changed under anesthesia at 4- to 6-week intervals.

SEPTIC ARTHRITIS

11. A 26-day-old premature infant seems to be unable to move the right lower limb. What may be the problem?

One must immediately rule out septic arthritis, particularly of the hip. Although uncommon in neonates, this devastating condition rapidly leads to loss of femoral head vascularity and dissolution of the hip. In addition to pseudoparalysis, one may find an irritable infant with swelling of the upper thigh. Vital signs usually are stable, and fever may not be present. The white blood cell count often is elevated, and the erythrocyte sedimentation rate (ESR) usually is quite high. Ultrasound may be used as an ancillary test , but an arthrotomy should be performed promptly if there is reasonable suspicion of a septic joint in a neonate. Multiple joints can be affected, and osteomyelitis of the adjoining metaphysis (in the hip, the upper end of the femur) is usually present in neonates. Severe injury to the growth plate can occur.

12. What causes septic arthritis? When is it most commonly seen?

Bacterial infection of joints can occur spontaneously by hematogenous spread; by direct inoculation, such as a puncture wound; or by extension from osteomyelitis in the metaphysis of an adjacent bone. *Staphylococcus aureus* is the most common organism in all age groups now that vaccination for *Hemophilus influenzae* is used. Group A streptococci are a frequent cause in children, as is *Streptococcus pneumoniae*. In neonates group B streptococci may be seen. Septic arthritis can occur throughout childhood but is infrequent in adolescence. In adolescents, gonococcal infection needs to be considered.

13. Describe the presentation of a child with septic arthritis.

The most frequently affected joints (in descending order) are the knee, hip, and ankle. Occasionally shoulder or elbow infections are seen. The presentation depends on the joint affected. The child with a lower limb sepsis may limp and then stop weight-bearing. The affected joint is held in a partially flexed position to reduce the intra-articular pressure. The patient appears unwell, is febrile, and guards the affected joint, complaining of severe pain with passive motion. Joint effusion may be seen if a peripheral joint, such as the knee, is affected.

14. What tests should be done?

Complete blood count, ESR, and blood culture should be ordered. Joint aspiration should always be done before treatment. Joint fluid should be sent for cell count, Gram stain, and cultures. Ultrasound may be useful for hip infections.

15. How do we distinguish toxic synovitis from septic arthritis?

Patients with toxic synovitis usually are well and have only a low-grade temperature. This self limiting condition occurs most frequently in the hip of 4–6-year-old children. Progressive worsening is the rule in patients with septic arthritis, whereas patients with toxic synovitis improve over time and are mobile. The white blood cell count is not elevated, and ESR is slightly elevated in patients with toxic synovitis. Serial examination is necessary. For some patients it is impossible to make the diagnosis clinically; aspiration is required.

16. What is the differential diagnosis of septic arthritis?

Osteomyelitis, toxic synovitis, juvenile rheumatoid arthritis, Lyme disease, and leukemia, among others.

17. How is septic arthritis in children treated?

The mainstays of treatment are decompression of the joint and adequate debridement, intravenous antibiotics, and early motion. Occasionally infections in smaller joints can be treated with aspiration and antibiotics, but there is a risk of cartilage loss and stiffness. Arthrotomy is the surest treatment to debride the joint fully and is required promptly in all cases of hip infection. Intravenous antibiotics may be switched to oral after 1 week in most cases; oral antibiotics are continued for 2 more weeks.

18. What happens if treatment is delayed?

Long-standing (more than 3–5 days) bacterial infection of joints produces erosion of articular cartilage. Avascular necrosis of the femoral head can result from increased intra-articular pressure. Septic dislocation of the hip can occur in infants. Associated osteomyelitis, frequently seen in infants, can result later in children. Joint stiffness and disability can result from untreated septic arthritis. Limb-length discrepancy or deformity can result if the growth plate has been damaged, especially in infants.

OSTEOMYELITIS

19. A 5-year-old boy with a 2-day history of knee pain and limping develops a fever of 39° C overnight. His knee joint is not swollen. What may be wrong? How can you make a diagnosis?

Acute hematogenous osteomyelitis (AHOM) of the distal femur or proximal tibia should be the primary consideration. For an early bone infection the diagnosis is clinical. The above history is typical. The child may have a history of trauma to the area or recent viral illness, appears unwell, has a fever, and guards the affected limb. There may be localized warmth, swelling, and erythema at the limb—in this case, the leg. Point tenderness at the metaphysis is virtually always present. Radiographs may show no abnormalities, or, if the disease has progressed for a few days, a radiolucency in the metaphysis and periosteal new bone may be seen. The white blood cell count usually is elevated with a left shift, and ESR is moderately to significantly elevated.

20. What is AHOM?

Infection of a bone can develop in children when blood-borne bacteria seed into the blood vessels within its metaphysis near the growth plate. The tibia or femur often is affected, but any bone can be involved. Pressure builds up within the bone, and pus tracks outward, elevating the periosteum from the cortex. As the infection spreads, it destroys bone and renders it ischemic. If the infection is left untreated, new bone (involucrum) forms around a segment of dead bone (sequestrum). Eventually the infection drains into a joint or externally via a sinus tract.

21. What needs to be done when the patient is first seen?

If AHOM is suspected, treat the patient with intravenous antibiotics until it has been ruled out or controlled. Blood cultures and bone aspiration need to be performed *before* starting antibiotics. Aspiration of the subperiosteal abscess, in addition to blood culture, yields positive cultures in 70% of cases. Consultation with an orthopedic surgeon is appropriate at the outset to aspirate the bone and follow the patient.

22. Why should surgery be involved?

Antibiotics alone cannot cure established bone infection because they cannot penetrate through pus or dead tissue. Once a significant abscess has formed, it expands relentlessly, destroying bone despite intravenous antibiotics. Surgical drainage of pus is a basic precept of medicine, often forgotten in the current era. Indications for surgery include failure to improve within 48 hours of treatment, worsening of the patient's condition or late presentation with abscess. Bone infection hurts. Early surgical intervention halts the progress of the bacteria, relieves the pressure of the pus from the bone, removes the bulk of the infected debris, and shortens the course of the disease.

CLUBFOOT

23. A newborn has one foot that points significantly inward. What may be wrong?

One possibility is clubfoot (congenital talipes equinovarus). The diagnosis is made by examination of the newborn.

24. What should the examiner look for?

The foot appears medially rotated and points downward, while the sole of the foot faces inward. The deformity is best appreciated by pointing the child's knee forward and inspecting the leg and foot. The calf is narrow, and a crease is seen posteriorly above the heel pad. The skin over the lateral aspect of the foot appears stretched, the lateral border of the foot is curved, and a crease may be seen at the sole of the foot. The heel pad feels empty because the os calcis is displaced proximally. Stiffness varies from case to case.

25. What is the incidence of clubfoot?

Idiopathic clubfoot occurs in about 1 of 750 births. The same deformity is seen in association with conditions that result in contractures (e.g., arthrogryposis, spina bifida); in such cases, it generally is more severe. It is twice as common in boys as girls and is bilateral in about one-half of patients.

26. Why does clubfoot occur?

The cause is unknown. Various theories include neurogenic and myogenic causes as well as limb deficiency. The risk is increased in families in which one member has a clubfoot. Clubfoot is not due to malposition and is established by the end of the first trimester of pregnancy. The deformity is complex and involves virtually all of the tissues from the knee downward. The muscles, tendons, and ligaments of the foot and leg are shortened and fibrotic. The bones of the foot are abnormally formed and grossly malpositioned. Even the vascular supply is affected.

27. Is the child able to walk?

Yes. Even untreated clubfoot does not prevent a child from walking. Surgeons who have participated in care of children in developing countries report that thousands of untreated people are indeed able to walk. Their main problems are foot wear and painful feet in adulthood.

28. What can be done?

Manipulation and serial casting are the mainstays of treatment in most centers. At each session, the deformed soft tissues are stretched gently, and the bones of the foot are repositioned. Then a cast is applied. Treatment needs to be started shortly after birth. The procedure is repeated twice weekly until correction has been achieved after about 3–4 weeks; then weekly-to-bimonthly casts are used to maintain correction for another 3–4 weeks. Some surgeons use heelcord lengthening at 3 weeks to complete correction.

29. How often does surgery work?

Results vary, depending on how stiff the foot is and from one center to another. In North America and Europe, surgical correction is performed for most cases of clubfoot. Surgery generally is done when the child is 6–12 months old.

BIBLIOGRAPHY

1. Lonstein JE, Bradford DS, Winter RB, Ogilvie JW: Moe's Textbook of Scoliosis and Other Spinal Deformities, 3rd ed. Philadelphia, W.B. Saunders, 1995.
2. Morrissy RT, Weinstein SL (eds): Lovell and Winter's Pediatric Orthopedics, 4th ed. Philadelphia, Lippincott, 1996.
3. Wenger DR, Rang M: The Art and Practice of Children's Orthopedics. New York, Raven Press, 1993.

76. NEUROSURGICAL DISEASE

Veetai Li, M.D., and Mark S. Dias, M.D., FACS

CRANIOSYNOSTOSIS

1. Describe the cardinal and variable features of common craniosynostosis syndromes.

Cardinal and Variable Features of Common Craniosynostosis Syndromes

SYNDROME	MODE OF INHERITANCE	COMMONLY INVOLVED SUTURES	ADDITIONAL VARIABLE FEATURES
Crouzon	AD	Coronal	Midface hypoplasia, shallow orbits, proptosis, strabismus
Apert	AD	Coronal	Midface hypoplasia, downslanting palpebral fissures, often complete and symmetrical syndactyly and polydactyly of hands and feet
Saethre-Chotzen	AD	Coronal	Facial asymmetry, low-set frontal hairline, ptosis, variable brachydactyly and polydactyly, normal thumbs
Pfeiffer	AD	Coronal	Proptosis, strabismus, hypertelorism, downslanting palpebral fissures, midface hypoplasia, broad thumbs and great toes, mild syndactyly
Carpenter	AD	All	Polysyndactyly of feet, variable syndactyly, genu valga, patellar displacement, mental deficiency (common)

AD = autosomal dominant.

2. Is craniosynostosis synonymous with premature closure of the cranial sutures?

No. Pathologic examination of the cranial sutures demonstrates complete obliteration of all or part of a cranial suture, which represents a completely abnormal process not encountered during normal sutural closure. Craniosynostosis is an abnormal process, not simply an acceleration of normal suture closure.

3. What are the types of craniosynostosis? What are the resulting head shapes?

There are a limited number of sutures—the coronal suture(s), sagittal suture, metopic suture, and lambdoid suture(s)—that can be abnormally closed, alone or in combination. Single suture closure is far more common in nonsyndromic cases. Single suture synostosis restricts calvarial growth along the closed suture, with compensatory growth along the other sutures; therefore, the resultant head shape can be predicted. Sagittal synostosis causes an elongated and narrowed head shape (scaphocephaly), metopic synostosis causes a triangular frontal head shape (trigono-cephaly), and unilateral coronal and lambdoid synostosis cause asymmetrical head growth (pla-giocephaly) with varying degrees of both frontal and occipital flattening on the affected side. Bilateral coronal synostosis causes a short head (brachycephaly).

4. Are some forms of craniosynostosis hereditary?

Yes. Numerous syndromes have been described, and in many various genetic mutations have been identified in fibroblast growth factor receptor (FGFR) gene loci. The table in question 1 lists a number of common genetic craniosynostosis syndromes and their clinical features.

5. What are the indications for surgery in children with craniosynostosis?

In most children, surgery is cosmetic. However, a secondary concern in some children (more commonly in children with multiple suture synostosis) is a more global restriction of calvarial growth, with increased intracranial pressure and resultant effects on brain growth and develop-ment. The incidence of elevated intracranial pressure varies from 7% (in isolated sagittal synos-tosis) to 33% or more (with multiple sutural synostosis).

6. Are children with craniosynostosis developmentally delayed?

Children with nonsyndromic synostosis generally are not delayed. Even among children with synostosis syndromes, developmental delays are quite variable and depend on the syn-drome. For example, almost all children with Crouzon syndrome are intellectually normal, whereas as many as 85% of children with Apert syndrome have developmental delays. Developmental delays uncommonly result from elevated intracranial pressure but are more likely related to uncertain genetic factors that have not yet been fully determined.

7. Does the child with a flat occiput have lambdoid synostosis?

Over the past decade, a growing number of cases of occipital flattening (or occipital plagio-cephaly) have been caused by laying children on their backs to prevent sudden infant death syn-drome (SIDS). The characteristic features are ipsilateral occipital flattening and ipsilateral frontal bossing with anterior deviation of the ispilateral ear and a parallelogram-shaped head. In con-trast, unilateral coronal synostosis and unilateral lambdoid synostosis most commonly produce a trapezoidal head shape with ipsilateral occipital and frontal flattening. The overwhelming major-ity of children with occipital plagiocephaly do not require surgery.

PEDIATRIC BRAIN TUMORS

8. Which are more common in children, supratentorial or infratentorial brain tumors?

The older literature emphasized that infratentorial tumors (located in the posterior fossa) were more common in children, but recent literature suggests that the distribution is more equal and in some series even favors a supratentorial location.

9. What are the three most common tumor types in children?

Astrocytomas (most of which are a specific benign type of astrocytoma called juvenile pilo-cytic astrocytoma), primitive neuroectodermal tumors (including medulloblastoma and other re-lated tumors), and ependymomas. In contrast, the most common tumors of adults are astrocytomas (most of which are malignant astrocytomas and glioblastoma multiforme), menin-giomas, and metastatic tumors.

10. What are the common presenting features of childhood brain tumors?

There are several patterns of presentation, depending on the age of the child. Infants with open fontanelles may present simply with enlarging heads, split cranial sutures, and bulging fontanelles without other symptoms. The older child usually has one of four presentations:

• The midline posterior fossa syndrome, with the triad of headache; anorexia, nausea, and vomiting; and papilledema. The symptoms are usually due not to the posterior fossa tumor per se, but to the resulting obstructive hydrocephalus. Often a misdiagnosis of a viral illness or otitis media is made until the symptoms progress or gait ataxia becomes apparent.
• Progressive neurological deficits are more common in children with brainstem tumors (pontine and medullary) and tumors of the cerebral hemispheres. The nature of the deficits reflects the location of the tumor.
• Seizures are more common in children with tumors of the cerebral hemispheres.
• Progressive visual loss and/or hypothalamic dysfunction sometimes is associated with diencephalic syndrome (a thin, emaciated child despite a reasonable appetite, often with paradoxical hyperactivity). Patients usually have suprasellar tumors, such as craniopharyngiomas and hypothalamic/optic pathway astrocytomas.

11. What is a primitive neuroectodermal tumor?

Primitive neuroectodermal tumors include a number of malignant central nervous system tumors, all of which share a common histologic pattern of small, round cells with scant cytoplasm, pleiomorphism, and mitotic figures. The most common is medulloblastoma, which occurs in and around the fourth ventricle. Other less common related tumors include pineoblastoma, retinoblastoma, and neuroblastoma. Neuroblastoma also is commonly found outside the neuraxis.

12. Are any brain tumors inoperable?

As surgical technology has improved, many tumors previously considered inoperable are now routinely removed. The only tumor that still is considered to be genuinely unresectable is the diffuse pontine glioma, which involves the entire pons in a nonfocal manner. Although some surgeons consider biopsy to exclude other diagnoses, biopsy is rarely done in children because the imaging features are so characteristic.

SPINAL DYSRAPHISM

13. What do the terms myelomeningocele, spina bifida, spinal dysraphism, and occult spinal dysraphism mean? Are they synonymous?

Although people often confuse these terms, they are not synonymous. **Myelomeningocele** refers to an open spinal cord malformation in which a portion of the caudal neural tube (the forerunner of the spinal cord) has failed to close properly. This portion of the spinal cord is therefore open (not skin-covered). **Spina bifida** generally refers to a myelomeningocele, although the term also has been used to refer to other spinal cord malformations. **Spinal dysraphism** refers to any developmental malformation involving neural tube closure and includes myelomeningocele as well as other related malformations such as spinal dermal sinus tracts, lipomyelomeningocele (spinal lipoma), diastematomyelia (also called split-cord malformations), and fatty filum terminale. **Occult spinal dysraphism** refers to a bony abnormality in which a spinous process and laminae have failed to fuse in the midline, usually without underlying spinal cord malformation. However, sometimes spina bifida occulta is associated with underlying occult spinal dysraphism involving the spinal cord.

14. What is a closed myelomeningocele?

Closed myelomeningocele usually refers to a full-thickness skin-covered spinal cord malformation. However, a closed myelomeningocele does *not* exist. Embryologically, a myelomeningocele forms when the neural tube fails to close properly. Therefore, the adjacent cutaneous ectoderm, which gives rise to skin, remains attached to the unclosed neuroectoderm, and the resulting lesion is, by definition, not skin-covered. Children with a large skin-covered sac usually have either a myelocystocele or a lipomyelomeningocele (spinal lipoma).

15. What problems do children with myelomeningoceles face?

Most children have varying degrees of paralysis and loss of sensation in their lower extremities, along with urinary incontinence (neurogenic bladder) and constipation. Orthopedic deformities of the feet and legs, hip dislocations, and spinal scoliosis, kyphosis, and lordosis may be present initially or develop later. The severity of the deficits depends on the size and location of the malformation; larger and more rostral malformations produce more severe deficits. However, a rare child may have relatively preserved sensorimotor function despite a high lesion. Moreover, children with cervical or high thoracic lesions paradoxically have relatively few or even no significant sensorimotor deficits.

16. What is the long-term outcome for children with myelomeningocele?

Most children with myelomeningocele survive to adulthood, and the life expectancy is not significantly different from the normal population. A shunt for hydrocephalus is required in about 80%. Eighty percent have normal intelligence, although 60% of these have some sort of learning disability. With aggressive treatments, 80% are socially continent of urine (most use intermittent bladder catheterization), and 60% of preteens are community ambulators (most use some sort of orthosis or bracing).

17. What are cutaneous stigmata of occult spinal dysraphism?

Patients with occult spinal dysraphism often have important skin markers that signify an underlying spinal cord malformation. Examples include midline hemangiomas; hairy patches (hypertrichosis); dimples; skin masses such as lumps of fat or other tissue, skin tags, or even appendages; and asymmetrical deviations of the rostral end of the gluteal cleft. These markers allow the spinal cord malformation to be identified and repaired before neurologic deterioration occurs.

18. What features distinguish a benign coccygeal dimple from a pathologic dermal sinus tract?

The **pathologic sacral dimple** is almost always well above the gluteal cleft on the flat region of the sacrum. Although the dimple may be tiny, there is often a surrounding hemangioma or a tuft of hair, skin tag, or other cutaneous marker of spinal dysraphism. In older children, there may be a history of neurologic, urologic, or orthopedic problems. The depth of the lesion is *not* a reliable feature to distinguish a benign from a pathologic dimple. Pathologic lesions must be repaired to prevent meningitis or deterioration from spinal cord tethering.

The **benign coccygeal dimple** is located at or within a couple of millimeters of the coccygeal tip, well within the gluteal cleft. Benign dimples may be deep, but their location and the lack of any associated features or neurologic, orthopedic, or urologic problems make them easy to identify. Coccygeal dimples are present in approximately 4% of normal infants and do not require treatment.

19. What is spinal cord tethering?

During the first month of embryonic life, the end of the spinal cord (the conus medullaris) normally is situated opposite the coccyx and connected to the end of the thecal sac by the filum terminale, a thin strand of undifferentiated neural tissue with no known function. During development, the conus rises, in part because of differential growth between the spine and spinal cord. As a result of this ascent, the conus ultimately lies opposite the disc space between the first and second lumbar vertebrae (the L1–L2 disc space). Spinal cords that lie significantly caudal to the L1–L2 disc space are said to be "tethered" and often are associated with an occult spinal dysraphic malformation. Most patients have a shortened filum terminale, which is thicker and infiltrated with fat—the so-called thickened or fatty filum. Patients with spinal cord tethering usually present with progressive neurologic, urologic, and/or orthopedic abnormalities. Treatment is to untether the spinal cord surgically.

HYDROCEPHALUS

20. What are the cardinal clinical features of an infant with hydrocephalus?

Accelerated head growth, full fontanelle, separation of the cranial sutures, sunsetting of the eyes.

21. What is the most common cause of macrocrania in infancy?

Benign extraaxial fluid collections of infancy, in which cerebrospinal fluid (CSF) accumulates excessively between the cortex and arachnoid layer (subarachnoid space). This process is self-limiting and is believed to reflect transient underdevelopment of the normal CSF absorption pathways (arachnoid granulations).

22. How do school-aged children with hydrocephalus present?

Common symptoms include headaches (particularly those that awaken the patient), vomiting, unexplained irritability, worsening in school performance, ataxia, and double vision. On examination patients may have papilledema and/or impairment of eye movements (especially difficulty with upward gaze).

23. What are the treatment options for hydrocephalus?

There are no good medical therapies for hydrocephalus. The classic surgical treatment is a ventricular shunt, an implantable silastic catheter with the proximal end in the cerebral ventricle and the distal end in the peritoneal cavity, heart, or pleural space. The shunt serves as an alternative pathway for drainage of CSF. An alternative treatment, suitable only for patients with noncommunicating hydrocephalus, is an endoscopic third ventriculostomy. An endoscope is navigated into the third ventricle, where a fenestration is made in the thinned-out floor, allowing CSF to escape the ventricular system and to flow directly into the subarachnoid space.

24. What are the most common problems with ventricular shunts?

Shunt malfunction is the most common problem; 50% of shunts fail by 5– 6 years after implantation. When failure occurs, shunt revision is necessary. The second most common problem is shunt infection, which occurs in 5–15% of cases.

CRANIAL AND SPINAL TRAUMA

25. What is a growing skull fracture (also known as a leptomeningeal cyst)?

It is an entity unique to children; 90% occur in children less than 3 years old. A diastatic fracture lies over a dural laceration, often with a region of parenchymal injury deep to it. The brain pulsations are thought to push the arachnoid and CSF into the cleaved fracture line, thereby further separating the bone edges. Surgical repair is required.

26. What is shaken baby syndrome? What are the classic features?

Shaken baby syndrome is a form of child abuse in which the child is violently shaken by the perpetrator and then sometimes thrown against an immobile object, often resulting in serious brain injury. Infants typically present with sudden onset of neurologic deterioration (often with an episode of apnea or seizure), retinal hemorrhage, subdural and/or subarachnoid hemorrhage on computed tomography (CT) scan of the head, and no reasonable explanation of how the injuries were sustained. Child protection services should be contacted when shaken baby syndrome is a likely possibility.

27. How do patients with posttraumatic migraines present?

Patients become combative or even lethargic within hours of a head injury (often a minor one). The clinical picture is similar to that of an expanding intracranial mass, such as an epidural hematoma, but the CT scan of the head is normal. Patients return to normal within 24 hours. Usually the patient or a family member has a history of migraines.

28. Can children have a spinal cord injury in the presence of normal spine radiographs?

Spinal cord injury without radiographic abnormalities (SCIWORA) is a well-described phenomenon unique to children, especially young ones. The most likely explanation for SCIWORA is transient displacement of the spine that spontaneously reduces; most likely it results from the accentuated elasticity of the ligaments of children.

29. Are the patterns of cervical spine and spinal cord injuries in children and adults the same?

No. Children (especially those younger than 8 years) have a much greater propensity for upper cervical (occiput to C3) injuries because of several features unique to this age group. Examples include a larger head-to-total body weight ratio, which makes the fulcrum of the spine higher; underdeveloped cervical musculature; wedge-shaped vertebral bodies; more horizontally aligned facet joints; and highly elastic ligaments.

BIBLIOGRAPHY

1. Albright AL, Pollack IF, Adelson PD: Principles and Practice of Pediatric Neurosurgery. Thieme, New York, 1999.
2. Cohen ME, Duffner PK:Brain Tumors in Children, 2nd ed. Raven Press, New York, 1994.
3. Dias MS, Li V: Pediatric neurosurgical disease. Pediatr Clin North Am 45:1539–1578, 1998.
4. Pang D (ed): Spinal dysraphism. Neurosurg Clin North Am, April 1995 [entire issue].

77. PEDIATRIC ENDOCRINE DISEASES

John G. Buchlis, M.D., Lou Ann Gartner, M.D., Jean-Claude Desmangles, M.D., and Margaret H. MacGillivray, M.D.

1. How do thyroid nodules present in children?

Thyroid nodules present as an asymptomatic, discrete mass in the thyroid gland.

2. What is the incidence of benign and malignant nodules?

The overall incidence of thyroid nodules increases with age. The actual prevalence is 4/1000 for benign nodules and 0.4/1000 for malignant nodules. The risk for malignancy in a solitary thyroid nodule is 10–15% in children who have never been exposed to radiation. Although functional thyroid nodules are believed to be benign, approximately 1–9 % are malignant. Hard, firm, fixated nodules with poor isotope uptake are suspicious for malignancy.

3. Describe the work-up of thyroid nodules in children.
- Thyroid function tests: thyroxine (T_4), thyroid-stimulating hormone (TSH), and thyroid antibodies.
- Basal serum calcitonin in patients with positive family history of medullary thyroid cancer (multiple endocrine neoplasia type 2 [MEN-2]).
- Fine-needle aspiration biopsy (FNAB) must be done by an individual with expertise. Limitations of FNAB include inadequate specimen (15–25 %) and false-negative results from sampling error (2%) Ultrasound-guided FNAB improves the accuracy of biopsy.
- Thyroid ultrasound distinguishes solid from cystic nodules. Hypoechoic nodules are usually solid and have a greater risk of being malignant. In contrast, cystic nodules are usually benign but up to 10% may be malignant.
- Radionuclide scanning: preferably with iodine 131 (I-131) because malignant tissue does not organify radioactive iodine.
- Thyroid suppressive therapy is of limited value because most benign nodules do not diminish in size and because 13–15% of thyroid cancers become smaller with thyroid hormone therapy.

4. Describe the treatment of thyroid nodules in children.

It is generally recommended that all nonfunctional (cold) thyroid nodules in children be excised. An intraoperative frozen biopsy is necessary to determine the extent of the thyroid surgery.

Opinions differ as to the surgical treatment for functional thyroid nodules. Nodules causing hyperthyroidism must be excised. In euthyroid patients, functional thyroid nodules are often monitored conservatively; however, some authorities advise removal for all thyroid nodules, regardless of results of radioiodine uptake studies.

5. Do children get thyroid cancer?

Thyroid cancer occurs in about 1 of 10,000 children and accounts for 1.5–2.1 % of all pediatric malignancies. The female-to-male ratio is 2:1. Children at great risk for developing thyroid cancer include those with prior exposure to ionizing radiation. No evidence suggests an increased risk in children who receive I-131 diagnostic thyroid imaging or I-131 ablation for Graves' disease.

The most common thyroid cancer in childhood is papillary carcinoma; other types are much less common and have a less favorable prognosis. They include follicular thyroid carcinoma, medullary thyroid carcinoma (MEN syndromes) and anaplastic carcinoma. A positive family history of medullary thyroid cancer, pheochromocytoma, hyperparathyroidism, or mucosal neuromas mandates screening for medullary thyroid cancer because it is inherited by an autosomal dominant mechanism. Baseline and pentagastrin-stimulated serum calcitonin levels as well as gene analysis identify affected children who must undergo total thyroidectomy to protect them from future development of medullary thyroid carcinoma.

6. How does thyroid cancer present in children?

The clinical presentation of thyroid cancer is a discrete, firm-to-hard nodule that may or may not be fixed to surrounding tissues. Vocal cord paralysis is a late complication. Palpable enlarged cervical lymph nodes, especially in the low anterior neck region, may be indicative of metastases. Rarely, thyroid cancer may present as a large metastatic cervical lymph node without a palpable thyroid nodule. Metastatic lesions in lymph nodes are usually movable, nontender, smooth, and discrete.

7. How is thyroid cancer diagnosed?
- Thyroid function tests: triiodothyronine (T_3), T_4, TSH, antithyroid antibodies
- Baseline serum thyroglobulin
- Baseline and post-stimulated serum calcitonin levels in patients with MEN
- Thyroid ultrasound, which identifies the character of the nodule: solid, cystic, or mixed
- I-123 thyroid scan, which identifies a nonfunctioning nodule but does not determine definitely whether the nodule is benign or malignant
- Optional studies: neck radiographs for calcifications
- Chest radiograph or computed tomography (CT) exam
- FNAB if performed and interpreted by an expert

8. How is thyroid cancer treated?

Surgery is the treatment of choice for thyroid cancer; the extent of the procedure has to be individualized. Total thyroidectomy is required for medullary thyroid cancer and large tumors that have metastasized. Total body scans using I-131 for metastases can be performed only in patients who have undergone total thyroidectomy and remnant ablation. Because the prognosis for papillary cancer is excellent, some centers perform lobectomy rather than total thyroidectomy.

9. What are the complications of thyroidectomy?

Hypoparathyroidism, iatrogenic hypothyroidism, recurrent laryngeal nerve injury, keloid formation, anesthesia risk, infection, bleeding, and death (rare).

10. What are the goals of thyroid replacement therapy?

The goals of thyroid replacement therapy are maintenance of a low normal TSH level and euthyroid state. Serum thyroglobulin is a useful marker of cancer recurrence and metastases. Baseline and pentagastrin-stimulated serum calcitonin levels are used to monitor medullary thyroid cancer. High-resolution neck ultrasonography is a sensitive method of detecting recurrence. Depending on the individual presentation, periodic chest radiographs or CT exams may be necessary.

11. What is the most common cause of hyperthyroidism in childhood?

The most common cause of hyperthyroidism in children is Graves' disease, an autoimmune condition caused by the production of an autoantibody that stimulates the TSH receptor. Signs and symptoms can be subtle or quite dramatic. The condition may respond to treatment early without complications or be very difficult to control.

12. What is the recommended treatment of juvenile hyperthyroidism?

Although I-131 ablation is considered the first line of therapy for Graves' disease in adults, most children are initially treated with antithyroid drugs. The two most frequently used drugs are **propylthiouracil** (PTU) and **methimazole** (MMI). PTU prevents the organification of iodine as well as the peripheral conversion of T_4 to T_3. MMI prevents the oxidation of iodide but does not inhibit the peripheral conversion of T_4 to T_3. The initial dose of PTU is 5–10 mg/kg/day (150–300 mg/m^2/day). MMI is given at a dose of 0.1–1.0 mg/kg/day. MMI can be given in two divided doses. Children with more severe hyperthyroidism and large goiters should be started on higher doses than patients with milder disease.

Because antithyroid drugs prevent synthesis of thyroid hormone but do not prevent release of preformed hormone, euthyroidism is not achieved until stored hormone is depleted. In a study by Gorton et al., the mean duration of PTU treatment before normalization of T_4 was 2.4 ± 1.9 months. If thyrotoxic symptoms are significant during this lag period, propranolol (0.5–2 mg/kg/day in divided doses given every 6–8 hours) can be used as adjunctive therapy. Propranolol should not be used in children with asthma, congestive heart failure, or insulin-dependent diabetes mellitus.

13. How are antithyroid drugs used?

Antithyroid medications typically have been used in two ways. Some clinicians titrate the dose in an attempt to maintain clinical and biochemical euthyroidism. Others intentionally overtreat to block thyroid function completely and then add L-thyroxine to maintain euthyroidism. Several methods can be used to taper or withdraw treatment, none of which shows a clearcut benefit over the others. Some practitioners gradually wean the medication as soon as improvement occurs. Others abruptly discontinue the medication when euthyroidism is achieved. Sometimes treatment is given for a predetermined period of 1 or 2 years after adjustments are made during the initial months of treatment. Prolonged treatment regimens result in higher remission rates, although the positive effect may be related solely to time.

14. What are the side effects of antithyroid drugs? How common are they?

The most common minor side effect are skin rashes, transient neutropenia, nausea, headaches, paresthesias, hair loss, and arthralgias. Persistence of neutropenia is best managed by discontinuation of drug treatment. In rare cases, agranulocytosis occurs, usually early in the course of treatment and with relatively high doses. Other significant side effects of antithyroid drug treatment are collagen vascular-like illnesses, hepatitis, and glomerulonephritis. Complete blood count and liver function tests should be drawn at baseline before the start of treatment and as needed in response to problems that develop. The rate of toxic effects of antithyroid drugs ranges from 5–32%, according to major pediatric studies.

15. What is the role of surgery in the treatment of juvenile hyperthyroidism?

Surgery is usually not the primary mode of therapy for juvenile Graves' disease. In the hands of an experienced pediatric surgeon, subtotal thyroidectomy continues to be an option for emergent treatment of severe thyrotoxicosis. Surgery is also an appropriate choice in some cases when medical treatment fails because of drug toxicity or noncompliance.

Surgery is the recommended treatment for thyrotoxicosis due to a solitary hyperfunctioning nodule in the thyroid gland. After removal of the nodule, the remaining thyroid tissue gradually regains function, and thyroid replacement is not necessary in the long term.

16. What are the endocrine causes of hypertension in children?

The most common causes of endocrine hypertension are disorders that involve the adrenal gland directly or indirectly. For practical purposes, the adrenal disorders are due either to abnormalities in the renin-angiotensin system or to intrinsic overproduction of mineralocorticoids from the adrenal cortex. In both situations the adrenal gland plays a pivotal role.

17. How do abnormalities in the renin-angiotensin system lead to hypertension?

Renin produced by the kidney hydrolyzes angiotensinogen derived from the liver, thereby changing it to angiotensin I. A converting enzyme from the lungs transforms angiotensin I into an octapeptide, angiotensin II. Angiotensin II causes vasoconstriction of the peripheral vascular system and also binds to cells in the zona glomerulosa of the adrenal cortex, leading to production of aldosterone. Children with normal or high renin hypertension are likely to have a renovascular abnormality, whereas children with low renin probably have overproduction of a mineralocorticoid from the adrenal glands or a volume-dependent form of hypertension.

18. How common is renovascular hypertension in children?

Renovascular stenosis is the most common cause of hypertension in childhood. It may be due to unilateral, bilateral, or segmental renovascular disease; Takayasu's disease; or, in occasional cases, neurofibromatosis. In young infants, renal vein thrombosis due to catheter placement should be investigated. Primary renal disease, including malformations of the kidney, also should be assessed.

19. How are renin-secreting tumors treated?

• Medical therapy using angiotensin I-converting enzyme inhibitors
• Surgical correction if medical treatment fails to control the hypertension

20. What is pill-mediated hypertension?

Adolescent girls who take oral contraceptive pills may develop hypertension. Estrogens cause an increase in renin substrate, but the precise mechanism leading to hypertension needs to be defined.

21. How does mineralocorticoid excess cause hypertension in children?

Overproduction of aldosterone or another mineralocorticoid produced in the adrenal gland causes hypertension, hypokalemia, and metabolic alkalosis. In rare cases, the mineralocorticoid receptor can be stimulated by glucocorticoids, leading to a low-renin hypertensive state. Aldosterone, secreted from the zona glomerulosa, is regulated primarily by angiotensin II, but adrenocorticotropic hormone (ACTH) and potassium also have an important stimulatory influence. Mineralocorticoids promote sodium and chloride retention in the renal tubule, which leads to water retention. Potassium and hydrogen ion excretion is stimulated by aldosterone. In certain circumstances, excess of atrial natriuretic factor overrides aldosterone, leading to high renal sodium losses even in the presence of elevated aldosterone.

22. What are the major types of mineralocorticoid excess?

• Primary aldosteronism
• Glucocorticoid-suppressive hyperaldosteronism (GSH)
• Cushing syndrome
• Hypertensive forms of congenital adrenal hyperplasia due to an excess of deoxycorticosterone (DOC)
• Deficiency of 11β hydroxysteroid dehydrogenase (11β OHSD)

23. What causes primary aldosteronism?

Aldosterone-producing tumors. Aldosterone-producing adenomas are rare in childhood, but when they occur, they usually affect girls. Aldosterone-producing adrenal carcinomas are even less common.

Idiopathic hyperaldosteronism (IHA). Bilateral adrenal cortical hyperplasia and unilateral nodular hyperplasia are milder forms of hyperaldosteronism that present with low renin, hypokalemia, and hyperaldosteronism. It is essential that the patient be on a normal or high sodium diet because low sodium intake falsely alters renal potassium losses. Urinary aldosterone output is elevated. Spironolactone leads to a rise in urinary aldosterone output in IHA but has no effect in patients with an aldosterone-producing adenoma. A dexamethasone suppression test is recommended to distinguish IHA from glucocorticoid-suppressible hyperaldosteronism. In IHA, aldosterone output is not reduced by dexamethasone. The medical treatment for IHA is spironolactone, whereas surgery is required for an aldosterone-producing adenoma.

24. What is GSH?

GSH is an autosomal dominant disorder in which aldosterone is stimulated by ACTH and suppressed by dexamethasone. The genetic defect involves a hybrid gene that is formed when the regulatory region of the steroid 11β hydroxylase gene (CYP 11β1), which is active in the zona fasciculata, becomes linked to the coding sequences of the aldosterone synthase gene (CYP 11β2), which is expressed in the zona glomerulosa. The encoded protein of this hybrid gene is able to synthesize aldosterone from DOC. The disorder is characterized by high aldosterone, hypokalemia, and low renin. Dexamethasone lowers aldosterone and alleviates hypertension. Maintenance low-dose glucocorticoid therapy corrects the hypertension in childhood.

25. What causes Cushing syndrome? How is it diagnosed?

In children younger than 7 years, Cushing syndrome results from adrenal adenoma or carcinoma. Hypertension is present in 70% of cases, and hypokalemia and renin levels vary. The cause of the hypertension is multifactorial: the action of cortisol on the mineralocorticoid receptor, an excess of renin-angiotensin substrate levels, activation of the renin-angiotensin system, enhanced vascular sensitivity to catecholamines, and prostaglandin inhibition. CT scan of the adrenal glands identifies the tumor. Measurement of morning and evening cortisol levels confirms loss of the normal diurnal cortisol rhythm. Quantitation of urine cortisol output over 24 hours is also diagnostic. Low- and high-dose dexamethasone tests confirm that cortisol output is autonomous and is not responsive to dexamethasone (i.e., not ACTH-dependent).

In older children, Cushing syndrome is more likely due to an ACTH-producing pituitary adenoma. The excessive ACTH causes bilateral adrenal hyperplasia. Cortisol excess tends to suppress with the high-dose dexamethasone test but not with the low-dose test. Sensitive magnetic resonance (MR) studies have identified the lesion in the pituitary gland, which usually is removed by transphenoidal neurosurgery.

26. What two enzyme deficiencies cause hypertensive forms of congenital adrenal hyperplasia due to an excess of DOC?

Deficiency of **17α hydroxylase** leads to diminished secretion of glucocorticoids as well as sex hormones. Overproduction of ACTH due to cortisol deficiency leads to elevated DOC production, hypertension, hypokalemia, and decreased aldosterone production. Males are underviriized because the 17α hydroxylase enzyme is present in the testis and adrenal gland. A deficiency of 17α hydroxylase leads to a lack of testosterone production in the 46XY fetus and female-appearing external genitalia. The uterus is absent because the testis produces antimüllerian hormone from the Sertoli cells, which function normally. The condition is inherited by an autosomal recessive mechanism. Genetic females with 17α hydroxylase deficiency fail to develop breasts or menstruation and are infertile. Treatment involves maintenance glucocorticoid therapy, which suppresses ACTH excess in both sexes and leads to normalization of blood pressure as DOC levels fall into the normal range. The previously suppressed levels of renin and aldosterone return to normal after administration of glucocorticoid therapy.

Deficiency of **11β hydroxylase** also is inherited as an autosomal recessive condition. The genetic female with this disorder has virilized genitalia at birth and often is assigned a male sex. Internally, the infant has ovaries and a uterus. If untreated, males and females experience progressive virilization from early childhood, leading to rapid growth, tall stature, advanced bone age, and early epiphyseal fusion with short adult height. The hypertension appears to result from DOC excess as well as an unusual sensitivity to DOC. Recently the 11β hydroxylase isoenzymes have been reported to be encoded by two genes located on chromosome 8. CYP11 β1 (11β hydroxylase β1) controls cortisol production in the zona fasciculata, whereas CYP 11 β2 (11β hydroxylase β2) synthesizes aldosterone in the zona glomerulosa. The diagnosis is made when low renin hypertension exists in the presence of high serum levels of 11 deoxysteroids (DOC, 11-deoxycortisol, or compound S) at baseline and after stimulation with ACTH, coupled with excessive androgen production. The treatment is glucocorticoid replacement to suppress the high endogenous production of ACTH, which leads to a fall in DOC and blood pressure and a gradual rise in renin and aldosterone production.

27. What causes a deficiency of 11β OHSD?

Syndrome of apparent mineralocorticoid excess (AMES). The major site of oxidation of cortisol to cortisone is in the kidney, where 11β OHSD catalyzes this conversion. Children with congenital 11β OHSD deficiency present with severe hypertension, hypokalemia, low renin, and unmeasurable aldosterone or other mineralocorticoids; hence, the name AMES. The cause is presumed to be a defect in the "cortisol to cortisone shuttle" whereby cortisol acts as a potent mineralocorticoid working through the renal type I mineralocorticoid receptors. Dexamethasone and spironolactone usually are effective in lowering cortisol production and blocking its mineralocorticoid action.

Licorice ingestion may cause acquired 11β OHSD deficiency. High doses of licorice administered to patients with peptic ulcers in the 1940s led to hypertension and hypokalemia. The metabolites of licorice inhibit the activity of 11β OHSD, leading to excessive cortisol accumulation and hypertension.

28. What is pheochromocytoma? How is it diagnosed and treated?

Pheochromocytoma is a rare tumor of childhood with peak incidence between 9 and 12 years of age. Bilateral and multiple adrenal tumors are more common in children than in adults. Malignant pheochromocytomas account for less than 10% of tumors. Affected children are more likely to have one of the MEN syndromes or a positive family history than are adults with pheochromocytoma. Both epinephrine and norepinephrine are elevated, but the latter is the predominant hormone produced. Other clinical findings include headache, excessive perspiration, tachycardia, palpitations, nervousness, emotional lability, constipation, polydipsia, polyuria, orthostatic hypotension, and vasoconstrictive phenomena.

Diagnosis depends on measurement of elevated norepinephrine, epinephrine, and metanephrine in a 24-hour urine collection. Urinary output of vanillylmandelic acid (VMA) is not diagnostic, nor are plasma catecholamine measurements. The tumor is localized by CT, ultrasonography, MRI, and metaiodobensyl-guanidine scintigraphy. During test procedures, the patient should receive alpha-adrenergic blockers to protect against hypertensive crises.

Surgical excision is the treatment of choice but should be undertaken only when the patient is protected by alpha-adrenergic blockade alone or in combination with beta blockade. Preoperative preparation and careful intra- and postoperative care are essential to a favorable outcome.

29. What is neuroblastoma? How is it diagnosed and treated?

Neuroblastoma is a common malignant tumor of early childhood. It may occur wherever sympathetic nervous tissue is found. The peak incidence is around 3 years of age. Metastases occur early. The tumor has the capacity to differentiate and mature into a ganglioneuroblastoma or ganglioneuroma. Neuroblastomas have the highest spontaneous regression rate of any tumor. Only 20% of children with neuroblastoma develop hypertension.

The typical findings are high urinary output of dopamine, norepinephrine, and/or their metabolites. Urinary VMA is not a useful screening test because VMA levels are normal in about 15% of patients. Treatment consists of surgical excision, radiation, and chemotherapy.

30. What other endocrine disorders may cause hypertension?

- Some patients with hyperparathyroidism develop hypertension ,presumably because parathyroid hormone (PTH) can activate the renin-angiotensin system.
- Hyperthyroidism causes systolic hypertension that resolves once the patient is rendered euthyroid.
- Acromegaly is associated with hypertension because excessive growth hormone leads to sodium and water retention.

31. How should infants with ambiguous genitalia be evaluated and managed?

At birth, an infant with ambiguous genitalia frequently is assigned a male sex in the delivery room based on the size of the phallus and the degree of external genital virilization. Under ideal circumstances, parents should be advised at birth that the physical appearance does not accurately identify whether the infant is a virilized female or an undervirilized male. If the gonads are palpable, the infant is more likely to be a male, but true hermaphroditism is still a possibility. Although the information is painful, most parents in retrospect appreciative being told that accurate sex assignment will depend on the results of diagnostic tests. This problem is a medical emergency because of the extreme anxiety that the parents experience.

The medical team should include professionals with expertise in genetics, psychological counseling, pediatric endocrinology, and pediatric genital surgery. They work closely with the parents, primary physician, and obstetrician. Parents should receive simplified explanations about genital differentiation during fetal life, the common origins of the structures that comprise female and male external genitalia (e.g., clitoris and penis, labia majora and scrotum), and the variable masculinizing effects of androgen on the external genitalia of either sex.

Although the final recommendation about sex assignment depends on the prognosis for satisfactory sexual functioning and reproduction, parents must be included as members of the team since they must be able to accept, support, and raise their child in the chosen sex. In some situations, sex assignment is independent of anatomic and functional variables; for example, parents whose religion mandates that 46,XY infants be reared as males regardless of the severity of the genital defect.

32. List the basic elements of sexual differentiation.

By week 7 of fetal life, the essential primordia are present:

Bipotential gonad—destined to be ovary or testis

Paired internal ducts—not bipotential
- Wolffian ducts become epididymis, vas deferens, seminal vesicles, and ejaculatory ducts
- Müllerian ducts become fallopian tubes, uterus, cervix, and upper third of vagina

Bipotential external genitalia
- Genital tubercle becomes clitoris or corpora/glans of penis
- Genital folds become labia minora or penile urethra
- Genital swelling becomes labia majora or scrotum

33. Describe the process of sexual differentiation.

Female sexual differentiation progresses normally in the presence or absence of the ovary (e.g., streak gonad) if the 46XX fetus is not exposed to androgens transferred from the mother or produced in the infant.

Male sexual differentiation is more complex. The testis is differentiated and functional by 7 weeks of fetal life. The two hormones produced by the testes control differentiation of the paired internal ducts as well as the male external genitalia, which are fully formed by 13 weeks. Leydig cells in the fetal testis produce testosterone, which acts directly and locally on the Wolffian ducts to stimulate differentiation. The Sertoli cells of the fetal seminiferous tubules secrete antimüllerian hormone (AMH), which also works locally to suppress the müllerian ducts, thereby preventing formation of the fallopian tubes, uterus, and upper third or the vagina. Testosterone must be converted to 5-alpha-dihydrotestosterone (5α-DHT) by 5α-reductase, an abundant enzyme in fetal genital tissues. Male external genital differentiation is controlled by

5α-DHT and its receptor (androgen receptor). Thus, testosterone is a prohormone that requires conversion locally in the genital tissues of the male. Defects in testosterone action result from deficiency of 5α-reductase or an absence or deficiency of the androgen receptor.

Normal male sexual differentiation is the consequence of a highly integrated cascade of genes. Many have been identified, but others are yet to be defined. The number of genes is increasing as we learn more about the pathways involved. For example, SRY on the Y chromosome controls testicular differentiation, and the WT1 gene is critical for development of the urogenital ridge from which the primitive kidney and primordial bipotential gonad are derived. Mutations in WT1 lead to renal and testicular dysgenesis and increased risk for Wilms' tumor. Other genes include:

- SF-I, which is essential for production of steroid hormones as well as AMH
- SOX9, which, if mutated causes testicular dysgenesis, sex reversal, campomelic dwarfism, and death in infancy.
- DAX-1, which is located on the X chromosome. Duplication of this gene in a 46XY male leads to testicular dysgenesis, sex reversal, and ambiguous genitalia. A double dose of DAX-1 in males has been referred to as DSS (double-dose sex reversal).
- Additional genes in 9p and 10q influence testicular differentiation by unknown mechanisms.

34. How are infants with ambiguous genitalia classified?

Virilization of genetic females (46XX) (female pseudohermaphroditism) may be caused by maternal androgens, ingestion or endogenous production of androgens, congenital adrenal hyperplasia, or aromatase deficiency.

Undervirilized genetic males (46XY) (male pseudohermaphroditism) may be caused by a deficiency of testosterone production (due to defects in testosterone biosynthesis, Leydig cell hypoplasia, or bilateral fetal testicular torsion) or defects in testosterone action (due to androgen resistance syndrome or 5α-reductase deficiency).

Chromosomal abnormalities and **abnormal gonadal differentiation** include mixed gonadal dysgenesis (45X, 46XY), true hermaphroditism, sex reversal syndromes, or pure gonadal dysgenesis.

Birth defects in the perigenital area include extrophy of the bladder and epispadias.

35. What is the most common cause of ambiguous genitalia?

The most common cause of virilization in the female fetus is congenital adrenal hyperplasia (CAH), which results from the lack of an enzyme necessary for cortisol production. Consequently, the fetal pituitary overproduces ACTH, causing hyperplasia of the adrenal cortex and overproduction of androgens in most affected infants. The fetal adrenal cortex is functional by 6 weeks of fetal life, and the fetal hypothalamic pituitary adrenal axis is autonomous and independent of the mother because of placental inactivation of maternal cortisol. Of the five enzymes that cause CAH, the most common deficiency is the 21-hydroxylase (21-OH) enzyme, which is essential for cortisol as well as aldosterone production. Of infants with CAH, 95% have 21-OH deficiency, and 75% of these are salt losers. In this autosomal recessive condition, females are virilized, but males are normal at birth. Affected infants are healthy until the second or third week of life when they gradually decompensate because of salt loss, hypovolemia, hypotension, hyperkalemia, weight loss, and (without treatment) shock and death. Females tend to be given a male sex assignment because the external genitalia are indistinguishable from 46XY males with hypospadias, chordee, and cryptorchidism. Males tend to be undiagnosed until they decompensate, and a significant number die without being diagnosed because they resemble infants with disorders such as bowel obstruction, gastroenteritis, and pyloric stenosis. The biochemical abnormalities that distinguish these CAH salt-losing males from other infants is the marked elevation of potassium in the presence of hyponatremia and metabolic acidosis.

36. What diagnostic procedures are appropriate for infants with ambiguous genitalia?

The following diagnostic procedures should be individualized based on the infant's presentation:

- Karyotype: gives information about genetic sex (46XX , 46XY, 45X/46XY). Because most true hermaphrodites have 46XX karyotype, they are not identified by karyotype testing.
- Electrolytes: low sodium, high potassium in salt losers.
- Renin: high in salt losers before decompensation.
- Serum 17-OHP is high in 21-OH deficiency.
- Baseline testosterone, follicle stimulating hormone (FSH), and luteinizing hormone (LH) in the first weeks of life give information about gonadotropin deficiency vs. primary Leydig cell dysfunction.
- Human chorionic gonadotropin (hCG) stimulation test: 100–200 U/kg is given intramuscularly on 3 consecutive days, and testosterone is measured on the fourth day. Testosterone and 5α-DHT measurements before and after the test identify 5α-reductase deficiency. The ratio of testosterone to DHT should be less than 10. Ratios above 10 suggest 5α-reductase deficiency.
- AMH measurement (not widely available).
- Pelvic ultrasound: gives information about the uterus and often the gonads.
- Genitogram: a small catheter is inserted into the genital orifice, and dye is administered to define the position of the urethra and to locate a connection to the upper vagina.
- Additional molecular studies (e.g., for presence of SRY, Y material in 46XX infants, SOX-9) require access to highly sophisticated genetic testing.

37. Describe the treatment of virilized genetic female infants.

Because 46XX infants with CAH have ovaries and uterus, female sex assignment is the standard recommendation. They are identified by elevated levels of 17-OHP, renin, and potassium and low levels of sodium with or without metabolic acidosis. Maintenance hydrocortisone (12–15 mg/m^2/day divided into 3 daily doses) and mineralocorticoid therapy (Florinef, 0.1– 0.2 mg/day) are used after a period of higher doses of hydrocortisone (60–75 mg/m^2/day) to suppress the elevated levels of ACTH, 17-OHP, and androgens. Written instructions for stress doses of hydrocortisone must be given to parents for use during acute illnesses.

Corrective surgery is usually postponed until 6 months of age. Currently, clitoral recession rather than clitoridectomy is the procedure of choice. The timing of vaginal surgery is important. Most young girls are not sufficiently mature to provide good postoperative self-care because they are uncomfortable using dilators to preserve vaginal width. We provide extensive counseling and detailed information about the patient's responsibility for postoperative care and rely on the girl to tell us when she is ready for the vaginal surgery. Usually we recommend that the operation be done in late adolescence (16–18 years of age), but opinions differ. In some centers, pull-through vaginoplasty is done at a very young age and may be a satisfactory option if a highly skilled surgeon is doing the procedure. The usual choices for vaginal construction are a skin graft or colon graft. Successful outcomes depend on the skill and experience of the surgeon and the competence of the patient, who is essentially responsible for the postoperative care after discharge from the hospital.

38. Describe the treatment of undervirilized genetic males.

Sex assignment in a 46XY male depends on the size of the phallus, its potential to enlarge when testosterone treatment is given, function of the testes, and parental preference. Males with isolated microphallus or a small phallus with hypospadias are treated with depot testosterone, 25 mg/month intramuscularly for 3 months. Most infants respond well. In infant males who need hypospadias surgery, we have sometimes given another one, two, or three injections of depot testosterone to augment the phallus and facilitate surgical repair.

The hardest decisions relate to assignment of sex in 46XY infants with almost no phallic tissue or with severe, complex abnormalities involving the bladder and genitalia. We provide the parents with all information about the potential risks and outcomes of male vs. female sex assignment, including the effects of the decision on reproductive potential and the need for future surgery and life-long hormonal therapy. We believe that the parents are part of the decision-making team. The critical missing element in such decisions is input by the infant. Some children have become outspoken adult critics of the medical profession because they believe that the surgical procedures were excessive, unnecessary, or even mutilating. Although we hope that this group is a minority, their unhappiness with decisions made in their early childhood should make all professionals sensitive to the possibility of patient disapproval and despair about treatment decisions made in good faith.

39. During a herniorrhaphy on a 2-year-old girl with normal external female genitalia, a testicle is found in the hernia sac. What should be done next?

This discovery is a crisis for surgeon and parents. Usually the surgeon leaves the operating room and informs the parents of the problem. An emergency consultation is requested of a pediatric endocrinologist, geneticist, and psychologist, who meet the family with the surgeon. The parents should be told that the gonad is a testicle and that additional tests are needed to determine the child's karyotype and the status of the uterus. They should be reassured that the child's sex of rearing will not be affected and that their daughter will have no confusion about her sexual identity if the family is supportive and accepting.

The likely cause is androgen resistance, which needs to be discussed with parents in simple terms, i.e., a hormone can work only if the receptor receives the message. Like a key opening a lock, the match must be perfect; if it is not, the message from the hormone is never received. The testicle functions normally and produces AMH, which suppresses müllerian development. Hence, the girl will have no uterus and will never menstruate, but she will develop breasts and have an entirely feminine body build. Psychologically, such girls identify as females and are romantically drawn to men.

Opinions differ about the timing of gonadectomies. We recommend bilateral orchiectomies at the time of discovery to eliminate the risk of gonadoblastoma at a later age. Starting at approximately 8 years of age, the girl should receive information about the need for estrogen replacement in her adolescent years so that she will develop breasts and strong bones. She also needs to know that she will not menstruate and that she will have to adopt children. When information is given at an early age, the patient is more accepting of her need to see a pediatric endocrinologist for hormone replacement. We usually do not tell children that the removed gonads were testicles. Instead, we tell the patient that the "ovary" was malformed and that the high risk of cancer made it essential to remove it at an early age. Such discussions should be carried out privately in a quiet office—not in a busy clinic setting. Privacy and honesty are essential if this girl is to preserve her self-confidence and trust in her parents and doctors. An individualized decision has to be made about when and how to give the patient information about the karyotype and the identity of the testis.

40. What should be done when an ovary is discovered in a boy?

A problem similar to the one above is presented when a boy with male genitalia and unilateral cryptorchidism is discovered to have an ovary during orchidopexy/hernia surgery. Probably the boy is a true hermaphrodite with 46XX chromosomes. Again, discussion with the family is essential to their understanding and permission for removal of the ovary. The testis is usually unable to produce sperm, but its ability to secrete testosterone varies. Gonadotropin levels are most helpful as the boy reaches peripubertal age.

41. Define precocious puberty.

Precocious puberty occurs when girls have breast development, pubic hair, and linear growth spurt before the age of 8 years. A recent study suggests that onset of sexual development after age 7 years in Caucasian girls and 6 years in African American girls can be considered within the normal range. Pubertal development typically occurs later in boys, and precocious puberty is diagnosed if signs of puberty are evident before the age of 9 years.

42. What causes precocious puberty?

Precocious puberty can be classified as gonadotropin-dependent or gonadotropin-independent. **Gonadotropin-dependent** precocious puberty is associated with evidence of maturation of the hypothalamic-pituitary-gonadal axis. Girls have both breast development and pubic hair, and boys have testicular enlargement, penile growth, and pubic hair. Production of pubertal hormones leads to acceleration of growth and advanced skeletal maturation.

In **gonadotropin-independent** or pseudoprecocious puberty, sexual development is not mediated by the hypothalamus. Other terms used to describe sexual development in such disorders are "isosexual" and "heterosexual." If development is isosexual, characteristics appropriate for the sex of the child are evident. Heterosexual development occurs if girls show evidence of virilization or if boys have evidence of feminization, such as development of glandular breast tissue.

Gonadotropin-independent precocious puberty in girls usually has an ovarian etiology. Benign follicular cysts are the most common cause. Other causes include granulosa-theca cell tumors, luteomas, or virilizing Leydig-Sertoli cell tumors. **McCune-Albright syndrome** is characterized by café-au-lait spots, polyostotic fibrous dysplasia, and gonadotropin-independent precocious puberty. The production of gonadal hormones is caused by an activating mutation in the signal G-protein system, which leads to continuous receptor activation. McCune-Albright syndrome is more common in girls.

Gonadotropin-independent precocious puberty in boys can be caused by stimulation of the Leydig cells by human chorionic gonadotropin (hCG), which can be produced by germinomas as well as hepatic or mediastinal tumors. CAH, adrenal tumors, and testicular tumors can lead to virilization without activation of the hypothalamic-pituitary-gonadal axis. **Familial testotoxicosis** is caused by an activation of the LH receptor, which causes continuous stimulation of testosterone production by Leydig cells. Hypothyroidism occasionally leads to thelarche in girls and testicular enlargement in boys. Longstanding, severe primary hypothyroidism in girls is associated with multicystic ovaries, which may present as an abdominal mass. Surgery is not indicated because thyroid replacement shrinks the mass and the cysts resolve. This is the only form of precocious sexual development associated with growth failure; hence, careful attention must be given to the child's height, growth velocity, and previous heights plotted on a standard growth curve.

Central precocious puberty is classified as **idiopathic** in about 95% of girls diagnosed with the condition. The trigger for the early initiation of pubertal events remains unknown. Organic causes for central precocious puberty are much more likely to be diagnosed in boys (50%). Intracranial lesions such as astrocytomas, optic gliomas, tuberculomas, germinomas, and pineal tumors may be involved. These tumors probably stimulate the onset of puberty by disrupting inhibitory tracts leading to the hypothalamus. Benign hamartomas may mimic the hypothalamus by producing gonadotropin-releasing hormone (GnRH), thus stimulating production of pituitary gonadotropins. Children with cerebral palsy, hydrocephalus, and neurofibromatosis type I are at risk for development of precocious puberty.

43. Describe the treatment for idiopathic gonadotropin-dependent precocious puberty.

Long-acting agonists of luteinzing hormone-releasing hormone (LHRH) are the most common treatment. This treatment causes downregulation of pituitary gonadotropin receptors by exposure to continuous rather than pulsatile secretion of GnRH. Most cases of precocious puberty caused by hormone-secreting hamartomas also can be treated successfully with LHRH agonists. The aromatase inhibitor, testolactone, is sometimes used to treat patients with McCune-Albright Syndrome or familial testotoxicosis. Spironolactone often is added to the treatment regimen in patients with familial testotoxicosis to block androgen receptors. Hypothyroidism is treated exclusively by thyroid hormone replacement.

44. Describe the evaluation of a boy with gynecomastia.

Gynecomastia is the enlargement of the male breast due to a proliferation of glandular tissue. Physiologic gynecomastia is common during the neonatal period, puberty, and advanced age. Causes of pathologic gynecomastia include testicular or adrenal neoplasms, ectopic hCG production by tumors, primary or secondary hypogonadism, androgen insensitivity, true hermaphroditism, hyperthyroidism, drug use, and excessive aromatase activity. Other associations include liver and kidney disease as well as starvation. Sex-cord tumors of the testes have been identified in several boys with Peutz-Jeghers syndrome.

Before initiation of extensive laboratory testing, an attempt should be made to differentiate true gynecomastia from adiposity or pseudogynecomastia. Asymmetric gynecomastia is commonly seen but necessitates evaluation for carcinoma, which generally presents as an eccentric, unilateral mass that is firm to palpation and fixed to underlying tissues. Mammography and fine-needle or surgical biopsy may be indicated in some cases. In normal pubertal boys, the incidence of gynecomastia is 50–75%. Breast enlargement typically occurs during mid-puberty at about 13 years of age and usually lasts from 6 months to 2 years. Pain and tenderness of the breast are common complaints. Pubertal gynecomastia is a physiologic condition that is thought to result from a temporary imbalance between estrogen and testosterone production. Extensive evaluation is not required if the remainder of the physical exam, including testicular exam, is normal. Reassurance about the transient nature of the condition should be given. If testes are small, karyotype should be done to rule out Klinefelter syndrome (XXY). Other forms of primary hypogonadism also should be considered. If hypospadias or cryptorchidism is present, syndromes of androgen insensitivity must be considered.

If gynecomastia occurs after the neonatal period and before puberty, careful evaluation is warranted. History should include questions about medication, drug use, or accidental exposure to estrogen-containing substances. Systemic and metabolic disease such as Peutz-Jeghers syndrome, hepatic dysfunction, and hyperthyroidism should be ruled out by physical exam and appropriate lab tests. Growth curve should be evaluated to rule out acceleration of linear growth due to chronic exposure to androgens or estrogens. Bone age should be obtained in boys with evidence of rapid growth. Physical exam should include a careful examination of the testes to rule out tumor. Tanner staging of the genitalia should be done. The initial lab workup often includes estradiol, testosterone, estrone, and beta hCG tumor marker. If evaluation yields normal results, idiopathic gynecomastia is diagnosed. Close follow-up is necessary.

45. How is gynecomastia treated?

Attempts have been made to treat both idiopathic and pubertal gynecomastia with several medications, including tamoxifen (antiestrogen), testolactone (aromatization inhibitor), and dihydrotestosterone. None has been shown to be consistently effective. If gynecomastia is persistent, mastectomy is sometimes indicated.

46. How is hyperparathyroidism in childhood classified?

Primary hyperparathyroidism
- Familial forms
   Familial parathyroid hyperplasia
   Neonatal primary hyperparathyroidism

   MEN-1   MEN-2
      Parathyroid hyperplasia   Parathyroid hyperplasia
      Pituitary adenoma   Medullary thyroid carcinoma
      Pancreatic gastrinoma   Pheochromocytoma
      Pancreatic insulinoma
- Sporadic forms
   Parathyroid adenoma (usually single)
   Parathyroid chief cell carcinoma (rare)

Tertiary hyperparathyroidism
- Hypophosphatemic rickets
- Chronic renal insufficiency

Other: inactivating mutation of calcium-sensing receptor
- Familial hypocalciuric hypercalcemia (FHH)
- Homozygous infant born to parents with hypocalciuric hypercalcemia
- Idiopathic infantile hypercalcemia of Williams syndrome

47 Define primary hyperparathyroidism.

Primary hyperparathyroidism, which is rare in childhood, is characterized by overproduction of parathyroid hormone (PTH). The condition usually is sporadic, but it may be familial due to autosomal dominant transmission or in association with MEN syndromes 1 and 2. The pathology is usually hyperplasia or adenoma of the parathyroid glands.

48. How is parathyroid hyperplasia diagnosed?

Parathyroid hyperplasia, which is caused by hyperplasia of all four glands, cannot be distinguished from parathyroid adenoma clinically. The condition is often familial and must be distinguished from FHH, which is inherited in an autosomal dominant pattern and does not require surgery. The two entities can be distinguished by the benign nature (serum calcium levels < 12 mg/dl, PTH in high normal range) and hypocalciuric characteristics (< 100 mg in 24-hr urine output) of FHH vs. the hypercalciuric state (> 200 mg calcium in 24-hour urine output) and medical complications of parathyroid hyperplasia.

49. How is parathyroid adenoma diagnosed?

Parathyroid adenoma is sporadic and presents between 3 and 13 years of age. Renal complications or bone disease lead to diagnosis. Ultrasound examination of the neck sometimes locates the adenoma. Kidney stones are diagnosed by hematuria, pain, and renal ultrasound. These tumors are believed to be monoclonal neoplasms resulting from somatic mutations in one parent's cells.

50. What causes MEN types 1 and 2?

MEN types 1 and 2 are autosomal dominant conditions. The MEN-1 gene is at 11q13, and the MEN-2 gene is on chromosome 10. Usually the clinical presentation is between 20 and 40 years of age (rarely in the first decade). Careful screening tests have identified children at risk for MEN-1 and MEN-2 based on molecular assessment of genes.

51. How is MEN-1 diagnosed?

About 90–95% of children with MEN-1 present with parathyroid hyperplasia or adenoma (which may be single or multiple). Tumors of the pancreas (30–80%), anterior pituitary gland (15–30%), and occasionally the adrenal gland are the main features. Pancreatic tumors secrete insulin, gastrin, pancreatic polypeptide, and occasionally glucagon. Excessive gastrin results in peptic ulceration (Zollinger-Ellison syndrome). The most useful test for screening family members is serum calcium because 95% of affected family members have hyperparathyroidism. Molecular diagnostic tests are even more specific for identifying family members at risk for MEN-1. The pituitary tumors may be either nonfunctional, causing pituitary insufficiency, or, more commonly, prolactinomas, causing galactorrhea-amenorrhea syndrome. Rarely a pituitary adenoma secretes growth hormone and results in acromegaly. The gene for MEN-1 normally functions as a growth suppressor. A mutated MEN-1 gene permits neoplastic transformation of cells in the parathyroid, pancreas, and pituitary glands.

52. How is MEN-2 diagnosed?

MEN-2 is characterized by two clinical syndromes that present with common and differentiating endocrinopathies. MEN-2a consists of medullary thyroid carcinoma, pheochromocytoma, and hyperparathyroidism (50%). MEN-2b is characterized by medullary thyroid carcinoma (97%), pheochromocytoma (30%), multiple mucosal neuromas, and Marfanoid habitus. Hyperplasia of the parathyroid is more common than adenoma and usually is not identified until the time of surgery. Medullary thyroid carcinomas secrete calcitonin, which becomes more elevated after pentagastrin testing. The high levels of calcitonin do not cause clinical symptoms.

53. What is Williams syndrome?

Williams syndrome is characterized by dysmorphic features, poor growth and short adult height, mental retardation, and cardiac abnormalities. In addition, 15% of patients have infantile hypercalcemia.

54. Describe the treatment of hyperparathyroidism.

Surgery is the treatment of choice for hyperparathyroidism, including excision of the adenoma or total parathyroidectomy and heterotopic autotransplantation of glandular tissue to the forearm of the nondominant hand.

Hyperparathyroidism in the neonatal period should be treated medically at first because affected infants often are dehydrated. Intravenous fluids (two-thirds or normal saline with 30 mEq/L of potassium) are used to correct dehydration, maximize glomerular filtration, and lower serum calcium concentration. Lasix (1 mg/kg IV every 6–8 hr) inhibits reabsorption of calcium as well as sodium and water. Prednisone (1–2 mg/kg/day) occasionally is added to the regimen. If medical treatment fails to correct the hypercalcemia, surgical treatment is required.

Tertiary hyperparathyroidism is unresponsive to medical therapy because the parathyroid gland no longer responds to serum calcium concentrations. Children with renal failure who are noncompliant with calcitriol therapy and patients with hypophosphatemic rickets who develop tertiary hyperparathyroidism from generous phosphorus therapy require parathyroid surgery for autonomous hyperplastic glands.

Homozygous infants born of parents with hypocalciuric hypercalcemia have life-threatening elevations of serum calcium. Emergency parathyroidectomy is needed for survival.

55. Define neonatal hypoglycemia. How common is it?

The definition of hypoglycemia in the newborn period is a blood sugar level < 40 mg/dl in infants older than 24 hours, regardless of gestational age. The incidence of symptomatic hypoglycemia is approximately 3 in 1000 live births. However, this figure is much higher in high-risk neonates such as small-for-gestational age (SGA) or premature infants.

56. What causes neonatal hypoglycemia:

Hyperinsulinemia (insulin level > 5 mU/ml with blood sugar < than 40 mg/dl)
- Transient hyperinsulinemia (most common cause)
  SGA infants: unknown mechanism
  Asphyxiated infants: islet-cell dysfunction
  Infants of diabetic mothers: fetal islet-cell hyperfunction and macrosomia caused by maternal hyperglycemia
  Erythroblastosis fetalis and Beckwith-Wiedeman syndrome: beta-cell hyperplasia
- Persistent hyperinsulinemia
  Genetic defects of beta-cell maturation
    Recessively inherited hyperinsulinemia (SUR/K ATP mutations)
    Autosomal dominant hyperinsulinism (activating mutation of glucokinase gene, activating mutation of mitochondrial glutamate dehydrogenase that causes hyperammonemia and hyperinsulinism, or unknown defects)
  Beta-cell adenoma (rare, usually sporadic except in families with MEN-1)
- Drug-induced hyperinsulinemia (factitious or accidental; rare in newborns)

Excessive tissue demands (infections, stress)

Impaired ketogenesis
- Fatty acid oxidation defects
- Inadequate fat stores (prematurity, SGA, malnutrition)
- Inadequate fat mobilization (hyperinsulinism, cortisol and growth hormone deficiencies)

Decreased glycogen stores (prematurity, SGA, malnutrition)

Deficiencies of counterregulatory hormones (cortisol and/or growth hormone may be deficient in congenital hypopituitarism)

Disorders of gluconeogenesis (galactosemia, fructose 1,6-diphosphatase deficiency, hereditary fructose intolerance)

Glycogen storage disease type I A (caused by a deficiency of glucose 6 phosphatase; most severe form, associated with hepatomegaly; presents in early infancy with severe hypoglycemia after short periods of fasting)

57. How is the cause of neonatal hypoglycemia diagnosed?
1. Draw a blood sample when the infant has a blood sugar below 40 mg/dl.
2. Send the sample to the laboratory for measurement of:
   - Insulin
   - Glucose
   - Growth hormone
   - Cortisol
   - Serum ketones
   - Lactate
3. Send a urine sample for measurement of ketones and reducing substances at the same time.

58. Describe the treatment of hypoglycemia.
The treatment of hypoglycemia is usually medical. Initial strategies include intravenous glucose or a frequent feeding schedule. If hyperinsulinism is documented in infants with persistent hypoglycemia that does not respond to the above treatment, the standard therapy is diazoxide (Proglycem), which suppresses insulin production (8–15 mg/kg /day in divided doses given every 8 hours). If hypoglycemia still fails to respond, surgery is indicated (i.e., partial pancreatectomy for diffuse islet-cell hyperplasia or excision of adenoma). Infants with hypopituitarism need hydrocortisone and growth hormone replacement.

59. What are the most common causes of obesity in children?
The most common causes of childhood obesity include excessive caloric intake, decreased energy expenditure, and familial predisposition. Exogenous obesity is always associated with normal or accelerated linear growth due to overnutrition.

60. What are the endocrine causes of obesity in children?
Endocrine-mediated obesity with growth deceleration and short stature
- Hypothyroidism: usually mild obesity.
- Growth hormone deficiency: truncal obesity, abdominal fat.
- Cushing syndrome (80–100 % of cases): obesity is usually generalized.
- Pseudohypoparathyroidism (Albright hereditary osteodystrophy): round face, short neck, and truncal obesity.

Other endocrine causes of obesity
- Primary hyperinsulinemia due to insulin receptor dysfunction. Tumor necrosis factor alpha is a potential mediator of insulin resistance.
- Leptin insensitivity with high leptin levels due to leptin receptor dysfunction.
- Leptin deficiency (rare); leptin is produced by adipocytes.
- Hypothalamic lesions (tumor, surgery, trauma); loss of satiety center leads to hyperphagic obesity.

BIBLIOGRAPHY

1. Arslanian SA: Nutritional disorders: Integration of energy metabolism and its disorders in childhood. In Sperling MA: Pediatric Endocrinology. Philadelphia, W.B Saunders, 1996, pp 523–547.
2. Braunstein,G. Gynecomastia. N Engl J Med 328:490–495, 1993.
3. Burch HB: Evaluation and management of the solid thyroid nodule. Endocrinol Metab Clin North Am 24:663–710, 1995
4. Donohoue PA, Parker KL, Migeon CJ: Congenital adrenal hyperplasia. In Scriver CR, Beaudet AL, Sly WS, Valle D (eds): The Metabolic and Molecular Bases of Inherited Disease, 7th ed. New York, McGraw-Hill, 1995, pp 2929–2966.
5. Foley TP Jr: Disorders of the thyroid in children. In Sperling MA: Pediatric Endocrinology. Philadelphia, W.B Saunders, 1996, pp 187–191.
6. Gartner, L, Poth M: Graves' disease in children and adolescents. Endocrinologist 5:422–430, 1995.
7. Gharib H: Current evaluation of thyroid nodules. Trends Endocrinol Metab 5:365–369, 1994.
8. Gorton C, Sadeghi-Nejad H, Senior B: Remission in children with hyperthyroidism treated with propylthiouracil: Long term results. Am J Dis Child 141:1084–1086, 1987.
9. Grumbach MM, Conte FA: Disorders of sex differentiation. In Wilson JD, Foster DW, Kronenberg HM, Larson PR (eds): Williams Textbook of Endocrinology, 9th ed. Philadelphia, W.B. Saunders, 1998, pp 1302–1425.

10. Harman CR, van Heerden JA, Farley DR, et al: Sporadic primary hyperparathyroidism in young patients: A separate disease entity? Arch Surg 134:651–656, 1999.
11. Lee P: Premature female sexual developmental disorders. In Lavin N (ed): Manual of Endocrinology and Metabolism. Boston, Little, Brown, 1994.
12. Low L, Wang C: Disorders of sexual development in the pediatric and adolescent Male. In Lavin, N. (ed): Manual of Endocrinology and Metabolism. Boston, Little, Brown, 1994.
13. Lteif AN, Schwenk WF: Hypoglycemia in infants and children. Endocrinol Metab Clin North Am 28:619–646, 1999
14. McClellan DR, et al: Thyroid cancer in children, pregnant women and patients with Graves' disease. Endocrinol Metab Clin North Am 25:27–46, 1996.
15. Milby J: Clinical review 1: Endocrine hypertension. Endocrine Rev 69:697–703, 1989.
16. Pollack MR, Chou Y-HW, Marx SJ, et al. Familial hypocalciuric hypocalcemia and neonatal severe hyperparathyroidism: Effects of mutant gene dosage on phenotype. J Clin Invest 93:1108–1112, 1994.
17. Rappaport R: Disorders of the gonads. In Behrman R, Kliegman RM, Jenson H (eds): Nelson Textbook of Pediatrics. Philadelphia, W.B. Saunders, 2000, pp 1752–1753.
18. Rosenfield R: The ovary and female sexual maturation. In Kaplan S (ed): Clinical Pediatric Endocrinology. Philadelphia, W.B. Saunders, 1990.
19. Rosenfield RL, Hochberg Z: Gynecomastia. In Hochberg Z (ed): Practical Algorithms in Pediatric Endocrinology. Basel, Karger, 1999.
20. Smith SR: The endocrinology of obesity. Endocrinol Metab Clin North Am 25:921–942, 1996.
21. Speiser PW, White PC: Congenital adrenal hyperplasia due to 21-hydroxylase deficiency. Clin Endocrinol 49:411, 1998.
22. Sperling MA, Finegold DN: Hypoglycemia in infants. In Sperling, MA: Pediatric Endocrinology. Philadelphia, W.B Saunders, 1996, pp 71–93.
23. Styne D: The testes: Disorders of sexual differentiation and puberty. In Kaplan S (ed): Clinical Pediatric Endocrinology. Philadelphia, W.B. Saunders, 1990.
24. White PC, Curnow KC, Pascoe L: Disorders of steroid 11 β-hydroxylase isoenzymes. Endocrine Rev 15:421–438, 1995.

78. PEDIATRIC ANESTHESIA

James M. T. Foster, MBBS, FRCPC, Doron Feldman, M.D., and Christopher Heard, M.B., Ch.B., FRCA

1. What is postoperative apnea?

Postoperative apnea is defined as a period of no ventilation during recovery after surgery and anesthesia. Brief apnea lasts from 6 to 15 seconds. Prolonged apnea lasts longer than 15 seconds or is associated with bradycardia. Apnea may be central, obstructive, or combined.

2. What are the risk factors for apnea in postoperative infants?

• Postconceptual age: The incidence is high in premature infants < 40 weeks and low after 50 weeks.
• Gestational age: The incidence is higher in infants born more prematurely for any given postconceptual age.
• Anemia: A hematocrit < 30 is associated with a higher risk.
• Surgical procedure: Minor procedures involve a lower risk.
• Anesthetic management: Apnea may occur after either general or regional anesthesia. The risk is less with regional anesthesia but increases if sedative agents are used.

3. What risks are associated with anesthesia in a child with an upper respiratory tract infection?

Potential problems secondary to either secretions or an irritable airway are laryngospasm, bronchospasm (with intubation), postextubation stridor, and hypoxemia.

4. Which patients are at risk of an allergic reaction to latex during anesthesia?

Children who have repeated exposure to latex-containing products are at risk, including those with spina bifida (15–65%), multiple surgical procedures, urogenital abnormalities, fruit allergy, and atopy or multiple allergies.

5. What are the presenting signs of an allergic reaction to latex?
- Hypotension
- Bronchospasm and wheezing
- Rash or urticaria
- Angioedema and stridor

6. How are allergic reactions to latex treated?
- Removal of antigen
- Epinephrine bolus (0.05 ml/kg of 1:10,000 epinephrine)
- Volume expansion (initially 20 ml/kg lactated Ringer's solution, repeated as necessary)
- Epinephrine infusion (if necessary)
- Bronchodilators (if required)
- Sample of clotted blood for diagnosis

7. Describe the management of postextubation stridor.

The child should be sitting up and comforted in an attempt to reduce anxiety. Humidified oxygen should be delivered by face mask or mist tent. If this strategy is insufficient, nebulized racemic epinephrine (0.5 ml of 2.25% solution in 3 ml normal saline) can be used. A response usually is seen within 20–30 minutes because of the vasoconstrictive effects on tracheal mucosa. The patient should be monitored for cardiac arrhythmias, which are rare. This treatment can be repeated several times. The patient should be observed for 4 hours after nebulizer use in case the edema recurs. Steroids are also useful; dexamethasone, 0.5 mg/kg (maximum of 10 mg), may be given every 6 hours for up to 24 hours. The use of a helium/oxygen mixture (30% oxygen) also improves the patient's symptoms because of decreased work of breathing from the less dense helium.

8. What is the appropriate management of a child undergoing emergency surgery for posttonsillectomy bleeding?
- Intravenous access
- Baseline hematocrit
- Fluid resuscitation
- Blood transfusion as necessary
- Supplemental oxygen
- Rapid-sequence induction with cricoid pressure to prevent aspiration of blood
- Empty stomach before extubation
- Fully awake patient before extubation

9. What are the premedication options for anxious children?
- Midazolam as an oral syrup or intranasal inhalation
- Fentanyl (may be given as a Elollipop)
- EMLA cream placed over potential intravenous sites
- Ketamine (useful intramuscularly for uncooperative patients)
- Rectal barbiturates (may be useful but are long-acting and unpredictable)

10. What are the anesthesia concerns for a child with Duchenne muscular dystrophy?
Respiratory concerns
- Muscle weakness and swallowing difficulties
- Recurrent pulmonary infections
- Restrictive lung disease due to scoliosis
- Postoperative respiratory insufficiency

Cardiovascular concerns
- Abnormal EKG at rest (90% of patients)
- Biventricular hypertrophy and sinus tachycardia at rest
- Heart block or arrhythmias (due to fibrosis of the conduction system)
- Heart failure in adolescents (may be asymptomatic because of limited exercise capacity)

Metabolic concern
- Risk of rhabdomyolysis with hyperkalemic arrest after the use of succinylcholine

Gastrointestinal concern
- Gastric hypomotility with increased risk for aspiration

11. What complications may be related to a mediastinal mass that occurs during anesthesia? How should such masses be managed?

Tracheobronchial compression may result in inability to ventilate, hypoxia, and cardiac arrest. The patient's position should be changed to lateral or semisupine. Resume spontaneous ventilation and attempt to pass a tracheal tube or rigid bronchoscope beyond the obstruction. Femoral-femoral cardiopulmonary bypass may be necessary.

Superior vena cava syndrome may lead to difficult intubation because of airway edema, difficult intravenous access, and increased bleeding in congested venous system. Elevate the head to reduce venous pressure.

Compression of the heart may impede venous return, causing hypotension and cardiovascular collapse. Pericardial effusion may lead to cardiac tamponade. A preoperative cardiac echocardiogram should be ordered to evaluate cardiac status. The patient should be positioned to minimize compression. Fluids, inotropes, and vasopressors may be used to treat cardiovascular collapse. Cardiopulmonary bypass may be needed; the groin should be prepared.

Cardiac arrest at induction may result from compression of the pulmonary artery due to changes in body position or critical reductions in preload.

A glandular tumor (pheochromocytoma, thyroid tumor) may secrete hormones. Do not forget about myasthenia gravis or myasthenic syndromes, because the patient may be highly sensitive to nondepolarizing muscle relaxants. If possible, a lymph node biopsy should be performed under local anesthesia to prevent these complications.

12. Name nine syndromes associated with difficult intubation.
- Pierre Robin sequence: mandibular hypoplasia, cleft palate
- Goldenhar syndrome: unilateral mandibular hypoplasia
- Hurler's disease: large tongue, obstructed nose, small jaw, atlantoaxial subluxation
- Down syndrome: large tongue, narrow nasopharynx, large tonsils/adenoids
- Still's disease: fused neck
- Treacher Collins syndrome: mandibular hypoplasia, cleft palate
- Kenny Caffey syndrome: mandibular hypoplasia, extreme dwarfism
- Tracheoesophageal fistula: tracheomalacia, difficulty in correct placement of the endotracheal tube (below the level of the fistula), gastric inflation
- Cleft palate: laryngoscope enters defect; airway obstruction after extubation

13. What methods can be used to prevent intraoperative hypothermia in infants?
- Increased room temperature (27–29°C)
- Warmer fluid for intravenous use or irrigation
- Circulating hot water blanket
- Overhead radiant warmer
- Forced hot air device (Bair Hugger)
- Wrap arms and legs in swaddling or cling film
- Knitted hat
- Warmed and humidified anesthesia gases

14. Why does the anesthesiologist keep the operating room so hot during surgery in neonates?

Full-term neonates start to become hypothermic at a room temperature of 23°C. Because anesthetized patients cannot increase activity to increase heat production and infants cannot shiver till at least 3 months, anesthetized infants are vulnerable to heat loss. The only mechanism to increase heat production is brown fat metabolism, which requires increased norepinephrine production. Brown fat metabolism has other effects, such as increased release of lipases, which leads to increased free fatty acids and glycerol, and increased cardiac output. The pulmonary vascular bed resistance increases, and skin perfusion decreases. These effects put the infant's transitional circulation at risk for shunting of blood across the foramen ovale and ductus arteriosus. It is better to avoid such problems by using all means at your disposal to prevent hypothermia.

15. What is the blood volume of a pediatric patient?

Premature infant	90–100 ml/kg
Newborn	80–90 ml/kg
3 months to 1 year	70–80 ml/kg
> 1 year	70 ml/kg

16. What are the guidelines for preoperative fasting?

The minimal fasting period before surgery is 2 hours for clear liquids, 4 hours for breast milk, 6 hours for infant formula, 6 hours for nonhuman milk, and 6 hours for a light meal. A light meal is a nonfatty meal such as toast and clear liquids. A fatty meal, such as fried meat, may require many more hours for gastric emptying. Clear liquids are those through which one can read newsprint when a clear glass is placed over a newspaper. Examples include carbonated beverages, pulp free juices, and jello.

17. What is cricoid pressure? What are the contraindications to its use?

Pressure is applied to the cricoid cartilage (some surgeons also place a hand behind the patient's neck) to occlude the esophagus and prevent passive regurgitation and possible pulmonary aspiration. Contraindications include active vomiting, unstable cervical spine, sharp foreign body in the esophagus or trachea at the level of the cricoid cartilage, Zenker's diverticulum, and fractured larynx.

18. What size endotracheal tube should be used? Should the tube have a cuff?

Adult males usually require a tube with an 8.0-mm internal diameter, whereas females require a 7.0-mm diameter. The appropriate size for a child is estimated by the formula, age + 16/4. These are guidelines, and tubes of various sizes must be readily available. There are no absolute rules for the use of cuffed tubes, but in all children over 8 years of age and in children requiring a 6.0-mm or larger tube a cuffed tube usually is used. High-volume, low-pressure cuffs should be used, but overfilling causes them to become high-volume, high-pressure cuffs and may impede the blood supply to the tracheal mucosa.

19. The child is wheezing in the preoperative assessment area. Why is a bronchodilator not used? Should the child be anesthetized as soon as the lungs are clear?

The issue of the wheezing child is an emotional one. Firstly, all that wheezes is not asthma. Other causes, such as aspirated foreign body, infection (pneumonia, bronchiolitis), or severe allergic reaction can present with wheezing. Less common causes, such as tracheal compression from tumors, vascular anomalies, and tracheal stenosis, also must be considered. Once nonasthmatic causes have been excluded by history and physical examination, a bronchodilator, such as albuterol, may be used. The next issue is whether the child requires emergency or elective surgery. The elective child can be rescheduled when the asthma therapy has been optimized, whereas the emergency patient needs maximal therapy for as long as possible with bronchodilators, steroids, and (potentially) antibiotics. Proceeding with an elective case in a poorly controlled asthmatic is potentially life-threatening. If it must be done, local and regional anesthetic techniques may avoid general anesthesia and the problems of exacerbating the airway irritability.

20. How should you manage endotracheal intubation in children with difficult airways?
The management of potentially difficult intubation at induction of anesthesia is controversial. There are several options: (1) awake intubation with a fiber optic bronchoscope; (2) general anesthesia with mask induction and spontaneous ventilation prior to laryngoscopy and intubation; and (3) local or regional anesthesia with avoidance of induction of general anesthesia. Paralyzing a patient after induction of anesthesia is potentially hazardous. Once paralyzed, some patients are impossible to intubate and ventilate, and they are at risk for severe hypoxia, cardiac arrest, and death. All of the available options include maintenance of spontaneous ventilation. If you cannot intubate a patient despite careful planning, call for help from colleagues and discuss rescheduling the case for another day or trying other options. Even in the setting of a full stomach or recently ingested meal, inhalational induction of anesthesia and intubation with direct laryngoscopy are an acceptable course.

21. Which children require a dextrose-containing intravenous fluid before coming to the operating room?
Neonates and preterm infants are at risk for hypoglycemia and may benefit from a 10% dextrose solution perioperatively because they have low glycogen stores and impaired gluconeogenesis. Critically ill children with burns and children on total parenteral nutrition also have increased caloric requirements.

22. What are the cardiac manifestations of Down syndrome in neonates?
• Complete atrioventricular canal
• Ventricular septal defect
• Patent ductus arteriosus
• Tetralogy of Fallot

23. What are the implications of these lesions for the conduct of general anesthesia?
These lesions may present with varying degrees of severity in the neonate with Down syndrome, but the conduct of anesthesia involves a number of issues. One hundred percent oxygen may exacerbate left-to-right shunting of blood, causing poor peripheral perfusion and acidosis. Hypoxia, hypercarbia, hypothermia, volume overload, and acidosis may cause right-to-left shunting. Air emboli, which may cause neurologic injury, must be avoided by de-airing the lines. Advice from a cardiologist about the nature of the lesion and the impact of altering systemic and pulmonary vascular resistances must be sought. These lesions are sometimes minor and require minimal interventions. Do not forget to give antibiotic prophylaxis. Affected children may not tolerate even low doses of volatile anesthetics, such as halothane, because of their myocardial depressant properties. Resuscitation drugs, such as epinephrine and phenylephrine, should be premixed and readily available.

BIBLIOGRAPHY

1. American Society of Anesthesiology Practice Guidelines: http://www.asahq.org/practice/npo/npoguide.html
2. Baum VC, O'Flaherty JE: Anesthesia for Genetic, Metabolic and Dysmorphic Syndromes in Childhood. Philadelphia, Lippincott Williams & Wilkins, 1999.
3. Berry FA, Steward DJ: Pediatrics for the Anesthesiologist. New York, Churchill Livingstone, 1993.
4. Cot CJ, Ryan JF, Todres ID, Goudsouzian NG: A Practice of Anesthesia for Infants and Children, 2nd ed. Philadelphia, W.B. Saunders, 1993.
5. Fletcher JE, Heard CMB: Management of the pediatric airway. Prog Anesthesiol 13, 1999.
6. Hall JK, Berman JM: Pediatric Trauma Anesthesia and Critical Care. New York, Futura, 1996.
7. Miller RD (ed): Anesthesia, 4th ed. New York, Churchill Livingstone.

79. MOLECULAR BIOLOGY FOR THE PEDIATRIC SURGEON

Scott C. Boulanger, M.D., Ph.D., Michael G. Caty, M.D., and Philip L. Glick, M.D.

1. Name the four bases that compose DNA and RNA.
DNA is composed of adenine (A), cytosine (C), guanine (G), and thymine (T). In RNA, thymine is replaced by uracil (U).

2. How do RNA and DNA differ chemically?
RNA contains a -OH group at the 2 position of the sugar moiety, whereas DNA has a -H (2-deoxy) at the same position.

3. How large is the human genome? How many genes are there?
The human genome contains approximately 6×10^9 base pairs. The genome is estimated to contain up to 100,000 genes.

4. What is a codon?
A codon is a three-nucleotide sequence (triplet) that codes for a specific amino acid during translation. Because there are only four nucleotide bases but 20 amino acids, at least three nucleotides are needed to code unambiguously for all amino acids. This hypothesis was proved in an elegant series of experiments (e.g., Nirenberg and Matthaei in 1961).

5. What is an intron?
An intron (intervening sequence) is a sequence of DNA that, although transcribed, is removed from mature RNA by splicing together of the flanking coding sequences (exons).

6. What modifications does an RNA molecule undergo to become a mature RNA?
Nascent RNA destined to become mature RNA (mRNA) undergo several posttranscriptional modifications. The 5' end of the mRNA is modified by creation of a methylated guanosine cap (7-methylguanosine). The 3' end is modified by addition of a polyadenylate tail (AAAA...). Introns also must be removed and exons joined by the process of RNA splicing. In addition, some RNAs undergo a process known as RNA editing. This process refers to the alteration of the RNA sequence at the RNA level. An example in humans is the apolipoprotein-B mRNA, in which a C is changed to a U in the RNA sequence, giving rise to a stop codon and, subsequently, a truncated protein.

7. Describe the structure of DNA.
DNA is a duplex of complementary chains that form a double helical structure. One DNA strand binds to a complementary strand by pairing between the nucleotide bases. This base-pairing follows strict rules. A pairs with T, and C pairs with G. The double-stranded molecule folds into a double helical structure. Watson and Crick made this observation in 1953 and in 1962 were awarded the Nobel prize in physiology for this observation.

8. What is PCR?
PCR stands for polymerase chain reaction. Developed by Mullis, this technique allows the amplification (copying) of a minute amount of a specific segment of DNA in vitro.

9. How is DNA replicated?
DNA is replicated in a semiconservative manner. The DNA helix unwinds, and each strand serves as a template for synthesis of a complementary strand. Each of the two newly created

double strands contains one strand from the original molecule and one newly synthesized strand; hence the term semiconservative.

10. Describe the steps in translation of RNA to protein.

The process of translation first involves transportation of the mRNA to the cytoplasm, where it binds with ribosomes. An aminoacyl-tRNA then binds the ribosome-mRNA complex at the A site. The growing peptide chain attached to the tRNA in the P site is then transferred to the A-site tRNA by peptidyl transferase. The ribosome shifts, placing the A-site tRNA into the P site and making room for the next aminoacyl-tRNA. This process continues in a 5' to 3' direction until termination.

11. How is DNA packed into a cell?

Double-stranded DNA is packed into nucleosomes by packaging with histone proteins. Nucleosomes are composed of a central core of proteins (called histones) about which a segment of DNA is wrapped. The nucleosomes are then arranged into the shape of a solenoid (coil of wire). Higher-order packaging allows the solenoids to condense into chromosomes.

12. Define promoter and enhancer.

A **promoter** is an element upstream of a gene that interacts with the RNA transcription machinery. It is, in part, responsible for transcription initiation, regulation, and tissue specificity. TATA boxes and CCAAT boxes are segments of DNA that are part of the promoter. They are involved in initiation and efficiency of transcription.

An **enhancer** is a DNA element that increases transcription of nearby genes. Enhancers can act over long distances and can be upstream, downstream, or even within a gene. Moreover, they can act even if inverted.

13. What is a restriction enzyme?

A restriction enzyme (endonuclease) is a bacterial protein that cuts double-stranded DNA at specific sequences. These enzymes leave either blunt-ended DNA strands or overlapping ends. Restriction enzymes are essential for gene mapping and cloning.

14. Can RNA be translated back into DNA?

Yes. A viral protein, reverse transcriptase, transcribes RNA back into DNA. This type of enzyme has been found in numerous organisms, including humans, in whom it plays a role in telomere formation. The Nobel prize for the discovery of reverse transcriptase was shared by Howard Temin and David Baltimore in 1975.

15. Are the genomes of all organisms based on DNA?

No. Certain viruses (i.e., retroviruses) are RNA-based organisms that rely on reverse transcriptase for their life cycle. Viroids are infectious agents that consist only of small circular RNAs. These elements cause disease in higher plants.

Scrapie is the agent responsible for causing Jakob-Creuzfeldt disease. Scrapie appears to consist only of a protein and is referred to as a prion. The prion protein, PrP, is encoded by a conserved mammalian gene expressed in normal brains.

16. What is a vector? Give examples.

A vector is an autonomously replicating segment of DNA. Vectors contain an antibiotic resistance gene that allows selection of the host cell containing the vector. Pieces of DNA can be cloned by insertion into vectors. The most common vectors are bacterial plasmids and phages. Retroviruses are important vectors for gene therapy.

17. Describe the Southern, Northern, Western, and Eastern blotting techniques.

First described by Edwin Southern, the Southern blot involves detection of specific DNA sequences after separation by gel electrophoresis. DNA is first digested by restriction enzymes and then separated by gel electrophoresis. The DNA is permanently transferred from the gel to a membrane. The membrane then is probed with a radioactive single-stranded segment of nucleic acid, which is specific for a DNA sequence. After washing away unbound probe, the membrane is exposed to x-ray film to obtain an autoradiograph.

Northern blots are similar to Southern blots except that RNA is separated by gel electrophoresis instead of DNA. Western blots, on the other hand, involve detection of protein. Protein samples, which have been separated by gel electrophoresis and transferred to membranes, are probed with antibodies to a protein of interest. The antibody–protein complex then is detected by a secondary antibody specific to part of the first antibody. The secondary antibody also carries a reporter enzyme capable of catalyzing a reaction that can be detected by photographic film.

Please note that Eastern blots do not exist.

18. What is a cDNA?

cDNAs are cloned segments of DNA originating from RNA transcripts. The RNA transcripts from genomic DNA are transcribed back into double-stranded DNA or complementary DNA (cDNA) and then inserted into vectors to create a library of DNA sequences (cDNA library).

19. What is cloning?

Cloning is a method of creating an unlimited amount of a particular segment of DNA. DNA is digested with a restriction enzyme and ligated into a vector, usually a bacterial plasmid containing an antibiotic resistance gene. The recombinant molecule is transformed back into bacteria. The bacteria containing the recombinant are selected for by growth on antibiotic plates that allow amplification of the plasmid.

20. Compare and contrast cloning with PCR.

PCR is an alternative to cloning that allows production of a nearly unlimited amount of a specific DNA sequence. PCR, however, is a completely in vitro method. It also requires some knowledge of the sequences flanking the region of interest; cloning does not.

21. How is DNA sequenced?

DNA usually is sequenced by the method of Sanger. DNA polymerase is used to create a sequence ladder of a particular segment of DNA. The ladder then is separated by high-resolution gel electrophoresis. In response to the needs of the Human Genome Project, rapid advances in automated sequencing have been made. Current devices allow the rapid handling of multiple samples simultaneously.

22. What is positional cloning? How is it done?

Positional gene cloning is a method of mapping genes when no biochemical information is available. The first step is to identify families carrying a specific trait and map the gene by linkage analysis using restriction length polymorphism. Candidate genes then are identified by sequence analysis of the region of the polymorphism (a task greatly simplified by the sequence data available from the Human Genome Project). A candidate gene is confirmed if it is found to be mutated in affected family members and normal in unaffected members.

23. Name three diseases that have been mapped to a specific gene by positional cloning.

Although there are numerous examples, three of the best known are Duchenne's muscular dystrophy (the first gene to be cloned), cystic fibrosis, and Huntington's disease. Duchenne's muscular dystrophy is an X-linked disease; mapping studies show that the gene resides at band p21. Many of the naturally occurring mutations are translocations or deletions. Huntington's disease was the first disease to be localized using restriction fragment length polymorphism. The gene resides on chromosome 4; mutation of the gene results from expansion of CAG triplet repeats. The cystic fibrosis gene is located on chromosome 7 and encodes a chloride channel. The most common mutation is a deletion of codon 508, which codes for a phenylalanine (ΔF508).

24. What is gene therapy?

Gene therapy is the treatment of human genetic disorders by introduction of recombinant DNA into the genome.

25. What is the difference between germline gene therapy and somatic gene therapy?

Somatic gene therapy involves introduction of DNA into somatic cells as opposed to germline cells in the ovaries or testes. Therefore, the effect of this DNA is not transmitted to offspring. Germline therapy does introduce DNA into germline cells, which can be passed to offspring.

26. Name three types of vectors used to introduce DNA into somatic cells.

The most common vectors for introduction of DNA in host cells are retroviruses, adenovirus and/or adeno-associated virus, and liposomes.

27. Which disease was studied in the first gene therapy trial?

The first disease to be studied was adenosine deaminase (ADA) deficiency, which results in severe combined immunodeficiency (SCIDS). The attractiveness of this disorder for gene therapy is based on its dismal prognosis, the fact that ADA deficiency can be cured by appropriately selected bone marrow transplantation, and the fact that replacement in the bone marrow compartment, even with low levels of expression, is sufficient for cure.

28. What two general strategies are used to introduce vectors into host cells?

In vivo therapy involves introducing the DNA directly into the patient. **Ex vivo therapy** requires removal of the target cells from the patient, introduction of the DNA into the cells, and replacement of the cells back into the patient.

29. Which disease was the first to be treated with in vivo gene therapy?

Cystic fibrosis. Several gene therapy trials for cystic fibrosis are under way. The studies use in vivo gene therapy, most commonly with engineered adenoviral vectors. The problems encountered in these studies were (1) transient expression of the cystic fibrosis gene and (2) inflammatory reaction to the virus.

30. Define oncogene and proto-oncogene.

An oncogene is an altered version of a gene whose products have the ability to transform eukaryotic cells into tumor cells. A proto-oncogene is the unaltered version of the oncogene.

31. Describe the difference between an oncogene and a tumor suppressor gene.

The fundamental difference between oncogenes and tumor suppressor genes is that oncogenes act in a dominant fashion. Tumor suppressor genes act in a recessive manner; in other words, both copies of the gene must be lost, or mutated, for transformation to occur.

32. Give two examples of tumor suppressor genes.

The best known tumor suppressor genes are *p53* and *RB*. Additional examples include *WT1*, which is responsible for Wilms' tumor, and *APC* which is responsible for familial adenomatous polyposis. The *p53* gene is implicated in numerous types of syndromes, including Li-Fraumeni syndrome. *RB* mutations result in retinoblastoma.

33. The oncogene *BCL* is involved in which cellular process?

BCL is involved in apoptosis (programmed cell death).

34. *ErbB* encodes which protein?

ErbB encodes EGF receptor kinase. This is an example of an oncogene involved in the signal transduction pathway, in this case a cell receptor. The viral homolog is found in the avian erythroblastosis virus.

35. *Ras* encodes which type of protein?

Ras encodes a glutamyl transpeptide-binding protein. In this case the oncogene encodes a different protein in the signal transduction pathway, a g-protein. G-proteins transduce the signal from cell surface receptors by activating an intracellular protein. Mutations in the *ras* gene constitutively activate it.

36. The *REL* gene encodes which type of protein?

REL encodes a transcription factor of the NF-kB family. This is an example in which an altered transcription factor induces tumorigenesis. The NF-kB transcription factor activates multiple genes.

37. Which gene is associated with improved prognosis in neuroblastoma? Worse prognosis?

High levels of expression of the gene *Trk* are associated with an improved prognosis, whereas *N-myc* is associated with a poor outcome.

38. The Wilms' tumor gene encodes which class of protein?

WT1 encodes a DNA-binding protein involved in transcriptional regulation. *WT1* is a tumor suppressor gene.

39. Multiple endocrine neoplasia type II and medullary thyroid carcinoma are caused by mutations in which oncogene?

The *RET* gene is responsible for multiple endocrine neoplasia (MEN) type II and medullary thyroid carcinoma. *RET* is a tyrosine kinase growth factor receptor.

40. Familial adenomatous polyposis is the result of mutation in which gene?

Mutations in the adenomatous polyposis coli (*APC*) gene result in familial adenomatous polyposis. This tumor suppressor gene appears to encode a protein that interacts with cell adhesion molecules. Mutations in *APC* are believed to occur early in the transformation to colon cancer.

41. Mutations in which gene have been linked to Hirschsprung's disease?

Mutations in the *RET* oncogene result in Hirschsprung's disease. Of interest, this gene is responsible for MEN type 2. Mutations that cause Hirschsprung's disease involve loss of function of the *RET* protein. Mutations that constitutively activate RET cause MEN type 2.

BIBLIOGRAPHY

1. Blaese RM: Development of gene therapy for immunodeficiency: Adenosine deaminase deficiency. Pediatr Res 33:49, 1993.
2. Blaese RM, et al: T-lymphocyte directed gene therapy for ADA-SCID: Initial trial results after 4 years. Science 270:475–480, 1995.
3. Boulanger SC, Caty MG, Glick PL: Molecular biology for the pediatric surgeon: A review. J Pediatr Surg [in press].
4. Gelehrter TD, Collins FS, Ginsburg D: Principles of Medical Genetics, 2nd ed. Baltimore, Williams & Wilkins, 1998.
5. Lewin B: Genes IV. New York, Oxford University Press, 1997.
6. Nakagawara A, et al: Association between high levels of expression of the trk gene and favorable outcome in human neuroblastoma. N Engl J Med 328:847, 1993.
7. Nirenberg MW, Matthei JH: The dependence of cell-free protein synthesis in *E. coli* upon naturally occurring or synthetic polynucleotides. Proc Natl Acad Sci USA 47:1588, 1961.
8. Rowe MI, O'Neill JA, Grosfeld JL, et al (eds): Pediatric Surgery. St. Louis, Mosby, 1998.
9. Sanger R, Nicklen S, Coulson AR: DNA sequencing with chain-terminating inhibitors. Proc Natl Acad Sci USA 74:5463, 1977.
10. Seeger RC, et al: Association of multiple copies of the N-*myc* oncogene with rapid tumor progression in neuroblastoma. N Engl J Med 313:1111, 1985.
11. Southern EM: Detection of specific sequences among DNA fragments separated by gel electrophoresis. J Mol Biol 98:503, 1975.
12. Tagge EP, et al: Molecular biology and the pediatric surgeon: Definitions and basic methodology. Semin Pediatr Surg 5:139, 1996.
13. Thomas PS: Hybridization of denatured RNA and small DNA fragments transferred to nitrocellulose. Proc Natl Acad Sci USA 77:5201, 1980.

14. Watson JD, Crick FHC: A structure for deoxyribose nucleic acid. Nature 171:737, 1953.
15. White TJ, Arnheim N, Ehrlich HA: The polymerase chain reaction. Trends Genet 5:185, 1989.

80. SPECIAL PROCEDURES

R. *Thomas Ross*, M.D., *and Mark C. Stovroff*, M.d.

VASCULAR ACCESS

1. What is a peripheral venous cutdown? When is it used?

Surgical venous cutdown is an alternate method of peripheral venous access. It involves an incision over a vessel (usually the saphenous vein) with isolation of the vein and subsequent venotomy. A cannula is inserted into the vessel, advanced, and secured in place. The technique has fallen out of favor because of its technical difficulties; however, venous cutdown remains useful in the emergency setting when attempts at percutaneous access have failed

2. What is an intraosseous catheter?

A needle is placed percutaneously into bone and advanced to the marrow space. Fluids then may be given into this space in lieu of direct venous access.

3. What is the preferred site for placement?

In infants and small children, the proximal tibia is considered optimal. The needle is inserted through the skin 1–3 cm below and just medial to the tibial tuberosity.

4. What is the anatomic course of intraosseous fluids?

The intraosseous route for vascular access is based on the presence of noncollapsible veins that drain the medullary sinuses in the bone marrow. This vascular network empties into the central venous circulation via nutrient and emissary veins.

5. What are the contraindications for intraosseous infusion?

Local infection, osteogenesis imperfecta, and osteoporosis.

6. What complications may occur?

Local cellulitis and/or osteomyelitis (less than 1% of cases).

7. What is a PIC line?

Peripheral intravenous central (PIC) catheters share attributes of central and peripheral venous access. A PIC catheter is a thin tube of biocompatible material that can be inserted percutaneously into a peripheral vein and advanced into the central circulation.

8. When should a PIC line be used?

PIC lines are suitable for intermediate vascular access for the infusion of hyperosmolar solutions (i.e., hyperalimentation fluids) or antibiotics. They are a mainstay of vascular access in the nursery, where access is difficult to obtain and maintain in preterm neonates. In older pediatric patients, they are commonly used for prolonged therapy (nutritional or antibiotic) in the hospital or home.

9. In the absence of peripheral vein access, how should vascular access be obtained?

Central venous catheters are a reliable means to administer large volumes of potentially irritating solutions. In addition, they can be used to collect blood samples and monitor hemodynamic variables.

Polyethylene catheters may be inserted into the subclavian, internal jugular, or femoral veins using the Seldinger technique. These catheters can be inserted electively or in emergent situations, usually without general anesthesia. Compared with other catheters, polyethylene catheters have a relatively high rate of infection and thrombotic occlusion. As a result, they should not be used for permanent access.

10. What is the Seldinger technique?
The Seldinger technique allows bedside access to the central circulation. After positioning, antisepsis, and local anesthesia, a needle attached to a syringe is guided subcutaneously toward the vessel while constant negative pressure is maintained on the syringe. Advancement of the needle is stopped as soon as venous blood is returned. Upon aspiration of venous blood, the syringe is removed and a guidewire is passed into the vessel. The needle is removed, and the catheter is threaded over the wire and into the vessel, thus avoiding losing the wire in the vessel. Once in place, all lumens are aspirated and flushed with heparinized saline, and the catheter is secured to the skin.

11. What maneuvers maximize successful percutaneous cannulation of the internal jugular and subclavian veins?
Trendelenburg positioning of the the bed and a Valsalva maneuver or holding the ventilator at end expiration for the ventilated patient.

12. For long-term access, what catheter should be chosen?
In children receiving chemotherapy or long-term parenteral nutrition, silastic catheters are preferred for long-term vascular access. Silastic catheters are constructed with relatively inert materials and offer increased pliability. They are associated with lower rates of infection and thrombus formation. Placed in a central vein and tunneled a distance from the access site to an exit wound, such catheters commonly are called Broviac or Hickman catheters.

13. What are the drawbacks of silastic catheters?
Infection, restriction of daily activities, frequent dressing changes, and altered body image.

14. Is there another alternative?
Implantable venous access devices or ports, which have a single-lumen or double-lumen injection port and a silastic rubber catheter. The entire device is placed surgically in the subcutaneous tissue at a site that is not apparent externally (commonly in the anterior chest wall). As with external silastic catheters, a port catheter is tunneled a short distance to a site adjacent to the central vein, where it is inserted via the Seldinger technique or direct cutdown. Because of its subcutaneous location, the port requires no local care and infrequent flushes; it does not restrict the activity of the child. Body image is preserved, and the infection rate is significantly lower.

15. Can umbilical vessels be used in the newborn?
In neonates the umbilical vessels may be accessed directly in the first few days of life. After several days, surgical cutdown may be necessary. An umbilical artery line may be used for blood pressure monitoring, blood sampling, and fluid or drug infusion. Umbilical vein lines may be used for central venous pressure monitoring, blood sampling, and fluid or drug infusion.

16. What are the major disadvantages of umbilical vein catheterization?
Catheter sepsis, catheter migration or misplacement, hepatic abscess, portal vein thrombosis, and perforation into the peritoneal cavity.

17. What complications are associated with central venous catheterization?
Acute complications
  Pneumothorax
  Vessel perforation with hemorrhage

Cardiac perforation with tamponade
Air embolism
Aberrant catheter localization
Long-term complications
Infection
Thrombotic occlusion of catheter or vessel
Pulmonary embolism
Catheter migration with extravasation of fluids
Superior vena cava syndrome

18. How is a pneumothorax treated?

Minor pneumothoraces do not require immediate evacuation as long as they are not associated with compromised ventilation or mediastinal shift. If they are of a significant nature, persist over time, or cause respiratory or hemodynamic compromise, a tube thoracostomy is necessary to evacuate the air.

19. What is the most common long-term complication of central intravenous catheters?

Infection. Although the rate and definition of catheter-related infection vary, an overall rate of 1.7 per 1000 days is generally accepted.

20. How can catheter infections be treated?

If applicable, immediate removal is the first choice. However, children with a catheter infection confined to the exit site or with bacteremia may be treated with local wound care and instillation of antibiotics through the infected line. This method can salvage the catheter with a good success rate. Clearly the best treatment for catheter-infected relation is prevention. Meticulous aseptic technique is required during insertion, catheter use, and site care.

21. What leads to catheter occlusion?

Thrombosis in or adjacent to the distal tip, precipitation of total parenteral nutrition constituents, chemotherapeutic agents, and inadequately placed catheters.

22. How can occlusion be treated?

Significant thrombosis requires removal of the catheter with systemic heparinization for 7–10 days. When catheter patency is reduced by partial thrombosis, immediate infusion of a volume of urokinase (50000 U) equal to catheter volume can improve potency in more than 80% of cases. Additional instillation of 0.1 n hydrochloric acid may restore patency in lines not successfully salvaged by urokinase.

23. What sites are used for arterial access?

Radial, axillary, femoral, posterior tibial, and dorsalis pedis arteries. The radial artery is used most commonly.

24. What is the Allen test?

The Allen test determines the adequacy of collateral flow to the hand before radial artery cannulation. Collateral flow is assessed by squeezing the wrist to occlude both the radial and ulnar arteries, resulting in blanching of the hand. Compression of the ulnar artery then is released. If the blanched hand flushes, adequate circulation to the hand via the ulnar artery is established.

INTESTINAL TUBES

25. What is a gastrostomy?

A gastrocutaneous fistula that is created surgically or percutaneously to allow feeding or decompression.

26. What are the indications for use of gastrostomy?

A gastrostomy is indicated for patients with a functional gastrointestinal tract who are unwilling or unable to consume sufficient nutrition for growth and development. Examples include children with alimentary anomalies, chronic diseases, central nervous system disorders, or developmental delays. It may be helpful as a route for string-assisted dilatation of esophageal strictures.

27. Why is gastrostomy tube feeding preferred over jejunal feeding?

Gastric feeding has a greater physiologic resemblance to oral feeding. It accommodates larger volumes and higher osmotic loads and avoids dumping syndrome.

28. In evaluating an infant for tube gastrostomy, why is it important to evaluate concomitant gastroesophageal reflux?

Because the placement of a tube gastrostomy frequently exacerbates preexisting reflux by downward displacement of the stomach and alteration of the angle of His.

29. How are gastrostomy tubes created?

A gastrostomy tube may be created by surgical, endoscopic, or radiologic (percutaneous) approaches. The two most common types are the surgically created Stamm gastrostomy and the percutaneous endoscopic gastrostomy (PEG).

30. How is the Stamm gastrostomy created?

The abdomen is opened through a midline or left paramedian incision. Double pursestring sutures are placed around a tube, producing a serosa-lined tract. The stomach then is attached to the anterior abdominal wall, creating a permanent connection.

31. What complications can occur?

Infection, perforation, formation of significant granulation tissue, and pyloric obstruction secondary to tube migration.

32. What is the PEG technique?

The PEG technique is a sutureless technique in which no operative incision is made to place the tube. Rather, the stomach is insufflated with air and transilluminated with an endoscope localized to a site within the stomach. A needle is placed percutaneously into the stomach. A guidewire is placed through the needle and endoscopically grasped and brought out through the mouth. A gastrostomy tube with bolster is tied to the guidewire and brought retrograde through the stomach and abdominal wall. Once visualized endoscopically, the tube is stabilized externally.

33. What are the complications of the PEG technique?

Intraperitoneal leakage, tissue necrosis, and gastrocolic fistula.

34. What precludes an attempt at PEG placement?

Aberrant anatomy, gastroesophageal reflux, or previous abdominal surgery.

35. When can gastrostomy tubes be changed safely to a new or skin-level gastrostomy device?

In the surgically created gastrostomy, this change can be done after 3 weeks. The PEG tube is best removed 12 weeks postoperatively to allow maturation of the tract.

36. When is a transpyloric feeding tube or feeding jejunostomy more advantageous than a gastrostomy tube?

In children with severe neurologic impairment (coma) or high risk of aspiration (gastroparesis or reflux).

37. What is the optimal position for the tip of a transpyloric feeding tube?
Just distal to the ligament of Treitz.

38. After what length of time should a temporary orogastric or transpyloric tube be converted to a formal surgical tube?
After 8 weeks.

39. How can a formal jejunostomy tube be created?
Via a needle jejunostomy, Witzel tube, or side-to-side jejunojostomy. The most important point in their construction is location at least 15 cm distal to the ligament of Treitz.

BIBLIOGRAPHY

1. Brokowski S: Pediatric stomas, tubes, and appliances. Pediatr Clin North Am 45:1419–1437, 1998.
2. Stovroff MC, Teague WG: Intravenous access in infants and children. Pediatr Clin North Am 45:1373–1395, 1998.

81. PRENATAL DIAGNOSIS AND FETAL THERAPY

Amanda J. McCabe, FRCS, and Philip L. Glick, M.D.

1. What tests are currently available for prenatal diagnosis?
Ultrasound examination: noninvasive direct imaging of normal and abnormal anatomy. The real-time image yields specific information about fetal movements and vital functions, such as heart rate variability and breathing movements, that reflect fetal well-being.

Amniocentesis: the gold standard with which all other invasive diagnostic tests are compared (chromosome and enzyme analysis of the amniotic fluid).

Chorionic villus sampling: a first-trimester test that biopsies the chorionic villi (mainly trophoblast) and is used to detect chromosomal abnormalities, inborn errors of metabolism, and X-linked disorders.

Maternal serum alpha fetoprotein (MSAFP): abnormal (increased or decreased) levels are a reliable indicator of fetal abnormality.

Fetoscopy: direct view of the developing fetus. In select cases it can be used to obtain fetal tissue samples such as skin and muscle.

Percutaneous umbilical cord blood sampling (PUBS): performed under ultrasound guidance. PUBS allows the diagnosis of rare congenital disorders (e.g., hemophilia, hemoglobinopathies), diagnosis of acquired fetal pathology (e.g., infections and immunologic disorders), and the study of biologic parameters and fetal physiology during pregnancy.

Ultrafast fetal magnetic resonance imaging: enhances the accuracy of prenatal evaluation.

Note: If MSAFP, ultrasound, and amniocentesis are performed, over 90% of all life-threatening birth defects will be detected prenatally.

2. What types of ultrasound examinations are described by the American College of Obstetricians and Gynecologists?
Basic: a brief survey of maternal pelvic organs and fetal anatomy. Major anatomic abnormalities may be identified. If the scan is suspicious or the pregnancy is at risk, a more detailed examination may be required. Basic ultrasound should document fetal number, presentation, cardiac activity, placental location, amniotic fluid volume, and gestational age, as well as survey for

gross fetal malformations or maternal pelvic masses. It should be performed or reviewed by an appropriately trained examiner.

Limited: used when the clinician needs specific information or when the ultrasound is performed during an urgent clinical situation. For example, limited ultrasound can be used to confirm fetal life or death; to assess amniotic fluid volume, fetal biophysical profile, amniocentesis, and localization of the placenta in antepartum bleeding; or to establish fetal presentation.

Comprehensive: used when an abnormality is suspected. This targeted ultrasound should be performed by an examiner with experience and expertise, and is usually performed in a center specializing in prenatal diagnosis of fetal abnormalities. In addition to the basic scan, it specifically looks for fetal abnormalities.

3. What are the common indications for amniocentesis?
- Advanced maternal age (35 years)
- Previous birth of a trisomic child
- Chromosome abnormality in either parent
- Women who are carriers of any X-linked recessive disorder (e.g., hemophilia)
- Family history of neural tube defects
- Carriers of inborn errors of metabolism

4. Does advanced paternal age pose any risk to the fetus?
Yes. Fetuses are predisposed to autosomal dominant diseases such as neurofibromatosis, achondroplasia, Apert's syndrome, and Marfan's syndrome. The risk rises exponentially with increasing paternal age, but evidence to provide a definite cutoff age for assessment is insufficient. Increasing paternal age also may be associated with spontaneous germline mutations in X-linked genes that are transmitted through carrier daughters to affected grandsons. The so-called "grandfather effect" includes disorders such as hemophilia A and Duchenne muscular dystrophy.

5. What risks are associated with amniocentesis?
- Spontaneous abortion occurs in up to 1% of cases.
- Fetomaternal transfusion causing later sensitization to Rh and other antigens.
- A small incidence of direct fetal trauma.
- Increased rates of respiratory distress syndrome (1.1 vs. 0.5%) and infant pneumonia (0.7 vs. 0.3%). The proposed mechanism is sudden subjection of fetal lung to a decrease in amniotic fluid volume.
- Some studies have reported a higher rate of hip dislocation (0.38 vs. 0.08%) and talipes equinovarus (0.46 vs. 0%).

6. What are the advantages of chorionic villus sampling over amniocentesis?
It is a *first*-trimester fetal cell sampling procedure (as opposed to a second- or third-trimester procedure) with a short culture time (24–48 hours) for cytogenetic studies. Final results can be obtained within 5–7 days. A rapid first-trimester diagnosis gives parents accurate information on which to base further decisions about pregnancy and possible termination. A diagnosis made before 12 weeks should reduce the emotional stress associated with waiting until later in the second trimester for results. The technique also can be useful after the first trimester in cases of oligohydramnios, when it may not be safe to perform amniocentesis.

7. What is the FISH test?
FISH stands for fluorescence in situ hybridization. Chromosome-specific DNA probes are available to detect the five most commonly seen chromosome aneuploidies: 13, 18, 21, X, and Y. The microdeletion syndromes presently available for analysis include cri-du-chat (5p), DiGeorge syndrome (22q), Kallmann syndrome (Xp), Miller-Dieker syndrome (17p), and Wolf-Hirschhorn syndrome (4p).

8. What is AFP?

AFP is a glycoprotein (similar to albumin) synthesized in the fetal liver, yolk sac, and gut. In the second trimester, when prenatal testing usually is done, amniotic fluid consists mainly of fetal urine that has been filtered by the fetal kidney. Fetal swallowing removes some of the amniotic fluid AFP, but a portion reaches the maternal serum transplacentally and transamniotically. AFP in fetal serum peaks (3 mg/ml) at around 13–15 weeks gestation, after which it declines. This decline is due to the expanding fetal circulatory volume rather than to decreased production. Fetal liver production of AFP reaches a peak at 22 weeks and maintains a steady output until 30 weeks, after which it also declines. The amniotic fluid AFP concentration, therefore, is relatively high early in the second trimester and thereafter declines steadily—a pattern that requires careful attention in defining the normal range of AFP values for each gestational week.

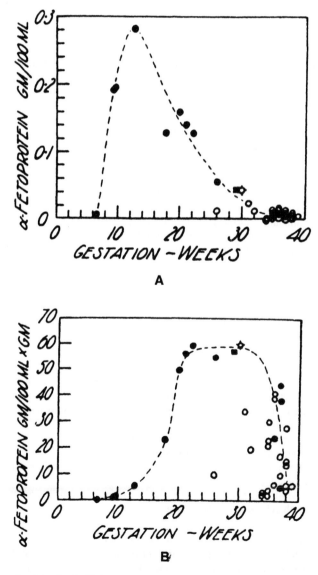

A, Gestational levels of AFP in fetal serum. *B*, Gestational fetal liver production of AFP.

9. What causes an abnormal MSAFP?

MSAFP varies with gestational age; therefore, an inaccurate gestational age can give falsely elevated or decreased levels.

Elevated levels: open neural tube defects, open ventral wall defects (gastroschisis and omphalocele), congenital nephrosis, cystic hygromas, gastrointestinal atresias, twin gestation (normal amniotic fluid AFP), sacrococcygeal teratoma, and some low-birth-weight infants (normal amniotic fluid AFP). The most frequent source of a falsely elevated amniotic fluid AFP is the presence of fetal blood cells in the amniocentesis sample.

Decreased levels: misdated pregnancy, molar pregnancy, fetal death, and some chromosomal abnormalities such as Down's syndrome and trisomy 18; also associated with congenital diaphragmatic hernia in some cases.

The AFP level is not diagnostic and must be viewed and weighted with other available information.

10. What are the basic aims of genetic counseling?

Medical facts: requires accurate information starting with the diagnosis of the affected family member and estimating the risk of occurrence or recurrence in future pregnancies.

Consideration of the information: aiding the counselees to rationalize the given facts into their own individual circumstances so that they can then choose an appropriate course of action.

Assessment of the family's emotional state: anxiety, hostility, guilt, depression, grief, and mourning may feature in the counseling forum. Recognition of these emotions helps communication between counselor and counselee.

11. Which fetal conditions may respond to prenatal medical treatment?
- Erythroblastosis fetalis: erythrocyte deficiency (intravenous transfusion)
- Pulmonary immaturity: surfactant deficiency (maternal glucocorticoids)
- Cardiac arrhythmias: supraventricular tachycardia (maternal digitalis/propranolol)
- Endocrine deficiency: thyroxine (transamniotic)

12. Which birth defects are currently considered for fetal surgery?

A number of life-threatening birth defects are candidates for fetal surgery, including congenital diaphragmatic hernia, congenital cystic adenomatous malformation of the lung, sacrococcygeal teratoma, and obstructive uropathy. Spina bifida, a non–life-threatening condition, is now considered for fetal intervention at some centers.

13. What are the selection criteria for candidates for fetal surgery?
- Singleton fetus (except congenital hydronephrosis, twin-twin transfusion syndrome, or fetus reduction procedures after in vitro fertilization)
- No concomitant anomalies using level II sonography and amniocentesis for karyotype, AFP levels, and viral cultures
- Family fully counseled about benefits and risks to mother and fetus
- Consent to treatment and long-term follow-up
- Plan for treatment by a multidisciplinary team and approval of a duly constituted institutional review board
- Access to a level-III high-risk obstetrical unit and neonatal intensive care unit
- Access to bioethical and psychosocial consultation

14. When was the first open human fetal surgery performed?

In 1981 the Fetal Treatment Program at the University of California, San Francisco, under the leadership of Dr. Michael Harrison, performed bilateral ureterostomies for bladder obstruction in a 22-week-old fetus without complication.

15. What is the most common cause of an abnormal mass in a neonate? What are the other possible causes?

Hydronephrosis is the most common cause and is readily detectable by antenatal ultrasonography. Other causes include ureteropelvic junction obstruction, ectopic ureterocele, and posterior urethral valves. Diagnostic care is mandatory, because small-to-moderate urine accumulations are commonly seen in the pelvis or infundibulum of normal fetal collecting systems.

16. Which fetuses with urinary tract obstruction are candidates for in utero intervention?

Fetuses with bilateral hydronephrosis that develop oligohydramnios during the last half of gestation predictably have renal damage and pulmonary hypoplasia and may benefit from early decompression. When the decompression is needed for a short period, a catheter shunt can be placed percutaneously; other cases, which present earlier, may require an open surgical cutaneous vesicostomy. Unilateral or mild bilateral hydronephrosis with evidence of good renal function does not require in utero intervention. Fetuses older than 32 weeks with bilateral hydronephrosis and oligohydramnios can be induced prematurely and delivered with a view to postnatal decompression.

17. What is the rationale for in utero intervention in a case of congenital diaphragmatic hernia?

The mortality rate of infants with congenital diaphragmatic hernia (CDH) has remained around 20–50% despite improvements in perinatal management and postnatal care. Death most often is attributed to the hypoplastic lungs. In infants that survive, pulmonary development is sufficient for postnatal survival, but a protracted course of ventilatory support may be required. Approximately 8% of fetuses die in utero or are stillborn. The real challenge is to identify this 8% and the 20–50% who will die despite optimal therapy. In such cases, fetal surgery should be seriously considered. Animal experiments have shown that the pulmonary hypoplasia associated with diaphragmatic hernia is partially reversible with in utero diaphragmatic repair or tracheal ligation. It is now possible to identify a poor prognostic group of fetuses with CDH that have liver herniation and a low lung-to-head ratio. A small number of such fetuses appear to benefit from temporary tracheal occlusion. However, further randomized clinical trials are needed to establish the efficacy of this treatment.

18. What in utero interventions have been tried in cases of CDH?

- Open fetal diaphragmatic repair: in a series of 14 repairs, 5 fetuses died intraoperatively from complications related to the reduction of the herniated liver or uterine contractions. In 9 patients repair was successful: 4 infants survived, 2 were born prematurely and died, and 3 died in utero within 48 hours of repair due to impaired umbilical blood flow.
- PLUG (plug the lung until it grows): tracheal ligation prevents the normal efflux of fluid out of the lungs. In experimental animal models this maneuver substantially enlarged the hypoplastic lungs associated with CDH and pushed the abdominal viscera back into the abdominal cavity. Videoendoscopic techniques have now enabled a FETENDO-clip to be successfully applied to the fetal trachea in utero. During caesarean delivery the infant is maintained on placental circulation until the airway is secured. Although animal studies document that tracheal ligation augments lung growth, lung maturation (i.e., surfactant production and antioxidant enzyme systems) is not similarly enhanced.

19. Does steroid therapy help the fetus with CDH?

Steroids can enhance endogenous surfactant production before term. In the nitrofen rat model of CDH, in which phosphatidylcholine is reduced, dexamethasone therapy increased the levels of this important surfactant lipid. The effect was enhanced when dexamethasone was given in combination with thyrotropin-releasing hormone. Intrauterine therapy with dexamethasone also has been shown to increase the compliance of CDH lungs. No human data yet support these animal studies.

20. Why do cystic adenomatoid malformations sometimes disappear?

The exact mechanism is not clear. Malformations may shrink as a result of decompression of fetal lung fluid through abnormal channels to the airway or gastrointestinal tract. It also is possible that they outgrow their blood supply and involute. Finally, it may be only an apparent shrinkage relative to the growing fetus.

21. How should the fetus with a cystic adenomatoid malformation be managed?

Counseling. The parents first should be counseled about medical facts. The natural history of prenatally diagnosed lesions is highly variable. Some large lesions disappear before birth.

Isolated cases with no hydrops. No antenatal intervention is deemed necessary; ultrasonic follow-up to term is performed. The delivery must be done in a facility with a level-III intensive care nursery and an operating room with extracorporeal membrane oxygenation capability.

Isolated cases with hydrops. The gestational age of the pregnancy as well as the mother's condition is considered. For fetuses older than 32 weeks, early delivery should be considered so that the lesion can be resected ex utero. Fetuses younger than 32 weeks with hydrops, benefit from placement of a double-pigtailed catheter shunt between the large lung cyst cavity and amniotic space. The shunt relieves compression around the fetal heart, great vessels, and normal lung tissue and reverses the hydropic state. This approach, however, is not suitable for microcystic lesions; one must make the difficult choice among no intervention, fetal surgery, or termination.

22. Define hydrops fetalis.

Hydrops fetalis is defined as a pathologic increase of fluid accumulation in serous cavities or generalized edema of soft tissue in a fetus. It may be recognized prenatally as scalp or placental thickening and pleural or pericardial effusion. It is characterized as immune-related (fetomaternal blood group incompatibility), or non–immune-related. The term *idiopathic* is used when no cause is identified.

23. What fetal conditions are associated with non–immune-related hydrops fetalis?

The causes are diverse. Up to 60% of cases remain idiopathic. Known causes include cardiovascular disorders (23%; anatomic defects and arrhythmias), chromosomal abnormalities (15%; Down's syndrome), recognizable syndromes (10%; osteogenesis imperfecta and achondrogenesis), and twin-twin transfusion (9%). Other broad categories include thoracic lesions, infections (cytomegalovirus, rubella), metabolic disorders (cystic fibrosis, Tay-Sachs disease), fetal anemia, and gastrointestinal disorders (meconium peritonitis, atresias and malrotation). Overall prognosis is poor, with a mortality rate between 50% and 98%.

24. What is the mirror syndrome?

The mirror syndrome is a maternal hyperdynamic preeclamptic state associated with fetal conditions that result in poor placental perfusion and endothelial injury. It is a life-threatening state for the mother and may be reversed by delivery of the fetus. The exact pathophysiology is unclear, but it may be due to the release of placental hormones, such as human chorionic gonadotropin (hCG), that stimulate thyroxin production at high levels or by direct release of vasoactive compounds from a tumor or the placenta.

25. What is the rationale for in utero treatment of fetal sacrococcygeal teratoma?

Sacrococcygeal teratoma (SCT) frequently causes fetal death by a tumor mass effect or by specific characteristics of tumor physiology. Mass effects include abnormal lie or dystocia secondary to tumor bulk and premature delivery. The tumor mass effect, with or without associated polyhydramnios, also may precipitate preterm delivery by uterine distention. The metabolic demands of the tumor depend on tumor size, rate of growth, ratio of cystic to solid composition, and tissue components of the mass. If demands are great, the tumor can steal blood flow from the placenta and fetus, usually by way of the middle sacral artery, which can become as large as the common iliac artery. Internal or external hemorrhage from the tumor also can render the fetus anemic and increase metabolic demands, leading to hydrops and fetal demise.

In cases of SCT with hydrops and placentomegaly, in which emergency delivery is not an option because of early gestation and lung immaturity, interruption of the blood supply to the tumor or resection of the mass may reverse the pathologic process.

An in utero ligation of the middle sacral artery or a debulking procedure for SCT is now possible in selected patients.

26. What is the significance of a missing gastric bubble on prenatal ultrasound?

More than 98% of normal fetuses have an identifiable gastric bubble below the left hemidiaphragm. Absence of this finding should lead the ultrasonographer to search for possible abnormalities, such as central nervous system lesions, esophageal atresia, tracheoesophageal fistula, CDH, and situs inversus.

27. Is polyhydramnios a significant sonographic finding?

Yes. It is a nonspecific indicator of a problem pregnancy and has a frequent association with serious congenital malformations. The pregnancy may be at risk of preterm labor or rupture of membranes. It also may be associated with maternal diseases such as diabetes, preeclampsia, anemia, and obesity. The greater the degree of polyhydramnios, the greater the likelihood that fetal anomaly is present and the higher the anticipated perinatal mortality and morbidity. The cause may be maternal, fetal, or idiopathic. According to reports, 15% are due to maternal factors, 13% to fetal factors, and 67% to unknown causes.

28. What are the causes of oligohydramnios?

Prerenal: placental insufficiency (preeclampsia, autoimmune disorders), fetal demise, maternal hypovolemia.

Renal: renal agenesis, polycystic kidneys.

Postrenal: bilateral ureteropelvic junction obstruction, megaureters, posterior urethral valves, urethral agenesis, preterm rupture of membranes.

BIBLIOGRAPHY

1. Adzick NS, Harrison MR: Fetal surgical therapy. Lancet 343:897–902, 1994.
2. American College of Obstetricians and Gynecologists Committee Opinion: Advanced paternal age: Risks to the fetus. Int Gynecol Obstet 59:271–272, 1997.
3. Harrison MR, Mychaliska GB, Albanese CT, et al: Correction of congenital diaphragmatic hernia in utero. IX: Fetuses with poor prognosis (liver herniation and low lung-to-head ratio) can be saved by fetoscopic temporary tracheal occlusion. J Pediatr Surg 33:1017–1023, 1998.
4. Harrison MR, Globus MS, Filly RA: The Unborn Patient. Philadelphia, W.B. Saunders, 1990.
5. Larmon JE, Ross BS: Clinical utility of amniotic fluid volume assessment. Obstet Gynecol Clin North Am 25:639–661, 1998.
6. Olutoye OO, Adzick NS: Fetal surgery for myelomeningocele. Semin Perinatol 23:462–473, 1999.
7. O'Neill JA, Rowe MI, Grosfeld JL, et al: Pediatric Surgery. St. Louis, Mosby, 1998.
8. O'Toole SJ, Sharma A, Karamanoukian HL, et al: Tracheal ligation does not correct the surfactant deficiency associated with congenital diaphragmatic hernia. J Pediatr Surg 31:546–550, 1996.
9. Suen HC, Losty P, Donahoe P: Combined antenatal thyrotrophin-releasing hormone and low-dose glucocorticoid therapy improves the pulmonary biochemical immaturity in congenital diaphragmatic hernia. J Pediatr Surg 29:359–363, 1994.
10. Tannuri U, Maksoud-Filho JG, Santos MM, et al: The effects of prenatal intraamniotic surfactant or dexamethasone administration on lung development are comparable to changes induced by tracheal ligation in an animal model of congenital diaphragmatic hernia. J Pediatr Surg 33:1198–1205, 1998.
11. Wagner RK, Calhoun BC: The routine obstetric ultrasound examination. Obstet Gynecol Clin North Am 25:451–463, 1998.
12. Wilcox DT, Karamanoukian HL, Glick PL: Antenatal diagnosis of pediatric surgical anomalies. Pediatr Clin North Am 40:1273–1287, 1993.

82. ISSUES IN HEALTH CARE REFORM

Arvin I. Philippart, M.D.

1. What does the phrase "health care reform" imply?
Originally based on the assumption that preventative measures would reduce health care costs, to date "reform" has been driven solely by control of the costs of health care.

2. Who are the driving forces behind health care reform?
Those who pay the bills: government through Medicare and Medicaid; employers who provide health insurance; and insurance companies.

3. Where is the patient in all this?
The term "patients" has been replaced by "consumers" or "customers," as in retail business. Therefore, patients have little input except to select the form of insurance coverage when, and if, employers provide options.

4. What options do employers provide?
Many large employers provide options based on cost: employees pay no additional cost for the least expensive option but additional payroll deductions are made for other options that allow "choice" of physician and hospitals.

5. Why not choose the least expensive option?
Most people do. The majority are healthy; their only risks are acute, self-limited illness (e.g., appendicitis, fractures) and pregnancy, both of which typically are uncomplicated.

6. Why do some people elect to pay more for "choice"?
There are a variety of reasons. Some have had prior acute or chronic illness, whereas others want to be able to choose "the best" (or favorite) doctors or hospitals or to have all treatment options available if they become ill.

7. Aren't all treatment options always available to everyone?
Sure—but under managed care and certain other insurances, some options are "available" only if the patient can pay for them.

8. Why would the patient have to pay for a treatment?
Managed care organizations mostly manage costs and restrict available treatment options to traditional therapies, excluding new scientific or technologic advances.

9. What was it like before health care reform?
Before the advent of Medicare and Medicaid in 1964, patient care services were provided by physicians and hospitals, and the patient was billed by each in the hope of payment. Many could not pay. Health care costs approximated only 5–6% of the gross domestic product.

10. How did physicians and hospitals stay in business?
First, health care was not considered a business. Physicians earned less and provided much care gratis or at reduced rates. Hospitals were poorly run, and hospital administrators frequently were unaware of revenue or collections. The poor often received a different standard of care than patients who could pay.

Second, hospitals stayed open because of support from the community (charitable contributions or local government support) and by cost shifting, in which patients who could pay paid more to cover losses incurred by the care of the indigent. To a much lesser degree, physicians also cost shifted.

11. What happened then?

- Medicare and Medicaid were created by the federal government to provide basic health care insurance for the elderly and the indigent.
- Employer-sponsored health insurance coverage increased because it was subsidized by tax deductions and helped to recruit employees in a growing economy after World War II.
- The explosion in medical technology beyond simple laboratory testing (complete blood count, urinalysis, and liver function tests) and plain film radiography greatly raised costs over an extended period and continues to raise them today.

12. What other changes affected health care?

The condensed version is: the expectations of the public changed. Medical science greatly increased life expectancy, and—for certain disorders—death became only one option rather than an inevitability, as before. Health care became a right rather than a matter of choice. Furthermore, because the public wanted all of this care close to home, the government greatly expanded the number of rural hospitals and supported a 50% expansion in the number of medical schools and students in the 1960s and 1970s on the faulty premise that it would make the public more content and reduce costs of physicians through competition.

13. What was the result of this boom in rural hospitals and in the number of physicians?

Care was more readily available, but costs rose rapidly—and specialty practice in the suburbs was more attractive than urban or rural general practice.

14. The concept of higher-quality care that is more accessible to more people sounds good— particularly if it is available without income considerations. What went wrong?

More and better care for a much expanded population costs a lot more money. When health care costs exceeded 10% of gross domestic product (GDP), there was a hue and cry for cost reduction. Health care costs now well exceed 15% of GDP, and simultaneously the economy has grown at a historically unprecedented rate.

15. You are implying that there will be a limit on the growth in costs?

Yes, but it is unknown where or when the public, through government, will decide.

16. Why are you so sure? Government doesn't seem to solve much.

Cynic! Whatever your perception, government in all its forms pays almost 50% of the current costs of health care. As the single largest payor, government will continue to drive change for better or worse. It already has had a major impact by embracing the managed care approach and by adopting the resource-based relative value scale (RBRVS).

17. What is the resource-based relative value scale?

Simply stated, it is a scale of relative value units (RVUs) that determines reimbursement for professional services paid by insurers who cover the majority of patients.

18. Are patients billed on the basis of RBRVS?

Not necessarily. First, a bill or charge may have little relationship to what reimbursement you receive from various payors, who pay whatever they determine is appropriate for that service. Second, RBRVS is a scale that values physician work in RVUs, not dollars. RVUs are converted to payment by multiplication of geographic adjustors for practice overhead and liability costs and then multiplication by a conversion factor in dollars. The conversion factor varies for each payor that utilizes RBRVS.

19. I still don't know how to bill a patient. For example, what would I charge for an inguinal herniorraphy?

All professional services are codified to a number or current procedural terminology (CPT) code. Over 7000 such codes and attendant RVUs are adjudicated and published annually by the American Medical Association in a book called *Current Procedural Terminology* after approval or adjustment by the Health Care Financing Administration. The CPT code for unilateral inguinal herniorraphy over 5 years old is 49505. Its RVU approximates 7. Your charge may be $500 or $5000. If the bill is paid by an insuror, the payment may range from $300 to $1500, depending on where you practice and what insuror pays the bill. Very few patients will pay the $5000 bill themselves. You won't be very busy if you expect that payment!

20. That isn't a very specific answer.

Understood and intentional. Now you understand how it was before RBRVS. Fee setting was individual, and the ranges were broad. Discrepancies existed between specialties and geographic areas.

21. How did RBRVS get started?

In the early 1980s, William Hsaio recognized the discrepancies and studied the feasibility of creating a scale that rated the work done by physicians providing a given service described by a CPT code. Using commonly performed codes, he was able to link a number of specialties onto a common scale. To compensate for the differences in costs of practice (office overhead, liability premiums, costs of training), adjustors were to be provided by payors to arrive at an RVU specific for any CPT code in any region of the country.

22. Why did the government get into the act?

The government wanted to control health care costs (the dollar conversion factor) as well as to reduce what were perceived as undue inequities between specialties and regions.

23. If the U.S. Congress adopted RBRVS only for Medicare, why is it so important?
- First, because of the large and growing number of Medicare recipients and the subsequent disallowance of the physician's ability to bill the patient for the difference between the bill and what Medicare pays.
- Second, in interval years states progressively adopted RBRVS for Medicaid reimbursement with smaller dollar multipliers.
- Third, because a number of national third party insurors, and even some managed care organizations, have adopted RBRVS. The result is that the large majority of physician reimbursement is now based on the RBRVS.

24. Why is RBRVS not a form of price fixing?

You can charge anything you want. Payment is fixed, not prices—and by government mandate, not a group of physicians.

25. Please clarify this alphabet soup: what is the difference between HMOs, IPAs, PPOs, and PHOs?

All are corporations created to negotiate contracts that enroll groups of patients. They differ in rules for the participation of patients, physicians, and hospitals. All fit loosely into the general category of managed care organizations (MCOs) because they limit one or more of the three interested parties.

HMO (health maintenance organization): an insurance product that emphasizes cost controls by restricting patient access to an approved list of physicians, hospitals, and therapies. HMOs come in two forms. Staff model HMOs utilize mainly physicians that they employ and salary. Group model HMOs utilize groups of physicians with whom they contract periodically.

IPA (independent practice association): a loosely organized group of physicians who fund a corporation to negotiate contracts for them with organizations representing groups of patients (e.g., employers).

PPO (preferred provider organization): similar to an IPA but often with more financial risk for physicians and a more selective physician membership.

PHO (physician-hospital organization): hospital and physicians contract and share risks and rewards.

26. How do I decide which to join?

You can participate in most or none. First, decide whether you want to be an employed, salaried physician, in which case your employer makes such decisions, or to establish your own practice, in which case you are compensated on the basis of productivity. With your own practice, you decide participation based on your need for more volume (patients) vs. the degree of discounted payments that you will accept. In some MCOs you must decide how much financial risk you will accept for the total health care bill for a group of patients, just like an insurance company.

27. The risk part is frightening!

Now you understand. Reflect some more, and you'll also recognize the inherent conflict between doing what is best for a patient and what it will cost you and/or the MCO.

28. I'd never pay attention to costs while considering a patient's treatment!

Wake up! Some MCOs do financial credentialing. You could be removed from their list of approved physicians and lose patient volume. If you generate excessive expense in caring for a group of patients, you may find yourself unpopular not only with MCOs but also with other physicians in your IPA or PHO. You will not fare well if you actively avoid any knowledge of the costs that you generate. Some knowledge of the real world is necessary, but it need not interfere with care decisions for a given patient.

29. Is this whole scene going to last forever?

Not clear. Many MCOs were profitable in the early 1990s. Only one-third were profitable in 1997. The extraordinary courtship of Wall Street and managed care is shaky right now.

30. What if I want to practice high-quality medicine and forget the rest?

Good for you! Quality patient care should be the goal of all—and can be cost-effective. The problem is the measurement of quality, which is in its infancy. Don't be afraid of the business side. You are smart, and this is not rocket science. You can learn it and, better yet, use it to your and your patients' benefit.

31. What do you think is the result of all this "reform"?

Health care inflation has slowed markedly in this decade, and a return of inflation at more moderate levels is anticipated. Administrative costs have risen remarkably, with a significantly smaller percentage of the health care dollars committed to patient care, education, and research. Problematic is the marked rise in the percentage of the population with no health care insurance, particularly children. The current system is cumbersome and faulty, with excessive administrative expense, but there is no consensus about future change.

BIBLIOGRAPHY

1. Bodenheimer T: The American health care system: Physicians and the changing medical marketplace. N Engl J Med 340:584–588, 1999.
2. Carrasquillo O, Himmelstein DU, Woolhandler S, Bor, DH: A reappraisal of private employers' role in providing health insurance. N Engl J Med 340:109–114, 1999.
3. Ginzberg E: The uncertain future of managed care. N Engl J Med 144–146, 1999.
4. Hsaio WC, Braun P, Dunn D, Becker ER: Resource based relative values: An overview. JAMA 260:2347–2353, 1988.

5. Iglehart JK: The American health care system: Expenditures. N Engl J Med 340:70–76, 1999.
6. Iglehart JK: The American health care system: Medicare. N Engl J Med 340:327–332, 1999.
7. Iglehart JK: The American health care system: Medicaid. N Engl J Med 340:403–408, 1999.
8. Kassirer JP, Angell M: Risk adjustment or risk avoidance? N Engl J Med 339:1925–1926, 1998.
9. Kuttner R: The American health system: Health insurance coverage. N Engl J Med 340:163–168, 1999.
10. Kuttner R: The American health care system: Employer-sponsored health coverage. N Engl J Med 340:248–252, 1999.
11. Kuttner R: The American health care system: Wall Street and health care. N Engl J Med 340:664–668, 1999.
12. Philippart A: Children and their surgeons. J Ped Surg 32:141–148, 1997.
13. Rosenbaum S, Frankford DM, Moore B, Borzi P: Who should determine when health care is medically necessary? N Engl J Med 340:229–232, 1999.
14. Wennberg JE: Understanding geographic variations in health care delivery. N Engl J Med 340:52–53, 1999.

83. HOW DO I BECOME A PEDIATRIC SURGEON?

Scott C. Boulanger, M.D., Ph.D., Michael G. Caty, M.D., and Philip L. Glick, M.D.

1. What is a pediatric surgeon?

A pediatric surgeon is a fully trained adult general surgeon who has completed a five-year general surgery residency and a two-year fellowship program in pediatric surgery at an approved program in the United States or Canada. Pediatric surgeons have passed certification examinations in both adult and pediatric surgery and hold a special certificate in pediatric surgery.

2. How many fellowships are available? How many fellows do they accept yearly?

Currently, there are 32 approved programs in the United States and seven in Canada. This number has grown recently. Most fellowships accept one fellow per year. Some of the 32 fellowships in the U.S. accept one fellow every other year. Information about fellowship programs can be obtained from the Frieda program, which is now on-line at www.frieda, or the Graduate Medical Education Directory (green book).

3. When do I apply for the fellowship?

Fellows are accepted approximately 16 months before starting. Applications are submitted in the fall approximately 20 months before starting (e.g., the fall of the fourth year of residency). Deadlines for completion of applications range from the end of September to November.

4. What are the typical application requirements?

All applications consist of a curriculum vitae, personal statement, and an application form. Most programs have adopted a standardized application form. In addition, some programs require copies of board and ABSITE scores and copies of medical school transcripts and deans' letters. Usually photocopies are acceptable. All completed applications require at least three letters of recommendation.

5. Who should write letters of recommendation? When should they be obtained?

It is highly recommended that at least one letter be from a pediatric surgeon. One letter should be from the department chairperson or program director. Some programs will not even offer an interview if they do not recognize the letter writers.

Since the earliest deadlines are the end of September, requests for letters should be made in early September at the latest. Offers for interviews generally are not granted until the application is completed, and often letters of recommendation are the last component to arrive. Ask early.

6. Does where I train affect my chances of acceptance?

Clearly the answer is yes. The vast majority of pediatric surgery fellows are from university residencies. In fact, the bias against residents trained in community programs is so strong that many programs do not even offer them interviews.

In addition, a recent survey of successful applicants found that some residency programs are more successful than others in placing people into fellowships. All are highly respected university programs that provide substantial access to research. Some recommend that counseling should begin while interested candidates are in medical school to steer them to appropriate residency programs.

7. Should I do research during residency?

Yes. Most successful applicants have done research as a resident, and the percentage has increased over the years as the match has become more competitive. They also tend to have published more than unsuccessful applicants. This trend, however, may change in the future as more programs are no longer able to offer research as an option. Of interest, the fact that so many pediatric surgeons did research as residents does not correlate well with active research as a pediatric surgeon.

8. What if my residency does not offer research as an option?

As this situation becomes more common, other options need to be found. One option is to work in a lab after completion of general surgery residency. The advantages are several-fold. First, one may have a greater number of research options, because one is not limited to the residency institution. In addition, working in a lab allows greater flexibility during travel about the country for interviews. The major disadvantage is that often you must interview at the beginning of your research experience. You probably will not have as many publications as if you had done research during residency.

Another option is to concentrate on clinical research. This often does not require taking a leave of absence, but it does require beginning early in residency.

9. How much do the application and interview process cost?

The answer depends on the number of interviews you have. You must underwrite the entire cost of each trip (i.e., transportation, food, accommodations). In addition, it is difficult to cluster interviews in an attempt to save money. Since most candidates go to most, if not all, of the interviews, you can anticipate spending as much as $10,000.

10. How many interviews should I go to?

As many as you can. Most viable candidates receive offers to visit all the programs. The more you visit, the better are your chances. Most general surgery residencies do not tolerate long absences to interview. Therefore, the actual number of interviews will be limited by money, time, and desire. Because the interview season extends from October to January, the weather also may take its toll on your interview schedule.

11. Are the interviews difficult?

In general, the actual interview is quite pleasant and often is no more than a polite conversation. Rarely you will encounter clinical or oddball questions. Be prepared to discuss your plans 5–10 years down the road, what you will do if you do not match (hint: you apply again), and what you are looking for in a program. The most important interviews are those with the chairperson and with the fellows. The fellows are usually the best source of information. In addition, questions about salary, working conditions, and insurance, should be directed to the fellows.

12. What qualities are programs looking for in an applicant?

A recent survey of program directors suggests that program directors place great emphasis on personality and ability to work with others. Because fellowship is more or less a two-year marriage between fellow and faculty, directors clearly wish to find residents who will fit in well. Directors also place great emphasis on letters of recommendation from and phone conversations with other pediatric surgeons before creation of a rank list.

Other factors considered important by training directors are the quality of the applicant's residency program, the applicant's technical and clinical ability, and the impression of the other pediatric surgical faculty and fellows.

Of interest, factors considered important by applicants in a previous survey often were not identified as important by training directors. Examples include number of publications and presentations.

13. How do I know if a program has an inside candidate?

Usually you do not know. Inside candidates do exist, but perhaps more often they are used as a measuring stick to compare other applicants. Programs that have committed to an internal candidate often withdraw from the match, thus saving you time and money. Be aware, however, that rumors abound on the interview trail about internal candidates, many of which are not true. It is common for residents to apply to the match from programs that have pediatric surgery fellowships. Do not allow that fact to keep you from applying, although most likely you will be compared to applicants from their general surgery program.

14. How many programs should I rank?

Unless you have a strong desire not to go to a particular program, you should rank every program you visit.

15. Who does the match favor?

Opinions vary greatly. In fact, the match is more or less neutral. Because many applicants believe that programs are favored, various strategies are used to create rank lists—for example, listing first programs in which they feel they have the best chance. Most pediatric surgeons recommend ranking programs in terms of where you want to go.

16. Is there any point to reapplying if I do not match?

Probably. A small percentage of people reapply. In a recent polling of a 7-year period, 16% of successful applicants were reapplicants. Perhaps one-third of reapplicants will match the second or third time. Most reapply in their chief year and spend the off year in a lab or some type of one-year fellowship (e.g., surgical intensive care unit or laparoscopy).

17. What aspects of a program should I evaluate most closely?

All programs maintain at least the minimal case load in order to keep the fellowship; nevertheless, caseload varies widely. You should be sure that there are enough cases to train you. In addition, you should try to determine the type of working environment. You will work with these attending physicians continuously for 2 years.

Programs also differ substantially in call schedules, location, salary, trauma and laparoscopic experience. There are also less tangible differences such as reputation and research exposure, which may influence future job choices and research. The most important aspect of training is the commitment of the faculty to resident education.

18. Do Canadian programs accept American applicants?

Yes. Some programs, however, are conducted in French-speaking hospitals.

19. How important are ABSITE scores?

The survey of program directors suggests that in-service scores are a minor consideration in choosing a fellow. But board scores are requested as part of the application process; low scores will be seen.

20. Who runs the matching process?

The process is now run by the National Resident Matching Program (NRMP), the same organization that oversees the residency match. As part of the application process you need to register with the NRMP and obtain an identification number. Without it you cannot participate in the match.

CONTROVERSY

21. Are group or individual interviews better for applicants?

For group interviews. Group interviews tend to be better organized. There is usually less waiting and a higher likelihood of meeting all the faculty, including the director and fellows.

Against group interviews. Group interviews tend to be fewer in number with a corresponding decrease in flexibility in scheduling. Often group interviews give the feeling of a cattle call. The amount of time that one can spend with individual faculty is often quite limited.

Individual interviews. Individual interviews usually allow greater flexibility in scheduling, but often one is not able to meet all the faculty. In addition, considerable waiting and late finishes can throw off travel arrangements. Perhaps the greatest advantages are more time with faculty and a better sense of the program.

BIBLIOGRAPHY

1. Hirthler MA, Glick PL, Hassett JM Jr, et al: Comparative analysis of successful and unsuccessful candidates for the pediatric surgical matching program. J Pediatr Surg 27:142, 1994.
2. Hirthler MA, Glick PL, Hassett JM Jr, Cooney DR: Evaluation of the pediatric surgical matching programs by the directors of pediatric surgical training programs. J Pediatr Surg 29:1370, 1994.
3. Hirthler MA, Glick PL, Allen JE, et al: Candidate's comments on the pediatric surgical matching program [letter]. J Pediatr Surg 247:413, 1992.
4. Lessin MS, Klein MD: Does research during general surgery residency correlate with academic pursuits after pediatric surgery residency? J Pediatr Surg 30:1310, 1995.

INDEX

Page numbers in **boldface type** indicate complete chapters.

Printed and bound by CPI Group (UK) Ltd, Croydon, CR0 4YY

03/10/2024

01040848-0013